Jade Remedies is an encyclopedia of therapeutic knowledge ... a highly thought-provoking discussion of Chinese herbal medicine. Peter Holmes is a creative voice in the development of East Asian botanical medicine in the west.
  Ted Kapchuk, O.M.D., author of *The Web That Has No Weaver*

Following *The Energetics of Western Herbs*, Peter Holmes has produced another unique gem that boldly explores herbal integration. Clear and enjoyable to read as it is detailed and comprehensive, this beautiful book offers us new maps for the journey towards the wise application of Chinese herbal medicine. It is a blessing that Peter Holmes' creative mind reaches out to make connections, where walls and separation tend to limit awareness and understanding.
  Randall Barolet, O.M.D., co-author of *Chinese Herbal Medicine: Formulas & Strategies*

Peter Holmes is a pioneer in the process of Western medicine integrating with traditional Chinese medicine. His new book, *Jade Remedies,* will be an essential resource for health practitioners in every branch of the healing arts. It will help those of us with a Western mind (just about all of us) understand the beauty and intricacies of Chinese medicine. This will enable more Westerners to tap into the rich storehouse of experience and knowledge refined over 5,000 years that is traditional Chinese herbal medicine.
  Christopher Hobbs, L.Ac., A.G.H., author of *Handbook for Herbal Healing*

Jade Remedies releases the Chinese materia medica from the shroud of Oriental mystique into a context that can be understood by the health care practitioner not trained in the nuances of Chinese medicine. Peter Holmes weaves a sensible new approach, synthesizing from both Eastern and Western traditions. The intrinsic nature of what works is presented in a format that brings the practical to the forefront. Most materia medicas are compilations of what has come before. Peter Holmes' thoughtful, fresh approach helps us look at Chinese herbs with new eyes and think about them as we never had before.
  Steven Foster, author of *Herbal Emissaries: Bringing Chinese Herbs to the West*

Finaly, a Chinese herbal materia medica that successfully merges the Western scientific with the Chinese energetic approach. With the inclusion of the chemical constituents of the medicinals this book helps to make Chinese remedies accessable to a Western practitioner as it also demystifies the Chinese theoretical idiom. New uses of the medicinals can now be incorporated, based on scientific research. With this book a welcome and timely perspective is created on an ancient form of medicine. This can only expand one's knowledge of single medicinals.
  Dagmar Ehling, D.O.M., author of *The Chinese Herbalist's Handbook*

JADE REMEDIES

A Chinese Herbal Reference for the West

Vol. 1

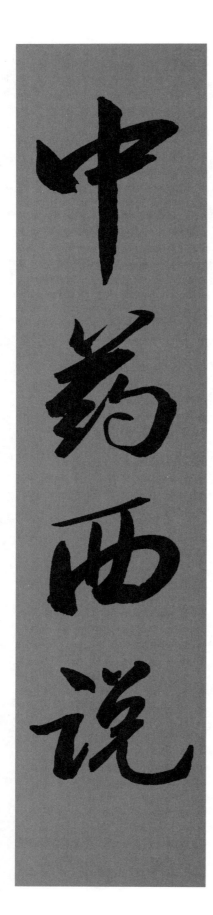

JADE REMEDIES

A Chinese Herbal Reference for the West

PETER HOLMES

Vol. 1

Snow Lotus Press ❦ Boulder

Important Notice

The information contained in this book is for educational purposes only. It is not intended to diagnose, treat or prescribe, and does not purport to replace the services of a trained practitioner or physician. The information presented herein is correct and accurate to the author's knowledge up to the time of printing. However, because herbal medicine, like everything else, is in constant development, it is possible that new information may cause future modifications to become neccessary.

Illustrations from *Zhi Wu Ming Shi Tu Kao* by Wu Qi-chun, 1848
Additional original illustrations by Mary Beth Jay
Oriental calligraphy throughout by Pan Hui-xiang, except for secondary remedy names by Chu Shi-xiong
Cover design by Peter Holmes and Vicky Londerville
Cover photographs by Paul Berg

FIRST EDITION
Copyright © 1996 Peter Holmes. All rights reserved.
Additional illustrations © 1996 Mary-Beth Jay
Front and back cover photos © 1996 Paul Berg

All rights reserved. No part of this book may be reproduced or transmitted in any form or by any means, electronic or mechanical, including photocopying, recording or by any information storage or retrieval system, without written permission from the author, except for the inclusion of brief quotations in a review.

ISBN 1-890029-28-9

Published by Snow Lotus Press, Inc., Boulder, Colorado, U.S.A.
Manufactured in the United States of America

For Betsy,
who guided me into the world of Oriental medicine

*In the end, all creatures return
to their distinctive roots.
That is called returning to one's destiny.*
Lao Zi, *Dao De Jing*

*Strive to get to the bottom of things,
and never follow word for word
the old methods of treatment*
Lan Oon, *Study on the Medicinal Source of the Sea*

*Knowledge begins with experience ...
theoretical knowledge is acquired through practice
and must then return to practice.*
Mao Zi-dong, *On Practice*

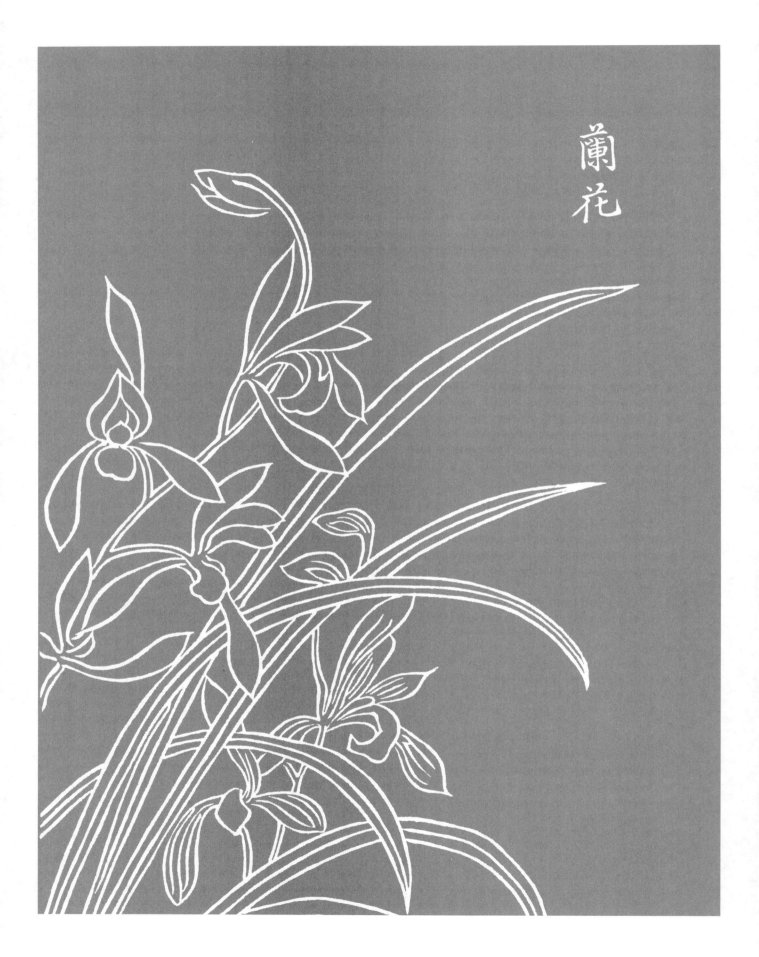

Contents

The Materia Medica   9
Acknowledgements   25
Making Best Use of This Book   27

PART ONE : Chinese Herbal Medicine in the West

Introduction   31

1 Ancient Medicine, Modern Medicine   36
Chinese Medicine in Transition   36
Chinese Medicine Renewed   40
Chinese Medicine as a Mirror   41
The Essence of Chinese Medicine   43

2 Redefining and Reclassifying Chinese Remedies   45
Science and Vitalism: The Two Pharmacologies   45
    Scientific Pharmacognosy   47
    Scientific Pharmacology   53
    Vitalistic Pharmacognosy   58
    Vitalistic Pharmacology   58
Traditional Greek Medicine and Beyond: The Western
    Vitalistic Tradition   59
    The Wise Woman Tradition   59
    Alexandrian Medicine: The Empirics   60
    Spagyric Medicine   60
    Homeopathic Medicine   61
    Vitalistic Herbal Medicine: Thomsonians, Eclectics
      and Physiomedicals   61
Connecting the Two Herbal Traditions: The Two Vitalistic Links   66
    The Four Remedy Actions   66
    The Symptom Picture   70
Reclassifying Chinese Remedies: The Anatomical Body Systems   75

3 The Remedy Presentation   80
The Primary Names   81
The Main Categories   82

Botanical Source	82
Pharmaceutical Name	84
Chinese Names	85
Other Names	85
Habit	85
Part Used	85
Therapeutic Category	85
Constituents	87
Effective Qualities	92
Tropism	106
Actions and Indications	107
Symptom Pictures	109
Preparation	110
Notes	111

PART TWO : The Materia Medica

	Remedies for the Nose, Throat and Eyes	115
	Remedies for the Respiratory System	137
	Remedies for the Cardiovascular System	191
	Remedies for the Gastrointestinal System	253
	Remedies for the Hepatobiliary System	319
	Remedies for the Urinary System	351
	Remedies for the Reproductive System	395
(Vol. 2)	Remedies for the Musculoskeletal System	451
	Remedies for the Nervous System	483
	Remedies for the Endocrine and Immune Systems	537
	Remedies for Infection, Toxicosis and Parasitosis	563
	Remedies for Tissue Trauma	623

PART THREE : Cross Indexes, Glossaries & Charts

Cross Index of Scientific Names
Cross Index of Pharmaceutical Names
Cross Index of Mandarin Names
Cross Index of Cantonese Names
Cross Index of Common Names
Glossary of Herbal Medicine Terms
Glossary of Latin Scientific Terms
Glossary of Cantonese Pronunciation
Symptom Picture and Disease
The Phytogeographic Regions of China
The Four Remedy Actions

Bibliography
Repertory
General Index

The Materia Medica

Remedies for the Nose, Throat and Eyes

Restoratives and Stimulants

REMEDIES TO RELIEVE NASAL CONGESTION AND PAIN, AND STOP DISCHARGE

➤ RELEASE THE EXTERIOR AND DISPEL WIND COLD WITH PUNGENT, WARM REMEDIES

Anticatarrhal nasal decongestants

Magnolia Xin Yi Hua : Yulan magnolia bud
Xanthium Cang Er Zi : Siberian cocklebur
Perilla Zi Su Ye : Perilla leaf
Angelica Bai Zhi : White angelica root
Allium Cong Bai : Fresh scallion bulb
Centipeda E Bu Shi Cao : Centipeda herb

Relaxants and Sedatives

REMEDIES TO REDUCE INFLAMMATION AND RELIEVE PAIN IN THE THROAT AND EYES

➤ RELEASE THE EXTERIOR AND DISPEL WIND HEAT WITH PUNGENT, COOL REMEDIES

Anti-inflammatories, analgesics, diaphoretics

Schizonepeta Jing Jie : Japanese catnip herb
Mentha Bo He : Asian fieldmint herb
Arctium Niu Bang Zi : Burdock seed
Morus Sang Ye : Mulberry leaf
Chrysanthemum Ju Hua : Chrysanthemum flower
Chimonanthus La Mei Hua : Wintersweet flower
Ilex Gang Mei : Rough holly leaf and root
Ilex Jiu Bi Ying : Round-leaf holly leaf
Tagetes Wan Shou Ju : African marigold flower
Sterculia Pang Da Hai : Sterculia seed
Oroxylum Mu Hu Die : Oroxylum seed
Lasiosphaera Ma Bo : Puffball mushroom
Borax Peng Sha : Borax
Buddleia Mi Meng Hua : Buddleia flower and bud
Celosia Qing Xiang Zi : Silver quail-grass seed
Equisetum Mu Zei : Horsetail herb
Eriocaulon Gu Jing Cao : Pipewort herb
Tamarix Xi He Liu : Chinese tamarisk tip
Evodia San Ya Ku : Bitter evodia root
Spirodela Fu Ping : Duckweed herb

Remedies for the Respiratory System

Restoratives
REMEDIES TO PROVIDE MOISTURE, PROMOTE SECRETIONS AND RELIEVE RESPIRATORY DRYNESS
➥ NOURISH THE YIN, GENERATE FLUIDS AND MOISTEN DRYNESS; CLEAR DEFICIENCY HEAT
Bronchial demulcents, mucogenic secretories, mucolytic expectorants
Ophiopogon Mai Men Dong : Dwarf lilyturf tuber
Asparagus Tian Men Dong : Shiny asparagus tuber
Anemarrhena Zhi Mu : Know mother root
Trichosanthes Tian Hua Fen : Snakegourd root
Lilium Bai He : Brown's lily bulb
Glehnia Bei Sha Shen : Northern sandroot
Adenophora Nan Sha Shen : Upright ladybell root
Fritillaria Chuan Bei Mu : Sichuan fritillary bulb
Heleocharis Bi Qi : Heleocharis herb
Lycium Di Gu Pi : Wolfberry root bark
Tremella Bai Mu Er : Silver ear mushroom

Stimulants
REMEDIES TO PROMOTE EXPECTORATION AND RELIEVE COUGHING
➥ WARM AND TRANSFORM PHLEGM COLD
Stimulant expectorants
Asarum Xi Xin : Asian wild ginger root and herb
Peucedanum Qian Hu : Asian masterwort root
Platycodon Jie Geng : Balloonflower root
Vitex Mu Jing Zi : Five-leaf chastetree berry
Pinellia Ban Xia : Prepared pinellia corm
Gleditsia Zao Jia : Honeylocust pod
Cynanchum Bai Qian : Prime white root
Zingiber Sheng Jiang : Fresh ginger root
Ardisia Zi Jin Niu : Marlberry root and herb

Relaxants
REMEDIES TO RELAX THE BRONCHI AND RELIEVE WHEEZING
➥ CIRCULATE AND LOWER LUNG QI
Bronchodilatant antiasthmatics
Perilla Zi Su Zi : Perilla seed
Aster Zi Wan : Tartary aster root
Prunus Xing Ren : Bitter apricot kernel
Stemona Bai Bu : Stemona root
Ephedra Ma Huang : Ephedra stem
Tussilago Kuan Dong Hua : Coltsfoot flower
Sophora Shan Dou Gen : Pigeon-pea root
Morus Sang Bai Pi : Mulberry root bark
Sargassum Hai Zao : Sargassum seaweed
Laminaria Kun Bu : Kelp seaweed
Inula Xuan Fu Hua : Japanese elecampane flower
Aristolochia Ma Dou Ling : Green birthwort capsule

Caragana Jin Ji Er : Caragana root
Haematitum Dai Zhe Shi : Hematite
Stalactitum E Guan Shi : Stalactite tip
Iphigenia Shan Ci Gu : Iphigenia bulb

REMEDIES TO RESTORE THE ADRENAL CORTEX AND RELIEVE WHEEZING
➥ TONIFY LUNG AND KIDNEY YANG, AND STOP WHEEZING
Adrenocortical restorative antiasthmatics
Juglans Hu Tao Ren : Walnut meat
Cordyceps Dong Chong Xia Cao : Chinese caterpillar mushroom
Gecko Ge Jie : Toad-headed lizard

Sedatives
REMEDIES TO PROMOTE EXPECTORATION AND REDUCE BRONCHIAL INFECTION
➥ COOL AND TRANSFORM PHLEGM HEAT
Anti-inflammatory antiseptic expectorants
Houttuynia Yu Xing Cao : Fishwort herb
Phyllostachys Zhu Ru : Black bamboo shaving
Eriobotrya Pi Pa Ye : Loquat leaf
Fritillaria Zhe Bei Mu : Zhejiang fritillary bulb
Belamcanda She Gan : Leopard flower root
Tricosanthes Gua Lou Ren : Snakegourd seed
Tricosanthes Gua Lou : Snakegourd fruit
Tricosanthes Gua Lou Pi : Snakegourd rind
Benincasa Dong Gua Ren : Waxgourd seed
Phragmites Lu Gen : Water-reed root
Momordica Luo Han Guo : Arhat fruit
Phyllostachys Zhu Li : Black bamboo sap
Phyllostachis Zi Zhu Gen : Black bamboo root
Plantago Che Qian Cao : Plantain leaf
Pumus Fu Hai Shi : Pumice
Cyclina Hai Ge Ke : Clam shell

Remedies for the Cardiovascular System

Restoratives
REMEDIES TO RESTORE CORONARY CIRCULATION AND RELIEVE CHEST PAIN
➥ VITALIZE THE BLOOD AND DISPERSE BLOOD STASIS IN THE HEART
Coronary restoratives
Ginkgo Yin Xing Ye : Ginkgo leaf
Crataegus Shan Zha : Asian hawthorn berry
Ligusticum Chuan Xiong : Sichuan lovage root
Salvia Dan Shen : Cinnabar sage root
Carthamus Hong Hua : Safflower
Pueraria Ge Gen : Kudzu root
Daphne Zu Shi Ma : Giraldi's daphne bark
Polygonatum Huang Jing : Siberian Solomon's-seal root
Ilex Si Ji Qing : Wintergreen holly leaf

REMEDIES TO PROMOTE ASTRICTION AND STOP BLEEDING
❧ STOP BLEEDING

Astringent hemostatics, styptics
Typha Pu Huang : Cattail pollen
Rehmannia Sheng Di Huang : Fresh rehmannia root
Sanguisorba Di Yu : Great burnet root
Agrimonia Xian He Cao : Furry agrimony herb
Cirsium Da Ji : Japanese thistle herb
Bletilla Bai Ji : Amethyst orchid root
Cynanchum Bai Wei : Swallow-wort root
Stellaria Yin Chai Hu : Stellaria root
Dioscorea Shu Liang : Dyer's yam root
Cephalanoplos Xiao Ji : Field thistle herb
Callicarpa Zi Zhu : Callicarpa leaf
Sonchus Ku Cai : Annual sowthistle herb
Dioscorea Huang Yao Zi : Potato yam tuber
Nelumbo Lian Fang : Lotus receptacle
Celosia Ji Guan Hua : Cock'scomb herb
Nelumbo Ou Jie : Lotus root node
Homo Xue Yu Tan : Charred human hair

Stimulants
REMEDIES TO PROMOTE CIRCULATION AND RELIEVE COLD
❧ TONIFY THE YANG, WARM THE INTERIOR AND DISPEL COLD; RESCUE DEVASTATED YANG

Arterial circulatory stimulants
Cinamomum Rou Gui : Cassia cinnamon bark
Cinnamomum Zhang Nao : Camphor flake
Aconitum Fu Zi : Prepared Sichuan aconite root
Bufo Chan Su : Toad venom
Thevetia Huang Hua Jia Zhu Tao : Peruvian thevetia leaf and seed

Relaxants
REMEDIES TO RELAX THE BLOOD VESSELS AND RELIEVE IRRITABILITY
❧ CIRCULATE HEART QI, RELEASE CONSTRAINT AND SUBDUE LIVER YANG

Hypotensive vasodilators
Clerodendron Chou Wu Tong : Forked glorybower leaf
Ilex Mao Dong Qing : Furry holly root
Chrysanthemum Ye Ju Hua : Wild chrysanthemum flower
Prunella Xia Ku Cao : Selfheal spike
Cassia Jue Ming Zi : Sickle senna seed
Rauvolfia Luo Fu Mu : Rauvolfia root
Catharanthus Chang Chun Hua : Madagascar periwinkle root and herb
Apocynum Luo Bu Ma : Lance-leaf dogbane root and herb
Salsola Zhu Mao Cai : Salsola root and herb

Sedatives
REMEDIES TO CALM THE HEART, SEDATE THE NERVES AND RELIEVE ANXIETY
➤ SETTLE AND CALM THE SPIRIT WITH HEAVY REMEDIES
Neurocardiac sedatives
Stegodon Long Gu : Dragon bone
Ostrea Mu Li : Oyster shell
Magnetitum Ci Shi : Magnetite
Pteria Zhen Zhu Mu : Mother of pearl shell
Fluoritum Zi Shi Ying : Purple fluorite
Calcitum Han Shui Shi : Calcite
Pteria Zhen Zhu : Pearl
Pinus Hu Po : Amber resin
Cinnabarum Zhu Sha : Cinnabar

➤ NOURISH THE HEART AND CALM THE SPIRIT WITH LIGHT REMEDIES
Neurocardiac sedatives
Scrophularia Xuan Shen : Black figwort root
Polygonatum Yu Zhu : Fragrant Solomon's seal root
Zizyphus Suan Zao Ren : Sour jujube seed
Cimicifuga Sheng Ma : Rising hemp root
Polygala Yuan Zhi : Thin-leaf milkwort root
Nardostachys Gan Song : Indian spikenard root
Biota Bai Zi Ren : Oriental arborvitae berry
Albizzia He Huan Pi : Mimosa bark
Nelumbo Lian Zi Xin : Lotus plumule
Polygonum Ye Jiao Teng : Flowery knotweed stem
Triticum Fu Xiao Mai : Wheat berry
Glycine Dan Dou Chi : Fermented soybean

Remedies for the Gastrointestinal System

Restoratives
REMEDIES TO RESTORE DIGESTION, PROMOTE ABSORPTION AND RELIEVE FATIGUE
➤ BENEFIT THE SPLEEN AND TONIFY THE QI
Sweet digestants, anastative nutritives
Codonopsis Dang Shen : Downy bellflower root
Panax Xi Yang Shen : American ginseng root
Atractylodes Bai Zhu : White atractylodes root
Dioscorea Shan Yao : Mountain yam root
Pseudostellaria Tai Zi Shen : Prince ginseng root
Campanumoea Tu Dang Shen : Java bellflower root
Codonopsis Yang Ju : Goat's tit bellflower root
Oryza Jing Mi : Rice grain
Hordeum Yi Tang : Barley malt sugar
Changium Ming Dang Shen : Bright changium root

REMEDIES TO MOISTEN THE INTESTINES AND RELIEVE DRYNESS AND CONSTIPATION
➥ MOISTEN THE INTESTINES AND UNBLOCK THE BOWELS
Gastric and intestinal demulcents, demulcent laxatives
Dendrobium Shi Hu : Stonebushel stem
Cannabis Huo Ma Ren : Cannabis seed
Prunus Yu Li Ren : Bush cherry kernel
Mirabilitum Mang Xiao : Glauber's salt

REMEDIES TO PROMOTE ASTRICTION AND STOP DIARRHEA
➥ RESTRAIN LEAKAGE FROM THE INTESTINES
Astringent antidiarrheals
Myristica Rou Dou Kou : Nutmeg seed
Terminalia He Zi : Myrobalan fruit
Papaver Ying Su Ke : Opium poppy husk
Sepia Hai Piao Xiao : Cuttlefish bone
Nelumbo Lian Zi : Lotus seed
Prunus Wu Mei : Black plum fruit
Elsholtzia Xiang Ru : Aromatic madder herb
Dolichos Bai Bian Dou : Hyacinth bean
Punica Shi Liu Pi : Pomegranate husk
Nelumbo He Ye : Lotus leaf
Halloysitum Chi Shi Zhi : Red kaolin
Limonitum Yu Liang Shi : Clay ironstone

Stimulants
REMEDIES TO PROMOTE DIGESTION, STIMULATE SECRETIONS AND RELIEVE FATIGUE
(No corresponding Chinese category)
Bitter digestants
Swertia Dang Yao : Asian green gentian root

REMEDIES TO PROMOTE DIGESTION, REDUCE COLIC AND RELIEVE ABDOMINAL PAIN
➥ WARM THE MIDDLE AND DISPEL COLD
Pungent analgesic digestants
Evodia Wu Zhu Yu : Evodia berry
Zingiber Gan Jiang : Dried ginger root
Eugenia Ding Xiang : Clove bud
Alpinia Gao Liang Jiang : Galangal root
Zanthoxylum Chuan Jiao : Sichuan peppercorn
Alpinia Cao Dou Kou : Katsumada's galangal seed
Ferula A Wei : Asafoetida resin
Litsea Bi Cheng Qie : Cubeb fruit
Piper Bi Ba : Long pepper fruit spike
Foeniculum Xiao Hui Xiang : Fennel seed
Trigonella Hu Lu Ba : Fenugreek seed
Diospyros Shi Di : Persimmon calix

REMEDIES TO PROMOTE DIGESTION, RESOLVE MUCUS AND RELIEVE ABDOMINAL FULLNESS
➥ TRANSFORM SPLEEN DAMP WITH AROMATIC REMEDIES
Pungent, dry digestants

Amomum Bai Dou Kou : Cluster cardamom pod
Areca Da Fu Pi : Betel husk
Raphanus Lai Fu Zi : Radish seed
Agastache Huo Xiang : Rugose giant hyssop herb
Atractylodes Cang Zhu : Black atractylodes root

REMEDIES TO PROMOTE DIGESTION, STIMULATE SECRETIONS AND RELIEVE ABDOMINAL FULLNESS
➥ REDUCE FOOD STAGNATION AND TRANSFORM ACCUMULATION
Enzymatic digestants
Hordeum Mai Ya : Sprouted barley grain
Gallus Ji Nei Jin : Chicken gizzard lining
Massa fermentata Shen Qu : Medicated leaven
Oryza Gu Ya : Sprouted rice grain

REMEDIES TO PROMOTE BOWEL MOVEMENT AND RELIEVE CONSTIPATION
➥ DRAIN DOWNWARD
Stimulant laxatives, purgatives
Senna Fan Xie Ye : Senna leaf
Ricinus Bi Ma Zi : Castor bean

Relaxants
REMEDIES TO RELAX DIGESTION, REDUCE COLIC AND RELIEVE ABDOMINAL PAIN
➥ CIRCULATE THE QI IN THE MIDDLE AND RELEASE CONSTRAINT
Intestinal spasmolytics, analgesics
Magnolia Hou Po : Magnolia bark
Amomum Sha Ren : Wild cardamom pod
Lindera Wu Yao : Lindera root
Curcuma E Zhu : Zedoary root
Melia Chuan Lian Zi : Sichuan bead tree berry
Santalum Tan Xiang : Sandalwood
Aquilaria Chen Xiang : Aloeswood
Citrus Fo Shou Gan : Finger lemon fruit
Aristolochia Qing Mu Xiang : Green birthwort root
Allium Xie Bai : Chinese chive bulb
Amomum Cao Guo : Cochin cardamom fruit
Litchi Li Zhe He : Lychee seed
Arca Wa Leng Zi : Cockle shell

Sedatives
REMEDIES TO REDUCE INTESTINAL INFECTION AND STOP DIARRHEA
➥ CLEAR DAMP HEAT FROM THE LARGE INTESTINE
Anti-inflammatory antiseptic astringents
Fraxinus Qin Pi : Korean ash bark
Pulsatilla Bai Tou Weng : Asian pasqueflower root
Galla Wu Bei Zi : Chinese sumac gallnut
Hemsleya Xue Dan : Hemsleya tuber
Portulacca Ma Chi Xian : Purslane herb

Pteris Feng Wei Cao : Phoenix-tail fern
Ailanthus Chun Pi : Tree of heaven bark
Gossampinus Mu Mian Hua : Silk cotton tree flower

Remedies for the Hepatobiliary System

Restoratives
REMEDIES TO RESTORE THE LIVER, PROMOTE ANABOLISM AND RELIEVE FATIGUE
➥ ENRICH LIVER YIN AND NOURISH THE BLOOD
Hepatic anastative nutritives, hemogenics
Rehmannia Shu Di Huang : Prepared rehmannia root
Lycium Gou Qi Zi : Wolfberry
Equus E Jiao : Ass hide glue
Zizyphus Da Zao : Jujube berry

Stimulants
REMEDIES TO PROMOTE UPPER DIGESTION, REDUCE LIVER CONGESTION AND RELIEVE EPIGASTRIC FULLNESS
➥ SPREAD LIVER QI, HARMONIZE THE LIVER AND SPLEEN, AND TRANSFORM ACCUMULATION
Liver decongestants, cholagogue laxatives
Citrus Chen Pi : Ripe tangerine rind
Citrus Qing Pi : Unripe tangerine rind
Saussurea Yun Mu Xiang : Wood aromatic root
Citrus Zhi Shi : Unripe bitter orange fruit
Curcuma Yu Jin : Turmeric tuber
Artemisia Yin Chen Hao : Downy wormwood herb
Artemisia Qing Hao : Celery wormwood herb
Eupatorium Pei Lan : Orchid-grass herb
Curcuma Jiang Huang : Turmeric rhizome
Citrus Zhi Ke : Ripe bitter orange fruit
Cucumis Tian Gua Di : Young cantaloupe stalk

Relaxants and Sedatives
REMEDIES TO REDUCE LIVER AND GALLBLADDER INFECTION AND INFLAMMATION
➥ CLEAR DAMP HEAT FROM THE LIVER AND GALLBLADDER
Anti-inflammatory and antiseptic hepatic decongestants
Gardenia Zhi Zi : Gardenia pod
Rheum Da Huang : Rhubarb root
Gentiana Long Dan Cao : Scabrous gentian root
Canna Mei Ren Jiao : Canna lily root
Lysimachia Jin Qian Cao : Asian moneywort herb
Desmodium Guang Dong Jin Qian Cao : Coin-leaf desmodium herb
Acanthus Lao Shu Le : Holly-leaf acanthus root
Sedum Chui Pen Cao : Stringy stonecrop root and herb
Dichondra Ma Di Jin : Dichondra herb
Hemerocallis Xuan Cao Gen : Tawny day lily root

Remedies for the Urinary System

Restoratives
REMEDIES TO RESTORE THE KIDNEYS AND BLADDER, RELIEVE UROGENITAL INCONTINENCE AND STOP DISCHARGE
➤ STABILIZE THE KIDNEY AND RETAIN URINE AND ESSENCE

Antieneuretics, antileucorrheals
Dioscorea Bi Xie : Long yam root
Euryale Qian Shi : Foxnut
Rosa Jin Ying Zi : Cherokee rosehip
Cuscuta Tu Si Zi : Asian dodder seed
Cornus Shan Zhu Yu : Japanese dogwood berry
Rubus Fu Pen Zi : Chinese raspberry fruit
Psoralea Bu Gu Zhi : Scurf pea berry
Alpinia Yi Zhi Ren : Sharp-leaf galangal berry
Allium Jiu Cai Zi : Asian leek seed
Astragalus Sha Yuan Zi : Flat milkvetch seed
Rubus Dao Sheng Gen : Korean raspberry fruit
Nelumbo Lian Xu : Lotus stamen
Paratenodera Sang Piao Xiao : Praying mantis egg case
Ephedra Ma Huang Gen : Ephedra root
Oryza Nuo Dao Gen : Sweet rice root

REMEDIES TO MOISTEN THE KIDNEYS AND BLADDER, AND RELIEVE URINARY IRRITATION
(No corresponding Chinese category)

Hydrogenics, urinary demulcents
Coix Yi Yi Ren : Job's-tears seed
Malva Dong Kui Zi : Musk mallow seed
Tetrapanax Tong Cao : Rice paper pith
Juncus Deng Xin Cao : Bulrush pith

Stimulants
REMEDIES TO DRY THE KIDNEYS, PROMOTE URINATION, DRAIN FLUID CONGESTION AND RELIEVE EDEMA
➤ BENEFIT THE FLUIDS AND DRAIN DAMP

Draining diuretics
Poria Fu Ling : Hoelen fungus
Alisma Ze Xie : Water plantain root
Imperata Bai Mao Gen : Woolly grass root
Polyporus Zhu Ling : Umbel polypore mushroom
Lobelia Ban Bian Lian : Rooting lobelia herb and root
Euphorbia Jing Da Ji : Peking spurge root
Knoxia Hong Da Ji : Knoxia root
Euphorbia Qian Jin Zi : Caper spurge seed
Phaseolus Chi Xiao Dou : Aduki bean

REMEDIES TO PROMOTE URINATION AND BOWEL MOVEMENT, DRAIN FLUID CONGESTION AND RELIEVE EDEMA
➥ EXPEL FLUIDS DOWNWARD

Purgative draining diuretics
Croton Ba Dou : Croton seed
Phytolacca Shang Lu : Asian poke root
Daphne Yuan Hua : Lilac daphne flower
Euphorbia Gan Sui : Sweet spurge root
Lepidium Ting Li Zi : Wood whitlow grass seed
Pharbitis Qian Niu Zi : Japanese morning glory seed

Sedatives
REMEDIES TO REDUCE URINARY INFECTION AND RELIEVE IRRITATION
➥ CLEAR DAMP HEAT FROM THE BLADDER

Anti-inflammatory urinary antiseptics and spasmolytics
Aristolochia Guan Mu Tong : Manchurian birthwort stem
Dianthus Qu Mai : Proud pink herb
Talcum Hua Shi : Talc
Polygonum Bian Xu : Knotgrass herb
Plantago Che Qian Zi : Asian plantain seed
Pyrrosia Shi Wei : Felt fern leaf
Lygodium Hai Jin Sha Teng : Japanese climbing fern herb
Akebia Bai Mu Tong : Akebia stem
Lopatherum Dan Zhu Ye : Bamboo grass leaf

Remedies for the Reproductive System

Restoratives
REMEDIES TO RESTORE REPRODUCTION AND RELIEVE INFERTILITY AND IMPOTENCE
➥ TONIFY THE KIDNEY AND FORTIFY THE YANG

Fertility and aphrodisiac restoratives
Epimedium Yin Yang Huo : Horny goat weed leaf
Curculigo Xian Mao : Golden eye-grass root
Cistanche Rou Cong Rong : Fleshy broomrape herb
Morinda Ba Ji Tian : Morinda root
Cynomorium Suo Yang : Lock yang stem
Cervus Lu Jiao : Mature deer antler
Cervus Lu Jiao Jiao : Mature deer antler glue
Stichopus Hai Shen : Sea cucumber
Hippocampus Hai Ma : Sea horse
Callorhinus Hai Gou Shen : Seal genitals
Actinolitum Yang Qi Shi : Actinolite

REMEDIES TO REMOVE UTERINE BLOOD CONGESTION AND RELIEVE MENORRHAGIA
➥ VITALIZE THE BLOOD AND DISPERSE BLOOD STASIS IN THE LOWER WARMER

Astringent uterine decongestants
Artemisia Ai Ye : Asian mugwort leaf

Rubia Qian Cao Gen : Heart-leaf madder root
Gossypium Mian Hua Gen : Cotton root bark
Paeonia Chi Shao Yao : Red peony root
Sophora Huai Hua : Japanese pagoda tree flower
Biota Ce Bai Ye : Oriental arborvitae tip

Stimulants
REMEDIES TO PROMOTE MENSTRUATION AND RELIEVE AMENORRHEA
➤ CIRCULATE THE QI AND VITALIZE THE BLOOD IN THE LOWER WARMER

Uterine stimulants, emmenagogues
Angelica Dang Gui : Dong quai root
Paeonia Mu Dan Pi : Tree peony root bark
Achyranthes Huai Niu Xi : White oxknee root
Vaccaria Wang Bu Liu Xing : Cowcockle seed
Impatiens Ji Xing Zi : Garden balsam seed
Saussurea Xue Lian : Snow lotus root
Rosa Yue Ji Hua : Moonseason rose bud
Caesalpinia Su Mu : Sappan wood
Campsis Ling Xiao Hua : Asian trumpet creeper flower
Cyathula Chuan Niu Xi : Hookweed root

Relaxants
REMEDIES TO RELAX THE UTERUS AND RELIEVE DYSMENORRHEA
➤ CIRCULATE THE QI IN THE LOWER WARMER AND RELEASE CONSTRAINT

Uterine spasmolytics
Cyperus Xiang Fu : Purple nutsedge root
Leonorus Yi Mu Cao : Asian motherwort herb
Paeonia Bai Shao Yao : White peony root
Sparganium San Leng : Bur-reed root
Prunus Tao Ren : Peach kernel
Lycopus Ze Lan : Bright bugleweed herb
Millettia Ji Xue Teng : Millettia root and stem
Manis Chuan Shan Jia : Pangolin scale
Trogopterus Wu Ling Zhi : Flying squirrel dropping
Litsea Dou Chi Jiang : Cubeb root and stem
Rosa Mei Gui Hua : Japanese rose flower

Remedies for the Musculoskeletal System

Restoratives
REMEDIES TO RESTORE THE SINEWS AND BONES, AND RELIEVE WEAKNESS
➤ TONIFY THE LIVER AND KIDNEY, AND STRENGTHEN THE SINEWS AND BONES

Musculoskeletal restoratives, detoxicants
Acanthopanax Wu Jia Pi : Five additions root bark
Eucommia Du Zhong : Eucommia bark
Loranthus Sang Ji Sheng : Asian mistletoe twig
Dipsacus Xu Duan : Japanese teasel root
Cibotium Gou Ji : Dogspine root

Stimulants and Relaxants
REMEDIES TO RELAX THE SINEWS, AND RELIEVE JOINT AND MUSCLE PAIN
➥ DISPEL WIND/DAMP/COLD, INVIGORATE THE COLLATERALS AND RELIEVE PAINFUL OBSTRUCTION

Diaphoretic and analgesic antirheumatics, antiarthritics
Ledebouriella Fang Feng : Wind-protector root
Cinnamomum Gui Zhi : Cassia cinnamon twig
Notopterygium Qiang Huo : Notopterygium root
Angelica Du Huo : Hairy angelica root
Clematis Wei Ling Xian : Chinese clematis root
Liquidambar Lu Lu Tong : Taiwan maple fruit
Dioscorea Chuan Shan Long : Nippon yam root
Piper Hai Feng Teng : Kadsura pepper stem
Sarcandra Jiu Jie Feng : Smooth sarcandra herb
Alangium Ba Jiao Feng : Alangium root
Sargentodoxa Da Xue Teng : Sargentodoxa stem
Chaenomeles Mu Gua : Chinese quince fruit
Luffa Si Gua Luo : Spongegourd
Morus Sang Zhi : Mulberry twig
Pinus Song Jie : Knotty pine wood shaving
Bombyx Can Sha : Silkworm dropping

Sedatives
REMEDIES TO REDUCE INFLAMMATION AND RELIEVE JOINT PAIN AND SWELLING
➥ DISPEL WIND/DAMP/HEAT AND RELIEVE PAINFUL OBSTRUCTION

Anti-inflammatory, analgesic, antipyretic antiarthritics
Stephania Han Fang Ji : Stephania root
Gentiana Qin Jiao : Large-leaf gentian root
Erythrina Hai Tong Pi : Asian coral tree bark
Tripterygium Lei Gong Teng : Yellow-vine root pith
Aristolochia Guang Fang Ji : Fangchi birthwort root
Cocculus Mu Fang Fi : Three-leaf cocculus root
Menispermum Bei Dou Gen : Siberian moonseed root
Trachelospermum Luo Shi Teng : Star jasmine stem
Lonicera Jin Yin Teng : Japanese honeysuckle stem and leaf
Periploca Gang Liu Pi : Silk vine root bark

Remedies for the Nervous System

Restoratives
REMEDIES TO RESTORE THE NERVES AND BRAIN, AND RELIEVE DEPRESSION
➥ TONIFY THE LIVER AND KIDNEY, AND BENEFIT THE ESSENCE

Antidepressant central nervous restoratives
Polygonum He Shou Wu : Flowery knotweed root
Ligustrum Nu Zhen Zi : Glossy privet berry
Morus Sang Shen : Mulberry fruit
Euphoria Long Yan Rou : Longan fruit

Eclipta Han Lian Cao : Field lotus herb
Centella Ji Xue Cao : Gotu kola herb
Sesamum Hei Zhi Ma : Sesame seed

Stimulants
REMEDIES TO STIMULATE THE NERVES AND BRAIN, AND REVIVE CONSCIOUSNESS
➧ OPEN THE ORIFICES AND REVIVE THE SENSES WITH AROMATIC REMEDIES
Analeptics, psychogenics
Acorus Shi Chang Pu : Rock sweetflag root
Liquidambar Su He Xiang : Storax resin
Dryobalanops Bing Pian : Borneo camphor
Moschus She Xiang : Musk
Strychnos Ma Qian Zi : Prepared vomit nut
Styrax An Xi Xiang : Benzoin
Securinega Yi Ye Qiu : Securinega shoot and root

Relaxants
REMEDIES TO RELAX THE NERVES AND STOP SPASMS
➧ EXTINGUISH INTERNAL WIND, STOP SPASMS AND CLEAR WIND PHLEGM
Spasmolytics, anticonvulsants
Gastrodia Tian Ma : Celestial hemp corm
Uncaria Gou Teng : Gambir vine twig
Cryptotympana Chan Tui : Cicada slough
Bombyx Jiang Can : Silkworm larva
Arisaema Tian Nan Xing : Prepared dragon arum corm
Chinemys Gui Ban : Tortoise shell
Amyda Bie Jia : Asian soft-shell turtle shell
Eretmochelys Dai Mao : Hawksbill turtle shell
Haliotis Shi Jue Ming : Abalone shell
Pinellia Zhang Ye Ban Xia : Pedatisect pinellia corm
Agkistrodon Bai Hua She : Multibanded krait
Zaocys Wu Shao She : Black grass snake
Elephe She Tui : Snake skin slough
Buthus Quan Xie : Scorpion
Scolopendra Wu Gong : Centipede
Chloris Qing Meng Shi : Chlorite

Sedatives
REMEDIES TO SEDATE THE NERVES AND RELIEVE PAIN
➧ CALM THE SPIRIT AND RELIEVE PAIN
Depressant analgesics and hypnotics
Siegesbeckia Xi Xian Cao : Hairy siegesbeckia herb
Typhonium Bai Fu Zi : Prepared giant typhonium root
Tribulus Bai Ji Li : Caltrop fruit
Corydalis Yan Hu Suo : Asian corydalis corm
Vitex Man Jing Zi : Seashore chastetree berry
Bupleurum Chai Hu : Asian buplever root
Ligusticum Gao Ben : Chinese lovage root

THE MATERIA MEDICA

Paederia Ji Shi Teng : Chicken dung vine root and stem
Cynanchum Xu Chang Qing : Panicled dogbane root and herb
Schefflera Qi Ye Lian : Taiwan schefflera leaf and stem
Aconitum Chuan Wu : Prepared Sichuan aconite root tuber
Aconitum Cao Wu : Prepared wild aconite root tuber
Sinomenium Qing Feng Teng : Sinomenium root
Citrus Ju He : Tangerine seed

REMEDIES TO SEDATE THE NERVES, REDUCE FEVER AND STOP SPASMS
➥ QUELL FIRE, EXTINGUISH WIND AND CALM THE SPIRIT
Depressant antipyretics and spasmolytics
Ursus Xiong Dan : Bear gallbladder
Bos Niu Huang : Ox gallstone
Saiga Ling Yang Jiao : Antelope horn
Bubalus Shui Niu Jiao : Water buffalo horn
Gypsum Shi Gao : Gypsum
Pheretima Di Long : Earthworm
Naja She Dan : Viper gallbladder
Phyllostachys Tian Zhu Huang : Tabasheer
Sus Zhu Dan : Pig gallbladder

Remedies for the Endocrine and Immune Systems

REMEDIES TO RESTORE THE ENDOCRINE GLANDS, INCREASE STRESS ADAPTATION AND ENHANCE IMMUNITY
➥ TONIFY THE RIGHTEOUS QI AND GENERATE THE PULSE
Endocrine restoratives, adaptogens, immune enhancers
Eleutherococcus Ci Wu Jia : Eleuthero ginseng root
Cervus Lu Rong : Velvet deer antler
Homo Zi He Chi : Human placenta
Panax Ren Shen : Asian ginseng root
Schisandra Wu Wei Zi : Schisandra berry
Ganoderma Ling Zhi : Reishi mushroom
Astragalus Huang Qi : Astragalus root
Glycyrrhiza Gan Cao : Ural licorice root

Remedies for Infection, Toxicosis and Parasitosis

REMEDIES TO REDUCE INFECTION, STIMULATE IMMUNITY, AND REDUCE FEVER AND INFLAMMATION
➥ DISPEL WIND HEAT AND DETOXIFY FIRE TOXIN
Broad-spectrum anti-infectives: immunostimulants, antivirals, antibacterials, antifungals, antipyretics, anti-inflammatories
Lonicera Jin Yin Hua : Japanese honeysuckle flower
Forsythia Lian Qiao : Forsythia valve
Dryopteris Guan Zhong : Shield fern root

Usnea Song Luo : Beard lichen thallus
Allium Da Suan : Garlic bulb

➤ CLEAR DAMP HEAT AND DETOXIFY FIRE TOXIN
Broad-spectrum anti-infectives: immunostimulants, antivirals, antibacterials, antifungals, antipyretics, anti-inflammatories
Andrographis Chuan Xin Lian : Heart-thread lotus leaf
Coptis Huang Lian : Chinese goldthread root
Scutellaria Huang Qin : Baikal skullcap root
Isatis Da Qing Ye : Woad leaf
Isatis Ban Lan Gen : Woad root
Phellodendron Huang Bai : Siberian cork tree bark
Berberis San Ke Zhen : Three-needle barberry root
Senecio Qian Li Guang : Climbing ragwort herb
Isatis Qing Dai : Woad pigment
Picrorrhiza Hu Huang Lian : Picrorrhiza root
Pyrola Lu Xian Cao : Asian wintergreen root and herb
Polygonum Huo Tan Mu : Chinese smartweed herb

REMEDIES TO REDUCE TOXICOSIS AND RESOLVE ECZEMA AND TUMORS
(No corresponding Chinese category)
Resolvent detoxicants: lymphatic decongestants, antitumorals, detumescents
Sophora Ku Shen : Yellow pagoda tree root
Taraxacum Pu Gong Ying : Mongolian dandelion root and herb
Solanum Long Kui : Winter cherry herb
Lithospermum Zi Cao : Purple groomwell root
Smilax Tu Fu Ling : Glabrous greenbrier root
Oldenlandia Bai Hua She She Cao : Snaketongue grass herb
Patrinia Bai Jiang Cao : Patrinia herb
Polygonum Hu Zhang : Japanese knotweed root and leaf
Dictamnus Bai Xian Pi : Dittany root bark
Viola Zi Hua Di Ding : Tokyo violet root and herb
Tinospora Jin Guo Lan : Tinospora tuber
Wikstroemia Liao Ge Wang : Wikstroemia root
Ampelopsis Bai Lian : Japanese peppervine root
Polygonum Quan Shen : Bistort root
Smilax Jin Gang Teng : China root
Echinops Lou Lu : Globe thistle root
Scutellaria Ban Zhi Lian : Barbed skullcap root and herb
Solanum Bai Ying : Climbing nightshade herb
Selaginella Shi Sheng Bai : Spikemoss herb
Momordica Mu Bie Zi : Cochin bitter melon seed
Paris Qi Ye Yi Zhi Hua : Paris root
Camptotheca Xi Shu : Happy tree root bark
Crotalaria Ye Bai He : Thin-leaf rattlebox herb
Lycoris Shi Suan : Red spiderlily corm
Cantharis Ban Mao : Cantharides

THE MATERIA MEDICA

REMEDIES TO CLEAR INTERNAL PARASITES
Antiparasitics: anthelmintics, antiprotozoals (antimalarials, antiamoebics)
Cucurbita Nan Gua Zi : Red squash seed
Areca Bing Lang : Betel nut
Quisqualis Shi Jun Zi : Rangoon creeper nut
Melia Ku Lian Pi : Bead tree root bark
Brucea Ya Dan Zi : Brucea berry
Dichroa Chang Shan : Feverflower root
Artemisia Huang Hua Hao : Annual wormwood herb
Torreya Fei Zi : Japanese torreya nut
Mylitta Lei Wan : Thunder ball fungus
Carpesium He Shi : Starwort fruit or seed
Agrimonia He Cao Ya : Furry agrimony winter bud
Aloe Lu Hui : Aloe resin

REMEDIES TO CLEAR EXTERNAL PARASITES
Antiparasitics, antifungals
Cnidium She Chuang Zi : Cnidium seed
Hibiscus Mu Jin Pi : Rose of Sharon root bark
Kochia Di Fu Zi : Kochia seed
Lithagyrum Mi Tuo Seng : Litharge
Realgar Xiong Huang : Realgar
Polistes Lu Feng Fang : Hornet nest
Sulphur Liu Huang : Sulphur
Hydnocarpus Da Feng Zi : Chaulmoogra seed
Alumen Ming Fan : Alum
Calomelas Qing Fen : Calomel

Remedies for Tissue Trauma

REMEDIES TO PROMOTE TISSUE REPAIR AND RELIEVE PAIN AND SWELLING
➥ DISPERSE CONGEALED BLOOD
Vulneraries, analgesics, detumescents
Panax San Qi : Pseudoginseng root
Commiphora Mo Yao : Myrrh resin
Boswellia Ru Xiang : Frankincense resin
Drynaria Gu Sui Bu : Boneknit root
Daemonorops Xue Jie : Dragon's-blood resin
Cissampelos Xi Sheng Teng : Ice vine root
Dalbergia Jiang Xiang : Asian rosewood
Eupolyphaga Tu Bie Chong : Cockroach
Hirudo Shui Zhi : Leech
Pyritum Zi Ran Tong : Pyrite
Ophicalcitum Hua Rui Shi : Dolomite
Calamina Lu Gan Shi : Calamine

Acknowledgments

I am deeply indebted to my teachers, mentors and friends who helped in my understanding of Oriental medicine. They include Naboru Muramoto, David Lee, Leung Kok-yuen, Henry Lu, Jean Schatz, Elisabeth de la Roche-Vallée, Claude Larre, John and Angela Hicks, Giovanni Maciocia, Ted Kaptchuk, Jacques Mora-Marco, Kathy Boisen, Michael Broffman, Randy Barolet, Dan Kenner, Cecile Levin and the many patients who over the years have come to me to help them untangle their particular disharmony.

I also gratefully acknowledge my teachers and mentors in Western herbal medicine and physiopathology, including Christopher Hedley, Simon Mills, Norman Easley, Michael Moore, Henri Verdier, Jean-Claude Lapraz, Josef Angerer, Josef Karl and Joachim Broy. In the vitalistic Thomsonian/Eclectic/Physiomedical tradition in particular, I am continuously inspired by the writings of John King, Finley Ellingwood, John Scudder, Herbert Webster, Joseph Thurston and A.W. and L.R. Priest. The pleomorphic researchers and practitioners past and present, especially Antoine Béchamp, Günther Enderlein and Thomas Rau, have also been highly influential.

To Brenda Cooke, Christopher Hedley, Roger Hirsch, Michael Barnett, Randy Barolet, Bonney Lynch, Lakshmi Lambert, Sarah West, Rachel Koenig, David and Ming Ming Molony, Rachel Lord, Julie Coughlan and my many students I am particularly grateful for moral support for my work and for indispensable soul food over the years.

Thanks also goes to those who assisted me practically in the creation of this book either through feedback or contribution of information: Rebecca Morris and J.P. Harpignes for careful editing, Alex Konn for assistance on terminology, Heidi Green for advice on academic correctness, Angela Longo-Spain for suggestions of clinical usage, Patrick Cunningham, Yan Pei-fen, Liu Yong, and Frances Lai for translation of Chinese material, Charles Chace for advice on remedy selection, Ma Xiu-ling for suggesting the Chinese book title, Pan Hui-xiang and Chu Shi-xiong for providing the remedy name calligraphy, Paul Berg for making available examples of his superb photography, Eric Silver for help with Cantonese language, Claire Joslin for compiling and correcting Cantonese remedy names, as well as the many nameless students of the American College of Traditional Chinese Medicine and the Traditional Chinese Medical College of Hawaii who over many years assiduously transcribed remedy names phonetics in Cantonese Chinese from their teachers.

Book production itself would not have been possible without the computer wizardry of Len Rubin, the trained page design sense of Bonney Lynch and Vicky Londerville, the careful graphics preparation of Gina Simpson-Li and the magical prepress work of Al Stone for the herb illustrations and calligraphies, and the front and back covers. Thank you all!

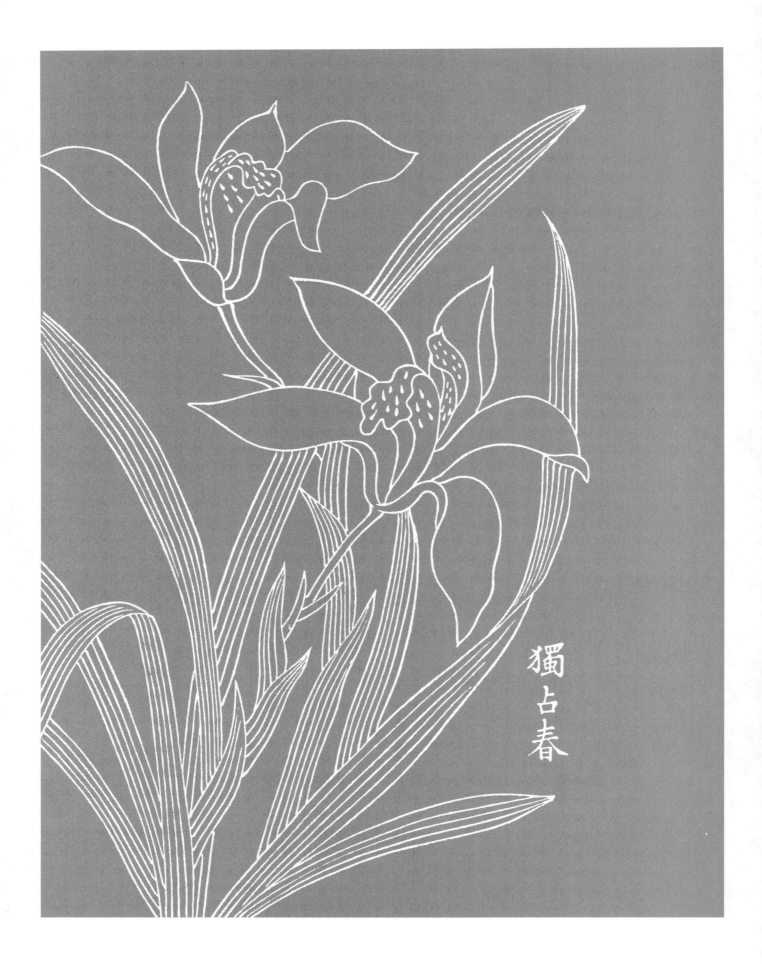

Making Best Use This Book

To get the most from this book, the following suggestions may be helpful. Whether you browse the text at random for casual reading or whether you want to obtain certain information about a remedy or treatment of a condition, keep in mind the following:

• Unless specified otherwise, all plant names are given in Mandarin Chinese first and foremost because it is the official language of the People's Republic of China. Mandarin is the Chinese default language throughout the text. However, the Cantonese names appear under "Chinese names" for each remedy and with other plants discussed under "Notes." There is also a separate Cantonese cross-index in Part Three at the back of Vol. 2. The Cantonese pronunciation will be useful for students of Cantonese teachers and apprentices of Cantonese doctors, as well as for anyone wishing to buy raw herbs in local Western stores and pharmacies. Likely as not, the owners or pharmacists will be of Cantonese or South Chinese descent.

• An upper case plant name refers to it as a remedy; lower case usage refers to the actual plant itself.

• Pathologies in upper case refer to syndromes based on the Chinese organ/channel networks, whereas pathologies in lower case refer to syndromes based on the physiological organs themselves. E.g., "Liver Yang rising" is a Chinese syndrome, wheras "adrenocortical deficiency" is a Western syndrome.

• References to authors and dates refer to literary sources listed in the Bibliography at the end of the book.

• The cross-indexes in Part Three allow you to find a remedy name in scientific Latin, pharmaceutical Latin, Mandarin, Cantonese, Japanese and English.

• For an explanation of unfamilar terms, such as the actions of remedies and the concepts of Oriental pathology, refer to the Glossary of Herbal Medicine terms in Part Three. Browsing the glossary now and then is a quick way for you to become familiar with the essential ideas and vocabulary of Oriental and Western herbal medicine. Technical terms only become more familiar with use—often more quickly than we realize.

• To find a remedy by its scientific or composite binomial name (as in the text), go to the General Index in either volume. To find remedies by therapeutic categories within the body systems, go to the outline of the whole Materia Medica that begins on page 9.

• The important information about the toxicity, safety and best use of Oriental remedies may quickly be accessed as follows. For the remedy in question, refer to two headings: "Therapeutic category" near the top of the presentation, and "Caution" under the Preparation section towards the end. Information on the three therapeutic categories is found in Chapter 3 on page 85.

PART ONE

Chinese Herbal Medicine in the West

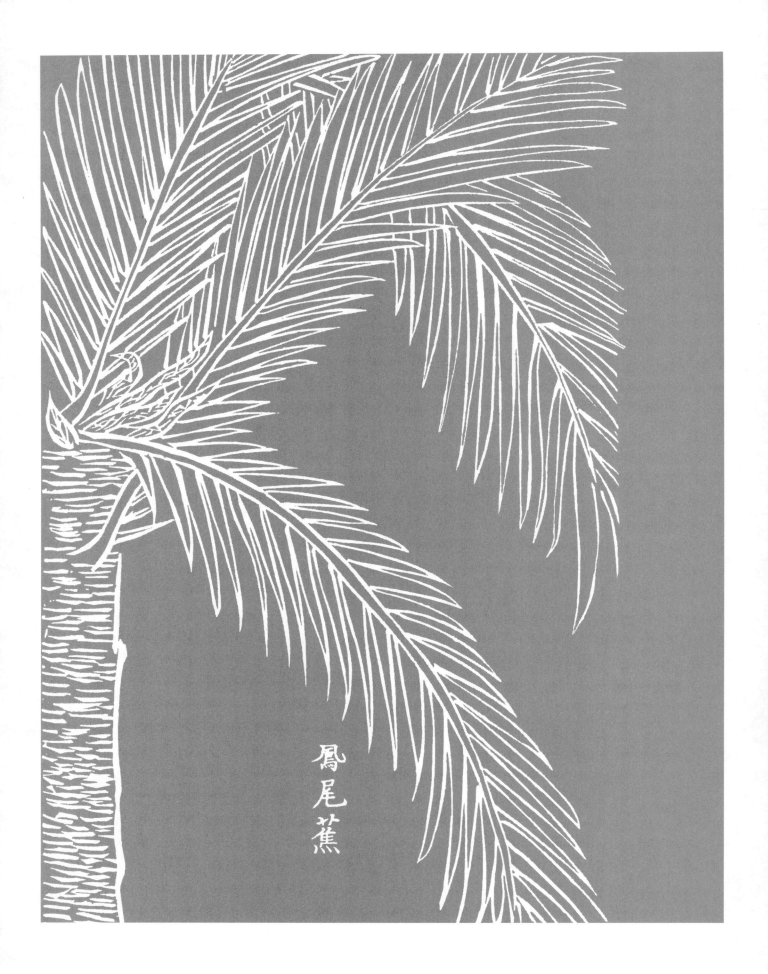

Introduction

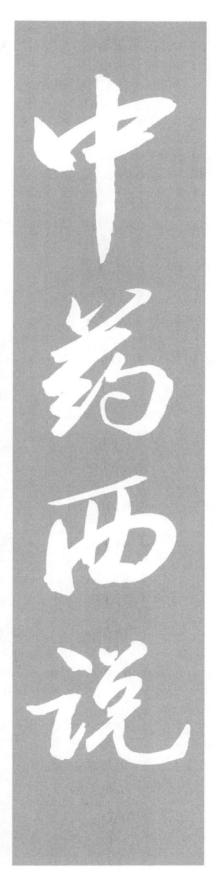

It was an overcast, wintery English morning much like any other. My mail that particular day in the early seventies contained a letter that proved to be a turning point in my life. It was from my friend Betsy in California. She was now studying with a Japanese herbalist in San Bruno and was writing to tell me about her amazing experiences with Oriental herbs. "You should come over and study herbs and medicinal foods with Muramoto," she advised, sage that she was. "It's changed my life."

    I trusted Betsy, and her gentle, glowing enthusiasm won me over. Two months later, at the dawn of spring, I was on a plane bound for San Francisco. Little did I realize that I was taking the first step of a journey that was to continue to the present day—my exploration of Oriental medicine. Through Muramoto Sensei I was first introduced hands-on to the sensuous, healing world of Chinese herbal medicine. Preparing his Shang Han Lun formulas—the mainstay of Japanese Kampo—acquainted me first-hand with the most widely used Chinese botanicals. I became familiar with the suave scent of the small pink rings of root bark called Botanpi, or Tree peony, used in Keishibukuryogan, one of the oldest Chinese prescriptions for menstrual problems; with the fresh, clinical spiciness of the spindly roots called Saishin, a key ingredient in Shoseiryuto, a classical formula for upper and lower respiratory infections; with the warm aroma of Kippi, ripe tangerine rind slices, and Binroji, betelnut quills, found in the Nine Taste Tea that regulates the intestinal flora.

    I assiduously drank various medicinal decoctions in ten-day courses and over time experienced relief from several minor ailments that I'd had for many years. And through Muramoto's practice I observed patients going through the most interesting physical and psychological changes. In addition to witnessing a reduction of their physical complaints, I also saw individuals

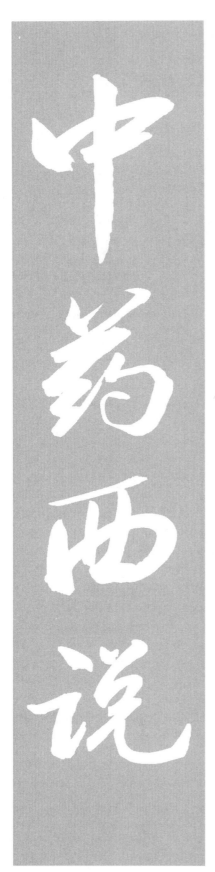

transforming into truer, deeper versions of themselves, shedding their old, hard skin for a softer, more vibrant one, dismantling their hard egos to allow a more flexible personality. My eyes opened to the power of Chinese medicine, my heart warmed to the gentleness of its way, and my senses basked in the aromatic delights that seemed inescapable, indeed essential to its herbal practice.

My exploration of Chinese medicine has continued to this day and along the way has produced this book. Initially it was the outcome of notes and files kept over many years on the various actions and indications of Chinese medicinals, drawn from a variety of oral and written sources, including my first teachers, Drs. Muramoto and David Lee. Eventually, compiling and organizing these notes became a way of producing a simplified, integrated and articulated Chinese materia medica.

Does the world need another Chinese materia medica? One may argue that this need has been adequately filled, seeing the whole range of texts now available, from the erudite to the popular, from the comprehensive to the simple. Today the presentation of Chinese remedies essentially divides into the traditional Oriental approach and the various contemporary Western approaches. In the traditional approach one studies translations and adaptations of Chinese texts that describe the nature, functions and uses of remedies purely in Chinese vitalistic medical terms. The modern approach is represented by scientific pharmacognosy, pharmacology, botany and statistical science, utilizing the language of modern chemistry, pharmacology, botany and statistics.

Two factors have always struck me as curious about this situation. First, to obtain truly comprehensive information from the available literature on Chinese remedies, one would have to be fully versed in Chinese medicine, chemistry and pharmacology. Second, there seemed no attempt in any of the current works to create links between the various approaches to Chinese remedies. There is the TCM (Traditional Chinese Medicine) approach which presents Oriental herbal medicine purely in terms of traditional vitalistic therapeutics (such as the two-volume *Chinese Herbal Medicine* by Bensky, Gamble and Barolet); there is the modern scientific approach which explains the efficacy of Chinese remedies in biochemical terms (such as the two-volume *Pharmacology and Applications of Chinese Materia Medica* by Chang and But); and there is the modern synthetic approach which (somewhat indiscriminately) mixes vitalistic and scientific terms (such as the *Oriental Materia Medica* by Hsu). Each type of approach is informed by a discrete, watertight system that excludes any other. The only exception to this is the *Barefoot Doctor's Manual,* which is a first step in creating a more integral presentation of remedies successfully combining ancient and modern perspectives.

The type of presentation I have always developed is neither purely Chinese medical, nor purely pharmacological or botanical. The traditional Chinese medical approach I found too unavailable for Western therapists untrained in its complex, fluid language and ignorant of its vitalistic basis. How are they to know that the Chinese Kidney is not the anatomical kidney at all, or the Chinese Liver not the anatomical liver? (They often don't.) How are they to understand the meaning of such terms as "phlegm fire," "internal wind" and "hidden Qi," even with the most vivid of imaginations and fervent of zeals? How would they even dream of using remedies that "clear heat and drain damp," "release the exterior," "invigorate the collaterals" or "subdue Liver Yang?"

Likewise, the approaches presented by biochemistry, pharmacology and botany seemed too specialized by themselves to contribute much of lasting value in the area of therapeutics. The biochemical knowledge that a certain plant contains various types of glycosides, for instance, in itself doesn't directly translate to a particular therapeutic action—although in relation to other factors such as other constituents, clinical trials or empirical usage, it may be a significant piece of information. In the area of botany, the fact that Chinese medicine uses five main species in the *Rosa* plant genus in itself doesn't tell us anything immediately therapeutically useful. Nor, for instance, does the fact that the remedy Bupleurum Chai Hu (Asian buplever root) is derived from several, not just one, species of *Bupleurum*. Nor does the fact that the remedy Cordyceps Dong Chong Xia Cao (Chinese caterpillar mushroom) is made up of the fungus *Cordyceps sinensis* with its host larvae *Hepialus armoricanus* or *Holotrichia koraiensis*. Of course the facts found by chemistry, botany and so on may be interesting in themselves, and they often are useful when put in relation with other facts and used to create a larger picture of the whole. However, from the purely therapeutic standpoint they offer little when presented as ends in themselves.

Essentially, I have attempted to develop a language that is readily accessible to us in the West while still retaining the depth of content and subtlety of meaning of the traditional world view from which it arose. To create accessibility in this text I have taken two basic steps. The first is to organize the Chinese materia medica according to the anatomical body systems, Western-style, instead of the traditional therapeutic classes. For instance, whereas traditionally the remedy Artemisia Yin Chen Hao (Downy wormwood herb) is classed among "remedies for draining damp," its Western body system category would be the hepatobiliary system: the remedy is a *liver decongestant* with classic *cholagogue, laxative* and *diuretic* actions. Releasing Chinese herbs from their traditional context immediately makes them available to Western practitioners, who think in terms of disorders of the body systems rather than imbalances among body energies and qualities.

The second step is to present the character and functions of Chinese remedies in the familiar terms of Western pharmacology rather than the unfamiliar corresponding Chinese terminology. Biochemistry and pharmacology are the cornerstone rationale for remedies in the West and the basis for remedy selection and combining. This completes the process and now makes Chinese remedies readily available.

Both these steps tend to make Chinese remedies, which for us are usually shrouded in a hoary Oriental mystique of incomprehensibility, much clearer to our understanding. This demystification is clearly a good thing. However, herein also lies the danger of reductionism that has plagued Western thinking for centuries. If presented on its own, this Westernized interpretation of remedies runs the danger of creating a quantitative simplicism that reduces qualitative details and fine textures to simple, uniform strokes: the clinical subtleties and individual nuances of the remedies become lost. Because of this, in both steps above I have taken care always to embed the Western information—the remedy actions and indications—in the context of Chinese vitalistic principles—the symptom pictures. For example, the remedy Tricosanthes Tian Hua Fen (Snakegourd root) is a good *mucogenic* and *bronchial demulcent* used for conditions of mucosal deficiency and dryness seen in various respiratory and febrile disorders, as well as in diabetes. Now, in certain herbal lineages this remedy is indicated by preference when the symptom of unquenchable thirst is present. This symptom is the fine qualitative detail that makes the usage of Tricosanthes Tian Hua Fen different from other *mucogenic bronchial demulcents*. It is what makes the remedy's specific symptom picture. As explained above, this process ensures that the Western

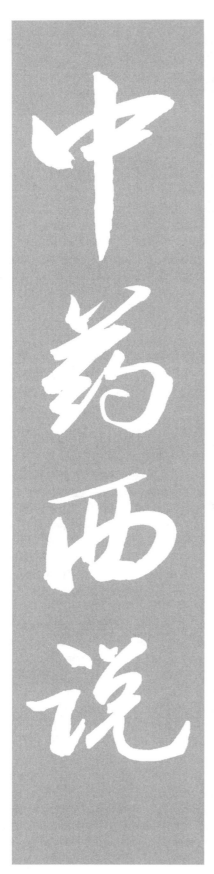

information remains part of a larger picture—literally; it encourages the practitioner to make links between the particular disease indications of a remedy and its more systemic symptom picture indications. Conversely, making this essential connection also enriches a remedy's traditional symptom picture use by providing valuable specific Western information.

In the process of searching for a more accessible terminology that would skirt these inherent dangers, I discovered a unique vehicle: the four basic treatment principles and remedy actions developed by the late nineteenth century Physiomedical herbalists, notably Cook and Thurston. The work of these practitioners represents one of the most recent examples of the Western vitalistic tradition. The terminologies that they developed specifically allow us to bridge the two streams of vitalistic Chinese herbal medicine and scientific Western botanical medicine. I realized that their basic principles of restore/relax, stimulate/sedate represent an ideal lynchpin able to hold together the Western remedy actions (e.g., *diaphoretic, diuretic, tonic,* etc.) and the principles of vitalistic herbal therapeutics (e.g., eliminating, restoring, relaxing, draining, etc.). These four principles have allowed me to make direct links between herb actions and treatment strategies, between pharmacology and therapeutics, and between plant chemistry and pharmacology. As a result, they have been key in making the large amount of scientific information available on Chinese remedies meaningful in relation to their traditional uses. Not just fascinating, but directly and crucially relevant! And conversely, they have provided the tool for the traditional remedy functions and indications to be clarified in the analytical terms of modern pharmacology. The net result of both these processes: remedy actions and indications that are much clearer, more precise and focused; and remedy profiles that approach homeopathic remedy pictures in their individuality and uniqueness.

In my striving to connect Chinese and Western herbal medicine, I found another common facet in these systems: the symptom picture. This is another key factor in any whole systems approach to therapeutics, and it is used in common by Chinese medicine (where it is called pattern of disharmony), Japanese Kampo herbal medicine (where it is called symptom conformation), the American Eclectic herbal medicine tradition (where it is called specific symptomatology) and European Homeopathy (where it is called symptomatology). Whereas in my *Energetics of Western Herbs,* the symptom pictures developed for each remedy by nineteenth century practitioners, such as Scudder, Ellingwood and King, helped me pinpoint their Chinese symptom picture uses, in this text they served as an important model for amplifying and refining the Chinese symptom patterns in light of today's disorders.

The four principles and the symptom picture represent tools for making most efficient use of traditional therapeutics and modern pharmacology combined. They open a dialogue between the vitalistic and the analytical approaches to healing. They thereby shed new light on the true nature and therapeutic potential of Chinese remedies—new light that we surely need in these times of chronic and degenerative disease, of advanced multifactorial conditions that sometimes seem to defy all untangling.

It is my sincere hope that developing this interactive language and synthesistic system for both my own satisfaction and use in actual practice will stimulate others to pursue the integration of diverse healing approaches. I believe that today this is necessary if we are to provide health care that is not only clinically more effective, but also truly holistic in the sense of supporting the individual growth of both patient and practitioner.

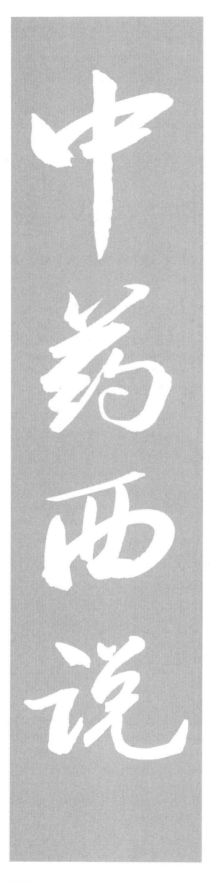

1

Ancient Medicine, Modern Medicine

Oriental medicine in the West is here to stay. Ever since its first tentative introduction to the West by Jesuit fathers in the sixteenth century, this ancient system of healing has demonstrated its effectiveness, its versatility and its profundity. Today Chinese medicine has developed beyond the confines of the Middle Kingdom, beyond the boundaries of East Asia, far beyond even the borders of the many Chinatowns found scattered worldwide. As an alternative medical system in the West, it has also been actively taken up by Western health professionals who are exploring and expanding its time-tested knowledge and applications. Its two main components, herbal medicine and acupuncture, are now widely accepted in the West as viable treatment modalities for ailments ranging from the simple and mundane to the complex and extraordinary. The use of patent remedies like Yin Qiao Jie Du Pian and Bi Yan Pian for simple colds, and Po Chai and Pill Curing for indigestion, for instance, are very widespread, while the use of acupuncture (in its many forms) and intensive Chinese internal herbal therapy for multifactorial disorders like ME (chronic fatigue syndrome) and AIDS have also become virtually standard in complementary health care. And a major type of Chinese herbal treatment, namely disease prevention and life extension through a regular program of Chinese tonic remedies, has become fairly popular. Remedies such as Asian ginseng root, Astragalus root, Wolfberry, Royal jelly and Deer antler are no longer household names in East Asia alone.

Chinese Medicine in Transition

It is not suprising that in this context Chinese medicine should currently find itself in a state of great transition as we try to understand it and use it for treatment of our contemporary diseases. What is the nature of this process of transformation that is everywhere in evidence?

About one third of the world's population, centered in East Asia, relies for its primary health care needs on Oriental medicine. The practice of Chinese herbal medicine is by far the largest aspect of this system, which is built on six millennia of cumulative experience in herbal prescribing. Herbal remedies are used in every social context from the lowest income household to the millionaire business tycoons; they are prescribed by every type of doctor from private physicians to street folk healers; and they are sold through a variety of different outlets from supermarkets to private pharmacies. Everyone in East Asia relies on crude herbs and their preparations for both medicine and food.

Throughout history, Chinese medicine has developed as an authentic continuous tradition that incorporates numerous lineages of teaching and practice, and that has freely exchanged medical ideas with neighboring systems of healing. Its paradox lies in that it is both a living tradition and a timeless paradigm of healing. As a living tradition it undergoes perpetual change and renewal, manifesting various styles of practice and therapeutic emphases throughout the centuries in those Asian countries where it is practiced, which include Korea, Japan, Taiwan, Vietnam and Malaysia. As a timeless paradigm of therapeutics it is based on immutable, constant and unquestioned assumptions regarding the nature of life, health and sickness.

Today Chinese medicine finds itself in a unique situation, namely, its momentous encounter with Western medicine. Ever since the gradual infiltration of allopathic Western medicine into major cities during the late nineteenth century, Chinese medicine has increasingly been unable to live out its existence in a timeless zone as it has for past millennia—self-sufficient, omniscient and incontrovertable—much in the way of traditional Greek medicine in its Islamic phase (800-1300 AD). Because Western medicine proved decisive in managing many of China's epidemiological conditions and in establishing modern hygiene, Chinese medicine finally found itself in a historical crisis. This crisis which began with the creation of the Republic of China in 1911 has continued through to the People's Republic of today. In addition, since the mid-twentieth century this crisis is also being played out in the West, notably in those countries where Chinese medicine is practiced most, France, the U.K. and the U.S. Essentially, there are two reasons for this current situation: the first epistemological, the second practical.

First, because Western medicine has taken over large sectors of health care throughout Asia, Chinese medicine for the first time has been forced into a position where it has to account for itself—where it has to explain its rationale and document its efficacy. It is true that throughout history Chinese medicine has been influenced by other systems—notably Tibetan and Ayurvedic medicine, as well as absorbing a large number of plant remedies from the Himalayan region, the Indian subcontinent and even Middle Eastern countries (*hu tao,* the walnut, means "Persian peach," for example, and numerous remedy names are simply phoneticizations of their Arabic, Persian, Sanskrit and other pronounciations). The system of the five elements itself, one that we consider archetypally Chinese, actually is a derivation of the four element-plus-one system used in traditional Greek and Indian/Ayurvedic medicine: Water, Fire, Earth, Air plus Ether (see Appendix B in Holmes 1989). Still, Chinese medicine in its core assumptions and methodology in the past has remained essentially unchanged; enriched in its concepts but not in any way challenged by other systems of medicine that share its vitalistic, empirical basis. The Greek medical diagnostic method of urine diagnosis, for example, that influenced Chinese medicine via Persian and Tibetan doctors during the Tang period, was merely another congenial tool for the Chinese physician to evaluate the patient's overall condition—alongside his native tongue and pulse diagnostics. It was simply another way for him to evaluate whether the condition was hot or cold, full or weak, external or internal. It certainly did not call into question the very model of this vitalistic system of diagnostics itself.

The current epistemological confrontation with Western scientific medicine, however, is unique. For the first time in history Chinese medicine is having its very assumptions questioned.

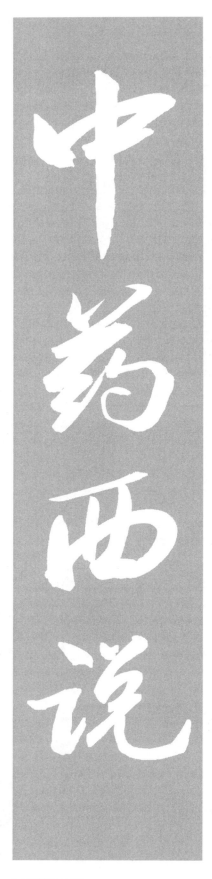

Its fundamental ontology—timeless and constant—is being challenged by the time-bound and ever-changing ontology of the West. Specifically, the vitalistic basis of Oriental medicine, with its entire pathologic, diagnostic and therapeutic methodology, is being questioned in light of Western science, including modern physiopathology, laboratory diagnostics and chemical and structural treatment techniques.

Second, the Western scrutiny that Oriental medicine is currently undergoing has a considerable practical counterpart. The confrontational encounter between the two systems is also being played out for reasons of sheer historical-cultural neccessity: the crisis within allopathic Western medicine itself. Because allopathic medicine is not based on a model of complete health, only on a concept of physical disease, it has become almost entirely a trauma or first-aid system on one hand, and an iatrogenic or drug therapy system on the other. As a result, it has left a conspicuous void in the successful managment of chronic disease as well as in preventive health care in general. Moreover, its crisis extends to the increased inability to cope with epidemic disease due to the overuse of antibiotics and the neglect of individual terrain diagnosis. Because nature abhors a vacuum, traditional systems of medicine that have endured and flourished over three millennia, such as traditional Chinese, Ayurvedic and Greek (Tibb Unani), have over the last hundred years increasingly been adopted by the West. The strength of all three systems is preventive medicine, the treatment of chronic conditions, constitutional and terrain diagnosis and a system of pharmacology using natural remedies relatively free of side-effects. These are precisely the elements missing from allopathic Western medicine.

This leaves us with a poignant paradox. On one hand, we in the West feel the innate urge to analyze Chinese medicine, to question its assumptions and methods—being very different from our own. On the other hand, we are experiencing an urgent need to supplement Western medicine with Chinese treatment methods, such as acupuncture and herbal medicine, that are proving effective and safe for managing chronic disorders. Although these two needs are not in themselves contradictory—they are still workable in actual practice—they nevertheless leave a legacy of unresolved issues in their wake. We may speculate about the ultimate result of this historical meeting between two systems as different from each other as night and day. Less ambitiously, we may ask, how is this confrontation currently presenting itself?

We can discern two major trends. On one hand, we can see Chinese medicine making small, almost imperceptible shifts of alignment with Western ideas and methods. The blurring of concepts that occurs in Chinese medicine as it is practiced in Japan, for instance, is an outstanding example. In colleges of acupuncture and shiatsu massage in particular, the twelve channels are always assumed to link specifically the organs that bear their name. The Liver channel thus is considered to have an energetic link with the anatomical liver, despite the fact that the Chinese name for that channel is "Foot Jue Yin," not "Liver," and regardless of the fact that in clinical practice the Liver channel acupoints are mainly used for urogenital disorders, not hepatic ones. This is simply cross-wiring of the channels, which are energetic by nature, with the internal organs, which are anatomical. This resultant confusion of concepts has spread to Europe mainly through French emissaries who in the early part of the twentieth century brought back certain aspects of Chinese medicine (primarily Song dynasty acupuncture methods). From there it has also pervaded, like a bedrock, the practice of Chinese medicine in the U.S.

Another case in point of this blurring is the almost ubiquitous assumption that the Chinese concepts *qi* and *xue* respectively refer to "energy" and "blood" as Western science defines these. Although nothing could be further from the truth, this blurring has actually led to a shift in alignment of contemporary Chinese medicine that has gone virtually unnoticed. When the term *qi* is translated as "energy," do we really know whether we mean energy as a scientific measurement or as a general "new age" concept of quality? Do we assume them to be one and the same, perhaps? Likewise, when a modern Chinese textbook talks about *xue yu,* is it refering to actual blood ecchymosis, blood sludging or hyperlipemia (take your pick!), or does it refer to a purely functional disorder that has no equivalent in the West? Amidst these uncertainties, the ultimate question here has to be, do we even attempt to look for a Western analogy or equivalent for these concepts?

On the other hand, the confrontation between the two medical systems is making us aware of the glaring discrepancy of approach, teaching and treatment method between them. For instance, in the area of physiology, whereas Chinese medicine looks primarily at function, Western medicine looks mainly at structure. This explains the difference between a pathology of gross functions as expressed in terms of syndromes, and a histological tissue pathology expressed in terms of bacteriology and microbiology. Equally, it is obvious, for example, that the pathology of the Liver (*gan*) in Chinese medicine involves primarily (but not exclusively) the nervous system, not the anatomical liver organ. About two-hundred years ago the medical researcher Wang Qing-ren devoted forty years of his life to exploring the differences between Chinese and Western anatomy and physiology, summarizing these in his 1831 text *Yi Lin Chai Cuo,* "Correction of Errors from Medical Literature." In the area of diagnostics, when a pulse is taken in Western medicine, the main information sought is any abnormality of rate and rhythm—quantitative information—whereas in Oriental medicine the qualitative sensations experienced by the practitioner is paramount: it is these that are classified into about twenty-eight different pulse qualities.

Examples could be continued endlessly. As regards therapy, Western allopathic medicine seeks mainly to alleviate symptoms and correct mechanical dysfunctions and, because it relies largely on synthetic medications, often ends up suppressing symptoms and generating negative side-effects. This is not to decry, of course, the value of Western medicine in emergency health-care, physical and epidemiological. Oriental medicine, on the other hand, attempts to treat the systemic condition in addition to alleviating symptoms (the common link) and, because it utilizes purely natural remedies, generally incurs no or minimal side-effects as it relieves symptoms.

As we become more aware of the fundamental differences in Oriental medicine in all its aspects, again the same paradox arises. In the very process of trying to understand Chinese medicine, the pragmatics of the Western health care situation usually intervene. We often end up using Chinese medical tools out of neccessity alone, without a satisfactory understanding of how they work either in Chinese or Western terms.

Challenged on one hand by the scrutiny of the Western analytical gaze, and on the other hand, paradoxically, by the West's immediate need for effective management of chronic disorders, Oriental medicine in its state of crisis is slowly, if imperceptibly, changing. In return, it is awakening in us the realization that its intrinsic nature is still profoundly different from our own medical system. What are we to do with this contradiction in terms of furthering a truly effective system of health care ?

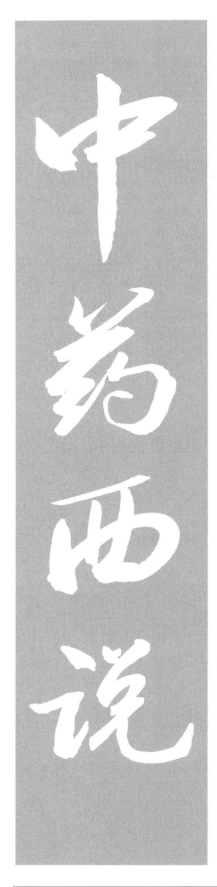

Chinese Medicine Renewed

A major reason for the perennial viability and therapeutic success of Oriental medicine is its adaptiveness, its versatility. Up to the present time, Oriental medicine has flourished because it has been able to adapt to a variety of different health care needs in various social settings in China and throughout East Asia. In Korea, Japan, Taiwan, Vietnam, Malaysia and California, it has developed to a greater or lesser extent a distinct flavor. In most of these countries new therapeutic ideas, new techniques and, of course, new herbal remedies have been developed in the practice of Chinese medicine. In Korea and Japan, for instance, completely distinct systems of acupuncture—the majority unknown in the West—have existed for almost a millennium. Japan in particular has developed a unique system of herbal medicine called *kampo,* with its own prescribing methods based on symptom conformation of standard herbal formulas. Traditional doctors, researchers and pharmacists in Taiwan and Japan have been leaders in the field of utilizing local plant resources, and over centuries have developed native plant equivalents to the standard plant sources of mainland China. In addition, in all those countries plant remedies not found on the continent, many of them highly effective, have been empirically researched and utilized. In some cases these are even imported back to the mainland. This adaptability to growth and modification is an intrinsic aspect of how Chinese medicine works, of its essentially dialectic nature. It is the source of its power and ability to survive.

No one would deny that the West's health concerns are somewhat different from those faced by less industrialized nations. Chronic and degenerative disorders are the current hallmark of countries in the "North." If Oriental medicine is to flourish in the West, it clearly needs to adapt itself to these conditions. It needs to grow new branches, based on its roots in the time-tested wisdom of the empirical dialectical paradigm. And, given its track record, Chinese medicine is most likely to succeed in this adaptation.

However, success is not primarily a quantitative thing: it is usually defined in terms of qualitative judgments. Moreover, Chinese medicine's adaptation to Western conditions can assume different forms. One form that it currently takes in the People's Republic itself is the tandem or cooperative situation, in which Chinese and Western medical treatment approaches are used concurrently. In this situation, practitioners when treating patients may make primary use of Chinese medicine, and secondarily of Western medicine, or vice-versa, depending on the requirements of the situation. It is often argued that the two therapies complement each other, and in a sense sometimes they do. *The Barefoot Doctor's Manual,* widely available in the West, is a classic example of a text based on the principles of mutual reinforcement of the two systems—although it may not be the best example of the New Medicine as promulgated in the early seventies by Maoist thinkers. In this practitioner's field manual Western social and personal hygiene practices are presented in clear detail; acupuncture points are here described just in terms of the symptoms and Western diseases they treat; therapeutic techniques include acupuncture, massage and Western methods of emergency treatment; and disorders are presented with both a Western and Chinese medical differential diagnosis.

Another form of adaptation currently adopted by Chinese medicine is the integrative trend. This approach, adopted mainly by pharmacologists and other researchers in the area of remedy pharmacology and acupoint biophysics and biochemistry, attempts to evaluate the therapeutic effects of herbal medicine and acupuncture in terms of scientific research. A particular remedy action may thus be explained by reference to the presence of one or more chemical compounds; the therapeutic effect of an acupoint may be clarified by noting its action on hormones, neurotransmitters and so on. For example, the salutory effect of the remedy Bufo Chan Su, Toad venom, in the treatment of circulatory collapse, hypotension and shock can be explained through its content in cardiotonic glycosides (called bufotoxins) and hormones (including epinephrine and serotonine). We must be careful here to discern the intent behind the integrative approach, however. This may be based on a cautious sense of reformism or a radical reformism (Unschuld 1985). In the first case, the idea is simply to enhance the credibility of a known therapeutic effect of a remedy, for instance, with scientific backup research. The confirmation of steroidal saponins in the remedy Dioscorea Chuan Shan Long, Nippon yam root, thus lends credence to, or scientifically validates, its traditional use in acute forms of arthritis. In the second case of radical reformism, the intent is rather to base the therapeutic applications of a remedy solely on biochemical research. Although the findings may be the same, here the empirical remedy uses are rejected as simply "unproven."

However, there are other possibilities involved in the process of adaptation. The most intriguing idea is that of a true interaction between Chinese and Western medicine, between a medicine based on vitalism and one based on analysis. This would bring it closer to the modern Chinese ideal of a New Medicine, entailing as it does a "dialectical synthesis of contradictory healing systems" (Unschuld). The materia medica in this book is based on the premise that this dialectical synthesis is possible. It is an attempt to promote Chinese medicine's adaptation in the West in a way that makes best use of the scientific approach in the context of Chinese vitalistic principles.

The key dynamic in such a dialectical integration is the Western vitalistic tradition because of its inherent ability to bridge the Western analytical approach and the vitalistic Chinese approach. Chapter 2 will show how the Western vitalistic system of pharmacology, based on the Eclectic and Physiomedical traditions of herbal medicine, can link us directly with Chinese pharmacology.

Chinese Medicine as a Mirror

Regardless of our belief about the nature and efficacy of Oriental medicine, about its present and future role in a Western health care setting, we may still ask ourselves the more pragmatic, bottom-line question: How can we as Westerners benefit from Oriental medicine? The clear answer is that Chinese medicine has demonstrably much to offer due to its efficacy in disease prevention and its effectiveness in treating chronic conditions—two areas in which Western allopathic medicine is relatively weak. Still, as shown by Unschuld (1985), not efficacy alone, but the cultural-ideological context also will determine to what extent a therapeutic system takes root and thrives in a particular society. Therefore, it is relevant to first take a step back and understand our own perception of Chinese medicine and consider how ultimately this perception affects its efficacy and viability in the West.

It is my belief that the West will reap the most benefits that vitalistic Chinese medicine has to

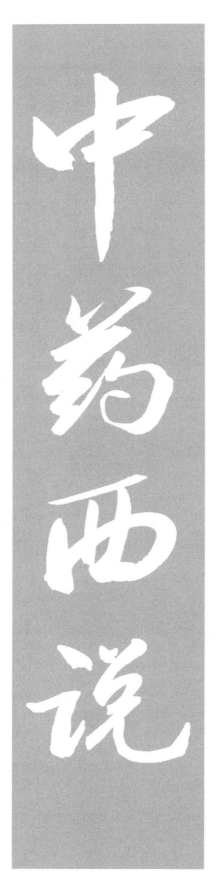

offer if we do not seek to impose our analytical science onto it, but instead use analytical science to enhance its empirical findings. The extent to which we accept Chinese medicine for what it is and can offer us in its own terms will largely determine its measure of success in the West.

Chinese medicine is based on a vitalistic system of logic, terminology and methodology. There is a difference between imposing the analytic method onto such a system and merely employing analytic terms to describe and inform it. By imposing we mean reducing the description of the methods and results obtained by Chinese medicine to scientific concepts alone, or reinterpreting these results in strictly scientific terms. This approach specifically relates to the "radical reformism" towards Chinese medicine that certain groups have advocated ever since the institutionalization of Western allopathic medicine in the early years of the twentieth century—a trend still prominent today.

The acupoint LIV-3, for example, is said by traditional acupuncturists to "pacify the Liver, regulate the Blood and open the channels." If we now say that LIV-3 works in this way simply because it is *anti-inflammatory, analgesic* and *tranquilizant,* we are effectively reducing the explanation of its effect to known physiological actions alone. Likewise in herbal medicine, if the remedy Fritillaria Chuan Bei Mu is understood to stop coughing and promote expectoration simply because it contains the *tranquillizing* alkaloids fritimine, sipeimine and others, this is a reductionist scientific rationalization of its overall therapeutic profile.

Using a non-imposing or descriptive approach, we rather use scientific data to elucidate the methods and results achieved by Chinese medicine. This relates directly to the "cautious reformism" approach towards Chinese medicine classically adopted by certain practitioners and organizations in the 1920s. In the non-imposing approach we may say that the acupoint LIV-3 relieves headache *and* it is known scientifically to possess *analgesic,* etc. activity. Here the relation between the therapeutic effect of the acupoint and the scientific fact is not causal but parallel. The scientific fact becomes an interesting enhancemement rather than a sole and ultimate rationalization. Similarly, when Fritillaria Chuan Bei Mu is known to relieve coughing and promote expectoration, we note the presence of *antitussive* alkaloids among its constituents, without claiming this to be the only explanation of its effects. The fact of alkaloids being present then becomes a useful enhancement of the remedy's complete picture rather than an all-consuming explanation.

There are other examples of reductionist reinterpretation that we believe are detrimental to our benefitting from Chinese medicine to the fullest extent. One such is the attempt, more common in China than in the West, to show scientifically that a certain class of Chinese remedies—for instance the Yang tonics, or the Blood tonics—share a common pharmacology or biochemistry. The analogy this conjures is the attempt of early European anatomists to find the seat of the soul by dissecting the human body. The point is this: analysis of the physical parts is not the right method for helping us explain the functioning of the whole—whether a class of remedies, a single remedy, an individual, whatever. The scientific approach by its very method starts with analysis of the parts, not the whole, whereas the vitalistic method always starts with a definition of the whole before proceeding to look at the parts. If we relax this scientific approach, however, and simply use analytical information to inform rather than explain the functioning of the whole, interesting observations then come to light. The class of remedies that "transform Spleen damp," for instance, mostly contain a high proportion of essential oils—which makes sense in terms of their "pungent taste quality" and their traditional use for digestive disorders. Equally, the remedy class that "nourishes the Yin and moistens dryness" is dominated (but not exclusively so) by remedies that contain saponins, which helps explain their *mucogenic, secretion-promoting* effect in dry respiratory conditions.

Clearly, it is how we use scientific information, rather than the information itself, that is crucial in letting Chinese medicine "breathe," rather than suffocating it beneath blankets of reductionist speculation. Our mindset, or intent, can snuff the life out of vitalistic Chinese medicine just as easily as it can turn it into an enhancement of Western health care. It is in this sense that Chinese medicine functions as a mirror to our own perception of it.

The Essence of Chinese Medicine

Every culture has an individuality, makes a distinct statement that is its own. This individual statement comes from its essence, is an expression of its spiritual essence. As cultural expression, Chinese medicine is no exception. Ultimately, we in the West will only benefit from Chinese medicine if we are open to the gift of its essence. Put into words, we may say that Chinese medicine is a search for balance in everything, as a statement of the unity of all life, for the benefit of all living things. Going to the essence of what Chinese medicine is, how it works and why it is effective, allows us to by-pass the confusion arising from looking merely at its form, its time-dependant mold. As Unschuld (1986) again evinces, its form down the ages has always changed. Its interpretations and representations have been equally numerous, leading right up to the modern interpretations of scientific pharmacology. Theories of pathology and pharmacology, models of diagnostics and therapeutics, all these—and then some—have come and gone ever since the dawn of time. Only by opening ourselves to its true gift, its timeless, individual spiritual essence, do we stand really to be enriched by it.

How would this process of enrichment actually occur? First, going to the essence of Chinese medicine allows us to adapt and utilize the perennial vitalistic wisdom that informs it according to our own Western understanding and current health needs. This is important if we are not to be enslaved by the conceptual forms and trappings that constitute Chinese medicine, as any other system. Second, going to its essence specifically allows us to reinterpret and adapt the structure and language that encases it without destroying its vitalistic basis. It means that we are able to freely and without damage adapt, or rework, the traditional conceptual structure of its pathology, diagnostics, pharmacology, etc., according to present-day knowledge in these areas.

For example, there is nothing in the actual content of Chinese medical physiopathology that is fixed or written in stone. As has been pointed out widely by different authors, the image of Oriental medicine as a homogenous, totally consistent, logical-to-a-T, unchanging conceptual system is absolutely illusory. Granted, it is hard for anyone trained in the current context of TCM (Traditional Chinese Medicine) education to see beyond this image. However, both the history and contemporary practice of Chinese medicine show that a bewildering plurality of models of physiology and pathology actually exist. Witness, for instance, the plethora of different ideas penned by countless authors down the centuries regarding the functions of the internal organs. If today we

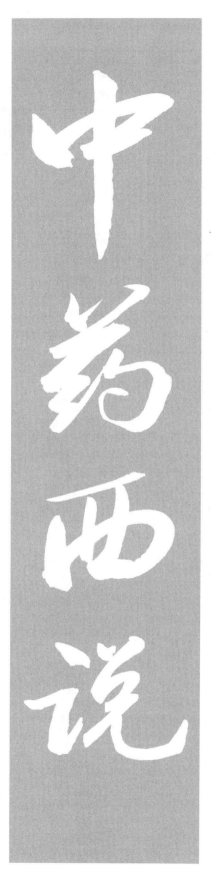

propose Chinese organ functions more in line with the anatomical organ systems, who is to say that this is not true Chinese medicine? A concept such as "nerve and brain deficiency," for instance, despite its initial ambivalent sound, may rightfully count as a Chinese syndrome of disharmony as long as it meets the criteria of vitalistic pathology. The fact that it uses the scientific-anatomic concept of the nervous system is incidental—being only the result of our current knowledge.

As another example, let us take the traditional Chinese syndrome "Liver Qi stagnation," which includes symptomatology we would ascribe to autonomic nervous and even hormonal imbalance. If we were to limit the definition of this condition in line with known physiologic liver dysfunctions, this would merely be a contemporary adaptation of a traditional syndrome. The redefinition of this syndrome would certainly be philosophically more authentic, terminologically less confusing and clinically more useful at the present time than pretending that Chinese Liver functions are the same as anatomical liver functions—which they clearly are not. Again, because it arises from its essence, the only absolute or constant in this process of adaptation is the vitalistic conceptual methodology used, not the details of the content itself. Those details, as history has shown, have changed throughout time. The essence is the key, not the details.

Another significant reason for the present timeliness of going to the essence of Chinese medicine is simply for the model of vitalistic medicine that it provides. Western medicine has been cornered for too long and too exclusively by science in general and by synthetic chemistry in particular. Chinese medicine by its mere presence shows us some possibilities of incorporating vitalistic principles and methods of therapy in Western allopathic medicine. The idea of prevention, not just cure, for example, which has always existed in the West—if we dig back far enough. The concept of natural remedies free of side-effects, which have been officially relegated to folklore. And so on. Because we find it easier in our need to seek help and inspiration from outside, from the East, rather than from the system of traditional Greek medicine in our own backyard, we have turned to Chinese medicine as a primary model of effective vitalistic medicine.

This materia medica is not only about Chinese remedies: it is also about the spirit of Chinese medicine. In the process of incorporating Western pharmacology and pathology in Chinese pharmacology and pathology, I have had to go to the essence of Chinese medicine and present it in a Western form. This text takes the jade of Chinese remedies and presents it to the West.

2

Redefining and Reclassifying Chinese Remedies

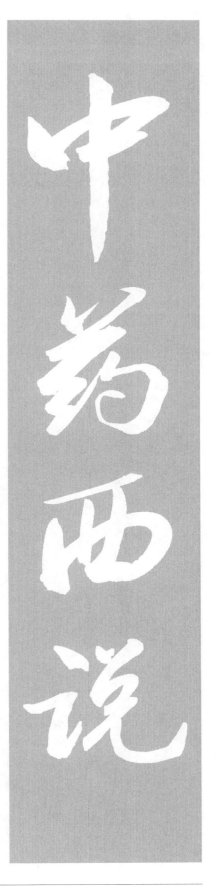

Having developed, adapted and survived for over 3,000 years, Chinese medicine is poised for yet another metamorphosis along its pleomorphic journey across the globe. This may be its most radical change yet: from an ancient, imperially sanctioned system of classical medicine to a viable system of health care in the West. We are drawn to wonder about the specific conditions that would make Chinese herbal medicine fully accepted and clinically effective in a Western context. Arguably, what is now required for us in the West is nothing less than a complete re-evaluation of this system if Chinese herbal medicine is to become an integral and recognized part of our society's health care options. This process is now possible as Oriental medicine has had a chance to settle down in the West and enough time has passed for us to feel more comfortable with it. The redefinition of its terminology in the language of Western medical systems, both allopathic and vitalistic, is now necessary if it is to fulfill its full potential as a healing modality on our shores.

Science and Vitalism: The Two Pharmacologies

Redefining Chinese herbal medicine entails stepping back and taking a hard, fresh look at its basic therapeutic tools, the remedies themselves. In order to work out the clinical details of Chinese herbology in Western terms, we first need to return directly to the essence of the Chinese remedies. Specifically, these need re-evaluating in both Western scientific and vitalistic terms. The nature of these terms will become clearer if we remember the two different essential approaches to obtaining knowledge that informs them. The now dominant scientific approach, based on reductionistic linear logic that relies on cause and effect observation, is governed by the need to

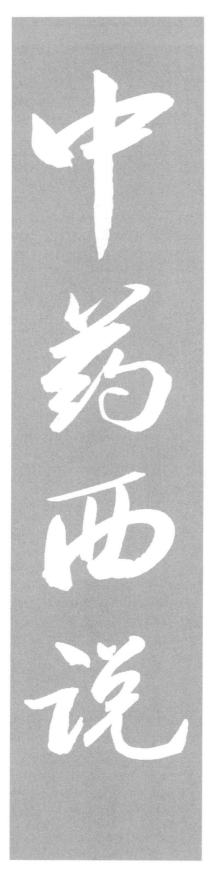

express facts in quantitative and mechanistic terms that can be measured, weighed or otherwise reduced to a mathematical formula; these facts must also be experimentally reproducible at any time anywhere, absolutely independent of the person observing them. The vitalistic approach, once dominant in indigenous and medical traditions, is based on systemistic spatial logic that relies on observation of correspondence and synchronicity, and is governed by the expression of facts in qualitative and living terms that relate directly to sensory experience in its infinite variety; these facts themselves are understood to undergo change over time and in space, as well as being relatively dependent on the person observing them, i.e., on the process of observation itself.

The point of interest here is this. The Western tradition of knowledge itself contains aspects of both analysis and vitalism. The traditional Greek medicine (TGM, for short) of antiquity combined the analytic/scientific and vitalistic/empirical approaches. TGM's and Greek philosophy's analytical stream ultimately led to Descartes' and Bacon's 17th century reductionism and has today resulted in Western allopathic medicine. The vitalistic stream, although running deeper than the scientific stream, has lost favor since the Renaissance. Nevertheless, it is still now mainly represented by homeopathic medicine (whose origins reach back beyond Hahnemann and Hering to the time of Paracelsus and his acolytes in the early 1500s), by spagyric medicine which goes back to the alchemical tradition of Valentinus, Van Helmont, Lulle, Weidenfeld and Becker, and by herbal medicine with its more recent revival by Eclectic and Physiomedical practitioners in North America and England such as Scudder, King, Ellingwood, Thurston, Cook and Priest. A large segment of the booming alternative medical movement has its roots in this Western vitalistic tradition.

It is this living presence of the rich tradition of vitalistic medicine in the West that can serve as a springboard for redefining and revitalizing Chinese herbal medicine. Because both systems of herbal medicine share a common empirical basis (as we will see below), Greek medical pharmacology actually allows us to reinterpret and redefine Chinese pharmacology in Western terms. True, there is certainly great potential for some aspects of Chinese herbal medicine to be accepted here through scientific validation alone. However, for it to come fully to fruition in the West in its whole form, I feel it will require revitalization through reinterpretation in the light of Western vitalistic principles, which are far closer to it than current allopathic constructs.

For those of you not interested in the scientific aspects of herbal remedies, please go directly to page 59 for a discussion of the Western vitalistic tradition and its connection to Chinese medicine.

Scientific Pharmacognosy

At least there should be no mystery about the best procedure for redefining Chinese remedies in scientific terms. It has three major aspects: pharmacognosy, pharmacology and remedy classification and therapeutics based on Western physiology. This third aspect is discussed separately at the very end of this chapter. The pharmacognosy of Chinese herbs, in its broadest sense, is already long underway, especially in China, Taiwan and Japan, and has seen a dramatic renaissance since the 1960s. The Chinese papers summarizing research in pharmacognosy since 1949 make it clear that much more energy is devoted to this field than even to pharmacology, and more than is done anywhere in the West (Cui 1979, Xu 1985 and 1989, Xu and But 1986). Areas such as remedy identification, naming, sourcing, production methods and chemical analysis are covered in meticulous detail, drawing on botany, mineralogy, zoology, phytochemistry, ethnobotany and history to produce a rich, multifaceted science.

Ethnobotany combined with chemical analysis, for example, has come up with a large number of folk remedies (mostly of plant origin) that yield significantly active compounds that are then repeatedly tested in live clinical trials for specific conditions. In some cases these studies validate traditional folk uses, and in other cases they do not. The active constituents in the root of *Salvia miltiorrhiza* (Dan Shen, cinnabar sage) were found in surveys to be higher in count in *S. trijuga* and *S. przewalskii*, which are not even considered official sources of the remedy Dan Shen (Jian Yang-hui 1989). In 1987 a new medicinal species was recorded in Anhui province, the orchid *Eria reptans*. Its pseudobulb is known as the remedy Pu Tao Mao Lan, and is used locally for its *antipyretic, antiseptic, analgesic* and *detumescent* effects (Shen Bao-an 1987). A study conducted on ten species of *Thalictrum* (meadow rue) collected from Northeast China showed that the root of *T. squarrosum* was highest (1.36%) in the *antitumoral* alkaloid thalidasine (Wang Zheng-tao et al. 1988). Another example of new potential sources of remedies is the numerous species of *Cordyceps* (Dong Chong Xia Cao, Chinese caterpillar mushroom). Through analysis of their habitat, chemical components and regional therapeutic applications, many species have shown the same *restorative* and *antiasthmatic* medicinal value as the original and primary remedy, *C. sinensis*. These species include *Cordyceps hawkesii, C. lianshanensis* (Tang Wan-quan 1980, Hu Ruo-ying 1983), *C. liangshanensis* and *C. militaris,* which is higher in amino acids than *C. sinensis* (Gao Hui-an et al. 1987).

On a more spectacular note, the originally obscure folk remedy from South China, Jiao Gu Lan, *Gynostemma pentaphyllum* (Cucurbitaceae), has found the limelight since the late 1980s. The remedy has evinced *adaptogenic* and *anti-aging* properties superior even to Eleuthero ginseng and cardiovascular actions superior to Asian ginseng. One experiment showed that the whole plant reduced or prevented experimental senility (Xu Fu-ben et al. 1989). Jiao Gu Lan is loaded with an array of over 82 saponin glycosides (incl. gypenosides and ginsenosides), 15 amino acids and numerous trace elements. Its actions are mainly neuroendocrine-immune (*adaptogenic, antiageing, immune enhancing*), hormonal (*gonadotropic, adrenocortical restorative, hypoglycemic*), metabolic (*liver-protective, protein synthesis promoting*) and neurocardiac (*neurocardiac sedative, hypnotic, analgesic, vasodilator, hypotensive, coronary flow restorative, antilipemic and hemodynamic regulator* (Chen Zai-zhi and Su Huan-qun 1989, Zhou He-ping 1988).

This identification and taxonomy process of the Chinese materia medica is a vast ongoing task. Of the 5,700 plus remedies traditionally used, 90% are of plant origin (But Paul-hui 1984). The plant remedies alone have been analyzed as deriving from 240 families, 1,544 genera and 4,941 species (But Paul-hui 1981), which respectively represent 84%, 52% and 19% of China's total flora of vascular plants. Historically, Chinese remedies have always been divided into classical remedies and folk remedies. Classical remedies are those that were officially entered into the imperial herbals, or *ben cao,* dynasty after dynasty, and are still used mainly by government-sanctioned doctors and pharmacists throughout the Chinese-speaking world. The twenty-seven volume Tang Ben Cao compiled by Su Ching in 659, for instance, contained 850 remedies (a number very comparable to the 882 remedies listed in the national pharmacopeia of 1978). Folk remedies are

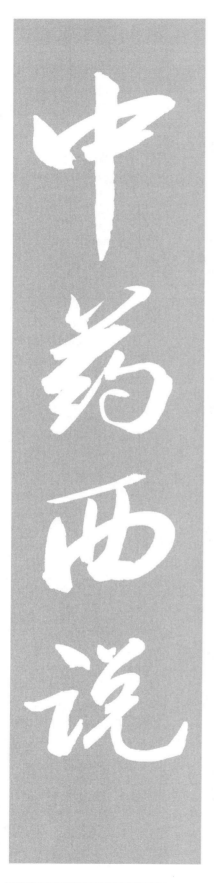

those used purely at the popular level (self-medication, family care, village folk healers, herb gatherers and farmers, etc.). It comes as no surprise that new species in use (or not yet in use) are constantly being discovered, and historical research is always coming to new conclusions as to the botanical identity of remedies presented in past herbals. The botanical source for the common digestive remedy Zhi Shi (Unripe bitter orange fruit), for example, classically was *Poncirus trifoliata* alone, not *Citrus aurantium* and spp., now commonly the case (Chen Zhong-ming 1981). The traditional botanical origin of the important *anti-infective* remedy Lian Qiao (Forsythia valve) is the fruit of *Hypericum ascyron*, as seen in the herbal Zhi Wu Ming Shi Tu Kao (which is the main source of illustrations in this book). In 1984 three new species of *Bupleurum* (*B. kunmingense, B. luxiense* and *B. polyelonum*) were identified, related to the commonly used species *B. chinense* and *B. falcatum* that represent the important *nervous sedative* and *anti-infective* remedy Chai Hu (Asian buplever root). Interestingly, their saponin count was found to be up to eight times that of the commonly used species (Pan Sheng-li et al. 1984). It was concluded in 1988 that the *diaphoretic* remedy Fang Feng (Wind-protector root) may originate in any of 10 different species of *Ledebouriella* (Wang Jian-hua 1988). Likewise, the *anti-infective* remedy Huang Lian is derived from the root of eight species and two varieties of *Coptis* (goldthread) (Wang Tian-zhi 1988). A survey from Beijing describes the evolution in the source plant as well as the plant part used for the remedy Yu Jin (Turmeric). Before the Ming dynasty, *Curcuma longa* was the only species used for Yu Jin. Since the early Qing dynasty, however, other species such as *C. aromatica* were also admitted for this remedy. Over time, the root tuber alone rather than the rhizome of these species became another definition for Yu Jin. Today, the tuber still furnishes Yu Jin and the rhizome Jiang Huang, although only *C. longa* (the original species) is used for Jiang Huang. The authors conclude that "from the viewpoint of resources exploitation and chemical and pharmacological studies, the use of the rhizome as medicinal part seemed more logical" (Chen Yu-heng et al. 1987, in Abstracts 2(3), Nov. 1988). The *anti-infective* remedies Ai Ye and Qing Hao normally and officially are derived from herb of *Artemisia argyi* (Asian mugwort) and *Artemisia apiacea* (Celery wormwood), respectively. In addition to possible derivation from other remedies such as Huang Hua Hao, *Artemisia annua* (Annual wormwood), Ai Ye and Qing Hao together have shown possibly to be derived from no less than 61 species and 11 varieties of *Artemisia*. Moreover, six species of the genus *Seriphidium* were also found to count for either Ai Ye or Qing Hao (see also the start of Chapter 3 for further *Artemisia* discussions) (Ling Yeou-ruen 1986).

The cultural and geographical pharmacognosy of the important tonic remedy Huang Qi, depicted on this book's front cover, should be of great interest to us in the West. It has certainly received extensive research attention in China. Two distinct genuses have historically served as source for the remedy Huang Qi: *Astragalus* and *Hedysarum*. A key study performed recently by five researchers shows that at least 20 different species of *Astragalus* are currently used, in one district or another, as source of this remedy (Sun San-sheng et al. 1990). Likewise, five species of *Hedysarum* are also commonly used for the remedy, making this truly a large two-genera family of Huang Qi. It is even thought by some researchers that the species referred to in classic texts up to the Ming dynasty belong in fact to *Hedysarum*, not *Astragalus*. However that may be, the fact is that today two main species of the genus *Astragalus* are officially recognized as source for Huang Qi—*A. membranaceus* and *A. mongholicus*—while *Hedysarum polybotrys* (the main species of that genus) is now more commonly called Hong Qi. Because of this, it is ironic to note that a rash of pharmacological studies have then proceeded to show that, as far as immune stimulation and polysaccharide content and activity go, the main *Astragalus* and *Hedysarum* species produce absolutely comparable results! (Shen Yu-qing et al. 1989, Mao Xiao-juan et al. 1988, 1988). Folk usage of relative interchangeability among members of the Huang Qi family seems thereby to be vindicated.

Clearly, the common Chinese practice of having several species (sometimes even more than one genus) as botanical origin of a remedy complicates the already complex field of taxonomy even further (see the next chapter for a full discussion of this). An outstanding case in point is the *anti-infective* remedy Guan Zhong, whose botanical origins was surveyed in two enlightening reports that contrasted the northwest and southwest Chinese taxa employed (Ai Tie-min et al. 1987). The northwestern sources of the remedy Guan Zhong were found to be mainly *Dryopteris filix-mas, Matteuccia struthiopteris, Lunathyrium vegetius, L. giraldii* and *Athyrium sinense,* whereas in the southwestern provinces Yunnan, Guizhou and Sichuan the species *Osmunda japonica, Woodwardia japonica, W. unigemmata, Dryopteris lepidopoda, Blechnum orientale* and *Cyathea spinulosa* are predominantly used. The morphological and anatomical differences of these plants and their rhizomes are clearly tabulated.

Studies of particular plant families and their pharmacological and therapeutic themes have also been carried out. Among the 220 genera and 2,250 species of composites found in China, 120 genera and some 500 species are used medicinally, about three-quarters of which have been scientifically evaluated in one way or another. Flavonoids, alkaloids, coumarins, essential oils, sesquiterpene lactones, acetylenic compounds, polysaccharides and organic acids are the main constituents found in the Compositae. Asterae, Inuleae and Senecionae are the main genera used in respiratory conditions by variously providing *expectorant, antitussive* and *bronchodilatant* actions. Cynareae are notoriously used for their *hemostatic* effect, while numerous taxa from many tribes and genera (including *Saussurea, Leibnitzia* and *Siegesbeckia*) bring various *antirheumatic* properties (Chen Lu-sheng 1987).

China also grows 94 genera, 505 species and 49 varieties of umbellifers, among which 46 genera, 141 species and 16 varieties are used in medicine. Predominant components include essential oils, coumarins, flavonoids, alkaloids and triterpenes, and the most common conditions treated with umbellifers as a whole are gynecological, hormonal, rheumatoid, upper respiratory and digestive (Yuan Chang-qi 1986).

But the materia medica consists of more than just plant remedies: It also includes fungal, mineral and animal remedies, which in turn subdivide. The latter, for instance, include important maritime as well as terrestial remedies. Maritime remedies alone include shells (clams, cockles, abalones, mother of pearls, oysters and turtles), bones (cuttlefish) and whole parts (sea horse, sea cucumber). Over 120 species of fungal remedies alone are also traditionally used, including various species of *Ganoderma* (reishi), *Armillariella* and *Cordyceps* (caterpillar fungus), as well as *Poria cocos* (hoelen), *Polyporus umbellatus* (umbel polypore), *Tremella fuciformis* (silver ear), *Fomitiporia punctata, Lentinus edodes, Irpex lacteus, Polystictus versicolor, Hericium erinaceus, Marasmius androsaceus, Hypocrella bambusae, Auricularia auricula, Shiraia bambusicola, Morchella* spp., *Pleurotus ostreatus* and the rare *Amanitopsis volvata*. Their chemistry and pharma-

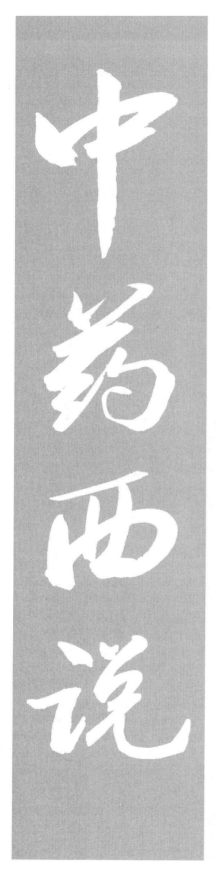

cology has been extensively researched (Lin Shu-qian et al. 1987).

Identification of plant remedies in Chinese medicine is made even more complex if we factor in the medicinal plants growing outside of mainland China in Vietnam, Taiwan, Japan and Malaysia. The island of Taiwan alone, for instance, has about 2,600 endemic plants, of which about 350 are used in Chinese medicine, but each includes several species. In addition, about another 1,000 of these (each with several species) are used as folk remedies. In Japan about 250 of the classical Chinese remedies are routinely used, although Japan too has a large number of endemic plants, many of which are used in folk medicine (Hsu Hong-yen 1987).

Physiochemical identification of remedies is another major aspect of pharmacognosy extensively conducted in China, and utilizes a wide range of methods such as UV, IR, TLC, HPTLC (very widely used), DCC, electrophoresis, polarography, spectrophotometry, fluorometry and plasma spectrometry. Examples of major chemical constituents found in Chinese remedies is given in Chapter 3. For instance, using HPTLC densitometry, the naphthoquinone contents of various genera and species that represent the *anti-inflammatory* remedy Zi Cao (Purple groomwell root) was shown generally to accord with the traditional classification of this remedy into five grades of quality—the highest count being 2.13-6.73% in *Arnebia euchroma,* the lowest being 0.13-0.81% in *Arnebia guttata, Onosma hookeri* and *O. paniculatum,* with the commonly used *Lithospermum erythrorhizon* coming somewhere in the middle with 0.39-1.8% (Fu Shan-lin et al. 1984). Atomic absorption spectrophotometry has been used to define the trace minerals and metalloids in the root of *Angelica sinensis* (Dang Gui, dong quai), 23 in all (Rui He-kai 1983). Trace elements seem to be the research fad of the 1990s, in fact. The content in the terpenoid iridoid geniposide of the fruit of *Gardenia jasminoides* (Shan Zhi Zi, gardenia) was evinced highest in the seed, and decreasingly in the fruit, fried fruit, charred fruit and fruit pulp (Tang Ying 1988). Another study from Sichuan conducted a mass comparison by both TLC and gas chromatography of 11 species of *Asarum,* all providing the respiratory remedy Xi Xin (Asian wild ginger). Their essential oil profiles were seen to be different, and their safrole and methyleugenol content was quantified. Also, their oil content ranged from as low as 0.40% in *A. tonjiangense* to a peak of 3.36% in *A. sieboldii,* which rightly should be considered the main botanical source for this remedy (Gu Yue-cui et al. 1987).

Through biochemical techniques, the well-known fact of plant remedy substitution has also been scientifically established. Substitution is a common practice in the herbal medicine trade, and is carried out both unknowingly, usually for lack of proper plant identification techniques on the part of plant collectors, and fraudulently, i.e. with the intention to adulterate. For example, in many provinces the botanical sources of the digestive remedy Shan Yao (Mountain yam root) go beyond the accepted species *Dioscorea batatas* and *opposita*. One study established through organoleptic inspection of the tubers and microscopic analysis of the starch grains that the species *D. persimilis, D. fordii, D. alata* and *D. japonica* are sometimes also used (Hang Yue-yu et al. 1987). In Liaoning the root of *Sphallerocarpus gracilis,* Mi Guo Qin, was found to pass as Codonopsis spp. (Dang Shen, downy bellflower) (Wen Jia-lun et al. 1985). The important *antirheumatic* remedy Wu Jia Pi, the root bark of *Acanthopanax gracilistylus* in the Araliaceae family, is often adulterated with that of *Periploca sepium* (Gang Liu Pi or Bei Wu Jia Pi, silk vine) in the Asclepiadaceae family. The *anti-infective* remedy Ma Lan Ye, the leaf of *Baphicacanthus cusia* (Assam indigo), may be adulterated by the species *Strobilanthes divaricatus, S. guangxiensis* and *S. penstemonoides*. Importantly, TLC analysis showed these substitutions to be devoid of the active component indirubin (Huang Xue-cai et al. 1988). Sha Yuan Zi, the seed of *Astragalus complanatus* (flat milkvetch, in the pea family), was determined through morphological and electrophoretic differentiation to be adulterated by the seed of *Abutilon indicum* (country mallow, in the mallow family) and the seed of *Crotalaria zanzibarica* (Zanzibar crotalaria, in the pea family) (Li Wai-wan et al. 1988). The remedy Jin Gui Lian, normally the root tuber of *Hemsleya giganthea, H. villosipetola* and *H. szechuanensis* in the Cucurbitaceae was found through microscopical identification to be adulterated by the tubers of *Stephania sinica, S. epigaea, S. excentrica* and *Tinospora sagittata* of the Menispermaceae, *Tricosanthes villosula, T. kirilowii* and *Thladiantha hookeri* of the Cucurbitaceae and *Phytolacca acinosa* (poke root) of the Phytolaccaceae. Because of its high value as a tonic and tissue trauma remedy, the root of *Panax notoginseng* (San Qi, pseudoginseng root) is sometimes substituteable with the roots of *Panax japonicum, Gynura segetum, Curcuma aeruginosa, C. kwangsiensis, C. wenyujin, Bletilla striata, Schizocapsa planta-ginea, Anredera cordifolia* and *Manihot esculenta* (Wen Sang-kai and Wei Jia-fu 1987).

A 1985 report on the crude remedies available on the Hong Kong market concludes that remedy adulteration is a fairly common practice (Liu Xin-chun et al. 1985). Many species offered for sale did not correspond to those established in the Chinese textbooks (or even to folk uses, for that matter). Wrong genera and species notably were found among the important remedies Cimicifuga Sheng Ma, Acanthopanax Wu Jia Pi, Paris Shan Ci Gu, Lithospermum Zi Cao, Erythrina Hai Tong Pi, Senecio Qian Li Guang, Pulsatilla Bai Tou Weng, Pinellia Ban Xia, Spirodela Fu Ping, Piper Hai Feng Teng, Trachelospermum Luo Shi Teng, Agkistrodon Bai Hua She, Buddleia Mi Meng Hua, Vaccaria Wang Bu Liu Xing and many others.

Clearly, there is a difference between accepting the fact that a single remedy may be derived from several botanical species, and the substitution of unacceptable species for a particular remedy. The fact is that every remedy has a clearly defined, commonly practiced and academically established botanical boundary that has been defined by thousands of years of therapeutic usage. Beyond the boundary of those well-defined botanical sources lies the practice of remedy adulteration. *This differentiation is crucial in the practice of Chinese herbal medicine.*

Chemical analysis has also proved useful in either confirming or disproving commonly held beliefs about the relative efficacy of various plant parts or the same part collected at various times of the day, month or year. The stem (rhizome) of Asian ginseng, Ren Shen Lu, from *Panax ginseng,* for example, was shown to have a high proportion of saponins (3.47%) relative to the main root (2.25-5.22%), and displayed no *emetic* effect—contrary to the old herbals. The implication is that the stem is equally valuable and should be used together with the root (Luo Shun-de 1983). In the root of the gynecological plant *Angelica sinensis* (Dang Gui, dong quai), the rootlets (the distal parts) contain 20% more ferulic acid than the main root, but less of the essential oil fraction ligustilide, while butylidene phthalide showed no distinct pattern of distribution (Rui He-kai 1983). "This difference in the contents of these active components may shed light on the different applications of the two parts in traditional medicine" (Xu and But 1986). The crude flavones and flavonoids syringin and isofraxidin in the root bark of *Acanthopanax* spp. (Wu Jia Pi, Five-additions) were shown to increase with drying and ageing (Xu Zheng-bin et al. 1984). The shell of *Chinemys reevesii* (Gui Ban, Tortoise shell) may be used as much as the plastron because

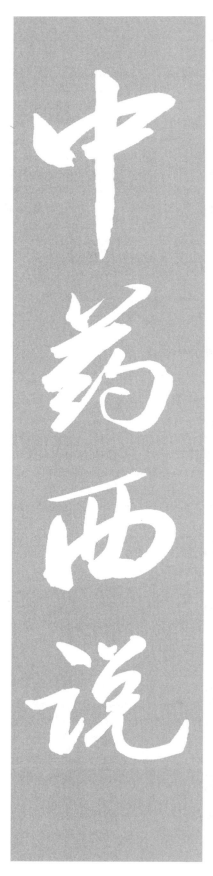

of its very similar composition and therapeutic action (Yang Mei-xiang et al. 1988). The alkaloidal content of the bulb of the *antitussive Fritillaria hupehensis* (Hubei Bei Mu, Hubei fritillary) has shown to be highest in mid-summer and reached its lowest level soon after, in mid-autumn (Guo Xin-fang and Li Jiang-zhen 1986). Likewise, in the day/night cycle the new bulb and herb of *Fritillaria pallidiflora* displayed their highest alkaloid levels at noon and their lowest levels, one-third the amount, at midnight (Zhang Deng-ke et al. 1988).

Geography is well known to slightly alter the chemical profile of plant constituents because of different soil and other environmental factors. The levels of the alkaloids tetrandrine, fangchinoline and cyclanoline found in the whole plant *Stephania tetrandra* (Hang Fang Ji, Stephania), from different regions varied respectively from 0.60 to 0.93, from 0.38 to 0.62, and from 0.25-0.54 according to TLC-densitometry (Yang Yi-fang et al. 1988).

Through biochemistry the various traditional processing methods can also be monitored for potential retention or loss of active components. The root bark of the peony, *Paeonia alba,* for example, is traditionally peeled off in the processing of the *spasmolytic* remedies Bai Shao and Chi Shao (White and Red peony root). Some researchers found that the discarded bark contained up to 2.27% of the monoterpene paeoniflorin (Quan We-guo 1987). This points to a questionable traditional practice, or at the very least, to the need for more pharmacological and clinical research. The root of Glehnia littoralis (Bei Sha Shen, northern sandroot) is similarly peeled of its bark, but the root bark was seen highest in the active coumarins imperatorin and isoimperatorin (Wang Jian 1987). Vinegar treating the corms of *Corydalis* spp. (Yan Hu Suo, Asian corydalis) causes a loss of the anti-anoxia quaternary alkaloids but an increase of the inactive tertiary alkaloids in this major *analgesic* remedy (Liu Cheng-ji et al. 1987). The same study also mentions that the raw root is preferred to the vinegar processed root in the treatment of coronary disorders. The traditional process of charring crude remedies by brief stir-frying, too, can lead to a diminution of active components. For instance, although the leaf of *Biota orientalis* (Ce Bai Ye, Oriental arborvitae tip) is traditionally charred to increase its *hemostatic* action, the concomitant loss of the *hemostatic* glycoside quercitrin may actually cause an inhibition of the desired action (Sun Wen-ji et al. 1987). The same loss of active *coagulant* or otherwise *hemostatic* constituents may lie behind the results of an extensive 1986 study on *hemostatics* in general. The conclusion was that the raw, unprocessed remedies significantly shortened bleeding time twice as effectively as the same charred remedies (Lu Hui-wen et al 1986). In the case of the *nervous sedative* effects of the seed of *Zizyphus spinosa* (Suan Zao Ren, sour jujube), the raw and fried seed have shown to be equally *hypnotic* and *anticonvulsant* (Lou Song-nian 1987).

On the positive side, the processed root of *Polygonum*

multiflorum (He Shou Wu, flowery knotweed) shows a 36.9% increase in phosphorus over the raw root (Chang Ming-xiang et al. 1988). Processing involves steaming the root in a decoction of black beans and wine until the decoction is dry. The processed root is an important *nervous* and *cerebral restorative* remedy and has shown greater *erythropoetic* and *hemopoetic* activity than the raw root (Shen Dao-xiu 1987). The essential oil and chlorogenic acid content of sulphur-smoked *Lonicera* spp. (Jin Yin Hua, Japanese honeysuckle flower) is higher than in the raw, steamed or fried remedy (Lu Ling-en 1987). Steaming of the corm of *Gastrodia elata* (Tian Ma, celestial hemp) prevents the alkaoid gastrodine from degrading into 4-hydroxymethy-phenol and destroys the beta-glycosidase (Sha Zhen-fang 1986).

Scientific pharmacognosy clearly has benefitted the practice of herbal medicine in many ways. Its findings will most likely continue to have a direct bearing on clinical practice. The Chinese scientific analysis of their own traditional materia medica is an unavoidable, neccessary and welcome part of Oriental medicine in transition.

Scientific Pharmacology

Like the various aspects of scientific pharmacognosy, the pharmacological analysis of Chinese remedies has also seen an enormous amount of effort since the early 1980s. Sometimes called biopharmaceutics, pharmacology studies the absorption, distribution, structural transformation and elimination of natural remedies or their isolated extracts. Whereas in the 1960s only five articles on pharmacology were published, in the 1980s there were over two hundred, and this figure is increasing exponentially every decade (Huang Jiao-cheng 1988). In tandem with the researchers, Chinese doctors on their part have not been slow to try out their findings both in conjunction with them (e.g., in statistical studies) and in their own clinical practice. This has resulted in numerous modern, experimental applications of Chinese remedies that have repeatedly proven effective. The number of experimental (i.e., non-classical, previously unrecorded) formulas making use of new pharmacological findings is also growing exponentially.

The main immediate references for information in this section are Zhu Da-yuan (1980), Xu Guo-jun and Wang-Zheng-tao (1989), Huang Jiao-cheng (1988), Chang and But (1987), Hsu Hong-yen et al. (1982) and Tang and Eisenbrand (1992), to which the reader is referred for further details. Numerous individual papers were also consulted in the references cited in these texts. The detailed monograph on each remedy is, of course, presented in the Materia Medica section in this text.

The most common approach taken by Chinese researchers is a very pragmatic one, namely to classify chemical compounds according to their pharmacological action—and we will follow suit. We should keep in mind, however, that the fact of pharmacological conclusions about a plant does not mean that it is neccessarily used in the way implied. The research may be congruent with traditional usage or it may not; if not, it may have already stimulated new applications, or it may not have. In many cases the scientific conclusions about a remedy simply promote a greater clinical emphasis on one or more particular well-known actions.

Important compounds working on the nervous system include alkaloids, glycosides, essential oils and various others. A large number of isoquinoline alkaloids have been defined in the corm of *Corydalis turtschaninovii* and spp. (Yan Hu Suo, Asian corydalis). They include corydaline, protopine and columbamine, the majority of which have shown *analgesic, hypnotic* and *muscle relaxant* activity. Terpenoid alkaloids of various kinds have been shown in the root structures of numerous *Aconitum* (aconite) species, which collectively furnish the botanical materials for three distinct remedies, Fu Zi, Wu Tou and Cao Wu. The alkaloids include aconitine, acetylaconitine, lappaconitine, mesaconitine, etc., and variously present *analgesic, anesthetic, anti-inflammatory* and *spasmolytic* properties. The triterpenoid schizandrol is one of many found in the berry of *Schisandra chinensis* (Wu Wei Zi, schisandra). It was found to be a potent inhibitor of central nervous functions, i.e., a *nervous sedative*. When the whole plant extract is used, however, this remedy is stimulant to various parts of the nervous system by operating directly on nervous tissue. The tubers of *Gastrodia elata* (Tian Ma, celestial hemp) have yielded the alkaloid

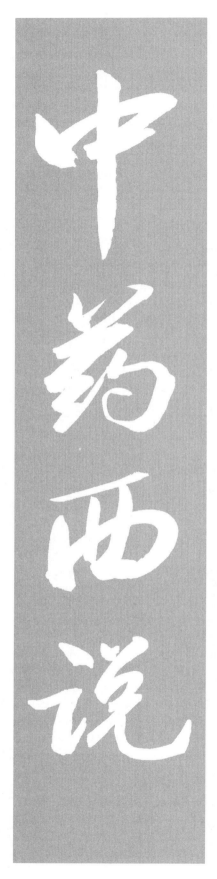

gastrodine (among others), which has proven *neuromuscular sedative, analgesic* and *spasmolytic* activities. Another compound in the tuber, vanilline, was found *hypnotic*.

Numerous compounds have been found to have a direct action on cardiovascular functions—the root of *Ligusticum wallichii* (Chuan Xiong, Sichuan lovage), for example. Its alkaloid tetramethylpyrazine (chuanxionqin, ligustrazine) has shown *anticoagulant* and *antilipemic* activity by inhibiting platelet aggregation and displacing calcium ions from platelet membranes. It is also *cardiotonic* and increases heart rate. Chuan Xiong also contains a highly aromatic essential oil with over 180 compounds, ferulic acid and phenolic compounds that separately and collectively have shown *capillary stimulant, systemic* and *coronary vasodilatory, hypotensive* and *spasmolytic* actions. The root and leaf of *Ilex pubescens* (Mao Dong Qing, furry holly) contain, among others, flavonoids with marked *coronary vasodilator* and *hypotensive* actions. The latter is thought to rely on peripheral vasodilation and to be related to cholinergic receptors. Tetrandrine is an alkaloid (one of several) found in the root of *Stephania tetrandra* (Han Fang Ji, stephania) that has shown consistent *anti-arrhythmia, antitachycardia, coronary dilatory* and *hypotensive* activities. The flavonoids in the flower of *Chrysanthemum indicum* (Ye Ju Hua, wild chrysanthemum) are known for their effective *hypotensive* activity, which relies on peripheral dilation, adrenergic blockade and possibly inhibition of the vasomotor center.

Plants with empirically known effectiveness against infections have been shown also to possess a wide range of active compounds that inhibit microorganisms. The glycoside forsythiaside, forsythol and rutin seen in the valve of *Forsythia suspensa* (Lian Qiao, forsythia) are experimentally known for their *antibacterial* activity, for example. Together with the plant's essential oil content, they can inhibit a large range of gram-positive and gram-negative microbes. Andrographolide, one of the main alkaloids in the leaf of *Andrographis paniculata* (Chuan Xin Lian, heart-thread lotus) has shown wide *antibacterial* activity. Artemisic acid isolated from the herb of *Artemisia annua* (Huang Hua Hao, annual wormwood) evinced inhibition of *Staphylococcus aureus* and *Shigella sonnei*. The plant's essential oil contains the ketone thujone which is known for its wide *antimicrobial* activity and esters known for their *antifungal* action. The leaf of *Isatis tinctoria* and *I. indigotica* (Da Qing Ye, woad) contain isatan B and the indole glycoside indican which have been found *antiviral* and *broad-spectrum antibacterial*. The root of *Coptis chinensis* (Huang Lian, goldthread) and other species has long been known for its high content in isoquinoline alkaloids. Chief of these is berberine (5-8%) which has evinced potent *antiviral, antibacterial* and *antifungal* activity.

Parasiticidal constituents have also been found among numerous Chinese medicinals. The phenol agrimophol, which is often used in extracted form, is seen in the winter bud of *Agrimonia pilosa* (He Cao Ya, furry agrimony); it was shown to kill the blood fluke *Schistosoma japonicum*. Quisqualic acid derived from the seed of *Quisqualis indica* (Shi Jun Zi, Rangoon creeper), showed the ability to paralyze earthworms. Artemisinine, a sesquiterpene lactone extracted from the herb of *Artemisia annua*, was found a potent inhibitor of *Plasmodium berghei* and *P. cynomolgi* (both resistant strains of malaria). The bitter compounds and glycosides from the fruit of *Brucea javanica* (Ya Dan Zi, Java brucea) have variously shown *anthelmintic, vermicidal, antiamoebic* and *antimalarial* activity.

Anti-inflammatory compounds also are numerous among Chinese remedies, and are often found in remedies treating conditions involving acute or chronic inflammation. Alpha-spinasterol, from *Bupleurum chinense* (Chai Hu, Asian buplever), has shown *anti-inflammatory* and *antipyretic* actions thought to be related to its inhibitory effect on the synthesis or release of prostaglandin E and bradykinin. The glycosides from the root of *Tripterygium wilfordii* (Lei Gong Teng, yellow vine), were shown to be strongly *anti-inflammatory*. The alkaloids baicalein and baicalin isolated from the root of *Scutellaria baicalensis* (Huang Qin, Baikal skullcap) were found both *anti-inflammatory* and *antiallergic;* the latter action was effected through inhibition of mercaptylase, responsible for the release of chemical mediators during antigen-antibody interaction. The alkaloids of the root of *Gentiana macrophylla* and species (Qin Jiao, large-leaf gentian), gentianine, gentianidine and gentianol, achieve an *anti-inflammatory* effect through neural pituitary-adrenal stimulation.

Chinese researchers have also placed much effort in identifying and extracting *antitumoral* (*antineoplastic*) plant constituents. For instance the leaf of *Baphicacanthus cusia* (Ma Lan Ye, Assam indigo), contains three agents, indirubin, tryptanthrin and qingdainone, that proved *antineoplastic* to a variety of carcinogenic tumors. Camptothecin and 10-hydroxycamtothecin isolated from the fruit and root bark of *Camptotheca acuminata* (Xi Shu, happy tree) have shown *antineoplastic* activity in various cancers. Many species of the genus *Rabdosia* have yielded important *antineoplastic* diterpenoid compounds. The herb of *Rabdosia rubescens* (Dong Ling Cao), for instance, contains the *antineoplastic* alkaloidal compounds oridonine and ponicidine, and the tetracyclic diterpenoids rubescensines A, B, C, D and E. The seed of *Brucea javanica* (Ya Dan Zi, Java brucea) contains bruceine, a quassinoid and oleic acid that have shown *antineoplastic* acivity both in vitro and in vivo.

Constituents that act as *immunosuppressants* in the presence of hypersensitivity disorders (types I through V) have also been identified. These include the alkaloid tripterine (celastrol) found in the root pith of *Tripterygium wilfordii* (Lei Gong Teng, yellow vine), which was shown to counteract a broad range of both allergic and autoimmune conditions; the polysaccharides in the fruiting body of *Ganoderma lucidum* (Ling Zhi, reishi), which evidenced activity against all types of hypersensitivity conditions; the glycoalkaloid solanine in the root and seed of *Solanum nigrum* (Long Kui, winter cherry), which was found active in immediate allergies; the polysaccharides from the root of *Glehnia littoralis* (Bei Sha Shen, northern sandroot) and the rhizome of *Dioscorea nipponica* (Chuan Shan Long, Nippon yam) that were shown effective in autoimmune disorders; the alkaloids from *Ephedra vulgaris* (Ma Huang, ephedra), which proved active in the presence of immediate allergies and autoimmune disorders with antibody-mediated cytotoxicity.

Various other plant remedies have presented *immunosuppressant* activity, although the constituents and mechanisms involved may not yet have been clarified. They include the root of *Angelica sinensis* (Dang Gui, dong quai), which was found effective in a wide range of immediate allergic conditions; the fruit of *Schisandra chinensis* (Wu Wei Zi, schisandra berry), which showed activity in allergic skin conditions; the root of *Glycyrrhiza uralensis* (Gan Cao, Ural licorice root), which is effective in both immediate and cell-mediated hypersensitivity disorders (including autoimmune conditions); the root pith of *Tripterygium hypoglaucum* (Kun Ming Shan Hai Tang), which has been found active in immune complex disorders and cell-mediated allergies; the fruit of *Ligustrum lucidum* (Nu Zhen Zi, glossy privet), which has proven effective in both immediate allergies and immune complex disorders.

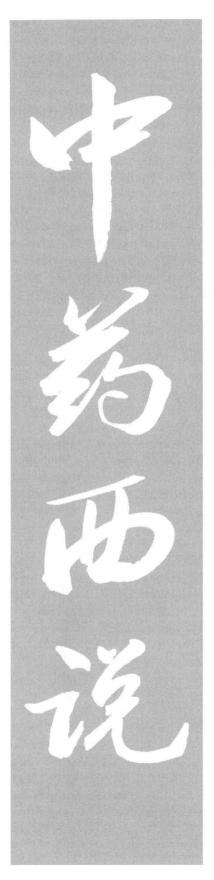

Components with *immunostimulant* activity, useful in a variety of immune-compromised conditions such as chronic/recurrent infection, radiation and cancer, include polysaccharides, saponins, flavonoids and oleanolic acid. In the case of protection from radiation, for instance, polysaccharides have been shown to work by variously protecting hemopoietic tissues, enhancing immune functions and reducing thymus atrophy. Polysaccharides in particular are seen to work in a number of different ways to fulfill their immune-stimulating function; some are better adapted at resolving chronic infectious conditions (e.g., subclinical "dormant" fungal and viral forms of microbial toxicosis), some better suited to radiation protection, and others best for forms of cancer. Major plants in which polysaccharides have been isolated include the root of *Eleutherococcus senticosus* (Ci Wu Jia, eleuthero ginseng), the root of *Astragalus membranaceus* (Huang Qi, astragalus), the flower of *Carthamus tinctorius* (Hong Hua, safflower), the leaf of *Epimedium saggitatum* (Yin Yang Huo, horny goatweed), the root of *Codonopsis pilosula* (Dang Shen, downy bellflower), the root of *Wikstroemia indica* (Liao Ge Wang, wikstroemia), the root of *Angelica sinensis* (Dang Gui, dong quai), the root of *Cynanchum auriculatum* (Bai Shou Wu, auricle dogbane), the root of *Apocynum venetum* (Luo Bu Ma, lance-leaf dogbane), the herb of *Lycopodium clavatum* (Shen Jin Cao, clubmoss), the lichen *Parmelia tinctorium* (Shi Hua, parmelia), as well as in various mushrooms such as *Ganoderma lucidum* (Ling Zhi, reishi), *G. japonica* (Zi Zhi, Japanese reishi), *Tremella fuciformis* (Bai Mu Er, silver ear), *Polyporus umbellatus* (Zhu Ling, umbel polypore), *Coriolus versicolor* (Yun Zhi), *Hericium erinaceus* (Hou Gu), *Cordyceps* spp. (Chong Cao, caterpillar fungus) and *Armillaria mellea* (Mi Huan Jun, armillaria polypore).

Just in the last ten years Chinese researchers have determined a number of constituents and whole plant remedies that yield *antioxidant* or free-radical inhibiting effects. These effects slow down the rate of cellular degeneration and promote integrity of cell function and structure. For example, the polysaccharide from the stem of *Sargentodoxa cuneata* (Da Xue Teng, sargentodoxa) was found to be a potent anti-free radical, followed closely by the naphthoquinone, tanshinone II, from the root of *Salvia miltiorrhiza* (Dan Shen, cinnabar sage). Sodium ferulate from the root of *Angelica sinensis* (Dang Gui, dong quai) was determined *antioxidant* as it prevented injury to red blood cells by the free radicals of peroxide, hydrogen peroxide, superoxide and hydroxyl; it also reduced tissue MDA concentration and increased superoxide dismutase activity.

Other plants that contain *antioxidant* compounds whose pharmacology may not yet have been elucidated include the berry of *Ligustrum lucidum* (Nu Zhen Zi, glossy privet), the herb of *Cistanche deserticola* (Rou Cong Rong, fleshy broomrape), the fruit of *Lycium barbarum* (Gou Ji Zi, wolfberry), the root of *Polygonum multiflorum* (He Shou Wu, flowery knotweed), the rhizome of *Atractylodes macrocephala* (Bai Zhu, white atractylodes), the cap of *Ganoderma lucidum* and spp. (Ling Zhi, reishi), the root of *Astragalus membranaceus* and spp. (Huang Qi, astragalus), the root of *Polygonatum sibiricum* and spp. (Huang Jing, Siberian solomon's seal), the herb of *Epimedium saggitatum* and spp. (Yin Yang Huo, horny goatweed).

Overlapping somewhat with the group of remedies called *adaptogenic,* yet distinct from them, are remedies that contain compounds that help protect from exposure to radiation (e.g., radiation therapy). In many cases, the exact *radioprotective* constituents and their pharmacology has not yet been elucidated. Remedies with a well-established *radioprotective* action include the root bark of *Eleutherococcus senticosus* (Ci Wu Jia, eleuthero ginseng root), which has shown the ability, for example, to increase leucocyte, erythrocyte and thrombocyte counts following X-ray irradiation; the root of *Panax ginseng* (Ren Shen, Asian ginseng), which enhanced resistance to radiation damage, improved nucleic acid and protein synthesis and protected hemopoiesis. The polysaccharides in the root of *Angelica sinensis* (Dang Gui, dong quai) proved *radioprotective* in that they reduced thymus atrophy and increased hemopoiesis. The total alkaloids in the root of *Sophora flavescens* (Ku Shen, yellow pagoda tree) showed *leucocytogenic* effect in both radiotherapy and chemotherapy. The polysaccharides from the mushroom *Tremella fuciformis* (Bai Mu Er, silver ear) provided protection from radiation by enhancing non-specific immune functions, for example by increasing plasma IgG levels and normalizing B-lymphocytes. They also treated the associated leucopenia by improving the recovery rate of hemopoiesis, increasing nucleated cells in the bone marrow and in endo-genous spleen colonies, and by boosting 3H-TdR uptake in the bone marrow and spleen. The total extracts of this remedy were also found effective in leukopenia from chemotherapy as well as from radiotherapy. Polysaccharides from the mycelia of the mushroom *Armillariella tabescens* (Liang Jun, armillariella polypore) was shown radioprotective by speeding up hemopoiesis, increasing leucocyte counts, CFU-s and 3H-TdR uptake in bone marrow cells, as well as by increasing the recovery rate of spleen weight.

Clearly, plant polysaccharides and alkaloids figure as prominently among constituents that afford protection from radiation as they do among immune-potentiating ones.

Compounds with a *contraceptive (antifertility)* action have also been found in plants traditionally used in both imperial and folk medicine for preventing conception. Examples include the alkaloids in the root of *Tripterygium wilfordii,* Lei Gong Teng (yellow vine), the phenolic glycoside gossypol in the root bark of *Gossypium hirsutum* (Mian Hua Gen, cotton), the essential oil fraction in the seed of *Daucus carota* (Hu Luo Bo, carrot) and the polypeptide trichosanthin in the rhizome of *Tricosanthes kirilowii* (Tian Hua Fen, snakegourd). Other remedies empirically known for their *contraceptive* effect but whose pharmacology has yet to be determined include the seed of *Impatiens balsamina* (Ji Xing Zi, garden balsam) and the root and herb of *Pyrola rotundifolia* subsp. *chinensis* and species (Lu Xian Cao, Chinese wintergreen).

These various aspects of scientific examination, separately and collectively, provide invaluable clues for understanding the dynamics, hitherto mysterious, of many Chinese remedies. By providing the necessary scientific explanation, scientific pharmacognosy and pharmacology help us in many cases come to terms with their historically and clinically validated uses. They thereby enable Western practitioners to reconcile the scientific analysis of Chinese remedies with their historical energetic effects. Moreover, looking into the future, these scientific procedures, as we have seen, may point to new and exciting avenues of therapeutic applications. Experimental, non-traditional uses of Chinese herbs have already yielded major clinical benefits in the relatively short timespan since science has been applied to them. The modern, taken-for-granted uses of Ginkgo Yin Xing Ye (Ginkgo leaf) for cardiovascular disorders, Astragalus Huang Qi (Astragalus root) for immune deficiency disorders and Tripterygium Lei Gong Teng (Yellow vine root pith) for autoimmune conditions all owe their existence to these avenues of approach. These extremely successful uses are completely contemporary and in most cases have no historical origin whatsoever. They are clearly an invaluable enrichment of the field of applications for numerous remedies, however, whether used in the crude or extracted form.

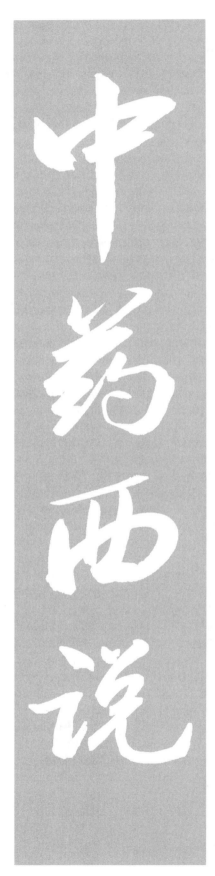

Vitalistic Pharmacognosy

The task of re-evaluating Chinese remedies in the vitalistic terms of energetic medicine today needs some clarification. Like the scientific procedures, this also divides into three aspects that correlate precisely with them: vitalistic pharmacognosy, or the analysis of effective qualities; vitalistic pharmacology, or clinical assessment of essential therapeutic actions; and remedy classification and therapeutics according to vitalistic principles. This Western vitalistic redefinition of Chinese herbs represents on my part an attempt to integrate the energetic pharmacological systems of traditional Greek and Chinese medicine. It is in a sense a return to the empirical clinical traditions of their origin, the approach that originally gave them meaning.

The vitalistic pharmacognosy of Chinese remedies is very well documented in numerous ben cao, or herbals, down past centuries. The effective qualities (popularly known as "energetics") of countless plant, mineral and animal remedies are clearly presented in terms of taste, warmth, movement and sometimes channel-entering properties. However, the language this information is couched in needs to be updated as much as the remedies themselves need scientific re-evaluation. The effective qualities need a modern reinterpretation if today we are to make intelligent use of this mass of empirical information. It would be to our great loss if it were conveniently relegated to "folklore" or "superstition" (those perennial dumping grounds of the Western reductionist mind). It is my conviction that for both historical and epistemological reasons this modern reinterpretation in the West can only be done on the basis of the vitalistic pharmacognosy that Greek medicine developed over twenty-five hundred years ago in the Eastern Mediterranean. Chapter 3 presents the basis of an integrated system of vitalistic pharmacognosy that is informed by aspects of both traditional Chinese and ancient Greek pharmacognosy.

Vitalistic Pharmacology

The situation is much the same concerning the vitalistic pharmacology (therapeutic actions) of Chinese remedies. In Oriental texts the effective qualities of taste, warmth and so on actually serve the criteria of both pharmacognosy and pharmacology: the latter two become indistinguishably one and the same. For example, an herb that is considered to possess pungent, warm and dispersing qualities (its pharmacognosy) is implicitly understood to be stimulating, dispersing and Qi and Blood vitalizing in effect (its pharmacology). When we then bring in the principles of traditional Greek pharmacology, again a more modern interpretation of a plant's essential therapeutic actions becomes possible. As will shortly be seen, it is the Eclectic/Physiomedical version of remedy pharmacology with its four principles of restoring/relaxing, stimulating/sedating, that can serve us most in a synthetic, integrated presentation of remedy pharmacology.

In any event, we have a long history of borrowing from other cultures' pharmacopoeias. After all, many common and well-researched so-called Western remedies were originally uniquely Chinese, or Asian, or South American. One of the most important Western spice remedies, for example, Ginger root, has always been imported from Nigeria, India or Southeast Asia. Peruvian bark, a key remedy for treating fevers for almost 300 years in the West, was originally brought from South America. The so-called China root, the much-touted specific remedy for one of the major Western disorders, syphilis, was for the most part the Chinese remedy Smilax Tu Fu Ling (Glabrous greenbrier root). Clearly, there is really but a thin and arbitrary dividing line between a Chinese and a Western remedy, especially now, in the "global village."

As explained in my *Energetics of Western Herbs,* there is also another option available that makes integrated use of both scientific and vitalistic systems of herbal medicine. This approach is to use the vitalistic aspect of herbal medicine and its dialectic process as a general basic context for working, while using scientific linear information as a specific discrete content. This approach would be analogous to the relationship between the medium and the message. At any rate, using this synthesistic approach with the initial priority given to vitalistic principles certainly allows one to modulate both systems, going back and forth between them as needed.

Traditional Greek Medicine and Beyond: The Western Vitalistic Tradition

Greek medicine is an ancient system of therapeutics indigenous to Western culture. We here define traditional Greek medicine as that system of medicine that has its roots in ancient Greece circa 600 BC, developed further in Rome and then in the Near East through medieval Islamic culture, where it was and is still known as *tibb-e al-yunani,* or *tib unani* in India (Ionian means Greek in Persian/Arabic), and continued in Renaissance Europe in the form of spagyrics, homeopathy and herbal medicine proper. The terms "Greek medicine" and "TGM" therefore refer to the country of its origin, as the term "Chinese medicine" does. Just as Chinese medicine is practiced not only throughout China but also throughout the Far East and important outposts worldwide, so Greek medicine also is still practised throughout the Middle East and India, and other places.

The Wise Woman Tradition
Given the contemporary dominance of allopathic and drug-oriented medicine, it may be hard to believe that the vitalistic tradition has historically been a more fundamental aspect of healing in the West, and that the analytical tradition came into its own barely 300 years ago. Vitalism is at the origin of traditional Greek medicine, predating the first analytical stirrings in the Hippocratic school that emerged in the fourth century BC. Western vitalism finds its source in the empirical tradition of "wise woman" healers, which also has its roots in the archaic shamanism found in all cultures. Women healers go back to prehistorical and historical matristic and post-matristic societies such as existed in Malta (c. 2000-3500 BC) and Crete (c. 1000-2000 BC). Wise woman medicine, as it is sometimes called, was still alive and well during the rise of Greek medicine in its dual aspects. This may be seen, for instance, in the documented ferocious legal battles between the traditional midwives and the male establishment medics that the city of Athens experienced throughout its early history. It is also present in the Greek temple cults where trancework, dreamwork and sacred sexual initiation were practiced. Wise woman medicine even survived into the modern era, but was almost snuffed out by the 300 odd years of Christian persecution of paganism, popularly called witch hunting. Because the wise woman tradition was and is an oral rather than a literate one, very little can be said about it today—except for one thing: We know it exists, we know its philosophy which (if its contem-porary proponents are anything to go by) is more Daoist and shamanistic than either (neo)platonic/hermetic or aristotelean/ rational. It has

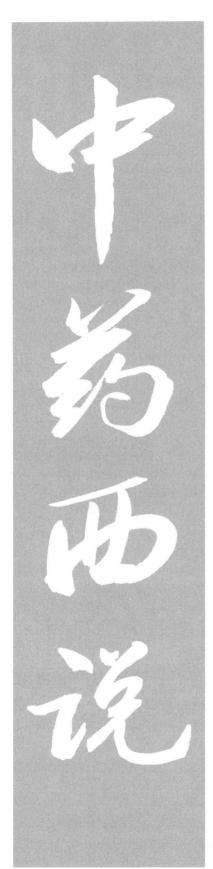

served as a largely silent undertow in the history of Greek medicine, periodically surfacing in many of its great as well as infamous moments.

Alexandrian Medicine: The Empirics

The Empirical school of Greek medicine, based in the major Greek cultural center of Alexandria between c. 200 BC and 200 AD, is the first major example of documented vitalistic herbal medicine practice in the West. It was a conscious effort to develop empirical observation, or medical phenomenology, to a more systemic and articulated phase. Empiric practitioners chose to avoid the speculation and rationalization about disease, remedies and the healing process that characterized the first formal school of Greek medicine, the Hippocratic school. They purposely eschewed the many hippocratic (and later galenic) theories about the four elements and four fluids in which disease was said to arise from an imbalance of the elements Water, Fire, Air and Earth, as well as unhealthy (injurious) combinations (*dyskrasios*) of the basic body fluids (*chymoi*), Mucus, Blood, Yellow bile and Black bile. On the contrary, the Empirics stuck as closely as possible to sheer observation without taking the next step of theorization. As a result, they developed the art of observing both pathological signs and symptoms and the action of remedies on the disease process with uncanny scrutiny. In corollary, they also experimented with empirical, previously untried remedy combinations and developed an astonishing body of effective herbal formulas for most types of conditions—not in spite of, but because they were unhampered by any theoretical dogma about the qualities of remedies and their codified actions on the elements and body fluids. Through simple empirical trial and error, the Empiricists noted which remedy combinations worked for a particular condition and which didn't.

Clearly, the Alexandrian school of Greek medicine represents a particularly pure example of vitalism unalloyed by any analytical tendencies. Greek Empirical medicine therefore has an important link with early systems of Chinese medicine as well as with modern homeopathy. On one hand it resembled early Chinese herbal medicine which also relied on empirical herb combining, as developed in the seminal work, the Shang Han Lun. On the other hand it mirrored homeopathy in that it also relied on the empirical process of remedy proving.

Spagyric Medicine

An offshoot of the ancient Western alchemical tradition, spagyric medicine has historically also been a significant part of vitalistic Greek medicine. Its medicinal preparations are based on crude plant parts and minerals that undergo lengthy protochemical processes using everything from simple distillation equipment to modern soxhlets. The final preparations achieved are either tinctures, elixirs, circulates or stones. With its Western origins in the alchemical works of medieval Persian alchemists such as ar-Razi and ibn Sina (both of whom are historically better known as TGM physicians), spagyrics in the West saw major development by Renaissance alchemist masters, including Marsilio Ficinus, Basilius Valentinus, Oswald Croll, Jan Van Helmont, Andreas Libavius and especially Raymond Lulle. By the nineteenth century, the division between traditional alchemy/spagyrics and scientific chemistry begun by the adventurous sixteenth century iatrochemists was finally completed. Still, the German spagyrist-chemists Weidenfeld and Christian A. Becker during the nineteenth century still were able to advance and refine time-worn spagyric remedies such as the Acetone of the Ancients and the Tincture of Gold. Today there are several small European companies as well as individuals producing simple spagyric remedies to the standards of the old masters. However, because of the all-consuming rise of modern coal tar chemistry in the late 1800s and its twentieth century offspring, the synthetic drug industry, spagyric medicine has ironically been reduced to as much a folk movement as wise woman medicine itself which it had once disdained as a primitive practice.

Homeopathic Medicine

Another important vitalistic system, homeopathic medicine, also has firm roots in the past. Leaning heavily on a blend of traditional alchemical and his own intuitive concepts, the Austrian physician and mystic Paracelsus in the early 1500s was an early proponent of the search for the *quinta essentia,* the quintessential energy, of each remedy. By a quirk of fate, this search was also the antecedant of modern chemistry. Paracelsus was followed by numerous emulators, including Johann F. Helvetius a century later, for example. At the turn of the nineteenth century, the German doctor and medical historian Samuel Hahnemann refined this search by developing the two techniques of succussion and dilution he considered necessary to let the genie (the quintessence) out of the bottle (the crude plant/mineral/animal remedy). Like his predecessors, Hahnemann saw this process as a revitalization of a remedy's dormant therapeutic energy, and so named it potentization. Remedies are said to be potentized to various decimal (x) powers. Because homeopathy involves the concept of life energy and is based entirely on the phenomenology of remedy provings operating by the law of similars, homeopathy is clearly yet another version of vitalistic medicine, a variant on the broad Western TGM theme. In fact, it is the most radical, since modern science finds it impossible to prove scientifically its modus operandi: After about the 3x potency, homeopathic remedies loose any detectable trace of their original physical substance, thereafter presumably operating entirely on an energetic or vibrational rather than on a physical or substantial level.

Vitalistic Herbal Medicine: Thomsonians, Eclectics and Physiomedicals

Clearly, herbal medicine as we know it in the West has both vitalistic and analytic roots. The analytic tradition is rooted in rationalistic Hippocratic medicine that sprang from the eastern Hellenic island of Kos. It was enriched and consolidated by Galen of Pergamon in Rome in a form that lasted to the threshold of the nineteenth century. The analytical stream was further developed by technique hungry Persian and Arabic doctors during the Middle Ages throughout the Islamic empire, eventually resurfacing in the protochemical practices of the iatrochemists in the early 1500s. With the experiments of Robert Boyle and somewhat later Antoine Lavoisier and then Friedrich Woehler, the modern chemistry was born that was to eclipse the vitalistic herbal tradition in the second half of the nineteenth century.

Based on its shamanistic origins in wise woman medicine and its first Greek development in Empirical medicine, the vitalistic tradition of herbal medicine has continued right up to the present day. This history is clearly traced in Harris Coulter's four-volume *Divided Legacy* and to some extent in Charles Lichtenthaeler's *Geschichte der Medizin,* for example. It received a boost with the establishment of the first European pharmacies in Italy and then Germany in the mid-fifteenth century and with the spread of essential oil distillation techniques in the early 1500s. The French alchemist and physician Arnald de Villanova had already discovered alcohol production in

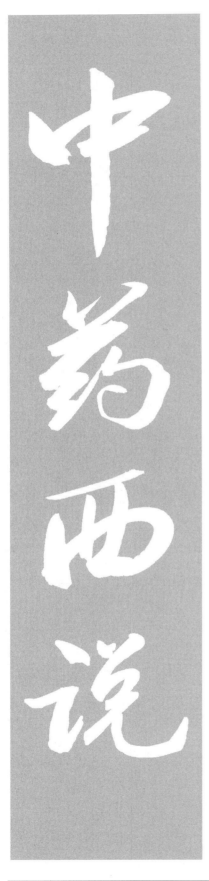

the 1200s and was the first to make alcohol-based tinctures and percolations. In another sense, the vitalistic tradition received a boost when herbal practitioners in the 1500s turned increasingly to local European plants as sources for medicine making rather than relying on imported Persian/Arabic formulas based on mideastern spices and Mediterranean herbs. Renaissance practitioners such as Paracelsus, Otto Brunfels, Hieronymus Bock and Walther Ryff all turned to wise women and folk healers in their attempt to salvage empirical herbal techniques. Each in their own way promoted a more holistic mode of herbal therapy based on local ecological wisdom combined with a reinterpretation of vitalistic Greek pharmacology and whole systems-based therapeutics. They were supported in this first by the renewal of botany (as distinct from botanical medicine) through plant researchers like Andreas Caesalpino, Charles de L'Ecluse, Conrad Gesner, the brothers Jean and Gaspard Bauhin and others; and second, by the renewal of holistic neoplatonic science by Galileo, John Dee, Johannes Kepler and Isaac Newton. Unfortunately, the rise of analytical science in the seventeenth century eventually diluted this central European "green" phase of herbal medicine, which then proceeded to go under in the eighteenth century Age of Enlightenment amidst intellectual squabbles about the ultimate nature of disease and matter.

The most recent resurgence of vitalistic herbal medicine occurred in North America in the nineteenth century and continued well into the twentieth. It was initially triggered by a New Hampshire farmer's son, Samuel Thomson, who in childhood had witnessed his own recovery from illness through the gentle herbal administrations of a certain widow Benton—at that time already a rare example of the vanishing breed of country herbal practitioners. In addition to acquaintance with the widow Benton and other "root and herb" doctors, Thomson was undoubtedly also able to observe Native American hygiene practices, such as sweatlodge ceremonies performed with indigenous botanical medicines. With this background Thomson put together simple yet effective empirical treatment methods that would serve everybody, regardless of the nature of their actual condition. His therapy essentially consisted of alternating courses of sweating and vomiting. These were implemented, respectively, by cayenne pepper drunk freely in a steam room and lobelia herb taken orally and by enema, and were always interspersed with lukewarm showers and periods of rest. Thomson's patented treatment program worked for the day and was widely popularized by his licensed practitioners (over 3 million in 1839). Their acceptance at the grassroots level was assured because of widespread dissatisfaction with heroic medicine (as it was then appropriately called) and its vicious treatment trio of drastic purging with *purgatives* like rhubarb, senna, jalap and castor oil, toxic salivation with calomel (mercurous chloride) and reckless bloodletting with the lancet.

The vigorous, vociferous Popular Health Movement of the 1820s and 1830s was more than mere middle-class disenchantment with kamikaze doctoring and russian roulette therapies: It was the only survival mode left to a population increasingly debilitated and decimated by iatrogenic causes as much as by natural ones. Note, in this connection, that the widespread cholera epidemics of 1831/2 and 1848/9 were the result of this genetic weakening, not its cause.

In the best of empirical traditions, the only rationale that Thomson claimed for his treatment methods was the restoration of the body's inner heat (which we can squarely equate with the Chinese concept of the Fire of Ming Men, or Kidney Yang). Taking just one of several Hippocratic medical principles to heart, he declared the pathogen of cold to constitute the basis for the progression of all illness, and spearheaded the use of cayenne pepper, the strongest of all *arterial circulatory stimulants,* to remove this cold. He liked to invoke Hippokrates to justify and rationalize his essentially naturopathic treament strategies which, as Priest correctly points out, foreshadowed those of the later German naturopathic and Nature Cure practitioners. Significant here is the fact that the Eclectic school of herbal medicine founded in 1827 by Wooster Beach (which in 1855 formalized as the National Eclectic Medical Association) and the Physio-Medical school founded in 1841 by the neo-Thomsonian Alva Curtis both had their roots and initial growth in Thomson's empirical methods. It was only gradually that theoretical and scientific considerations were encouraged among practitioners busy practising vitalistic medicine.

The Eclectic medics John King and John Scudder were the first to take a decisive step away from using botanical remedies simply as vehicles for generating warmth and causing elimination through sweating and vomiting. They jointly developed the concept of "specific medication," which means nothing more than the selection of a single particular herbal remedy for a certain condition, to be based on actual differential diagnosis rather than singular blanket assessment. The Eclectic duo also produced botanical remedies that utilized only the "concentrated principles" found in plants—a dream that only became true reality in the hands of the brilliant biochemist John Uri Lloyd who joined their enterprise from 1870 onwards. Later on, Physiomedical practitioners also researched along more theoretical and scientific lines. Based on Beach's concept of "equalizing the circulation," William Cook, for instance, in the 1870s began to correlate the functions of the circulatory and nervous systems, and introduced the idea of over-contracted and over-relaxed tissues. Joseph Thurston in the 1890s went on to explore the role of autonomic nervous functioning behind local pathology—an approach once again made modern by practitioners as seemingly different as Jean-Claude Lapraz and Michael Moore.

The burgeoning alternative practice of homeopathy, too, made a radical move away from eliminatory strategies that were empirically derived. An increasing number of astonished patients were discovering the delights of a form of vitalistic therapy that was not only safer than the current heroic treatment meted out by the regular doctors, but also gentler (and genteeler) than Thomsonian fuss and drama. Specifically, homeopathy developed the idea of using natural remedies in energetic and small-dose form, namely in potentized form, rather than in large-dose form. Samuel Hahnemann's idea was to utilize the inherent energy of remedies as much as possible, rather than their physical chemical constituents—because, he reasoned, the purpose of those constituents was none other than to physically hold or contain their energies. However, instead of adding scientific explanations (as did the Eclectics and Physiomedicals) to an empirical system that already worked well as it was, homeopaths enlarged on the phenomenological aspect of their practice. By observing the signs and symptoms that resulted from giving minute, potentized doses of natural substances (which they called "proovings"), homeopaths developed a large repertoire of remedies from the botanical, mineral and animal kingdom. In turn they took careful note of the whole, unique symptom-sign complex that each patient presented when they took a case history. Early practitioners and researchers such as Hans Gram and Constantine Hering in the 1830s and 1840s were thereby able to fine-tune the symptomatology of remedies to include mental and emotional, as well as physiological, symptoms—a unique feat in the domain of herbal medicine.

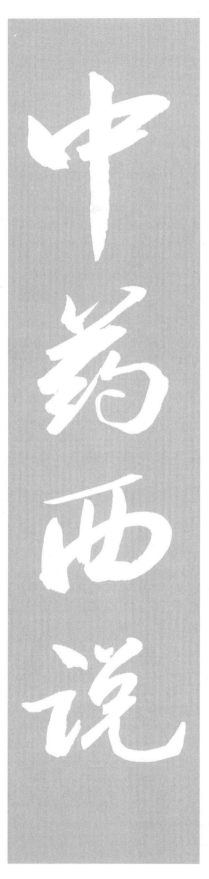

More than the Thomsonian school, however, it is the Eclectic, Physiomedical and Homeopathic schools of herbal medicine that can now be seen as the true successors to the Alexandrian Empirics of middle Greek medicine. Instead of being locked into a fixed routine of a treatment system, early Eclectic practitioners such as Wooster Beach and John King were constantly being alerted to a variety of Native American plant remedies by the Philadelphia botanists Jacob Bigelow and William and Benjamin Barton. In the true Frontier spirit of those days, they and their colleagues happily used botanicals on a trial and error basis on their many patients, always monitoring their actions by close observation. Through this empirical practice they developed clinically effective uses for indigenous remedies such as Blue flag root, Helonias root, May apple root, Sumac root bark and many others. Eventually, as the Eclectic circle grew with pioneers like John Scudder, Herbert Webster, Finley Ellingwood and Harvey Felter, these practitioners built up an extensive and high quality herbal materia medica that hasn't been surpassed since. This body of plant remedies today is still at the core of Western herbal medicine practice, regardless of the theoretical orientation of its various practitioners. Exactly the same can be said of homeopathic doctors, whose live proovings of many thousands of natural substances, alternating with skillful clinical practice, gradually built up a vast arsenal of effective remedies still in use today.

Like the Alexandrian Empirics, the Eclectic and Physiomedical practitioners developed empirical vitalism in a systemic and articulated way. This is because the semiological, diagnostic and therapeutic basis of their practice was the European system of clinical medicine then dominant, which was based on pure phenomenological observation (clinical medicine immediately preceded Koch's bacteriological medicine). Moreover, the Eclectics were aided in applying herbal remedies to their clinical approach by the homeopathic system of medicine which, as it happened, was gaining momentum at exactly the same period as Eclectic herbal medicine itself. Homeopathy provided the Eclectics with the therapeutics-related tools of specific symptomatology, symptom pictures and keynote symptom differentiation. To a minor extent, homeopathy also influenced the symptomatologies of herbal remedies themselves. Unlike the ultra-observational Empirics and modern Homeopaths, however, Eclectics chose not to avoid rationalizing the actions of remedies on the disease process. Still, their remedy rationales still involved systemic observations, as when they discussed *anticatarrhal, antidyskratic, astringent, stimulant, sedative* and similar herb properties. And on this basis the Eclectics and Physiomedicalists later reduced all remedy effects to three and later four basic actions: *astringing, relaxing, stimulating* and *sedating*. And like the Homeopaths, Empirics and Chinese doctors, they made a direct relationship between a remedy action and disease syndromes rather than speculating about the intrinsic properties of the remedy itself. That exercise had been worked to a sophistic death by the medieval Persian physicians who based their work more on Galen than on anyone else.

Clearly, of all the currents within the Western vitalistic stream of healing, it is herbal medicine that provides the most direct links with Chinese herbal medicine. The use of plants in relatively simple preparations such as infusion, decoction, compress and bath goes back to prehistory. In the Greek and Roman civilizations (500 BC to 400 AD) herbal medicine was vigorously developed by several schools of medicine as well as by the *rhizotomoi,* the herb collectors and herbal products vendors of the market squares in towns and villages. Herbal medicine in the West has never seen more widespread use than in that era. In tandem with the empirical methods adopted by early Chinese doctors, the Empiric practitioners of Alexandria were the first systemic proponents of the specifically empirical approach.

However, in the Greek medical tradition of the West, vitalism has always been accompanied by the simultaneous development of the complementary analytical approach, and vice versa. One has never dominated for too long before it has been gradually superseded by the other. The vitalism of classic Greek medicine eventually was replaced by the analytical dominance of the Persian/Arab doctors. Thomsonian vitalism gradually ceded to Physiomedical analysism. In China, on the other hand, there simply never was any analytical development. Chinese medicine historically is an exercise in variations on a single theme—the theme of vitalistic medicine. A prominent example, currently extant, is the Japanese *kampo* school of herbal medicine which—true to its sources in the Shang Han Lun—relies solely on the process of matching the patient's symptom profile with that of the formula. This ultra-empirical conformation, or confirmation, procedure in turn is identical to classic homeopathic treatment protocol! In its essence, Chinese medicine has always remained as empirical as the Empirical, Thomsonian and Homeopathic systems of natural medicine. This despite the various elaborate theories that numerous schools of Chinese medicine constructed over the centuries to explain and to rationalize their pathologic perceptions and therapeutic procedures. Today, Chinese medicine is as active as ever in the process of developing experimental herbal and acupoint formulas for the whole gamut of modern disease conditions. Since the cultural revolution even more so, perhaps, than at any other time in the history of Chinese medicine. And here is the exact area in which Western researchers and practitioners, with their more theoretical/analytical approach, have a difficult time. The inability of current allopathic schools of Western medicine to accept the empirical schools of medicine (rather than vice versa) lies at the crux of the contemporary struggle between the analytic and vitalistic approach. The struggle itself, however, clearly goes back to the roots of the Greek medical tradition itself.

In retrospect, it may be reasonably asked, why should Chinese remedies require scrutiny from the vitalistic perspective at all? Surely this is exactly the contribution of traditional Oriental medicine to herbal medicine today? However, again it is my belief that Chinese vitalism, if it is to adapt and survive in the West, can only do so by connecting with Western vitalism. Ultimately it is our own Western vitalistic herbal tradition that will provide the tool that will help us realize the full potential of Chinese herbal medicine in the West. Who knows, perhaps even Chinese herbal practitioners will benefit from this cross-fertilization. After all, the Chinese themselves point out that a living tradition is one that constantly undergoes creative development through change and variation: if it does not, it becomes a stagnant, fossilized tradition that relies on formal mannerism at the expense of essential content. It is the pharmacology and therapeutics of our own traditional Greek medical system, therefore, that allow us to reinterpret and redefine Chinese energetic pharmacology. The common empirical basis of both medical traditions makes this very possible.

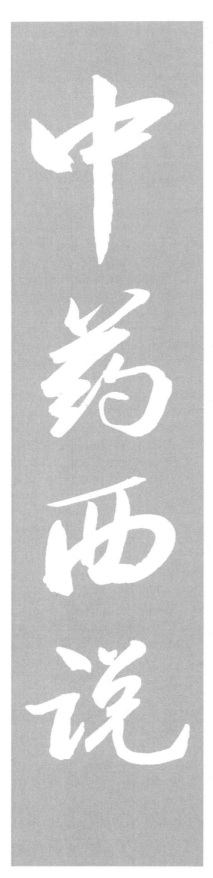

Connecting the Two Herbal Traditions: The Two Vitalistic Links

Vitalistic medicine in the West, which includes herbal medicine, possesses two interesting theoretical aspects that underlie its practice: the concept of fundamental remedy actions and the concept of symptom pictures. These two concepts are traditionally found in textbooks discussing pharmacology, diagnostics and therapeutics. They interest us here particularly because they can help us understand the vitalistic principles of Chinese herbal medicine on one hand and, to some extent, the analytical aspects of the Western tradition on the other. In other words, the two concepts create a bridge allowing us to pass in one direction of research or the other.

On a practical level, the four remedy actions in particular allow us to take the final step of classifying Chinese remedies in terms of the anatomical body systems. From the therapeutic point of view, assigning remedies to the body systems only makes sense once we have somehow differentiated the remedies in terms of their essential, generic nature and function. We need to explore the different options available to us in our search for generic remedy actions tbefore applying them to each and every body system.

The Four Remedy Actions

Western herbal practitioners, like their Chinese counterparts, have always searched for ways of simplifying the many therapeutic effects demonstrated of natural remedies and of classifying them according to their simplest, broadest therapeutic effects. The motivation behind this search is as pragmatic as it is theoretical: the large number of remedies used in any period when herbal medicine has flourished has always needed to be organized in a way that is manageable in clinical practice. Moreover, when all is said and done about their nature and functions, the remedies ultimately remain just expressions of a few basic treatement principles. Both Oriental and Western doctors, on the whole, have followed the therapeutics-driven approach of classifying remedy actions, which is to classify them according to the treatment of a basic number of disease conditions. The remedy classification of Cheng Zhong-ling, for instance, still used today, is a good example. This early eighteenth century physician divided remedies into eight fundamental types according to the therapeutic actions of causing sweating, causing vomiting, purging, harmonizing, warming, clearing, tonifying and reducing. Another classification, found in the twelfth century text Shen Ji Jing (Classic of Sagacious Remedies), is similar, although based more on the nature of the remedies themselves. Here, remedies and prescriptions are organized according to their ability to disperse, unblock, tonify, purge, make slippery, astringe, dry, moisten, lighten and make heavy. The classic example in the West is the text Peri Kraseos

Kai Dynameos Ton Haplon Pharmakon (*On the Mixture and Effective Qualities of Simple Remedies*) written in about 165 by the Greek physician Claudios Galenos (Galen). This work also lists remedies according to their basic natural qualitative actions of warming, cooling, drying, moistening, astringing, softening, restoring and relaxing (Holmes 1993). Later practitioners such as Lémery, Ettmueller and De Tournefort extended these categories to include the more therapy-oriented remedy actions of causing sweating, causing urination, causing expectoration, causing menstruation and a few others.

However, just a few practitioners in both East and West went beyond even these basic remedy classifications, distilling all remedies further to two or three template types. Zhang Zi-he reduced Cheng Zhong-ling's eight treatment methods down to just three—causing sweating, causing vomiting, purging (all to be understood in their most broad sense). Likewise, a Roman physician, a contemporary of Cornelius Celsus, classified remedies according to whether they tightened or relaxed tissues, i.e. heightened or decreased tissue tone. John Floyer in the early 1700s viewed remedies primarily as either warming or cooling, and later Thomsonian practitioners and Eclectic and Physiomedical physicians of the early nineteenth century generally classified remedies as *stimulants* or *relaxants*. Historically, the common denominator in Western herbal medicine came to be the twin categories of *warming/stimulating* remedies and *cooling/relaxing* remedies, which crystalized during the Eclectic era of herbal medicine in North America.

In both East and West, there exist several variations on the theme of essential remedy actions and treatment strategies. What they all have in common is one, two or more complementary/opposite pairs: *warming* versus *cooling, tightening* versus *relaxing, moistening* versus *drying, raising* versus *sinking, stimulating* versus *sedating,* and so on. Some remedy actions are based purely on tissue states, such as the astringing/relaxing dyad of the early Physiomedicalists (Cook, Thurston) and the closely related consolidating/dispersing dyad used in some traditions of Chinese herbal medicine. The latter pair of actions, although it is also based on the effects of remedies on tissue states, is ultimately more broad in practice because it includes functions based on energy as well as tissue changes. Other remedy actions are based on autonomic nervous activity, such as the stimulating/sedating pair of Physiomedicalists (Thurston, Priest). Some are based on circulatory dynamics, such as Floyer's warming/cooling axis, also expressed in Chinese medicine as dispelling cold/clearing heat. Others again are based on the cycle of assimilation and rejection, such as the tonifying/eliminating (restoring/purging) pair used in both Chinese and Galenic-Greek medicine.

For the purposes of organizing the Chinese materia medica according to a set of simple dyads, it was decided to develop a modified version of the twin dyad established by Thurston and Priest: restoring (contracting, astricting)/relaxing and stimulating/sedating (refer to the chart immediately before the Repertory). A.W. and L.R. Priest in their text *Herbal Medication* describe this fourfold group strictly in terms of nervous system dynamics. These concepts, however, have historically clearly always been more widely applicable. *It was therefore decided to define these four remedy actions more generically and put them on a completely vitalistic or energetic basis.*

The four Physiomedical actions of *restoring, relaxing, stimulating* and *sedating* take on a new light when used as vitalistic remedy actions, like those of Chinese medical pharmacology. Rather than representing particular physiological actions related to tissue state, circulation and innervation, each with their specific and limited applications, the four actions can become more generic and therefore more widely applicable. At the same time, their multivalency can represent both remedy actions and treatment strategies. For instance, each of the four actions can be systemic or local, functional or structural, describe tissue or energy. *Restoratives* to the circulation, for example, include a variety of different herb types, including *coronary restoratives, hemostatics* and *venous decongestants,* while *restoratives* to the nervous system are only one in kind, *central nervous restoratives*. As another example, from the physiological point of view, the fundamental action of stimulation can involve either circulatory or nervous stimulation. Circulatory stimulation divides into arterial, capillary and venous stimulation. Nervous stimulation divides into autonomic/

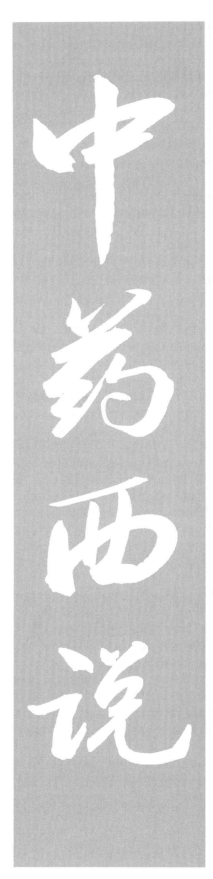

smooth muscle and neuromuscular/striped muscle. As far as herbal therapeutics is concerned, moreover, stimulation can result in a large number of therapeutic effects, each of which is useful for a particular systemic, organ or local condition. Stimulation of the arterial circulation alone can be used in treatment methods such as causing sweating, reducing cold conditions, treating rheumatic conditions, relieving nervous tension, promoting digestive functions, stimulating menstrual flow, etc.

Simply stated, what is proposed here is not yet another physiological definition of a basic set of remedy actions, as we find in the history of Western herbal medicine, especially during the last 200 years. What is needed is a new interpretation of these actions, a new approach to their use. In other words, a whole systems model of remedy actions that, through its multivalency, can serve a variety of different diagnostic and therapeutic goals.

The four basic actions of remedies consist of two pairs or dyads.

- The **restoring/relaxing** dyad is regulating, and remedies with either action gently bring function and/or structure back to normal balance by working in conjunction with the person's own vital energy.
- The **stimulating/sedating** dyad is directional. Remedies with either action functionally and/or structurally cause an alteration by directing the person's vital energy in a particular way.

Each action addresses a primary type of pathological condition which in practice can assume numerous presentations. Each action is embodied by a large number of remedies acting in various ways on diverse body functions and exercising different pharmacological actions. The section on effective qualities in Chapter 3 also describes in some detail these basic remedy actions (qualities) with respect to their particular body systems.

- The **restoring** action is used to treat deficiency conditions, marked by weakness, atonicity, hypofunctioning, etc. of function/structure. Restoring remedies are on the whole sweet or moderate in their taste, warmth and moisture qualities. Examples of *restoratives* would be Rehmannia Shu Di Huang (Prepared rehmannia root), Codonopsis Dang Shen (Downy bellflower root), Angelica Dang Gui (Dong quai root) and Dioscorea Bi Xie (Long yam root). Western equivalents include Nettle herb, Hawthorn berry and American ginseng root. *Restoratives, astringents, nutritives and demulcents* are restoring types of remedy actions.
- The **relaxing** action is used to treat excess conditions, characterized by tension, hypertonicity, hyperfunctioning, etc. of function/structure. Relaxing remedies are generally pungent

or moderate in their taste, warmth and moisture qualities. Examples of *relaxants* would be Ligusticum Chuan Xiong (Sichuan lovage root), Chrysanthemum Ju Hua (Chrysanthemum flower), Magnolia Hou Po (Magnolia bark) and Uncaria Gou Teng (Gambir vine twig). Western equivalents include Camomile flower, Skullcap herb and Black cohosh root. *Spasmolytics, anticonvulsants* and *muscle-relaxants* are examples of the relaxing types of herb action.

- The **stimulating** action is used to treat deficiency conditions that present the pathogens of cold or damp. Stimulating remedies are generally warm, pungent, dry and dispersing in quality. Cinnamomum Gui Zhi (Cassia cinnamon twig), Ledebouriella Fang Feng (Wind-protector root), Peucedanum Qian Hu (Asian masterwort root) and Saussurea Yun Mu Xiang (Wood aromatic root) are good examples of *stimulants*, while Western examples include Rosemary leaf, Juniper berry and Wormwood herb. *Diaphoretics, diuretics, laxatives, expectorants, emmenagogues, emetics, arterial stimulants, antirheumatics* and *digestive stimulants* all belong to the stimulating type of remedy action.
- The **sedating** action is used to treat excess conditions that present the pathogens of heat or damp. Sedating remedies are generally cool, bitter or salty, dry and consolidating. Scutellaria Huang Qin (Baikal skullcap root), Taraxacum Pu Gong Ying (Mongolian dandelion root and herb), Gypsum Shi Gao (Gypsum) and Stegodon Long Gu (Dragon bone) are good examples of *sedatives*, while Western examples include Hops flower, Goldenseal root and Echinacea root. *Refrigerants (antiphlogistics), anti-inflammatories, antipyretics* and *most anti-infectives* are the main sedating types of remedy actions.

A general advantage of understanding the rubric of restoring/relaxing, stimulating/sedating as generic vitalistic remedy effects rather than as specific physiological remedy actions is that the Chinese remedy actions easily fit into this basic framework. In this way the four basic remedy actions pull together the large number of Western pharmacological actions on one hand and the fairly large number of Chinese herb actions on the other.

- *restoring* — tonifying Qi, nourishing Blood, enriching Yin, moistening fluids, benefitting Essence, stabilizing Kidney, tonifying Liver and Kidney
- *relaxing* — circulating Qi, subduing Liver Yang, extinguishing internal wind, releasing the exterior
- *stimulating* — tonifying Yang, warming the interior, transforming damp, draining damp, removing accumulation, dissolving food stagnation, dispelling wind/damp/cold, releasing the exterior
- *sedating* — clearing heat, clearing damp heat, clearing toxic heat, calming Spirit

In this text, the four remedy actions are used in conjunction with the physiological body systems, so that each system comprises *restorative, relaxant, stimulant* and *sedative* types of remedies. In every body system, each type will have particular actions unique to that system. These actions are fully described in the introduction to each body system in Part Two, and are also found in synopsis form in the materia medica outline that follows the table of contents. For example, *restoratives* to the upper respiratory system (the first, Nose, Throat and Eyes section) are specifically *nasal decongestants* with *anticatarrhal, antiseptic* and sometimes *diaphoretic* actions. *Restoratives* to the lower respiratory system (the section following) are specifically *bronchial demulcents* with *mucogenic, mucolytic* and *expectorant* actions.

This fourfold organization of the materia medica according to four essential remedy actions has two practical advantages. On one hand, the remedies within each body system are clearly differentiated, making choice of remedies for particular conditions much easier in actual practice. On the other hand, the great number of remedy actions in each system are reduced to four basic groups, thereby facilitating the selection of particular remedy actions.

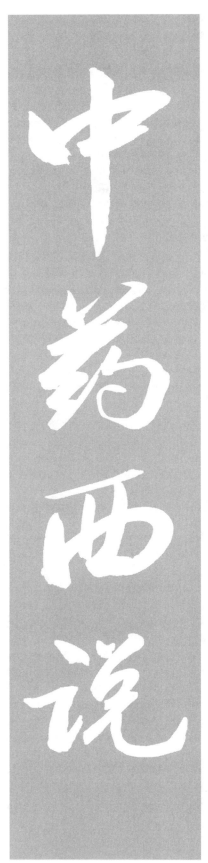

The Symptom Picture

The second link that interests us in the practice of herbal medicine is the concept of the symptom picture. There are three main vitalistic traditions that utilize this concept: Oriental herbal medicine, Greek herbal medicine, Homeopathy and Eclectic herbal medicine.

In the same way that traditional doctors devised systems of basic remedy actions to simplify and organize the countless herbal remedies used in practice, so they also worked out ways of simplifying and classifying the numerous signs and symptoms that patients presented. And the symptom picture was born. This concept historically preceded the concept of disease, and has gone under many other names. Greek medicine coined the word syndrome; Chinese medicine uses the word *zheng*, denoting a pattern of disharmony; Japanese doctors talk about *sho*, the symptom conformation; Eclectic doctors spoke of specific symptomatology. The essential idea is the same throughout: a group of signs and symptoms that collectively define a condition of illness.

A more technical definition of the concept of symptom picture or syndrome has been given as "a group of similar symptom-sign presentations of unknown origin, or of various known origins, which are not clearly distinguished from others." This may usefully be contrasted with the concept of disease, which conversely is "a group of similar symptom-sign presentations of a single origin, which indicate a deviance from homeostasis and which may be caused by definite endogenous or exogenous pathogens" (Leiber and Olbrich 1981, in R. Gross 1985). The differences between these two basic concepts of illness is tabulated at the end of the book immediately before the Repertory. The main point about the symtom picture is this. In contrast to the disease concept where signs and symptoms are thought to be caused by specific pathogens, such as toxins, bacteria, viruses, etc., in the symptom picture interpretation, signs and symptoms are seen to be both cause and effect of the illness at the same time. In fact, one could go so far as to say that the phenomenal observation of signs and symptoms itself defines the symptom picture. Contrast this with the concept of disease which is defined solely by analysis of the physiological mechanisms of pathogenesis underlying the signs and symptoms. It becomes clearer why the term "symptom picture" is particularly appropriate for describing the concept of syndrome: It is the particular pattern of physical, emotional and mental symptoms presented by the individual that creates the whole gestalt, the complete profile of an illness.

This syndrome approach to defining an illness is far older than the disease approach, which has only been developed systematically for about three hundred years. Symptom pictures are described in textbooks of Greek medicine in Greek, Arabic, Persian, Hebraic, Latin and ancient European languages, and in Chinese and Ayurvedic medical works. They appear later on in the West in the guise of remedy symptom picture in the Homeopathic and Eclectic medical traditions, where illness is essentially classified by the remedies used to treat them.

It is very likely that the Eclectic doctors John King and John Scudder (see above) were influenced by homeopathic practitioners of their day when they developed the concept of "specific medication." First and foremost, this simply denoted selecting a specific single remedy for certain conditions, rather than using the then current Thomsonian and Galenic treatment methods. These generic methods were based on using herbal remedies as vehicles for either eliminating treatment strategies—e.g., causing sweating through herbal *stimulants* like Cayenne along with steam baths, purging with "vegetable purges," causing vomiting with Lobelia herb or Ipecac bark, etc.—or sedating strategies through the use of *sedatives* such as opium and laudanum. In other words, what King and Scudder were anxious to see was their colleagues taking a more thorough case-history—not unlike the homeopath's first patient intake—and then choosing the one main remedy that most closely matched this symptomatology—the specific medication. To this end, they also devised the term "specific symptomatology," which conversely is the complete, condensed symptom picture or profile treated by a particular remedy. Throughout the second half of the nineteenth century, a hardy handful of Eclectics assiduously observed the patterns of signs and symptoms that patients brought into their practice, which included tongue, pulse, stool, urine and complexion observations. Through this empirical process the specific symptomatology of most known remedies was established: They became specific medications in the hands of skilled, consciencious doctors. They can still be found in reprints of trusty Eclectic texts such as *King's American Dispensatory* (King, Felter and Lloyd) and *American Materia Medica, Therapeutics and Pharmacognosy* (Ellingwood). It makes complete sense to us nowadays why the use of single remedies should be successful—because successful this tailored prescribing approach was. The Eclectic remedies were prepared in highly concentrated alcoholic extracts which to some extent engaged the same energetic laws as homeopathic remedies themselves, while at the same time still maintaining the more generic influence of the remedies in water extract form.

The same methodology is adopted by Japanese *kampo* practitioners when they search for the "symptom conformation" of well-established formulas. Instead of prescribing a single remedy in tincture form, *kampo* doctors prescribe an herbal formula in decoction (water extraction) form—one of many formulas from the oldest surviving complete Chinese herbal medicine text, the Shan Han Lun classic.

Prescribing according to symptom pictures or syndromes is endemic to most traditions of herbal medicine in China, Taiwan, Malaysia, etc. Here a patient's illness is assessed in terms of zheng, the pattern of disharmony, and a standard or free-style formula is prescribed. Again the approach here is observational and imagistic. Although Chinese medicine does have various theories about the origins and progression of illness (always based on functional and energetic aspects), on the whole it devotes more attention to the current configuration of a condition in the here and now. More important than discussions of etiology to Chinese doctors are exploring ways of defining a patient's current presentation. And in their syncretic approach, there is nothing wrong with considering several possible explanations of a condition. Clearly, more than anything else, Chinese medicine is poised in the clinical moment preceding treatment.

Unsurprisingly, therefore, Chinese doctors also describe herbal remedies and formulas in terms of the conditions for which they are used. And herein lies the key to understanding remedies with respect to symptom pictures. Every remedy can be as accurately described, from the therapeutic point of view, in terms of the symptom picture it treats as in the way that it acts, i.e., in terms of specific symptomatology rather than pharmacology. In Homeopathy and Eclectic medicine there is one single overall symptom configuration particular to a remedy, whereas in Chinese medicine, a remedy's indications are broken down into several specific symptom pictures. In all cases, however, the underlying principle of remedy differentiation and treatment remains the same. The patient's specific symptom configuration—the unique, specific pattern of symptoms and signs—needs to be matched against that of a single remedy or formulation. The one with the best

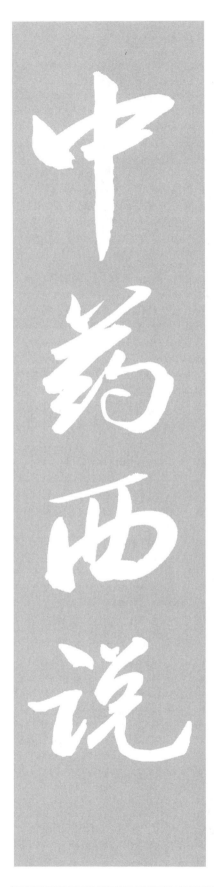

match is prescribed. This process of comparing the two symptom pictures involves attention to their overall profile on one hand and their particular, unique signs on the other.

For instance, a patient may complain of a sore throat and a cough, may be irritable and have a rapid pulse. Looking at this symptom picture as a whole, we would say that this person is presenting the syndrome lung wind heat. So far so good. Turning our attention now to the particular symptoms, we find out that the patient's throat is also dry and itchy, that the voice is somewhat hoarse and that there is some wheezing with slight chest pain. These are symptom details unique to this condition which also should be considered in our choice of remedy or formula. The first choice of single remedy would be Platycodon Jie Geng (Balloonflower root). In terms of remedy actions, Platycodon Jie Geng is a *respiratory stimulant* with *expectorant, demulcent* and *anti-inflammatory* actions combined. However, it is only one of several *respiratory stimulants* that address lung wind heat. It is only through consideration of the whole symptom picture that this particular remedy clearly becomes choice number one. Other possible, but less ideal, remedy choices for the symptom picture presented would have been Belamcanda She Gan (Leopard flower root), Arctium Niu Bang Zi (Burdock seed), Tagetes Wan Shou Ju (African marigold flower), Sterculia Pang Da Hai (Sterculia seed) and Oroxylum Mu Hu Die (Oroxylum seed).

There are several advantages to using herbal remedies in this way. The first is that it allows one to match the patient's presenting symptoms with a remedy in a purely observational or phenomenological way. It becomes possible to make a rational and accurate selection of a remedy without having to undergo the whole process of understanding both the pathology dynamics of the condition and the pharmacology dynamics of the matching remedy. It short-cuts this process that some practitioners find tedious and others interesting, depending on their preference. The key to working with the symptom pictures of remedies is thorough knowledge of these and keen observation—the kind of calm, unbiased, mirror-like observation that Oriental artists, poets, meditators—and doctors—have cultivated for millennia. Observing natural phenomena in this way, noticing the transformations that symptoms undergo, is different from trying to look for their mechanism of disharmony and understand their cause. It is simply cool observation that is dynamically polarized between a unifying overview of the whole picture and a differentiating attention to specific details. These are the qualities of observation required to successfully match up the symptomatology presented by the patient with that of appropriate remedies.

The other advantage to working with symptom pictures when selecting remedies is that one is not limited to the realm of physiology alone. Mental and emotional symptoms, if they are present, are also taken into consideration. This is usually not the case when remedy selection is done on the basis of herb actions and physiological disorders. In the symptom picture approach the concern is not assessing physical disorders or defining a disease, but with obtaining a comprehensive composite picture of the illness—which often includes mental and emotional aspects. The reality of illness is such that as patients we rarely present physical symptoms alone: More commonly, we complain of a particular mixture of physical, emotional and mental signs and symptoms.

There is a bewildering variety of syndromes used in Chinese medicine. This is for two reasons. First, because Chinese medicine includes two major herbal traditions, the Shang Han Lun and the Wen Bing traditions. What these traditions have in common is the fact that all syndromes are based on energetic conditions in relation to the location (interior/exterior, three Warmers, four levels), nature (hot/cold, six evils), status (full/empty, four injuries) and direction (rising/ sinking, dispersing/consolidating) of the condition. It is the large number of possible permutations among these four essential parameters of illness that generates the many syndromes described in traditional textbooks, and still used by Chinese herbalists today.

Second, the variety of symptom pictures used is large because relatively recently, syndromes according to the *zang fu,* the organ-channel networks, were devised. These syndromes have no history prior to the 1950s: The therapeutic strategies they embody are not found in any of the classical literature in traditional Oriental medicine. They were created mainly for political reasons in order to develop a compromise system of herbal medicine whose design was to facilitate integration of traditionally trained doctors into a conventional Western hospital setting. Today, the *zang fu* syndromes dominate Chinese medical pathology taught in colleges of traditional Oriental medicine in the West. The *zang fu* syndromes possess the advantage of greater specificity of pathology than the more systemic traditional syndromes, and so often provide the greater detail necessary for the individualized type of Western health care. However, by the same token, their very specificity also possess the disadvantage of making them unsuitable for treating systemic and terrain conditions, especially if the aim is preventive treatment or if the Western biomedical diagnosis isn't clear. Be that as it may, for us in the West the *zang fu* syndromes have another serious drawback: The energetic organ-channel networks have an extremely confusing relationship to the Western anatomical organs. And the names we give these energetic networks do not help either: As mentioned in Chapter 1, naming the *gan* organ-network, for example, by the same name as the anatomical liver organ, and then naming this a "liver syndrome," is a bad case of cross-wiring. This term confuses the Chinese concept of *gan,* an energetic matrix or orb, and the concept of liver, a physiological organ. Because of the inevitable overlap between the functions of the energetic organ-channel networks and the anatomical organs, it has become increasingly difficult to separate the two.

In this text, the position adopted was the following: If a Chinese symptom picture could be said to involve the anatomical organ implied in its name, then the name of the organ is put in lower case. This syndrome then becomes a physiologically based one, rather than a purely energetically based syndrome. Cases in point are syndromes such as "intestines damp heat" (whose symptoms directly involve the intestines), and "lung Qi constraint" (whose symptoms indirectly involve the lungs). If a Chinese symptom picture does not involve the anatomical organ implied in its name, the name of the Chinese organ-channel concerned goes into upper case. In this case the syndrome remains purely energetic by definition, and in that sense belongs to the traditional Shang Han Lun/Wen Bing lineages. Examples of this type of syndrome are "Liver Yang rising" (whose symptoms do not involve the anatomical liver, but rather the nervous system), "phlegm damp Heart obstruction" (whose symptoms do not involve the heart but the central nervous system) and "Pericardium fire" (whose symptoms do not involve the pericardium but again the nervous system). In many cases there is no organ name to confuse us, as in the clear-cut energetic syndromes "wind/damp/cold obstruction," "external wind heat" and "wind phlegm obstruction." The syndromes involving the Chinese concept *xue,* usually erroneously translated as "blood," makes interpretation of "Blood stagnation," "Blood deficiency," Blood level heat," etc.,

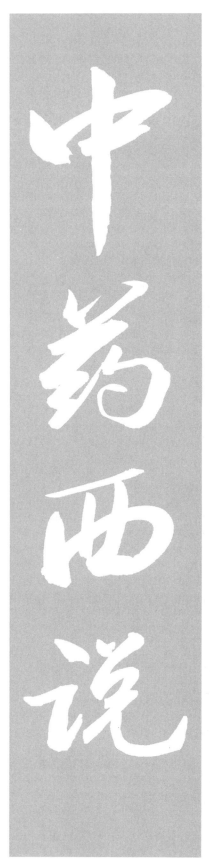

very difficult. These in this text are usually left untouched—except that "blood" becomes "Blood"! However, it was decided in any event to give priority to the use of syndromes based on physiological organ functions whenever possible.

In order to show the tie-in between the Chinese remedies and body system functions, the emphasis in this text is to put as many of the syndromes indicating the use of the remedies on a physiological basis. As a result, it was sometimes neccessary to create new or alternative syndrome terms where previous terms were insufficient for this purpose. The syndrome "nerve and brain deficiency" is therefore a modern rendering of the more traditional term "Liver and Kidney Essence deficiency," while "musculoskeletal deficiency" is a modern description of "Liver and Kidney depletion," "liver and adrenal Yin deficiency" that of "Blood and Qi deficiency," "stomach and small intestine Qi deficiency" that of "Spleen Qi deficiency," "intestines Qi constraint" that of "Liver/Spleen disharmony," and so on. Despite unavoidable ambiguities and overlaps here and there between energetic and physiological functions, the absolute criteria used in all cases of modern syndrome renderings is again the following: the organ name begins with a lower case in the case of physiological functions, and with an upper case in the case of energetic functions.

Clearly, the concept of the four remedy actions and the symptom picture are typical of Western systems of vitalistic medicine, especially Eclectic and Physiomedical herbal medicine, and Homeopathy. Nevertheless, the same principles of remedy organization, pathology organization and herbal prescribing are also found in Chinese medicine. Again, this is to be expected from two systems of herbal medicine that share the vitalistic and largely empirical approach. Because Western herbal medicine still retains a close connection with the scientific approach—and we saw how this is already being implemented in modern-day China—it can build a bridge between the vitalistic and scientific aspects of Chinese herbal medicine. The thesis of this chapter is that it provides that crucial missing link.

Chinese herbal medicine clearly has the potential for remarkable growth in two important ways. First, through the close connection with Western/Greek vitalistic herbal traditions, the re-evaluation of its vitalistic pharmacology and therapeutics. Second, through the connection with Western bioscience, the reinterpretation of its pharmacognosy and pharmacology in scientific terms. Of these two possibilities, the first process is the one currently in most need of attention, and arguably the more important. In this way, I believe, Chinese medicine stands a chance of becoming an integral, recognized and distinct system of modern health care in the West.

Reclassifying Chinese Remedies: The Anatomical Body Systems

A major practical therapeutic consequence to redefining Chinese remedies in Western terms, whether these are scientific or vitalistic, is that we begin to think about them in terms of body system functions rather than purely energetic functions. The materia medica in this text specifically realocates them to particular body systems and presents their physiological actions according to their known functions and dysfunctions. To the best of my knowledge, this procedure has not yet been attempted. Yet from the clinical perspective it is currently the most important consideration, because it gives the remedies their primary definition within a Western therapeutic framework.

The advantages of taking this step are obvious. The information about each remedy's functions and uses become easily accessible to the Western practitioner—given that these are also presented in the Western physiopathological terms. Moreover, simply assigning remedies to particular body systems is not the only consideration. More important first of all is to characterize them (as we just saw) by their dominant essential remedy action, namely restoring, relaxing, stimulating or sedating. Their main action will define them as belonging to one of these four treatment categories. Alisma Ze Xie, for example, is mainly used in the treatment of various urinary disorders, and so clearly belongs to the urinary system. But is the herb primarily a *restorative, stimulant, relaxant* or *sedative?* This important remedy actually is both a *urinary stimulant*, in that it causes diuresis and relieves edema, and a *urinary sedative* in that it addresses acute urinary tract infections. (It finally ended up as a *urinary stimulant*, mainly because there are so many other fine *urinary sedatives* available.)

Once each remedy has been characterized by its fundamental action on a particular body system and assigned to one of the four treatment categories, the challenge then becomes seeing the remedy in a completely new light. We need to take a completely fresh look at its functions and indications in physiopathological terms. The problem here is that these may have nothing to do with the traditional treatment category the remedy came from or even the main way it is was used in pre-twentieth century Chinese medicine.

The umbelliferous remedy Bupleurum Chai Hu (Asian buplever root) is a fascinating case in point. This remedy is traditionally classed as a pungent-cool agent for releasing the exterior because it addresses Shao Yang stage conditions presenting alternating chills and fever, irritability, etc. These are mainly infectious conditions which, in times prior to modern hygiene, usually occupied the largest portion of a doctor's practice. However, looking today at its overall profile of physiological actions and indications, it becomes clear that Bupleurum Chai Hu acts predominantly on the nervous system as a *sedative*. The remedy possesses significant *analgesic* and *spasmolytic* properties that are used in treating various types of pain arising from spasm, inflammation and infection, ranging from headache through to dysmenorrhea, cholangitis, colitis and influenza. In traditional terms, Buplever root spreads Liver Qi and thereby relieves chest and flank pain, epigastric and abdominal pain and menstrual pain. Moreover, it does not possess the typical *diaphoretic* action of remedies associated with releasing exterior conditions. Granted, research has shown that it possesses *anti-infective* actions (including *antiviral, antibacterial* and *antigenic* activity), and because of this, the remedy is a definite candidate for the remedies that reduce infection in the last section of this materia medica. (It would have gone under the herbs to dispel wind heat.) However, a look at Bupleurum Chai Hu's general gestalt of indications will reveal that its tropism for the nervous system is predominant and that its application for a variety of disorders involving neurological hyperactivity (mainly pain, spasm and inflammation) is greater. In contrast, its *anti-infective* nature is not nearly as broad-spectrum as those *anti-infective* remedies it would have rubbed shoulders with: *Bupleurum* is simply not used for the great variety of infectious conditions as are the likes of Forsythia Lian Qiao and Dryopteris Guan Zhong. Interestingly, two other remedies traditionally classed as surface-releasers also ended up in this text as *nervous sedatives:* Cimicifuga Sheng Ma and Cryptotympana Chan Tui.

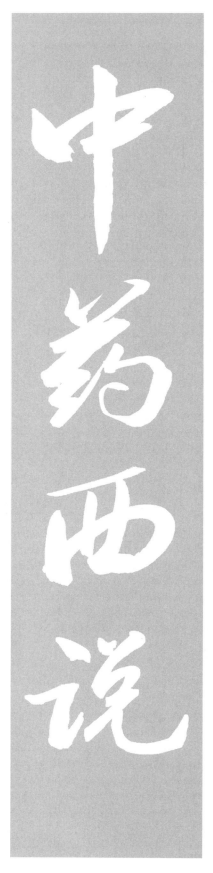

The key to determining the appropriate class of body system for each remedy is to find both its main contemporary usage and the therapeutic function at which it seems to excel. We tend to assume that these two factors always coincide, but this is not neccessarily the case. Among the hundreds of remedies that have been tested in China, Taiwan and Japan for reducing hyper-sensitivity, very few have emerged that in terms of clinical applications possess an *immune-regulating* action first and foremost. The majority of these remedies still fulfill other primary functions while secondarily also possessing *immune-modulating* effects.

The vast differences of terminology alone between Chinese and Western medicine poses the single biggest obstacle in our ability to see a remedy's main Western physiological function clearly. Terms that seem identical in both Chinese and Western medicine, such as organ names (e.g., "Spleen," "Liver," "Kidney"), the terms "Blood," "Phlegm" and so on, in fact point to completely different clinical realities. This is because, as we saw in Chapter 1, the approach of each system is very different, one being energetic, the other tissue-based.

A simple example of terminological differences can be seen in those remedies that address the syndrome known as Liver and Kidney depletion. These remedies fundamentally treat such symptoms as weak, sore lower back, knees and legs, possibly with general weakness. While in physiology it is the connective tissue that weakens and causes these symptoms, in Chinese medicine this process is seen as a severe deficiency, a "depletion" of Liver and Kidney organ/channel energies. Obviously, these Chinese medical functions are different from the liver and kidney functions known to Western physiology. Instead of trying to create connections between two different functions just because the names used to describe them are the same, each function should be examined separately for its own clinical meaning. So in Chinese pathology, as the Liver weakens it fails to nourish the sinews, and as the Kidney weakens it fails to nourish the bones. In Western herbal medicine, however, this condition instead is seen to involve a weakening of the connective tissue with a tendency to endogenous toxicosis (toxin retention from meta-bolic faults) as the interstitial fluid-soaked connective tissue, acting as a transit zone for nutrients and wastes, increasingly soaks up superfluous toxins that eventually erode the integrity of the host tissues. So, important remedies like Eucommia Du Zhong (Eucommia bark) and Acanthopanax Wu Jia Pi can be seen either as "tonifying the Liver and Kidney, and strength-ening the sinews and bones" or as restoring the connective tissue and resolving metabolic toxicosis. The point here is this. Explained either way, the clinical reality is that these remedies relieve the above-named symptoms, and so presumably the same underlying pathological condition, which is often seen in relation to rheumatoid arthritis, rheumatic disorders, muscular atrophy, osteoporosis and so on.

If there is to be an end to the current rampant confusion of Western and Oriental medical terminologies, the crying need to see beyond words to the clinical condition treated by each remedy becomes nothing less than self-evident. Another striking example of language's deceptive veil is the challenge posed by the traditional herb class for "vitalizing the Blood" (*huo xue*), particularly those remedies among them that are used for dysmenorrhea. The confusion arises more from the Chinese term *xue*, usually translated as "Blood," than from the verb *huo*, meaning to "vitalize" or "activate." While menstrual pain for the most part arises from uterine cramping, this in Chinese medicine is generally termed "Blood stasis," and the great majority of remedies employed are "Blood vitalizers that disperse Blood stasis." (The main exceptions to this are Cyperus Xiang Fu and Lindera Wu Yao, which are said to relieve dysmenorrhea by "circulating Qi.") The simplest explanation for this interpretation of dysmenorrhea is that menstruation involves bleeding, and so any cramping pain must involve a stasis of the Blood (*xue*). Now, it is a fact that dysmenorrhea can be differentiated into various other conditions such as cold damp congealing, Blood and Qi deficiency, Liver and Kidney exhaustion, Kidney and Liver Yin deficiency, etc. However, the interesting historical fact remains that the remedies themselves used to treat painful menses invariably are described as doing so because they "vitalize Blood and disperse Blood stasis." Western herbal medicine, on the other hand, describes uterine cramping as a spasmodic condition of the smooth muscles, for which smooth muscle *relaxants/ spasmolytics* are used. This in Chinese medicine relates directly to conditions of constrained Liver Qi, which typically involve pain arising from smooth muscle spasm. It would make sense, therefore, to view menstrual cramping primarily as a condition of Qi constraint in the Lower Warmer. We would then define the appropriate class of remedies for this condition as "circulating Qi and releasing constraint." However, as just noted, the majority of remedies that treat dysmenorrhea are traditionally described as treating Blood stasis rather than Qi stasis. It follows that these remedies should be squarely redefined as "circulating Qi in the Lower Warmer." This is the logical conclusion, in this particular case, of seeing beyond the confusion arising from concepts that appear to be similar but in reality are different—in this case Blood (*xue*) and blood (the body fluid). By acknowledging terminological differences, the clinical reality behind the phenomenon of dysmenorrhea is allowed to become apparent.

Once remedies are examined from a Western perspective, we saw how a remedy like Bupleurum Chai Hu is used today in rather a different way than it was centuries ago when infectious disease was rife. We also saw how the remedies for dysmenorrhea are traditionally called "Blood vitalizers" even though they treat spasmodic menstrual conditions that do not involve a pathology of the blood itself. Both these are problem issues. However, there are cases where the remedies' modern uses remain essentially identical to their traditional uses (with or without variational and additional uses), despite the terminological differences used to describe them. Happily, this is more often than not the case. The remedy Uncaria Gou Teng, for instance, in Western terms is seen as a *nervous relaxant* with its *spasmolytic* and *anticonvulsant* actions that treat spasmodic nervous disorders such as infantile seizures, tremors and stroke. Again the only consideration, from the Western practitioner's point of view, is that in traditional terms the remedy is described as "extinguishing internal wind" and "clearing wind phlegm." But in itself this description is not a problem, and diversity is invariably positive. The point is that despite differences of interpretation and linguistic description, the clinical reality of Uncaria Gou Teng is that the remedy treats one and the same set of symptoms, and therefore the same underlying condition. In the hands of Chinese physicians it has done so for thousands of years.

Traditional and contemporary uses of numerous remedies that treat respiratory conditions are also identical. Asarum Xi Xin and Pinellia Ban Xia, for instance, are both classic remedies used for coughing with production of copious sputum, symptoms typically seen in bronchial infections. In traditional language these remedies "warm and transform phlegm cold," while in biomedical terms they stimulate the bronchi and promote sputum expectoration—*bronchial stimulants* that exert an *expectorant* effect: *stimulant expectorants,* for short. Because their clinical use with

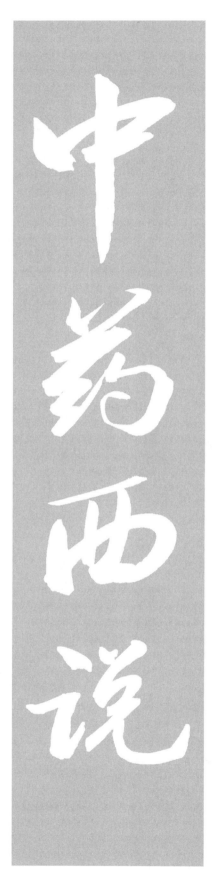

respect to the symptoms they treat is the same, we can posit an absolute equivalence between the two terminological interpretations of their effect and so the two remedy classes they belong to. The same goes for those remedies that treat chronic diarrhea, for instance. While Oriental textbooks discuss using these remedies to "restrain leakage from the intestines," Western textbooks advise their use in causing astringency, naming them *astringent antidiarrheals*. Their clinical use is identical.

There is another way of stating the challenge involved in reorganizing the remedies in a physiological framework. That is, that to be successful, the physiological categories would have to represent the exact meeting point of the Chinese energetic remedy functions and the Western biomedical remedy actions. In other words, using the articulated skeletal framework of the body systems and the four remedy actions, is it possible to fill in the substantial content of the remedy actions themselves? For the most part, this again poses no major difficulty as long as the clinical condition (including signs and symptoms) addressed is one and the same. For example, the intersecting point of Chinese remedies that "dissolve food stagnation and remove accumulation" and Western remedies with an *"enzymatic digestive"* action is remedies such as Hordeum Mai Ya, Massa Fermentata Shen Qu and Gallus Ji Nei Jin because they treat epigastric fullness and distension, nausea and so on. The meeting ground (improbable though it may seem) of remedies that "disperse congealed Blood and relieve pain" and remedies with *"vulnerary (tissue-repairing), analgesic* and *detumescent actions"* is such remedies as Panax San Qi, Drynaria Gu Sui Bu and Commiphora Mo Yao: These treat the pain, swelling and redness caused by tissue trauma. The intersecting point of herbs for "clearing damp heat from the liver and gallbladder" and *"hepatic decongestants* with *antiseptic* and *anti-inflammatory"* actions is seen in Gardenia Zhi Zi, Lysimachia Jin Qian Cao and Canna Mei Ren Jiao, for instance, as they address congestive (sub)infectious conditions of the liver and associated parts.

In other instances, however, the meeting ground of the energetic functions and the biomedical actions has to be carefully thought out. This is the case with the many types of remedies used in Chinese medicine for treating infectious conditions. Here there is no one-to-one equivalence. Whereas the West is used to treating infection essentially through the principle of promoting tissue asepsis, Chinese medicine prefers to address infection in terms of its many manifestations, such as hot or cold conditions, including various types of hot conditions such as damp heat, full heat, toxic heat, and so on. *Anti-infective* remedies are simply not a bottomless black liner-bagfull of *antivirals, antibacterials, antifungals* and *lymphatics* as modern Western textbooks sadly would have us believe. *Anti-infectives* still require differentiating, if an intersection between the two systems is to be found. One middle-of-the-road solution is to establish a small number of remedy classes for infection that are still based on the traditional differentiation of its main patterns of presentation—namely wind heat, damp heat, toxic heat and fire. However, because most remedies that resolve wind heat and damp heat also clear toxic heat (fire toxin), this text compresses *anti-infective* remedies into essentially two categories. One, *anti-infectives* that dispel wind heat and detoxify fire toxin, and two, *anti-infectives* that clear damp heat and detoxify fire toxin. While the bulk of them are found in the Infection and Toxicosis section, the wind heat *anti-infectives* are also in the Nose, Throat and Eyes section (where they specifically relieve nasal congestion and pain), and the damp heat *anti-infectives* are also in most body systems under *sedatives* to those systems.

In a few cases there is no meeting ground to be found between the energetic and the biomedical remedy actions. The remedies that reduce toxicosis in particular, the *detoxicants* of Western herbal medicine, have no equivalent as such in Oriental medicine. Within a body system-based framework they play an important role in the dynamics of both tonifying and draining principles of treatment, and become especially relevant to chronic, dormant or preclinical infectious conditions. It is therefore logical to include remedies for toxicosis alongside the *anti-infectives* and *antiparasitics*. This latter category itself is a problem in the sense that all infection involves microorganisms that by definition are already parasitic in their behavior. Infection only arises when normally symbiotic microbes turn parasitic on their host rather than remaining eubiotic (positive). However, because a remedy class to reduce "parasitosis and toxicosis" fails to express the idea of acute infection, it is neccessary to add the category of infection within this section. Note also, in this connection, that the Western concept of toxicosis or toxins (in the plural) bears no relation whatsoever to the Chinese concept of fire toxin (in the singular). Toxicosis is a tissue state created by toxins, whereas fire toxin or toxic heat is a particular energetic state of heat (alongside damp heat, wind heat, etc.). The most that could be said is that fire toxin is just one possible end-result of chronic toxicosis among many (hardening and deposition are examples of two others). However, the important point here is that although there is no actual intersection between *detoxicant* remedies and a Chinese treatment category, taking the remedies for Infection, Toxicosis and Parasitosis as a whole, there is clear evidence of interaction among these three subsections as well as among the *anti-infectives* in particular.

It is interesting to note also that the Chinese materia medica contains remedies of a type that is hardly ever considered to form a separate category to itself: the *adaptogens* that restore the endocrine glands and enhance immunity. These "harmony remedies" or "imperial remedies" are the pride of Oriental medicine and have virtually no equivalents in the West. They epitomize everything about Chinese medicine—indeed about Chinese culture—that has to do with prevention of disease, with enhancement of the individual's inborn terrain and with the pursuit of harmony and longevity in life.

Looking at the distinction between Chinese remedies that have herbal, mineral and animal substances as their source, it is interesting to see in which classes these now fall. A total of nine minerals belong to the section of *neurocardiac sedatives,* and five to the section of topical *antiparasitics,* while a smaller number are found in the *vulneraries* for tissue trauma, the *antiasthmatics,* the *antidiarrheals* and the *CNS spasmolytics*. The majority of animal remedies, on the other hand, are found among the *nervous system relaxants* and *sedatives*. In general, because of the difference between the traditional and body systems categorization of remedies, the remedy placements are sometimes (but not always) very different from the traditional categories in which they are found. The patterns of organization of the remedies are different, fresh. Nevertheless, or perhaps because of that, they make complete sense from the Western physiological point of view.

It is hoped that this reclassification of remedies will do more than allow therapists in the West access to intelligent, informed usage of Chinese remedies. It is hoped that ultimately it will contribute to the successful continuance of Oriental medicine as a unique, viable, vital tradition of healing in the West.

3

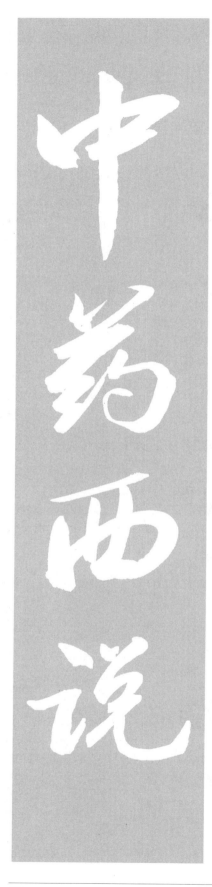

The Remedy Presentation

The materia medica is the major reference section in this book, and consists of primary and secondary Chinese remedies. The primary remedy has a longer presentation that includes an illustration of the natural plant, mineral or animal from which it is prepared. The secondary remedy, because it is less commonly used, and because of space limitations, is given a more condensed presentation without an illustration.

Two factors guided my choice of main remedies in this text. First, they are the most commonly used medicinal items in classical Chinese medicine, the ones most likely to be found in an Chinese doctor's prescription in any major Chinese population center, such as Shanghai, Beijing, Hong Kong, Singapore, Taipei, San Francisco, etc. Second, special consideration is given to remedies frequently employed in the People's Republic and the West today—even though they do not belong to the main 300 or so traditional remedies that constitute the backbone of Chinese medicine. Gossypium Mian Hua Gen (Cotton root bark), often used for female reproductive disorders on the mainland, and Ginkgo Yin Xing Ye (Ginkgo leaf), routinely given for circulatory problems in Europe and the U.S., are two such remedies.

The only criterion that makes a remedy secondary is if its functions are completely covered by a primary remedy. The actions of Oroxylum Mu Hu Die (Oroxylum seed), for example, although in themselves excellent for throat inflammation with pain, are more than adequately covered by Arctium Niu Bang Zi (Burdock seed). Nor, taking the practice of Chinese medicine as a whole, is Oroxylum Mu Hu Die very widely used for this condition, in contrast to Arctium Niu Bang Zi. Another criterion to consider is simply a remedy's availability. The more regional a remedy, the less likely it becomes available elsewhere, especially in the West. This classifies it as secondary.

Remember, though, that while the secondary remedies are,

on the whole, less frequently used in Chinese medicine, any one of them might be an important component in an herbal prescription. It's all a question of relativity. A highly effective secondary, regional herb, when used in the locale of its growth, is actually not a minor herb. In that setting it is then a primary, frequently used remedy by practitioners in that area. Furthermore, there are some "secondary" regional remedies that are routinely used all over China, Taiwan and Hong Kong only for managing certain conditions. Schefflera Qi Ye Lian (Schefflera root and herb), for instance, is noted for its highly effective *analgesic* and *nervous sedative* action, while Sarcandra Jiu Jie Feng (Smooth sarcandra herb) is often selected for its specific *antitumoral* effect in many types of cancer. Once again, these remedies are often given a shortened presentation because they are less commonly used by the mainstream of Chinese practitioners as a whole, not because they are any less effective.

In chapter 2 we considered how the repertory of Chinese remedies, like any repertory, has a cyclical nature. At any given period in history, there are certain remedies that are on the wane; the kind of remedies that everyone knows and reads about in books, but tends not to use in actual daily practice. Then there are the "up-and-coming" remedies that hold greater promise for effectiveness. Today it is often hard to get more information about these other than the desirable actions claimed by the promotional literature of nutritional supplement companies. Yet it is these remedies that are considered "hot" items among practitioners and, soon after, the public at large. At the time of writing, for example, Turmeric root, Ginkgo leaf and Coleus root are examples of this type.

This materia medica attempts to strike a balance between a core body of important traditional, time-tested Chinese remedies—the same ones taught in Chinese medicine schools in the West—and a small array of remedies rapidly vaulting into prominence through biochemical research and contemporary clinical practice.

In presenting each remedy in the Materia Medica section in a detailed and comprehensive way, my aim was to allow one not only to choose specific information at will but, equally important, to gain a broad, overall perspective of the remedy. An in-depth understanding of herbal remedies and a detailed knowledge of their specific actions and indications are both essential to the practice of herbal medicine.

The presentation of the main remedies in the materia medica attempts at comprehensivity in several ways. First, the materia medica includes both scientific and empirical information. The scientific information is primarily concerned with the plant's chemical constituents and pharmacological actions; the empirical information is expressed in terms of the plant's effective qualities and uses according to traditional symptom pictures. This presentation reflects the integrated analytical/phenomenological approach pursued throughout the text.

Second, the materia medica generally includes a very wide range of information about each remedy, including its botanical, mineral or zoological sources and its habit, its chemical constituents, energetic qualities, various types of actions on body systems, organs and tissues, symptom picture uses, preparation forms, doses, methods of use, and cautions and contraindications. Third, this tabular information is enriched with notes that not only highlight the remedy's main functions and uses, but also areas of particular contemporary interest.

The Primary Names

In order to facilitate identification, every remedy in this text is given two primary names at the top. The first one is the clinical name; the second one is the common English name.

The clinical name is a composite name that consists of two parts: the botanical genus followed by the Mandarin Chinese name, which is phoneticized in Pinyin. For example, the plant *Polygonum multiflorum,* known as He Shou Wu in Mandarin Chinese, bears the clinical name Polygonum He Shou Wu. This binomial naming system was introduced by Jake Fratkin in the

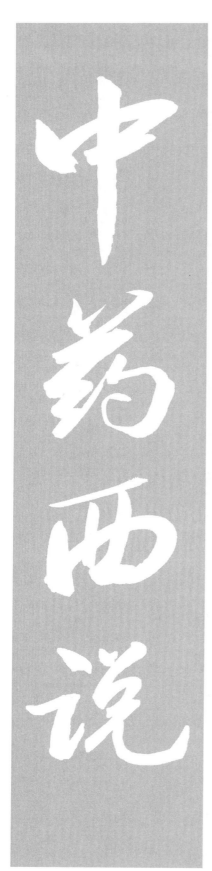

mid-1980s. It is mainly used in practitioners' and students' circles and provides the easiest way to identify a particular remedy.

The plant's common name consists of the English name and the part of the plant used (whether root, herb, berry, etc.). The common name equivalent to Polygonum He Shou Wu, for example, is Flowery knotweed root. A remedy's common name may be derived from a variety of sources, including traditional names for the plant, literal translations of its botanical species name, and translations of one of its Chinese names. Where no common plant name existed, it was necessary to create an original name. In this case, the English name is asterisked.

The Main Categories

Botanical Source

For botanical identification purposes it is important for us in the West to know the exact plant species that provide the raw material for Chinese remedies. However, when we consider the sheer variety of species actually used as source material for a single Chinese remedy, it becomes disarmingly clear that we are not justified in designating just a single species to represent each remedy. In North America, for instance, the remedy Echinacea root is represented by three main species: *Echinacea purpurea, E. angustifolia* and *E. pallida.* Modern botanical identification of the plant materials used in Chinese medicine has shown that it is the rule rather than the exception that more than one plant species is used for a single herbal remedy. In a few cases, even species of different genera are used for a single remedy.

The main genus and various species currently used are given first, and the other possibilities are listed in order of decreasing importance. If more than four species are used for a remedy, the words "and spp." are added. Please note that this list of vicariad sources is usually not, and in fact cannot ever be, exhaustive or definitive. Local plant usage throughout the Chinese-speaking world and botanical research are both in a state of constant slow evolution.

The *anti-infective* remedy Da Qing Ye is an extreme example of a remedy that has both different genera and species as its botanical source. The main genera used for this remedy are *Isatis* and *Baphicacanthus*; the secondary ones are *Clerodendrum* and *Polygonum.* In the *Isatis* genus, the main two species used are *Isatis tinctoria* and *Isatis indigotica.*

Another good example of botanical polymorphism is the remedy Jin Qian Cao. Two main genera/species furnish the raw materials for this important biliary and urinary remedy: *Lysimachia* spp., and *Desmodium styracifolium,* while in some areas certain species of *Glechoma* and *Hydrocotyle* also count for Jin Qian Cao. We should also note that in some cases a qualifier is added for more local versions of a remedy. This is why Jin Qian Cao derived from *Desmodium styracifolium* is often called

Guang Dong Jin Qian Cao (literally "Jin Qian Cao from Guangdong province.") It would of course be botanically ideal if every local genus/species version of a remedy had a qualified name indicating the locality of origin. In practice, however, this is simply not how the Chinese go about naming their herbs. A consistent system of this kind would be extremely difficult to establish, mainly because of the sheer size of the country, the diversity of its population and the very number of plant names in existance all over the country. The primary remedy name in one area might be a secondary or even a very minor name in another part of China. Alone agreement on a primary name for each remedy would be very difficult to establish.

The absence of a one-to-one correspondence between the remedy name and its botanical source may seem unfortunate. However, it simply results from the different aims of herbal medicine, which is healing through plants, and botany, which is naturalistic plant classification. Given the sheer number of botanical genuses, species and varieties currently ennumerated, it is actually not surprising that botanical plurality for each remedy is the rule rather than the exception.

In actual practice, one plant genus/species may be used predominantly and others secondarily, or several genuses/species may be used with more or less equal frequency. Alternately, one genus/species may be used mainly in one area of China, while other genus/species may be used in other areas. This is especially true of remedies used in Taiwan and Japan, where a large number of local genuses/species are used to represent the main remedies.

The consistent botanical plurality of Chinese remedies underscores just one point: The dominant concept here is the remedy, not the plant of origin. The standard used in Chinese medicine is the concept of the remedy, with its own particular therapeutic profile of actions and indications—not the botanical source. Herbal medicine defines a remedy by a set of specific pharmacological actions and clinical indications, not plant morphology. The remedy then becomes a therapeutic archetype that transcends the realm of botany, manifesting at different times and in different places in the guise of various species and genera. The archetype is clearly pleomorphic by nature. The original archetype, however, crucially remains the same. Thus, the remedy Wu Tou is the prepared central taproot derived from several species of aconite. Although Wu Tou is often differentiated into more specific remedies such as Bei Wu Tou, Cao Wu and Chuan Wu in various parts of China, they are still all called Wu Tou because they all represent its therapeutic essence. The original archetypal concept of Wu Tou thereby remains untouched and constant.

A further complication occurs when botanists—striving either for taxonomical accuracy or botanical immortality—call a certain plant by one name, and doctors—bound by tradition and habit—call the same plant by another name. Currently the most complex case in point has to be the taxonomical debates surrounding the *anthelmintic* remedy *Artemisia annua*. Should we call these the *Artemisia* wars?

In Chinese medicine, the species *Artemisia annua* is generally known as Qing Hao. The same name, however, is also given to the species *Artemisia apiacea*. Because these species are now being clinically used in somewhat different ways by progressive doctors, a valiant effort to differentiate them is underway. Botanists, schools of botanical pharmacy and the more progressive doctors are now tending to call *Artemisia annua* Huang Hua Hao, not Qing Hao. However, past literature and many contemporary texts published by traditional medical schools confusingly still refer to this species as Qing Hao. Traditions die hard—especially in China.

Predictably enough, problems of identification of *Artemisia* species now compound these taxonomical arguments. It is ironical that at least one researcher into the history of the Chinese materia medica now believes to have determined that the original source of the remedy Qing Hao in ancient Chinese medicine was indeed *Artemisia annua*, not *A. apiacea* as was believed all along.

From the therapeutic point of view it is clearly important for *Artemisia annua* to have a separate common name from *Artemisia apiacea:* only the first species is a good *anti-infective* with *antiparasitic* and *antiprotozoal* actions. However, the effort of botanists, pharmacists and doctors to forge a separate identity for *Artemisia annua* is constantly being undermined by the seemingly ineradicable usage of the name Qing Hao, especially at the local and popular level, for

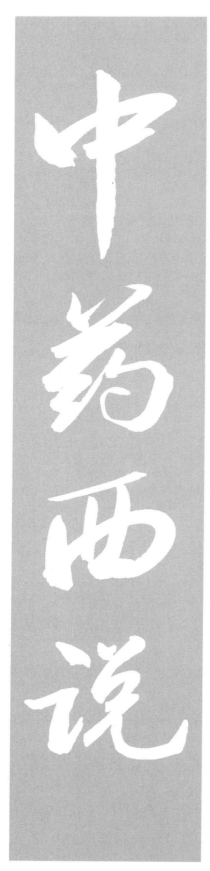

several species of *Artemisia*, not just the two in question.

The point here is this. Just because Chinese medicine is based on botanical plurality does not mean that we shouldn't take advantage of botanical definition and greater specificity of pharmacological action when this is desirable. Another major example of where it actually becomes crucial to know the species of the remedy being used is the remedy Wu Jia Pi. In the past Wu Jia Pi was derived from the root of *Acanthopanax* species such as *spinosus, gracilistylus, senticosus* and *sessiliflorus*. The species *senticosus*, however, has shown to possess *adaptogenic* properties that extend the range of its therapeutic applications way beyond that of all other species. This may be partly why the botanist Maximowicz renamed the plant *Eleutherococcus senticosus,* and this is why its modern name is now Ci Wu Jia, commonly known as Eleuthero or Siberian ginseng.

Pharmaceutical Name
The pharmaceutical name is a standard name for a remedy, derived from its botanical genus and the part of the plant employed. This naming system is used in the People's Republic of China more than anywhere else. Although the pharmaceutical name has the advantage of giving the specific plant part used as remedy, e.g. radix (root), semen (seed), herba (herb), etc., it does not provide the same degree of completeness and ease of identification as the composite clinical name at the top.

The latin terms used to create a pharmaceutical name include animal and mineral parts used in Chinese medicine. They are identical to the names given in the Chinese Pharmacopeia, with the exception of a few changes made for the sake of accuracy. For example, the remedy Xin Yi Hua, literally "Yulan magnolia flower," is better rendered in pharmaceutical Latin as "Gemma Magnoliae" rather than "Flos Magnoliae." The medicinal plant part used is the unopened flower bud, which is "gemma," not the opened flower, "flos." Likewise, the correct pharmaceutical name for the remedy Yin Yang Huo is "Folium Epimedii" rather than "Herba Epimedii:" the actual part used is the large leaf, characteristically tightly tied together in small bundles.

In other cases, for the sake of consistency and precise morphological identification, it was necessary to alter the traditional pharmaceutical name. In this text the pharmaceutical names are based directly on the actual botanical/zoological/geological name, not on an unrelated, different name entirely. Thus, by renaming the remedy Zhu Ru "Caulis Phyllostachis" instead of "Caulis Bambusae," or the remedy E Jiao "Gelatium corii Equii asini" instead of "Gelatinum Asini," consistency and clarity is achieved in the pharmaceutical naming of Chinese remedies.

A glossary of latin botanical, mineral and zoological terms is found at the back of the book.

Chinese Names

Chinese remedy names divide into Mandarin and Cantonese, the two most common languages found throughout the Chinese-speaking world. Mandarin is presently the official language of the Chinese people. Listed here are the remedy names in their official Mandarin and Cantonese form of pronunciation. The phoneticization system used is Pinyin for Mandarin and Yale for Cantonese. The glossary of Cantonese pronunciation in Part Three will help with Cantonese remedy names.

Here again, this list of Chinese names is by no means exhaustive, especially as regards Cantonese pronunciation, which has numerous variations throughout South China, Hong Kong, the U.S. and wherever Cantonese doctors practice Chinese medicine.

Other Names

Given here are alternative English names for the remedy, sometimes a literal translation of the main Chinese name, and its main Japanese name.

Habit

Here appears a brief type-description of the main plant genus from which the herbal remedy originates, its preferred, most common place of growth and the morphology and appearing time of its flowers. These key characteristics are designed to make plant identification, growing and collecting easier for the prospective grower or wildcrafter.

Part Used

The exact, most commonly used part of the plant, mineral or animal that provides the remedy is given here. It is always used in dry form (not fresh) unless specified otherwise.

Therapeutic Category

The most essential question for understanding the nature of a remedy is its therapeutic category or status. Is the remedy mild, medium strong or strong? The fundamental therapeutic nature of a remedy is defined by these three categories and, besides their theoretical value, also have wide practical implications. By providing a comprehensive safety framework for each remedy, the three therapeutic categories directly affect factors such as remedy selection and usage. By far the majority of remedies in the Chinese pharmacy, as in the Western, belong to the mild category, but several stronger, slightly toxic ones also exist.

This three categories system was formulated in the 1930s by the German medical herbalist Rudolf Weiss. The three therapeutic categories themselves, in different ways, reflect the traditional Chinese and Greek medical categorization of remedies.

Mild remedies. These have very structive or Yin therapeutic effects, being gentle, slow-working, cumulative and often trophic, or nutritive. They can be more nutritious and food-like, and include weeds and medicinal foods such as Alfalfa herb, Nettle leaf, Ginger root and Hawthorn berry. The Chinese pharmacy also includes some animal remedies in this category; for example, Velvet deer antler, Tortoise shell and Antelope horn. Remedies of the mild category should be taken over long time-periods for their full healing potential to unfold; they can be used daily. Side effects or negative reactions are minor or nonexistent, and so these remedies are said to possess minimal or no chronic cumulative toxicity. Their final therapeutic effect is either *restorative* (tonifying) or *relaxant,* but never *stimulant or sedative* as remedies of the medium-strength and strong categories are.

Mild remedies are used both preventively and curatively. They are particularly well suited to the treatment of chronic and systemic deficiency conditions when the vital forces, or Righteous Qi, need tonifying. Their nutritive value is essential when vitality is depleted. Also, children and elderly people often rely exclusively on remedies in this category for any complaint. All traditional longevity formulas and elixirs consist entirely of plant (and some animal) remedies in this category.

Most remedies in the Chinese pharmacy have mild therapeutic status. Understand that mild

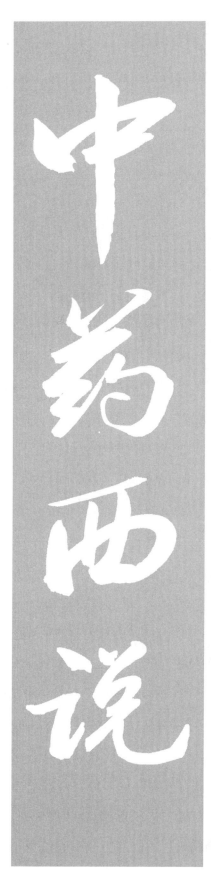

simply means they have structive effects as opposed to active effects. It does not mean that they have no effects. Nor does it mean they are "simply foods." A mild remedy is not ineffective because it does not contain strong, potentially toxic constituents such as alkaloids. In fact, structive, nutritive and subtle physiological changes account for at least 80 percent of all remedy actions.

Strong remedies. These have very active or Yang effects, which are strong, rapid and immediate. Being more drug-like, they should be taken rarely, and then once only. They cause immediate side effects and negative reactions and, therefore, are defined as possessing acute toxicity. Because strong remedies mostly cause powerful stimulation or sedation, they are therapeutically draining and are often used for the symptom treatment of severe or advanced conditions.

Remedies in the strong category are most appropriate in severe acute or local conditions where pathogenic elements have to be dealt with directly and immediately. As a result, the individual's vital force has to be robust enough to cope with the negative side effects of such remedies. Strong remedies should be avoided where the vital force is weak, as well as in younger and older people. They should only be used when the exact conditions are known that call for their use, when the safe dosage is known, how often they should be taken and what, if any, side effects might occur.

The Chinese pharmacopeia contains virtually no remedies in the strong category because of the way that toxic plants, in their crude state, are prepared in order to reduce or annul their toxicity. A good example of an remedy that has strong status in its raw state is Aconitum Fu Zi, Sichuan aconite root. But, once Aconitum Fu Zi is subjected to various processes, it is rendered absolutely nontoxic. Prepared Sichuan aconite root, therefore, belongs to the mild therapeutic category. It has been used as such in complete safety for thousands of years.

Medium-strength remedies. These have both structive (or Yin) and active (or Yang) effects; these effects are intermediate between the mild and strong types. Because medium-strength remedies have some characteristics of those in both the mild and strong categories, they may cause slight negative side effects to occur. They are therefore defined as possessing some chronic toxicity, i.e., a toxicity that slowly accumulates over time—but only if the remedy is ingested every day. For this reason, they are typically used for one to three weeks at a time and then discontinued. Because remedies are rarely used on their own (especially in Chinese medicine), their low-level cumulative toxicity is mitigated when they are used in small dosage levels within formulas. In rare cases, the low toxicity of medium-strength remedies may even be annulled entirely when used in combination with certain other remedies. Chinese herbal texts are full of examples of cancelling effects between remedies.

Chinese remedies of the medium-strength category are

found in all body systems' sections where a variety of treatment methods are performed. Typically, medium-strength remedies either stimulate or sedate, and are routinely used in both acute and chronic conditions of many kinds. An example of the use of a medium-strength remedy is the animal remedy Buthus Quan Xie (Scorpion), which is used in formulas for acute conditions, such as the onset of convulsions, rather than for long-term treatment.

Constituents

The remedy's main chemical constituents known to date are listed here. Unless otherwise noted, these always refer to the first plant species given under "botanical source." When two distinct species or genuses furnish materials for a single remedy, the constituents of each are usually listed separately.

The usefulness of knowing a plant's chemical components lies in the application of scientific pharmacognosy and pharmacology—respectively, the scientific/analytic approach to understanding plants and their effects on living beings.

In general, there are only two ways of obtaining information about a remedy's nature and potential use for healing, the first traditional, the second modern. The first is to determine these through direct sense perception and intuition using the trial and error process of live experimental usage. This may include tasting, smelling, touching and observing the plant, mineral or whatever in addition to observing its effects when given to patients for certain conditions. This experiential, empirical approach has led over the millenniums to the accumulation and codification of very complex and accurate therapeutic information. It is today known as vitalistic or energetic pharmacognosy and pharmacology. This is the basis for all traditional systems of herbal medicine, including the Chinese, Ayurvedic and Greek systems.

The other way of finding out about a plant's potential use is to analyze a remedy through various scientific laboratory techniques. This is the modern way which demands scientific proof of traditional plant uses. Some of the techniques of analysis currently used are the HPLC method, TLC densitometry, UV absorption spectrophotometry, gas chromatography (used mainly for essential oils), preparative column chromatography, acidic dye colorimetry (used for alkaloids), electrophoresis and polarography. With these tests, researchers can determine what type of bioche-mical constituents comprise each remedy. This analytical, theoretical approach is known as biochemical or scientific pharmacognosy and pharmacology.

It would not be a difficult exercise to classify Chinese remedies according to those chemical components that are presumed primarily active. Chinese medicinal plants are extraordinarily rich and diverse in their constituents. The efficacy of many of the numerous compounds they contain has been proven through *in vivo* (live) clinical trials in hospitals, as well as through *in vitro* (laboratory) experiments. Researchers work both with the actual plant, mineral or animal, in a water or alcohol preparation, and with its extracted compounds. The scientific credibility which this research has brought to the practice of Chinese medicine is not negligible, and is continuously on the increase.

The sheer number of remedies used in East Asia for healing is vast, if we include those used by local folk-healers in villages on one hand and medical doctors in modern clinics on the other. As a result, although researchers in the People's Republic of China, Taiwan and Hong Kong together have analyzed more plant remedies than the Western nations combined, and although many of these have undergone extensive biochemical analysis, there are still many plants that have hardly been investigated at all. This fact, as well as the emphasis on research in general, accounts for the different quantity and quality of information that is available on the chemistry and pharmacology of various Chinese remedies.

Not surprisingly, in both Chinese and Western herbal medicine the same types of constituents form the basis for certain remedy actions. We will highlight some of the more interesting constituents found in Chinese medicinals and briefly indicate their role in shaping the remedies' therapeutic actions.

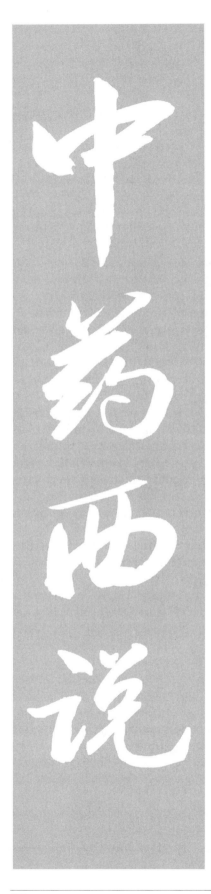

- **Essential oils** are found in high quantities in plants such as Angelica Dang Gui (Dong quai root), Atractylodes Cang Zhu (Black atractylodes rhizome), Asarum Xi Xin (Asian wild ginger root), Cinnamomum Zhang Nao (Camphor flake) and Saussurea Mu Xiang (Wood aromatic root). For the most part, these remedies are stimulating and relaxing by nature and owe their predominantly *stimulant, spasmolytic, anti-infective, anti-inflammatory* and *analgesic* actions to essential oils. Most plants have numerous, complex and unique essential oil combinations. Ligusticum Chuan Xiong (Sichuan lovage root), for example, has shown over 180 different essential oil molecules.

- **Vitamins,** with their many health-giving properties, are abundant in numerous herbal remedies. Those containing vitamin E, for instance, with its benefits for the skin and cellular performance, include Angelica Dang Gui (Dong quai root), Salvia Dan Shen (Cinnabar sage root) and Epimedium Yin Yang Huo (Horny goat weed). Vitamin A, invaluable for immunity, growth and vision, occurs in botanicals such as Magnolia Xin Yi Hua (Yulan magnolia bud) and Atractylodes Cang Zhu (Black atractylodes rhizome). Vitamin P (including rutin) is an active component in the *capillary restorative* effect of remedies such as Sophora Huai Hua (Japanese pagoda tree flower), Ginkgo Yin Xing Ye (Ginkgo leaf) and Forsythia Lian Qiao (Forsythia valve).

- **Trace minerals,** essential to every metabolic reaction, are found in almost all plants. Sargassum Hai Zao (Sargassum seaweed), Coptis Huang Lian (Goldthread root) and Panax Ren Shen (Asian ginseng root) are particularly good sources of trace minerals. The Chinese in recent years have devoted increasing research time to identifying and pharmacologically justifying the numerous trace elements found in Chinese remedies.

- **Minerals,** such as calcium and magnesium in one form or another, are primarily found in animal and mineral remedies. The first category includes several maritime remedies such as Ostrea Mu Li (Oyster shell), Pteria Zhen Zhu Mu (Mother of pearl shell), Haliotis Shi Jue Ming (Abalone shell) and Sepia Hai Piao Xiao (Cuttlefish bone). Minerals, especially electrolytes, also occur plentifully in animal horns, such as Saiga Ling Yang Jiao (Antelope horn) and Bubalus Shui Niu Jiao (Water buffalo horn), in other shells such as Chinemys Gui Ban (Tortoise shell) and Amyda Bie Jia (Asian soft-shell turtle shell), as well as in the fossil remedy Stegodon Long Gu (Dragon bone).

  In the second mineral category are found actual mineral remedies like Gypsum Shi Gao (Gypsum), Magnetitum Ci Shi (Magnetite) and Chloris Qing Meng Shi (Chlorite). Regardless of their origin, the majority of all these mineral remedies have a *central nervous sedative* action, often coupled with a *spasmolytic* one.

- **Polysaccharides,** highly complex sugar chains, are the key ingredients of several immune stimulating/enhancing remedies. These include Ganoderma Ling Zhi (Reishi mushroom), Polyporus Zhu Ling (Polyporus mushroom), Astragalus Huang Qi (Astragalus root), Codonopsis Dang Shen (Downy bellflower root), Bupleurum Chai Hu (Asian buplever root) and Epimedium Yin Yang Huo (Horny goat weed). Much current pharmacological research is being conducted on plant polysaccharides.

- **Amino acids,** with their nutritive, tissue-building and various other anabolic effects, are found in botanicals such as Codonopsis Dang Shen (Downy bellflower root), Panax Xi Yang Shen (American ginseng root) and Rehmannia Shu Di Huang (Prepared rehmannia root). They are also found in high concentration in many animal remedies, including Cervus Lu Rong (Velvet deer antler), Chinemys Gui Ban (Tortoise shell), Pheretima Di Long (Earthworm), Sepia Hai Piao Xiao (Cuttlefish bone), Paratenodera Sang Piao Xiao (Praying mantis egg case) and Cryptotympana Chan Tui (Cicada slough).

- **Organic acids** have a cooling, *anti-infective* effect, as shown in the remedies Prunella Xia Ku Cao (Selfheal spike), Carthamus Hong Hua (Safflower) and Crataegus Shan Zha (Asian hawthorn berry).

- **Bile acids** (cholic acid, deoxycholic acid, etc.) are available in the animal remedy Gallbladder with bile, obtained from the bear, pig, ox and—in South China—various reptiles (especially vipers). Bos Niu Huang (Ox gallstone) is also a good source of bile acids. Remedies containing bile acids have always been used for their excellent digestive and heat clearing effects.

- **Enzymes** occur in remedies such as Crataegus Shan Zha (Asian hawthorn berry), Gallus Ji Nei Jing (Chicken gizzard lining) and Hordeum Mai Ya (Sprouted barley grain). By facilitating enzymatic digestion, these remedies are useful in various digestive disorders, especially those arising from pancreatic deficiency.

- **Alkaloids** possess a variety of potential actions, notably *anti-infective, spasmolytic, anti-inflammatory* and *antitumoral* ones. Some Asian plants whose alkaloids have been isolated include: Sophora Ku Shen (Yellow pagoda tree root), which to date has been found to contain eight alkaloids, including matrine, oxymatrine and sophocarpine; Ligusticum Chuan Xiong (Sichuan lovage root), containing tetramethylpyrazine (also known as ligustrazine); Dichroa Chang Shan (Feverflower root), which contains the *parasiticidal* dichroin and changrolin; Corydalis Yan Hu Suo (Chinese corydalis root) with its *analgesic* corydaline and many other alkaloids; the highly *anti-infective* Coptis Huang Lian (Goldthread root), containing numerous alkaloids such as berberine, palmatine and magnoflorine; and Fritillaria Zhe Bei Mu (Zhejiang fritillary bulb), an important *lymphatic decongestant* and *antitussive remedy,* containing peimine, peimitidine and numerous others.

Several animal remedies owe at least part of their therapeutic action to the presence of alkaloids. So Moschus She Xiang (Musk, the secretion of the Asian musk deer) contains up to 2% of the alkaloid muscone, for example.

- **Saponin glycosides** are contained in many important *Qi and Blood tonics* that enhance digestion, promote nutrient assimilation and increase weight gain. These restorative botanicals include Astragalus Huang Qi (Astragalus root) which (among others) contains daucosterin, astramembrannins and soyasaponins; Panax Xi Yang Shen (American ginseng root) with its content in ginsenoside and panaxoside; and Codonopsis Dang Shen (Downy bellflower root), containing codonopsine and codonopsinine.

Some remedies, such as Dioscorea Bi Xie (Long yam root) and Achyranthes Huai Niu Xi (White ox-knee root), contain steroidal saponins that exert *anti-inflammatory* and in some (but not all) cases *hormonally stimulating* actions. Saponins are also largely responsible for the *mucolytic expectorant* effect of *respiratory demulcents* such as Ophiopogon Mai Men Dong (Dwarf lilyturf root), Polygala Yuan Zhi (Thin-leaf milkwort root) and Polygonatum Yu Zhu (Fragrant Solomon's seal root).

- **Anthraquinone glycosides,** known for their *stimulant laxative* effect, occur in the widely-used Rheum Da Huang (Rhubarb root) and Cassia Fan Xie Ye (Senna leaf). Anthraquinones are also seen in other remedies not primarily employed for treating constipation, such as Polygonum He Shou Wu (Flowery knotweed root), Morinda Ba Ji Tian (Morinda root) and Rubia Qian Cao Gen (Heart-leaf madder root). In some of these remedies the glycosides also exert an important

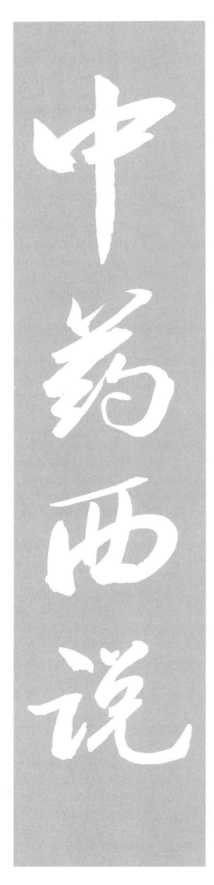

urinary stone-dissolving effect.
- **Coumarin glycosides,** with their *blood-thinning* effect, are the main active agent in several *anticoagulant* remedies, including Daphne Zu Shi Ma (Giraldi's daphne bark) and Angelica Du Huo (Hairy angelica root). In these two particular plants the coumarins also possess *antitumoral* and *platelet-inhibiting* activities.
- **Flavonoid glycosides** exert a restorative action on the circulation and heart, along with *spasmolytic, anti-inflammatory* and *diuretic* effects. Flavonoids are significant in such plants as Ilex Mao Dong Qing (Furry holly root), Ginkgo Yin Xing Ye (Ginkgo leaf), containing ginkgetin, bilobetin and quercetin; Scutellaria Ban Zhi Lian (Barbed skullcap root); Scutellaria Huang Qin (Baikal skullcap root), with its woogonin, oroxylin and skullcap flavanoids; and Pueraria Ge Gen (Kudzu root), containing isoflavonoids.
- **Cardiac glycosides** that exhibit restorative effects on the cardiac circulation are active in such botanicals as Polygonatum Yu Zhu (Fragrant Solomon's seal root), containing quercitol and kaempferol; Salvia Dan Shen (Cinnabar sage root), containing tanshinones and danshensu; Pueraria Ge Gen (Kudzu root), containing puerarin and daidzenin; and Scutellaria Huang Qin (Baikal skullcap root), containing scutellarin.

Bufo Chan Su (Toad venom) is an important *cardiovascular stimulant* remedy because of its notable content in cardioactive glycosides, called bufogenins and bufotoxins.
- **Tannins** possess an inhibiting effect on discharges, including diarrhea, leucorrhea and hemorrhage, as well as mild *antiseptic* and *anti-inflammatory* actions. Remedies such as Agrimonia Xian He Cao (Furry agrimony herb) and Rubia Qian Cao Gen (Heart-leaf madder root) contain high levels of tannins.

At their best, scientific pharmacognosy and pharmacology provide detailed, specific information about certain plant constituents and their theoretical activity on human tissues. This is usually in complete alignment with the traditional uses of remedies. Moreover, an even greater advantage can be obtained from pharmacognosy: the possibility of coming up with new clinical applications of traditional herbs. This leading-edge area of pharmacology in the relatively short time of its existence has already yielded positive results. Among the many hundreds of remedies researched in Hong Kong, China, Taiwan, Japan and Germany over the last forty years, many have yielded information that has proven extremely useful in clinical practice. As a result, a handful are now well known in the West, including Ginkgo leaf, Reishi mushroom, Eleuthero ginseng root and Asian ginseng root. But there are many dozens of others waiting in the wings that have also experienced substantial research, that cry out for clinical application in the West and about which—for a variety of reasons—very little is yet known. Here are just three such examples.

Sophora Huai Hua (Japanese pagoda tree flower) is traditionally widely used as a *hemostatic* in conditions of Blood heat causing hemorrhage. Its new application for stagnation of the venous circulation causing varicose veins, hemorrhoids, etc., is due to the findings of flavonoids (rutin, quercetin and others) and triterpenoid saponins (betulin and sophoradiol), both known for their *anti-inflammatory* and *restorative* actions on blood vessels.

Bupleurum Chai Hu (Asian Buplever root), an important classical botanical traditionally used as an *antipyretic* in intermittent fevers and *analgesic anti-inflammatory* for various types of pain and inflammation, has yielded special triterpenoid saponins, polysaccharides and phytosterols among its interesting components. These have variously shown to exert significant actions on the immune system and on enhancement of the body's defenses in general. This mainly comprises an *immunostimulant* effect (mainly antigenic activity) useful in both viral and bacterial infections in general, and an immune-regulating effect (mainly *antiallergic*) applicable in immediate allergies such as hayfever, middle ear infections and bronchial asthma. The defense-enhancing profile of Bupleurum Chai Hu would not be complete without mention of its *interferon-inducent, liver-protectant* and *radiation-protectant* activities.

Tripterygium Lei Gong Teng (Yellow vine root pith), a traditional remedy used just locally in Guangdong for acute arthritis and dermatitis, on investigation showed the presence of highly active alkaloids, glycosides and diterpenes, which include three different classes of alkaloids (tripterygium, macrocylic and sesquiterpene alkaloids) and two kinds of diterpenes (epoxiditerpenes and diterpenes). Consequently, the remedy's clinical uses have mushroomed to utilize its potent immune-regulating, antitumoral, dermatropic and renal restorative actions (among many others) in the treatment of such disorders as autoimmune conditions of many kinds (including rheumatoid arthritis, lupus, psoriasis and glomerulo- and purpuric nephritis), cancerous conditions (especially of the uterus and breast) and skin conditions (including most forms of dermatitis, intractable pruritus, pityriasis and alopecia aerata).

Having noted the advantages of scientific pharmacology, we may ask: How does scientific pharmacology relate to vitalistic pharmacology? Essentially, the first is more specific and detailed, whereas the second is more general and broad-based (see below). Each system of pharmacology, being entirely logical and clinically relevant in its own right, fulfills different functions in helping us understand the therapeutic nature of medicinal plants. On the whole, therefore, the two systems complement each other.

It is crucial to realize here that the functions of each pharmacological system is simply *different* from the other, not more or less effective. Effectiveness has to do with the degree of clinical application of a system, not with a theoretical comparison with another system. It is this factor that evidentially accounts for the relative effectiveness of *several* systems of traditional herbal medicine currently practiced worldwide.

Nevertheless, regardless of how sophisticated or effective it may be, every system has weak aspects: this is the natural limitation of any conceptual system. So, biochemical and vitalistic pharmacology both tend to suffer from certain disadvantages in actual practice. Arguably, we have now reached a point in global health care where the explanations given for remedy actions by one system alone are insufficient by themselves. It is becoming clearer that by taking the biochemical and vitalistic approaches to plant pharmacology together, a larger, more accurate remedy profile may be obtained (see also Holmes 1989).

Biochemical pharmacology is strictly based on scientific methodology. Its disadvantage is that it tends to isolate and divide data, and therefore has difficulty building up a picture of the whole. Strictly speaking it can only make statements about the different chemical parts of a remedy, never about the whole remedy. Western pharmacology therefore cannot truly explain the probable interactions of plant constituents among themselves, nor can it fully predict their interaction with and utilization by the body. It is these two facts that explain why biochemically similar plants often have different therapeutic effects, and why, conversely, biochemically different plants often achieve identical therapeutic effects.

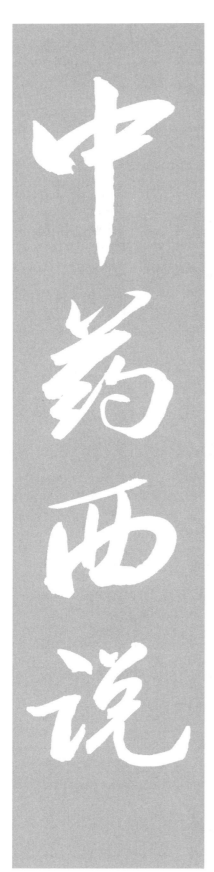

A more accurate perspective on a remedy's therapeutic profile can therefore be obtained when we place the findings of biochemistry in the context of those of traditional empirical pharmacology, or at least combine the findings of both. The presentation in this text of the remedy's constituents followed by its effective qualities aims to achieve just that.

Effective Qualities
The remedy's effective qualities listed here belong to the system of vitalistic pharmacology, the traditional empirical approach to understanding and classifying the many therapeutic effects of natural remedies. They describe a remedy's most fundamental, systemic effects on the individual. Put another way, they are the immediate, experienced characteristics that a remedy exerts on the human organism (rather than the biochemical information obtained about it). They thereby provide the most immediate and general information about the nature, functions and uses of a remedy.

Called *qi* in Chinese pharmacology and *dynameis* in Greek (Tibb Unani) pharmacology, effective qualities over millennia have been continuously refined and codified by practitioners and empirical researchers into both general and specific therapeutic actions. The terms *qi* and *dynameis* translate as "effective qualities," because these plant properties have dynamic energy-altering and potentially therapeutic effects on human physiology. They help us determine almost all of an herb's actions and uses.

The effective qualities divide into primary, secondary and tertiary qualities.

• The fifteen primary qualities are based on a remedy's taste, warmth and moisture effect on the body.
• The seven secondary qualities are based on a remedy's effect on tissue tone, stimulation, hydration and nutrition.
• The ten tertiary qualities are based on a remedy's further effects on tissue and energy movement.

There are two main values to knowing the effective qualities of a botanical, mineral or animal remedy. First, the qualities help us understand the remedy as whole therapeutic agent rather than a mere collections of chemical constituents (each with their discrete theoretical pharmacology). By unifying the many bits of therapeutic information about a remedy, they provide us with a complete rather than fragmented perspective. This whole perspective is necessary in actual treatment if we wish to address the whole condition presenting, not just a particular body tissue or system. Remember, though, that there a times when one approach is necessary above the other—depending on diagnostic factors such as whether the condition is acute or chronic, local or systemic, etc.

Second, the effective qualities link us directly and specifically to a remedy's therapeutic uses. According to the laws of vitalistic pharmacology, a remedy with pungent, warm, dry qualities, such as Ephedra herb, for example, is known to have *stimulant, diaphoretic* and *drying* functions that are useful at the onset of a cold or flu with respiratory mucus congestion and discharge. This holds true, of course, regardless of the actual chemical constituents present in the plant—although we *can* also make certain primitive links between qualities and constituents (see below).

Whereas biochemical pharmacology gives us a specific chemical explanation for some of the plant's particular functions and uses, vitalistic pharmacology allows us to understand it as a systemic therapeutic agent. Once we understand their overall character, we can begin to relate to remedies much like individuals with their strengths, weaknesses, likes, dislikes and habits—all those elements that constitute a personality. This is essential for knowing their therapeutic applications from the inside out rather than by rote. It is particularly important for using them in free-form herb prescribing, where an herbal formula is individually built up—as opposed to relying on standard fixed formulas.

Chinese pharmacology is entirely vitalistic, or energetic, by nature. It brings to bear on the mere century-and-a-bit of modern biochemical research the cumulative weight of thousands of years of empirical pharmacological experience. In general, the majority of Western pharmacological research supports the traditional uses of remedies for particular conditions and disorders. However, there are certain remedies in which modern lab results seem to shed no light on their traditional empirical usage. In this case we can only rely on the empirical historical validation for their use. In most cases where science cannot "explain" the traditional purported actions of a remedy, this points to the limitations of science and our own knowledge rather than any inadequacies of empirical usage. In some cases, when more tests are performed, and with the advance of testing methods, often a traditionally reported remedy action will finally be revindicated after all.

The **primary effective qualities** are taste, warmth and moisture.

Taste

A plant's quality of **taste** is broken down into a total of eight separate (sub)tastes—sweet, pungent, salty, sour, bitter, bland, astringent and oily. Each taste has specific energetic effects on the body, both locally and globally, immediate and long-term. Experiments with each taste's properties and physiological actions have been conducted, exhaustively recorded in pharmacology manuals and continuously refined in Chinese medical practice for many millennia. Here is how the tastes work:

- **The sweet taste** harmonizes, calms, cools, slows down, thickens, moistens and restores. The sweet-tasting Ophiopogon Mai Men Dong (Dwarf lilyturf root) is a prime example of these actions. Its *respiratory demulcent restorative* action helps dry, hot and irritated lung conditions accompanied by thirst, dry cough, hot spells, unrest and dehydration.
- **The pungent taste** activates, energizes, warms, speeds up, dries and disperses. The pungent, aromatic herb Asarum Xi Xin (Chinese wild ginger root and herb), for instance, has *respiratory stimulant,* i.e., *stimulant expectorant,* properties. These properties are perfectly adapted to treat congested, cold, catarrhal and damp bronchial conditions presenting a full, moist cough, coughing up with expectoration of white sputum, cold hands and feet, and general congestion or aches and pains.
- **The salty taste** moistens, softens, sinks, drains, dissolves and resolves. Sargassum Hai Zao (Sargassum seaweed) is a good illustration of a marine botanical with a primarily salty taste. The energy of this taste engenders a *draining diuretic* action that is useful for edema, and a *resolvent* effect that divides into *detumescent, lymphatic decongestant, anticoagulant* and *antilipemic* actions. These effects are appropriate for conditions such as goiter, lymph gland swelling, nodules, blood clots, fatty deposits and tumors.
- **The sour taste** coagulates, tightens, stimulates and decongests. A case in point is the sour-tasting Cornus Shan Zhu Yu (Japanese dogwood berry). Its *genital astringent, coagulant hemostatic* and *anhydrotic* actions apply to discharges such as profuse mentrual bleeding, seminal

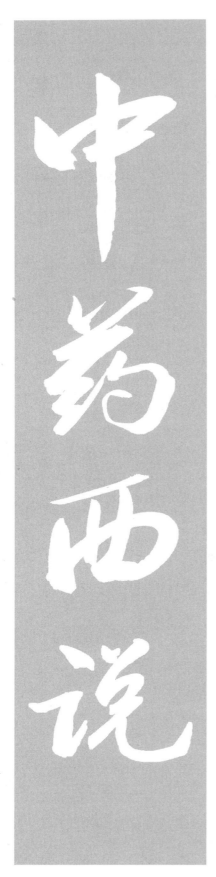

incontinence, uterine bleeding and excessive sweating.

• **The bitter taste** strengthens, grounds, drains, cools, detoxifies and dries. Stephania Han Fang Ji (Stephania root) is a bitter remedy with resultant *draining, cooling, relaxing* and *detoxifying* effects. These actions are beneficially put to use with congestive, hot, tense, damp and toxic conditions such as edema, high fevers, inflamed stiff joints, high blood pressure and chronic boils.

• **The bland taste** drains water and dries damp, as does, for example, Polyporus Zhu Ling (Polyporus mushroom). The energy of its bland taste causes fluids to drain downwards and the amount of urine eliminated to increase. Its *draining diuretic* action relieves water retention with edema and ascites.

• **The astringent taste** solidifies, tightens, dries, decongests and slows down. Rubia Qian Cao Gen (Heart-leaf madder root), whose astringent taste has a *uterine decongestant* effect, treats pelvic blood congestion accompanied by heavy menses; it also has a *hemostatic* action with hemorrhage.

• **The oily taste** slows down, moistens, thickens, makes heavy and warms. Rehmannia Shu Di Huang (Rehmannia root), more than any other remedy, perhaps, represents the oily taste. The *warming, moistening, secretory* effects engendered by the taste qualities of this remedy are useful for such conditions, among others, such as blood deficiency, thirst and dehydration.

Not only do the taste qualities generally explain the functions and uses of remedies, they specifically becomes an important consideration when remedies are combined into a formula—when two or more herbs are combined, in other words. This is not so much of a problem when ready-made, pre-existing formulas are used, but is a major factor when herbs are individually prescribed.

For example, when *restorative* remedies of a sweet taste quality are combined for treating a Yin and fluids deficiency condition, it becomes important not to spoil this tonifying and moistening effect by including remedies with an excessive pungent taste or very dry quality. This would go directly against the energetic effects of the sweet remedies. Likewise, because too much sweet quality can have an oily effect which may upset digestion, it conversely becomes important to mitigate any oiliness through the inclusion of a few remedies mildly possessing other tastes.

Each taste quality can have negative side-effects when used excessively or when applied to the wrong condition. The bitter and pungent tastes in particular can have too drying, draining or dispersing effects when badly handled. In the majority of individual formulations, herbs with these two tastes must be carefully combined with remedies possessing other tastes.

Warmth

Warmth occurs in a remedy as an effective quality because remedies are said to have warming or cooling effects on the body. This is determined on the basis of both a person's subjective reaction to a remedy (a symptom) and the herb's ability to cause signs of heat or cold. Many factors, including the time of year, month and day, the weather, climate, etc., as well as the condition itself of the individual taking the remedy, combine to determine whether a particular plant will exhibit warming or cooling properties. In general, it is important to know whether a remedy is warming or cooling because it has to oppose the warmth factor of the condition being treated.

Energetic pharmacology divides a remedy's warmth factor into grades—hot, warm, neutral, cool and cold. Cinnamomum Rou Gui (Cassia cinnamon bark), for example, is considered a hot-natured remedy because its *circulatory stimulant* action treats deficiency and cold conditions involving cold skin, cold extremities and exhaustion. It is defined in Chinese medicine as "warming the interior and clearing cold." The *circulatory stimulant* effect of Cinnamomum Gui Zhi (Cassia cinnamon twig), on the other hand, is additionally *diaphoretic* and is used for the onset of colds and flus; hence, this remedy is defined rather as warm. It is a "pungent warm remedy that dispels wind cold."

Senecio Qian Li Guang (Asian ragwort herb) is a case in point of a very cold remedy, being used for many kinds of acute infections with high fever and acute inflammation; it is said to "clear heat and dry damp." Patrinia Bai Jiang Cao (Patrinia herb), on the other hand, is only considered cool rather than cold. It mainly treats acute local infections with inflammation and purulence rather than systemic fever; it is described as "clearing fire toxins."

A case where it is crucial to know the warmth quality of a remedy is, for example, with the onset of a cold or flu. *Diaphoretics*, i.e., sweat-inducing remedies, are the treatment of choice in these conditions. However, not all *diaphoretics* work in the same way. Where sneezing, chills, shivers, etc., announce the start of an infection, the condition is called external wind cold. It is treated with *warming diaphoretics,* such as Cinnamomum Gui Zhi (Cassia cinnamon twig) and Ledebouriella Fang Feng (Wind protector root). If fever and no fear of cold predominate, the same infection is defined as external wind heat. It is remedied with *cooling diaphoretics,* such as Schizonepeta Jing Jie (Japanese catnip herb) and Morus Sang Ye (Mulberry leaf).

In cases where there is a difference between the initial warmth effect of a remedy when taken and its subsequent warming or cooling effect, or if the remedy shows both warming and cooling properties simultaneously—as with Cinnamomum Zhang Nao (Camphor flake)—this is noted. Discrepancies among these various aspects are explained in terms such as "warming or cooling potential."

Moisture

As an effective quality, moisture refers to the moisturizing or drying property of a remedy on tissues. The qualities dry and moist, together with those of hot and cold, belong to the principal four effective qualities or *dynameis* of Greek medicine and are considered equally important in Asian medicine. Adenophora Nan Sha Shen (Upright ladybell root) is considered moist because it not only moistens dry coughs and relieves thirst with its sweet taste, but because it also softens and liquifies hard bronchial sputum. Ephedra Ma Huang (Ephedra herb) is defined as drying not mainly because it relieves allergies with nasal discharge, but because it tends to dry out the body tissues by causing sweating and urination with its pungent, somewhat bitter and warm qualities (which disperse the body fluids towards the periphery).

The moisture quality of a remedy can be critical in choosing remedies. A good example would be with chronic bronchitis in the context of a lung phlegm cold condition. Asarum Xi Xin (Chinese wild ginger root and herb), Pinellia Ban Xia (Prepared pinellia tuber) and Platycodon Jie Geng (Balloonflower root) are all equally good for this condition—all are *stimulant expectorants* that, from the Western perspective, will treat bronchitis. However, taking the moisture quality into account, the overall effect of these remedies is not at all the same. The first remedy has a very drying nature because of its pungent, somewhat bitter taste, its hot warmth quality and systemic *stimulant* nature. It must not be used for treating bronchitis with signs of dryness or heat present.

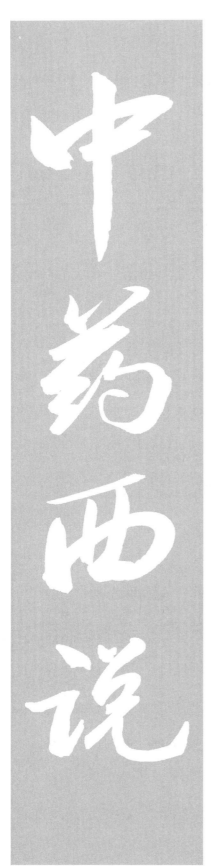

The second botanical, with its pungent, somewhat astringent and warming effective qualities, is only moderately drying. It may be used for bronchitis with both damp and dry, hot and cold conditions. The third remedy, however, because of its sweet taste, is moistening. It is therefore particularly suitable for treating the kind of bronchitis that presents dry cough, dry throat and hoarseness.

The Secondary Qualities
A remedy's secondary and tertiary effective qualities describe a remedy's more specific effects than the primary qualities. These qualities apply to solid and fluid body tissues as well as to energetic movements, to structure as well as to function. The secondary and tertiary qualities can be said to lie halfway between the primary qualities and the specific actions of a remedy. In this sense, they are both general quality, such as sweet, warm, moist, and specific effect, such as *diaphoretic, expectorant*. They are the more specific and active aspects of the primary qualities, as well as the general precursors of the specific remedy actions. Taking the example of Perilla Zi Su Ye (Perilla leaf), its stimulating, dispersing and relaxing secondary/tertiary qualities are based on its primary pungent, warm, dry qualities. These, in turn, form the basis for its *stimulant diaphoretic, digestive stimulant, bronchial relaxant* and *fetal relaxant* actions.

Note that the first two pairs of secondary qualities, restoring/relaxing and stimulating/sedating, are one and the same as the four fundamental remedy actions that organize the remedies within each body system.

There are three pairs of secondary effective qualities, which describe tissue tone, stimulation and hydration, respectively—plus one single extra quality that has to do with nutrition.

- *restoring/relaxing*
- *stimulating/sedating*
- *moistening/decongesting*
- *nourishing*

Restoring/relaxing. This first pair of qualities refers to the tone of the tissues and their functional integrity, as well as to their manifestations of deficiency/weakness and excess/stress. Restoring and relaxing are the most gentle of the secondary effective qualities, and remedies possessing them invariably achieve a balancing effect on the part or system they treat. This explains why remedies with either of these two qualities are so widely used.

The restoring quality treats deficiency conditions by enhancing the function and structure of an organ, tissue or part. Deficiency conditions are typified by weakness, inadequacy or looseness. In Chinese medical terms the restoring quality "tonifies the Qi" or "nourishes the Blood" of the whole system or any organ. It is generally signaled by sweet or somewhat bitter effective qualities. Remedies with a restoring quality are "tonics" in the true sense of the word. Because of the misuse of that word, however, we prefer the term "restoratives" to descibe them.

The sweet tasting Codonopsis Dang Shen (Downy bellflower root), for instance, has a restoring effective quality that works on both the small intestine and the blood. This *gastrointestinal restorative* is used for weakness or Qi deficiency of the stomach and small intestines (Chinese Spleen functions) and blood deficiency (in both a Chinese and Western sense), resulting in fatigue, pale complexion, weight loss and slow digestion, for example.

Eucommia Du Zhong (Eucommia bark), on the other hand, has a restoring effect on the whole connective tissue. As a *musculoskeletal restorative* it addresses deficiency of the musculoskeletal system (Chinese Liver and Kidney functions) accompanied by muscular weakness, fatigue, and lumbar and knee weakness.

Schisandra Wu Wei Zi (Schisandra berry) is representative of a botanical with a significant restorative action on the nervous system. It treats central nervous system deficiency conditions, manifesting as mental and physical fatigue, mental stupor, loss of sensory acuity, chronic depression, insomnia, etc. It is classed as a *nervous restorative*.

The sweet, oily tasting Rehmannia Shu Di Huang (Prepared rehmannia root) is known to have a *liver restorative* effect (which includes liver protection). In Chinese medicine the remedy "enriches liver Yin," thereby generating stamina and promoting endurance. As such, Rehmannia Shu Di Huang is clinically used for hepatic deficiency conditions involving inadequate glycogen, glucose and protein storage, presenting loss of stamina, weight loss and evening fatigue.

The restorative effect of Magnolia Xin Yi Hua (Yulan magnolia bud), on the other hand, is exerted on the nasal mucosa. The *anticatarrhal* action of this remedy relieves mucosal deficiency conditions, such as frequent head colds with nasal discharges and sinus congestion. It is classified as a *nasal restorative*.

Remedies with a relaxing effective quality treat tense conditions characterized by constraint, tightness or spasm found throughout the system, or in a particular organ or part. They relax, loosen and decompress tense conditions functionally and structurally. In Chinese medicine *relaxant* herbs are variously defined as "circulating the Qi," "releasing constrained Liver Qi" and "moving Qi stagnation." They generally possess pungent or somewhat bitter taste qualities.

Magnolia Hou Po (Magnolia bark) exemplifies a *relaxant* remedy with a tropism for the intestinal tract. Its concerted *spasmolytic, analgesic* and strong *anti-infective* actions address tense or Qi constraint conditions of the small and large intestines, presenting such symptoms as irregular stool, diarrhea under stress and abdominal pain. Magnolia Hou Po is an important *intestinal relaxant*.

The relaxing effect of Aster Zi Wan (Tartary aster root), on the other hand, is focused on the respiratory system. Its *bronchodilatant* action relaxes the bronchi—"circulates lung Qi" in Chinese medical terms—and so relieves the wheezing, chest constriction and spasmodic coughing of bronchial asthma. It is classed as a *respiratory relaxant*.

Artemisia Liu Ji Nu has a relaxing quality that eases tension and Qi constraint conditions in the female reproductive organs. Through *spasmolytic* and *analgesic* actions, this *reproductive relaxant* relieves the menstrual cramps of spasmodic dysmenorrhea.

The relaxing effect of Plantago Che Qian Zi (Asian plantain seed) affects the urinary tract that, in conditions of tension, produces urinary irritation and difficult, obstructed urination. Plantain seed is an important *urinary relaxant*.

Ilex Mao Dong Qing (Furry holly root) has a relaxing effect on the cardiovascular system, treating tense heart Qi constraint or Liver Yang Rising conditions. Its *cardiovascular relaxant* action relieves palpitations, dizziness, ringing ears, etc.—often seen as a result of hypertension, for instance.

Finally, the relaxing effect of Uncaria Gou Teng (Gambir vine twig) affects the entire nervous system that is in a state of tension or constraint. This remedy is a *nervous system relaxant*

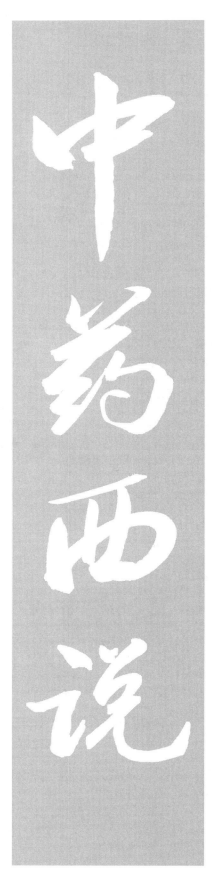

with *spasmolytic* and *anticonvulsant* actions that treats signs of unrest, tremors, spasms and convulsions—a condition known as "internal wind" in Chinese medicine.

Stimulating/sedating. As a rule, the this dyad of effective qualities treats conditions with either cold or heat involved, respectively. This pair of qualities has to do with the degree of stimulation and its immediate manifestions of warmth or lack of warmth, i.e., coldness. It is easier to misuse remedies with these two qualities as they are stronger and act more quickly than the restoring and relaxing types. Herbs with stimulating or sedating qualities tend to push the natural functions of an organ or tissue somewhat beyond its normal limits—thereby producing warmth or coldness.

Remedies with stimulating qualities tend to possess pungent, warm, dry, primary effective qualities with a net energizing, warming effect. They address deficiency conditions characterized by cold, weakness or hypofunctioning, and work by stimulating energy and blood circulation to the organ or part affected. Chinese medicine describes stimulants in terms such as "warming the channels and collaterals."

For example, Peucedanum Qian Hu (Asian masterwort root), with its content of aromatic essential oils, has a *stimulating* action on the bronchi that "warms and transforms phlegm cold." In physiological terms it is a *stimulant expectorant* with an *antibacterial* action. This *respiratory stimulant* is used for cold, mucousy/catarrhal conditions of the lungs presenting productive coughing, cold hands and feet, etc. This may be seen in chronic bronchitis or emphysema, for example.

The stimulating effective quality of Cinnamomum Rou Gui (Cassia cinnamon bark), on the other hand, acts directly on the arterial circulation to "tonify the Yang, warm the interior and clear cold." It is an important *arterial circulatory stimulant* for removing internal cold arising from Yang deficiency, accompanied by chills, cold skin and fatigue.

In the case of Agastache Huo Xiang (Rugose giant hyssop herb), the stimulating effect is centered almost entirely on digestive functions. Excess mucus is cleared and intestinal dyspeptic conditions are relieved as this *intestinal stimulant* "transforms damp" in the small intestines with its pungent, warm, dry primary qualities.

Citrus Chen Pi (Ripe tangerine rind), although similar to the last remedy, specifically stimulates bile production and flow. Because this much-used cholagogue relieves upper abdominal distension and pain, indigestion and constipation, it is said to "spread Liver Qi and harmonize the Liver and Spleen:" it is a classic *hepatobiliary stimulant*.

The remedy Alisma Ze Xie (Water plantain root) illustrates the stimulating quality influencing kidney and bladder functions. As excess fluid is drained from the tissues and urination is increased, edema and obstructed urination are relieved.

The highly effective diuretic action of this common *urinary stimulant* remedy is described as "draining damp."

In the case of Carthamus Hong Hua (Safflower), the stimulating effect primarily affects the uterus, causing an *emmenagogue* action. As *uterine stimulant,* Safflower relieves difficult, delayed, scanty menses; it is said to "vitalize the Blood."

Remedies with a sedating (calming) effective quality act to treat excess conditions involving heat (i.e., inflammation or fever) as well as simple hyperfunctioning. By calming and slowing down hyperactivity and reducing the amount of stimulation to the part concerned, these remedies are traditionally known to "clear heat," "quell fire" or "calm the spirit." Sedating remedies on the whole possess bitter and cool primary qualities that contribute to their secondary sedating and cooling effect.

Pulsatilla Bai Tou Weng (Asian pasqueflower root) is a classic example of a sedating remedy with bitter, cold qualities that act on the intestinal tract. It is an *intestinal sedative* operating through *anti-infective, anti-inflammatory, spasmolytic* and *analgesic* actions that relieves acute infectious damp heat conditions of the intestines presenting diarrhea, mucousy or bloody stool and urgent defecation.

On the other hand, a systemic sedating effect through the central nervous system can be seen in Siegesbeckia Xi Xian Cao (Siegesbeckia herb). This botanical's *nervous sedative* action—traditionally described as "calming the Spirit"—is *analgesic* and *inhibitant* to the *sympathetic nerves*—useful with various types of pain and hyperactivity.

The sedating action of Houttuynia Yu Xing Cao (Fishwort herb), although useful in a variety of infections, excells in hot, infectious lower respiratory conditions (lung phlegm heat syndrome), including lung abscesses. We may class the remedy as a *respiratory sedative* that physiologically operates through *anti-infective, detoxicant* and *anti-inflammatory* actions in concert.

Canna Mei Ren Jiao (Canna lily root) illustrates the sedating effective quality applied to the liver. It is a *hepatic sedative* with *liver decongestant, cholagogue* and *liver protective* actions that treats acute hepatitis with jaundice, irritability, right flank pain, etc.—known by the symptom complex "liver damp heat."

For the urinary tract, Dianthus Qu Mai (Proud pink herb) has a sedating action that relieves painful, irritated, burning or difficult urination, including the infectious type, through a combination of *diuretic, antibacterial, anti-inflammatory* and *analgesic* actions. This *urinary sedative* addresses syndromes of "bladder damp heat."

Moistening/decongesting. The last dyad of secondary qualities we need to consider, moistening/decongesting, refers to the amount and quality of hydration, as well as its direct manifestations of dryness and dampness. The moistening/decongesting pair of qualities therefore addresses conditions entailing either dryness or congestion, respectively. Remedies with these qualities are both easy to use and misuse. They may be either cloying and congesting or, conversely, cleansing and draining—effects that someone in fairly good health should not sustain for too long as they may produce congestion or deficiency, respectively.

Remedies with moistening qualities are used to treat conditions of dryness. Dryness often involves a compromised mucous membrane, causing local irritation and other symptoms depending on location, and a tendency to systemic dryness as a sign or symptom. By physiologically moistening the mucosa and hydrating tissues, moistening remedies are described as "nourishing and moistening the Yin," "generating fluids" and "moistening dryness." On the whole, moistening remedies are sweet or bland tasting, and neutral to cool in warmth. They are known as *demulcents* in Western herbal medicine.

Lilium Bai He (Brown's lily bulb) exemplifies the moistening quality primarily affecting the respiratory mucosa. This simple *demulcent* is used for dry bronchial conditions presenting dry cough and dry scratchy sore throat. It "moistens the Lungs."

Tremella Bai Mu Er (Silver ear mushroom) is a culinary example of the moistening effect.

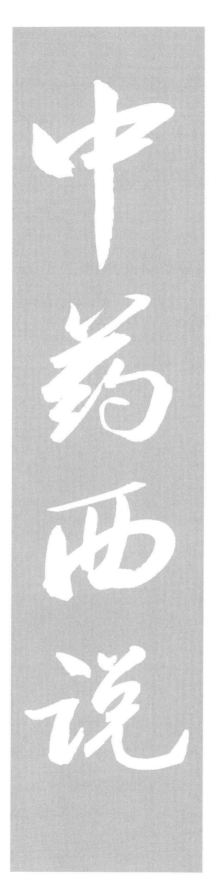

This medicinal food is useful not only for counteracting local respiratory dryness with dry cough, but also helps systemic Yin-deficient conditions presen-ting dehydration and thirst. (It is also *nutritive* because of its trace element content, and *immune stimulant* because of its polysaccharides).

A good example of the moistening quality affecting (paradoxically) the urinary tract is Coix Yi Yi Ren (Job's tears seed). This remedy is *demulcent* to the urinary mucosa and *hydrating* to the whole system in cases of metabolic acidosis, thereby relieving symptoms as scanty, irritated urination, thirst, dry itchy skin, and so on.

The moistening effect of Zizyphus Da Zao (Jujube berry) is directed primarily at the stomach. This *gastrointestinal demulcent* treats the syndrome stomach dryness with indigestion and epigastric or abdominal pain.

Remedies possessing the decongesting effective quality tend to be either pungent, bitter or bland by taste. Because they promote the breakdown and elimination of excess substances in the body, they can treat an excess of congested fluids, such as blood, interstitial fluids, sputum and lymph. Chinese medicine variously defines *decongestant* remedies as "vitalizing the Blood and removing Blood stasis," "draining damp," "transforming phlegm," "transforming Spleen damp," depending on the body system affected.

Alisma Ze Xie (Water plantain rhizome), for instance, has a decongesting quality that entirely affects the body's waterworks. The net result is a *decongestant* or *draining diuretic* action. With its bland, mild taste it "benefits the fluids and drains damp," i.e., promotes urination, drains fluid congestion and thereby relieves edema.

For remedies with a decongesting effect on the circulation, we must look to *venous decongestants*. An important remedy for reducing venous blood congestion is Sophora Huai Hua (Japanese pagoda tree flower), which works on systemic and pelvic congestion, thereby relieving varicose veins, congestive dysmenorrhea and so on. It would be accurate to define this remedy in this sense as "vitalizing the Blood and clearing Blood stasis."

A remedy such as Cynanchum Bai Qian (Prime white root) exemplifies a decongesting effect on the bronchi. The pungent, warm primary qualities are typical for this *stimulant expectorant* that "warms and transforms cold phlegm," thereby relieving the productive cough or difficult expectoration of congestive catarrhal bronchial disorders.

Nourishing. Remedies with a nourishing quality are naturally sweet tasting, and they often actually satiate hunger. By providing substantial nutrients to a system, organ or part, they treat the type of deficiency condition characterized by insufficient nutrition and wasting (hypotrophy). The term *"trophorestorative"* was coined by Physiomedical practitioners in the last century to describe this remedy effect. Although Chinese medicine has no exact definition or classification of these nutritive remedies, they would logically be described as *restoratives* that "generate the pulse."

The sweet tasting Ophiopogon Mai Men Dong (Dwarf lilyturf root) can be considered nourishing to the lungs. It is a *respiratory trophorestorative* with a *demulcent* effect that provides moisture and promotes mucus secretions with its "Yin nourishing, fluids generating" action, relieving dry cough, thirst and weakness.

Like the Western hawthorn berry, Crataegus Shan Zha (Asian hawthorn berry) has a nourishing effect on the heart muscle. It is an important *cardiac trophorestorative* remedy that strengthens the heart and improves cardiocirculatory functions over a long time span. It can be considered to "generate the pulse."

Lycium Gou Ji Zi (Wolfberry) has all the hallmarks of a *liver trophorestorative*, although this yet has to be proven in Western pharmacology. As liver and *metabolic restorative, liver protective, anastative nutritive* and *antioxidant* it can improve various chronic hepatic, metabolic and nutritive deficiencies (in which liver functions are crucial), such as malassimilation, glycogen storage disorders, anemia, malnutrition, hepatitis, etc.

Polygonum He Shou Wu (Flowery knotweed root) illustrates the nourishing quality affecting the brain and whole nervous system. It is a *nervous* and *cerebral trophorestorative* that can relieve chronic depression, sleep loss, absent-mindedness and general weakness. In traditional terms this remedy is considered to "tonify Kidney Essence."

A typical nourishing quality for the musculoskeletal system is contained in the animal remedy Chinemys Gui Ban (Tortoise shell), which can be considered a *musculoskeletal trophorestorative*. Its high mineral and keratin content provides nutrition to promote delayed skeletal development in children, as well as to relieve a gamut of hypotrophic conditions of the bones, muscles and sinews—conditions for the most part attributed to "Liver and Kidney Depletion" in Chinese medicine.

The Tertiary Qualities

A remedy's tertiary effective qualities are five further, more specific dyadic subdivisions of its secondary qualities. Again, they apply to both the physical/substantial and energetic aspects of a remedy. The first three pairs are more concerned with body substance, while pairs four and five have more to do with energetic movement in the body.

The first three pairs of tertiary qualities are:

- *astringing/eliminating*
- *solidifying/dissolving*
- *thickening/diluting*

Astringing/eliminating. The first pair of tertiary qualities generally has to do with the circulation and metabolism of body fluids. If their metabolism is disturbed, they will either tend to abnormally discharge or get stuck. Either way, they then change from being beneficial to being injurious in character. Herbal medicine in all traditions has recognized remedy categories of *astringents* and *eliminants* based on these two fundamental qualities. The first stage of disease often involves attempted body eliminations such as mucus, sweating, diarrhea, coughing, and so on. These should either be encouraged with *eliminants* (if the elimination is unsuccessful due to weakened vital force) or inhibited with *astringents* (should they become counterproductive, e.g., excessive or continuous).

Remedies with the astringing quality essentially address discharges, and for this purpose they usually possess a dry primary quality. By tightening and ultimately strengthening tissues, *astringents* are able to arrest various types of discharges, such as mucus in the stool, vaginal mucous, expectoration of sputum, loose stool, sperm loss, excessive sweat, excessive menstrual

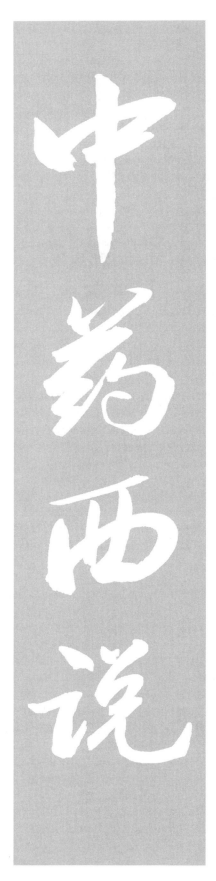

blood and bleeding. Secondarily, their astringing quality is invaluable for promoting tissue repair in the case of tissue trauma such as injuries, and sores and ulcers both topical and internal. Finally, astringing remedies are useful in managing skin and mucosal inflammation and/or infection.

Biota Ce Bai Ye (Chinese arborvitae twig), for example, we may consider to have an important astringing quality. Apart from its tannic, dry, astringent taste, it also stops hemorrhage (a *hemostatic*), repairs wounded tissue (a *vulnerary*) and treats peptic ulcer and diarrhea (an *anti-diarrheal*). It is good all-round *astringent*.

Terminalia He Zi (Myrobalan fruit) is another significant *astringent* remedy that originates in Ayurvedic medicine and is extensively used in Chinese medicine. Its astringing quality works best on digestive and urinary functions, and is excellent for chronic diarrhea of many types, blood in the stool and male and female genital incontinence. In Chinese terms it "restrains leakage from the intestines, stabilizes the Kidney and retains urine." In addition, this remedy is also *anhydrotic* in conditions of excessive daytime or night-time sweating.

Commiphora Mo Yao (Myrrh) is another often overlooked remedy that presents an excellent astringing quality. This is essential in contributing to the remedy's premier *vulnerary* character—*tissue healing, astringing, detergent, anti-inflammatory*, etc.—for treating a wide range of tissue trauma.

An unusual *astringent* remedy for the West is Sepia Hai Piao Xiao (Cuttlefish bone). Affecting mainly the digestive and urinary tract, its astringing effect treats diarrhea, urinary incontinence and spermatorrhea. The remedy's additional *antacid* and *antisecretory* action in the stomach makes it beneficial for hyperacid and ulcerative peptic conditions. Topically the astringing quality is seen in its good *styptic* and *tissue healing* actions.

Remedies that are eliminating in quality/effect essentially treat stagnation of a pure or impure body fluid. With their generally pungent and stimulant qualities, *eliminants* can break up stasis of the interstitial fluids causing edema, stasis of sweat causing skin rashes, menstrual stasis causing difficult, sluggish or absent menses, stasis of the stool causing constipation, stasis of bronchial sputum causing cough, as well as stasis among metabolic functions in general.

Asarum Xi Xin (Asian wild ginger root) is a classic wide-acting *eliminative* remedy. Its pungent, warm, eliminating qualities cause sweating, opening of the nasal passages, expectoration of sputum and diuresis, and are mainly put to use in respiratory infections. It is used to "release the exterior, dispel wind cold, and warm and transform plegm cold."

Angelica Du Huo (Hairy angelica root) is another good example of an *eliminant* remedy in action. By promoting fluid and toxin elimination from muscles and joints via diaphoresis, this remedy focuses on the treatment of rheumatic and rheumatoid arthritic conditions. It "dispels wind/damp/cold and relieves painful obstruction." Like many a good eliminant, this species of Angelica also stimulates the uterus, promoting menstruation in case of amenorrhea.

The eliminating quality with respect to the liver, gallbladder and whole digestive tract is demonstrated in the primarily *stimulant* remedy Saussurea Mu Xiang (Wood aromatic). By promoting hepatic and intestinal eliminations (bile and stool), this remedy relieves biliary and gastrointestinal congestion with biliary and gastric dyspepsia, and constipation. The remedy "spreads Liver Qi and removes accumulation."

Solidifying/dissolving. This second teriary dyad addresses conditions of excessive softness and hardness, respectively. Both these conditions involve metabolic disruption in the connective tissue, with the possible generation of toxic metabolites. Reckeweg calls this the Impregnation stage of illness where the vital force tries to absorb toxins into the connective tissue, thereby causing softening or hardening manifestations.

Remedies with a solidifying quality are used to address pathological conditions of tissue softness. *Solidificants* work primarily on connective tissue to strengthen soft bones and teeth—where they can help prevent and treat fractures and osteoporosis, for example—and also benefit the body's entire system of sinews, the tendons, ligaments and muscles. On these they act over time to address conditions of prolapse, sublaxations, joint hypermobility, herniation and topical injuries.

The solidifying quality can readily be seen in a remedy such as Eucommia Du Zhong (Eucomia bark). This botanical generally solidifies muscles and bones and—again by strengthening connective tissue—also reduces urinary and seminal incontinence. It "fortifies the Kidneys, tonifies the Liver and strengthens the bones and tendons" with its solidifying effect.

Chinemys Gui Ban (Tortoise shell) has outstanding solidifying qualities that operate on musculoskeletal tissues. It thereby specifically strengthens bone, muscle and cartilage, addressing a wide range of disorders arising from weakness of these—conditions summarized as Liver and Kidney depletion in Chinese medicine.

The dissolving quality can readily be seen in remedies that are used to soften hardness or dissolve congealed substances that precipitate onto or into tissues. Examples include hardened mucus (e.g., impacted intestinal mucus, hardened bronchial sputum), hardened stool causing dry constipation, swelling and hardening of the lymph glands, mineral deposits causing stones (gallstones, urinary stones) or bone spurs, tissue fibrosis causing fibroid tumors, cysts, polyps or fibrocystic breasts, and tissue sclerosis such as liver sclerosis ("cirrhosis") and lung sclerosis. *Dissolvents* clearly are important in addressing the Deposition stage of disease where the body attempts to remove toxins by precipitation.

The dissolving quality is displayed, for instance, in Polygonum He Shou Wu (Flowery knotweed root). Prime examples of this quality are its *antifibrotic, deposit-dissolving, lymph gland swelling-reducing* actions. In this respect, Polygonum He Shou Wu can be considered a *dissolvent* in such conditions as fibrocystic breasts, lymphadenitis and, most likely, urinary stones.

Rubia Qian Cao Gen has an important dissolving quality acting on the bile duct and the bladder, where it is used to treat mineral deposits, i.e., stones. Like the last-mentioned remedy, Rubia Qian Cao Gen also contains anthraquinones that are active in its *dissolvent* action.

Ursus Xiong Dan (Bear gallbladder), with its various bile acids, also has important dissolving qualities, this time specifically on gallstones.

Mirabilitum Mang Xiao (Glauber's salt) is a prime example of the dissolving quality affecting the large intestine. As a salty tasting, dissolving *saline laxative,* it mainly addresses constipation from hardened or impacted stool.

Thickening/diluting. The third pair of tertiary qualities addresses conditions of excessive thinness or, conversely, excessive thickness among the body's fluid tissues. Rather than involving the functions or metabolism of fluids like the first tertiary pair of qualities, this pair affects their

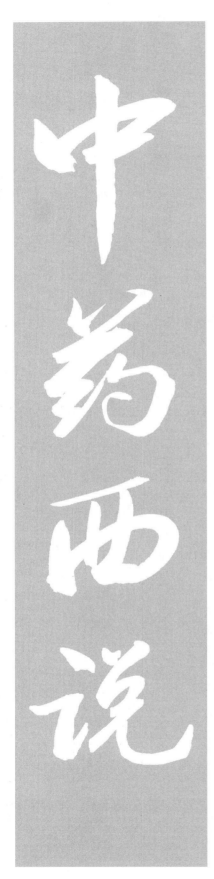

substantial structure. Because Greek and Roman doctors were especially aware of body fluid pathology, they took any observed fluid thickening or thinning proccess very seriously, prescribing *attenuants* (also called *dilutants*) or *inspissants*, respectively.

Remedies that contain a thickening quality address pathological thinning of one of the righteous body fluids—blood, interstitial fluid and mucus. Often sweet, sticky and dense by nature, these *inspissant* herbs primarily treat deficiency conditions involving lack of nutrition, dryness, hypotrophy, such as forms of chronic malabsorption, weightloss, anemia and malnutrition. *Inspissants* can be essential in any chronic or degenerative condition entailing a weakening of fluid tissue structure.

Codonopsis Dang Shen (Downy bellflower root) has an important thickening effect on blood and fluids—a significant aspect of its overall *restorative* primary effect. The root's very sweet, sticky tasting *hemogenic* (blood-building), *anastative* (metabolically up-building) actions are used to treat various blood, liver and nutritive deficiencies (including anemia, malabsorption, fatigue, etc.). Chinese textbooks define it as "strengthening the Spleen," and nowadays might add that it "enriches liver Yin and nourishes the blood."

The thickening effect of Dendrobium Shi Hu (Stonebushel stem) acts mainly on the gastric mucosa. This *inspissant* acts as a *mucosal restorative* and *mucogenic* to thicken and moisten gastric mucosa that has become sleazy through bacterial dysbiosis, local hyperacidity, stress, etc. The remedy "nourishes the Yin and moistens the stomach."

The thickening effective quality is evident in Typha Pu Huang (Cattail pollen). This remedy possesses a fast-acting thickening quality that causes increased blood coagulation, making for a good *hemostatic* and *styptic* for a variety of hemorrhage or bleeding.

Lycium Gou Ji Zi (Wolfberry), on the other hand, has a more long-term thickening effect on blood serum . It works on the liver with its *hepatic nutritive* effect, enhancing serum quality, which ultimately generates stamina, improved resistance and weight gain. This thickening effect is part of what is traditionally known as "enriching Liver Yin."

Remedies with a diluting quality can treat hyperviscosity among the fluids. Blood has a notorious ability to congeal, forming clots, or to become too fatty, causing hyperlipidemia. Interstitial fluids, too, can become heavy and thick from toxicosis of most kinds, and the same with lymphatic fluids, which then cause swelling of the lymph glands. *Attenuants* generally address endogenous toxicosis of a metabolic and microbial nature, as seen in atherosclerosis, thromboses, hyperlipidemia, lymphadenitis, arthritis, rheumatic disorders and viscous sputum or intestinal mucus.

The diluting quality is manifested by Salvia Dan Shen

(Cinnabar sage root). By diluting or thinning fluids and blood and thereby decreasing blood clotting factors, it treats true congealed blood phenomena such as thrombosis and menstrual clots. This *attenuant* remedy is traditionally classed as "vitalizing the Blood and clearing Blood stasis." *Dilutants* that work at the blood and fluids level have a *detoxicant* effect that can reduce various forms of endogenous toxicosis—especially metabolic—which is the basis for eczematous, rheumatic and arthritic conditions. Salvia Dan Shen is here no exception.

With its content in saponins, the sweet, moist-natured Asparagus Tian Men Dong (Shiny asparagus root) is said to have a diluting quality. By diluting hardened bronchial sputum it achieves a *mucolytic* effect that in turn causes expectoration. Although this species of asparagus is a well-known *bronchial demulcent,* it is also an important *mucolytic expectorant* as a result of its *dilutant* action on bronchial mucosa.

The final two pairs of tertiary effective qualities are concerned with energetic movements in the body. In Chinese medicine, they are also known as the four movements (*si qi*). These pairs are:

- *raising/sinking*
- *stabilizing/dispersing*

Raising/sinking. This pair has to do with vertical movement of energy in the body, and is concerned in particular with a deficiency or excess of energy in the brain. In physiological terms, insufficient cerebral circulation or, conversely, any tendency to cerebral blood congestion are pathological conditions that require the opposite tendency to be resolved.

Remedies with a raising quality bring more energy to the brain in terms of either nervous/cerebral activity or cerebral circulation. Traditional herbal texts refer to this raising effect as the "clear Yin rising upwards"—an effect also associated with the Yin Qiao extra channel and its master point Kd 6.

Ligustrum Nu Zhen Zi (Glossy privet berry) illustrates the raising movement quality well. This remedy brings energy to the head and brain, relieving symptoms such as poor concentration, dizziness, ringing ears and premature hair graying.

The much-researched remedy, Ginkgo leaf, has now become another classic raising type of remedy. Ginkgo leaf can thereby correct cerebral deficiency of both nervous and circulatory origin, with symptoms such as memory and concentration loss, ringing in the ears, premature senility and chronic depression.

Remedies with a sinking quality bring down excess energy from the brain in terms of either nervous/cerebral activity or cerebral circulation. This includes remedies that reduce cerebral congestion arising from fever. The sinking movement is linked to the Yang Qiao extra channel and its master point Bl 62.

The intensely bitter tasting Coptis Huang Lian (Chinese goldthread root) has a sinking movement. It removes excess energy from the head and brain, and clears the heat of fever (by lowering blood from the head). It "quells fire."

Remedies with a strong bitter taste, a primary quality, in general possess a sinking energetic movement. This includes Scutellaria Huang Qin (Baikal skullcap root) and Gentiana Qin Jiao (Large-leaf gentian root).

Stabilizing/dispersing. The second pair of tertiary movements has to do with movement away from or towards the body's center. It is related to the astringing/eliminating dyad, the first of the tertiary qualities, which describes the tissue rather than movement aspect of this phenomenon.

Remedies possessing a stabilizing movement bring energy inwards towards the body's center, thereby counteracting a tendency of solid or fluid tissues to move or collapse outwards and downwards. Stabilizing remedies can reduce body discharges and, equally important, prevent and treat tissue and organ prolapse.

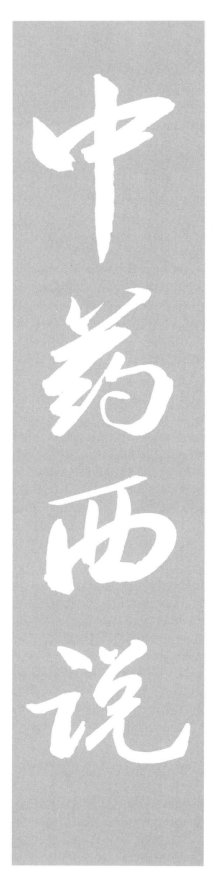

Cimicifuga Sheng Ma (Rising Hemp root) has an important stabilizing effect that will help in prolapsed conditions of the intestines, rectum and uterus.

The stabilizing action of Stegodon Long Gu (Dragon bone), on the other hand, can primarily be seen in its effect on reproductive organ discharges, diarrhea, uterine bleeding and excessive sweating.

Remedies with a dispersing movement disperse energy away from the body's center, thereby counteracting a tendency for fluid tissues to contract inwards and congest. Dispersing remedies treat insufficient elimination and deficient skin metabolism. Remedies with a dominant pungent taste, a primary quality, automatically possess the dispersing movement.

The pungent Notopterygium Qiang Huo (Notopterygium root) is a case in point. By causing fluids to move outwards towards the periphery, this dispersing remedy "releases the exterior" by stimulating circulation, causing sweating and relieving pain in the muscles and joints.

Tropism

Tropism designates the body systems, organisms, organs, tissues, body parts and energetic systems—such as channels and chakras—with which a remedy has an affinity, bias or resonance. The phenomenon of tropicity has also been verified experimentally with essential oils and can be inferred from experimental herbal research. It is also used daily in electroacupuncture, for example.

Listed first of all are the body systems affected by the remedy. In the Greek herbal-medical tradition, each remedy has a definite effect on certain body systems, tissues or parts. The main system it treats determines its categorization in this Chinese materia medica. For instance, although also working on the urinary, musculoskeletal and digestive systems, Cistanche Rou Cong Rong (Fleshy broomrape herb) primarily affects reproductive functions. It is more frequently used for disorders such as sexual disinterest, impotence and infertility than for any other kind. Likewise, although profoundly affecting digestive, cardiovascular, reproductive and nervous system functions, Panax Ren Shen (Asian ginseng root) essentially works on the endocrine glands. Because it regulates a number of hormonal secretions, it is found under remedies for the endocrine and immune systems.

Tropism is the rationale behind traditional Western remedy classifications such as *cordials* (going to the heart and circulation), *pectorals* (going to the chest and lungs), *hepatics* (going to the liver), *digestives* (affecting digestive organs), *cephalics* (going to the head and brain), *nervines* (going to the nerves) and *hysterics* (going to the uterus [*hysteros* is Greek for uterus]).

In a similar way, in Chinese medicine, a remedy is said to "enter" certain meridians or channels throughout the body in such a way that each taste quality has an affinity or tropism for certain tissues (e.g., saltiness "travels" to the bones, sweetness to the flesh, and bitterness to the heart). The channels comprise a comprehensive, articulated network of energetic frequencies studded with "points" of lower electromagnetic resistance. The remedy Magnolia Xin Yi Hua (Yulan magnolia bud), for example, enters the Lung and Stomach channels because it addresses disorders caused by energetic imbalances of those channels.

In traditional Greek medicine, a remedy is also said to affect larger systems of organization called the four bodies, which are the warmth, air, fluid and physical body. The four bodies not only correspond to the Greek four elements of Fire, Air, Water and Earth as they are found in the natural world, but also embody them, incarnate them, in the individual human being.

The **Warmth body** is housed in the blood, mediated through the cardiovascular system and controlled by the hypothalamus and pituitary endocrine glands. It deals in every respect with the body's active warmth and the individual's functions of integration, organization and homeostasis. *Refrigerant* remedies that clear heat, reducing inflammation or fever, such as Gardenia Zhi Zi (Gardenia seed) and that create warmth through circulatory stimulation, such as Zingiber Gan Jiang (Dried ginger root), clearly affect the Warmth body.

The **Air body,** with its primary substrate the nervous system, is mediated by the kidney/adrenal system and controlled by the thyroid gland. It deals with functions characterized by sensitivity, response and movement. Relaxant remedies that reduce tension and constraint, such as Cyperus Xiang Fu (Nutsedge root), and remedies that build energy and strength, such as Glycyrrhiza Gan Cao (Ural licorice root), operate on the level of the Air body.

The **Fluid body** is housed in the connective tissue, mediated by the various body fluids and governed by the liver and adrenal cortex. It deals with transformation or metabolism, both anabolic (upbuilding) and catabolic (breaking down). Artemisia Yin Chen Hao (Downy wormwood herb), through its hepatic activity, organizes the body fluids and reduces water retention. Ophiopogon Mai Men Dong (Dwarf lilyturf root), with its *secretory*, systemic *hydrating* effect, by fostering body fluids reduces dehydration and thirst. Both these botanicals clearly manage the Fluid body.

The **Physical body,** which is the structive body substance itself with its many tissues types, is supervised by the thymus and spleen, and mediated in particular by the lungs. All remedies, in one way or another, affect the Physical body, since this is the foundation on which all physiological transformations occur.

Actions and Indications

This section of the presentation gives information on the remedy's primary therapeutic functions, organized according to Western physiological actions and therapeutic indications. The actions include most currently well-known actions, such as *"nasal decongestant"* and *"expectorant,"* as well as less common ones, as *"interferon inducent."* All therapeutic actions used in this text may be found in the Glossary at the book's end.

The first remedy action given is the main action on the body system to which the remedy belongs. In general, the remedy actions and indications begin with the most important and end with the least important. The main exceptions are actions related to microorganisms, such as *antibacterial, antiviral,* etc., and functions primarily for external use, such as *vulnerary, detumescent,* etc. These are always listed last, except with remedies for infection and tissue repair. Remember, though, that some remedies are equally good in almost all their functions—Salvia Dan Shen (Cinnabar sage root), for example.

While some of the remedy actions are more obvious, well-researched and well-known, others are less apparent, more recent and have received less attention. Although my aim was to be as comprehensive as possible and include every action known about a remedy, often one or more minor actions were omitted because of insufficient available evidence either pharmacological or clinical. Still, it should be emphasized that, in terms of Western pharmacological actions, most contemporary Chinese remedy uses revolve around three, at the most four, actions per remedy.

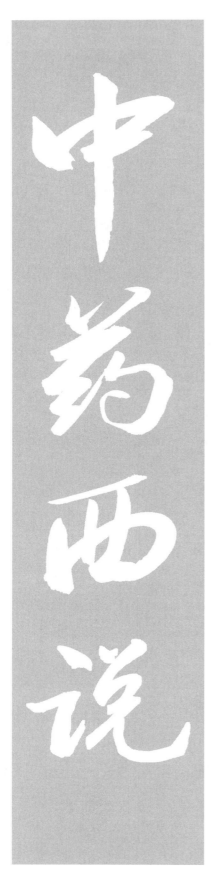

The typical number of actions per remedy given in this book is over twice that. Because of the nature of this text and space limitations, references to research papers, with a few exceptions, are not included. The major primary and secondary available sources for this information may be found in the bibliography.

There are essentially three types of remedy indications given in this section: symptom/sign, condition and Western disease indications. Examples of symptom indications include headache, constipation, diarrhea, jaundice. Condition indications are, e.g., congestive dysmenorrhea, respiratory tract infections, catarrhal conditions, parasitic infestations and autoimmune conditions. Disease indications include such terms as anemia, pelvic inflammatory disease, diabetes and essential hypertension. Clearly, these three types of indications often overlap. Herbal remedies may be chosen for any type of indication, depending on whether symptom relief or more systemic treatment is being sought—in turn always related to the specific requirements of the condition being treated.

For example, one may select a remedy uniquely because of a certain action that it carries out or a specific symptom that it relieves. Polygonum He Shou Wu (Flowery knotweed root) might be indicated in a condition purely for its *trophorestorative* effect on the brain; Carthamus Hong Hua (Safflower) solely because of its excellent *coronary decongestant* and *anticoagulant* actions. Conversely, Angelica Bai Zhi (White angelica root) may be found in a formula simply because it is one of the best remedies for headaches at the crown of the head; or Dioscorea Bi Xie (Long yam root) because it treats the symptom of cloudy urine, whatever the underlying cause.

On the other hand, many remedies are applied for the totality of their actions and indications. Some conditions require the inclusion of a remedy simply because of its overall therapeutic gestalt. Here the general profile of the condition is perfectly matched by that of the remedy, i.e., the remedy is said to have a good conformation. Cyperus Xiang Fu (Nutsedge root), for instance, is very much needed when the condition Qi constraint is dominant in a woman, causing tension and pain in cardiovascular, reproductive and digestive functions. This remedy's systemic *relaxant* action, especially with symptoms of restlessness, palpitations, menstrual cramps and abdominal pain, completely matches the condition of systemic Qi constraint.

Likewise, a practitioner might select a remedy because of its usefulness with a certain disorder. In the People's Republic, remedies such as Oldenlandia Bai Hua She She Cao (Snaketongue grass herb), Scutellaria Ban Zhi Lian (Barbed skullcap root) and Solanum Bai Ying (Climbing nightshade root and herb), for example, are frequent ingredients in herbal formulas that treat various types of cancer. Schizonepeta Jing Jie (Japanese catnip herb), Mentha Bo He (Fieldmint herb) and Cryptotympana Chan Tui (Cicada slough), on the other hand, are much used for treating eruptive fevers such as measles and chickenpox. Ganoderma Ling Zhi (Reishi mushroom) and Tripterygium Lei Gong Teng (Yellow vine root pith) are often relied on in both allergic and autoimmune disorders for their *immune regulating* action. Gastrodia Tian Ma (Celestial hemp root), Uncaria Gou Teng (Gambir vine twig) and Bombyx Jiang Can (Silkworm larva) can find much usage with peripheral nervous system disorders because of their combined nerve *relaxant/sedative* action.

If the indicated symptoms, diseases and conditions of a remedy are all present together in a person's overall condition, then a remedy is all the more called for. Theoretically, an individual presenting, say, a cough, muscle aches and coronary disease with high blood lipid levels at the same time would be well served by the remedy Dioscorea Chuan Shan Long (Nippon yam root). Its *stimulant expectorant, analgesic neuromuscular relaxant, coronary decongestant* and *antilipemic* actions would address this person's whole imbalance at the same time.

Symptom Pictures

As we saw in Chapter 2, the traditional way of using herbal remedies and formulas in Chinese medicine hinges around symptom pictures. These are also variously known as patterns of disharmony, symptom complexes or syndromes (this word comes from the Greek *syndrome*, meaning a combination). Symptom pictures are simply snapshots of ways in which imbalance or illness actually manifest. Symptom pictures include not only the one or several primary symptoms from which a person may be suffering, but also other, secondary symptoms which, together with the primary ones, make up the whole symptom picture. Matching the symptom picture of a remedy with that of the patient is the simplest and one of the oldest methods of using remedies. It certainly is also the most holistic.

Symptom pictures show how an herbal remedy can be used in the phenomenological, symptom-related way, as opposed to an analytical way based on actions and indications (see the chart just before the Repertory in Part Three). Symptom pictures portray the more pragmatic use of a remedy in a typical, real-life, clinical situation, based on the image of the syndrome with its many typical symptoms. Rarely do we treat a single symptom, rarely does an illness present only one symptom, and rarely does a remedy treat one symptom alone. In actuality, several symptoms usually occur at the same time, whether part of a single illness or not. Organized by the mind in a meaningful way, these symptoms become pictures or patterns. Likewise, the many symptoms relieved by a remedy, when seen as a whole, form a typical symptom picture. Traditional Chinese and Greek medical symptom pictures have been refined over millennia by empirical observation, and today they are being still further refined with input from the Western physiological perspective.

The symptom pictures listed in this section of the remedy presentation represent the main, but not the only, ones for which it is used. The advantage of using symptom pictures for guidance in remedy selection lies in that it is relatively easy to use while retaining a high degree of accuracy. A remedy might be chosen because it treats a certain symptom pattern exhibited by the patient, because the match between the remedy's and the patient's symptom picture is a good one. Scrophularia Xuan Shen (Black figwort root), for example, is ideal for the symptom picture **heart Qi constraint and nerve excess,** consisting of typical signs and symptoms such as restlessness, irritability, anxiety, sleeplessness and palpitations. The same remedy is also used for the syndromes **Yin and fluids deficiency,** and **Blood and Nutritive level heat.** If a person's symptomatology consisted of a combination of these three symptom pictures, then Scrophularia Xuan Shen would be indicated all the more; most likely, it would then become the main constituent of an herbal fomula for that person. Alternately, it might be used on its own if a tincture is preferred.

Although one may select a remedy purely because it possesses a certain action, treats a specific disease, or addresses a certain symptom picture, one may equally well choose a remedy for a variety of characteristics. Ultimately, every remedy is unique, consisting of actions, indications and symptom picture uses particularly its own and unlike any other (this is true even of remedies that are similar). Likewise, every person is unique, presenting different subclinical or clinical

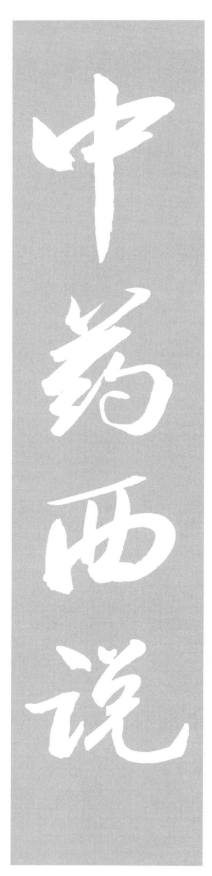

symptoms, imbalances and syndromes at any given moment in their life. A remedy such as Polygonatum Yu Zhu (Fragrant Solomon's seal root), therefore, could be theoretically chosen to treat someone with a unique symptom configuration such as chronic thirst, dry coughs, hot spells, unrest, loss of sleep, cold hands and feet, depression, palpitations, giddyness and tremors of the fingers—symptoms caused by dry lungs, autonomic nerve imbalance and circulatory deficiency at the same time. Here the concerted actions of the remedy Polygonatum Yu Zhu—*respiratory demulcent, secretory, neuromuscular relaxant* and *cardiac stimulant*—are all engaged as they treat the particular gestalt of this case.

Preparation

Use

In Chinese medicine, most remedies are traditionally prepared in water by decoction, and are usually combined with a smaller or greater number of other remedies to create a formula. However, like Western herbs, Chinese herbs can also be taken in the form of an alcohol extract, such as a tincture or fluid extract. Very occasionally, a tincture may be a less appropriate administration form than the decoction, and this is indicated. On the other hand, being alcohol based, a tincture is capable of extracting a larger spectrum of constituents than water alone, and in addition has an enhanced energetic action. Because of these two factors, it is often a superior form of administration. In practice, the tincture can treat a wider range of disorders than water preparations, and is usually preferable when a remedy is given as a simple—a single remedy—or combined with only a small number of other remedies.

Note that herbs containing a high proportion of essential oils should be infused rather than decocted to prevent their evaporation. This is the case with aromatic leafy or flowery Chinese items such as Chrysanthemum Ju Hua (Chrysanthemum flower), Mentha Bo He (Asian fieldmint herb) and Schizonepeta Jing Jie (Japanese catnip herb). With those essential oils containing remedies that are roots, the roots should be sliced or ground finely and the decoction time, if possible, reduced. The overnight cold water infusion is an excellent alternative preparation for soft roots containing essential oils: Ligusticum Chuan Xiong, Angelica Dang Gui, Saussurea Yun Mu Xiang and Ephedra Ma Huang are four examples that stand to benefit from this method.

Most remedies can be prepared for external applications as well as taken internally. The basic preparation, whether decoction, infusion or tincture, is then applied to the skin with cotton—a swab—or a piece of cloth—a compress—etc., or used to prepare a gargle, mouthwash, vaginal sponge, douche or whatever. For full details on remedy administration, internal and external preparation forms and methods of use, see the author's *Energetics of Western Herbs,* Vol. I.

Chinese pharmacy excels at altering the properties of remedies through numerous processing techniques that include dry-frying, honey-frying, boiling in water, alum or other liquids, steaming and various other methods. The purpose of this is to direct the therapeutic action of the herb in a certain way, to enhance one or more of its properties. Many remedies are generally available *only* in prepared, not crude form: Prepared pinellia corm, Prepared Sichuan aconite root and Prepared dragon arum corm are classic examples. Only the more important of these processes are mentioned in this part of the presentation. For reliable information on the processing and preparation methods of Chinese remedies, the reader is referred to *Chinese Herbal Medicine: Materia Medica* by Bensky and Gamble.

Dosage

The usual dosage range is here indicated for both water preparation (decoction or infusion) and alcohol-based tinctures. The dosage range allows flexibility for differences in age, body weight, etc. of the person as well as the specific condition being treated.

The decoction, infusion and powder dosage is given in grams, indicated by g; tincture dosages are given in milliliters, indicated by ml.

Caution

Cautions relate to both the nature of the remedy and the way it should or should not be used. In the first case, remedies of the medium-strength therapeutic category are the main consideration. Remedies in this class should only be used for a certain period of time, especially if used alone, very frequently or at high dosage. This caution is always mentioned in case the remedy is ever used as a simple—in tincture form, for example—despite the fact that it is traditionally hardly ever administered on its own. Even a medium-strength remedy is frequently found in Chinese decoction formulas at a low proportion, in the context of which it can be used for weeks and months on end without in itself causing the slightest side-effects.

In the second case are therapeutic cautions that include such things as usage during pregnancy, in specific conditions of pathology and under special circumstances.

Contrary to the cautions, the contraindications or "forbiddens" are absolute.

Notes

These self-explanatory notes serve mainly to highlight those actions and indications of a remedy that are generally considered the most effective. It prioritizes primary from secondary herb functions, and relates them first, to their symptom pictures uses, and second, to their chemical constituents (when this relationship is known).

This summary is particularly useful if large numbers of remedies need to be memorized. Rule-of-thumb tags for each remedy, such as an outstanding symptom, disorder or syndrome indication, can facilitate learning and memorization. This is especially useful in clinical practice for formula building. Knowledge of certain chemical components in the remedies can likewise serve as springboards for memorization and therapeutics.

For example, although Curcuma Jiang Huang (Turmeric root), is an excellent *stimulant* to hepatobiliary functions, it is traditionally remembered in Chinese medicine—and clinically more often used—as *the* remedy for shoulder pain. Today we would also select this remedy for its *anti-inflammatory, antioxidant* and *antitumoral* actions. Likewise, Ledebouriella Fang Feng (Wind-protector root) is seen by many skilled Chinese herbalists not so much as a remedy for rheumatic disorders (wind/damp/cold obstruction conditions), but as *the* remedy for causing diaphoresis when dryness, or fluid deficiency, is present. It is a rare *moist diaphoretic* that will not injure the body fluids and reduce internal moisture. Now we also know that this essential oil remedy also contains polysaccharides that make it an excellent choice for treating infections in general.

PART TWO

The Materia Medica

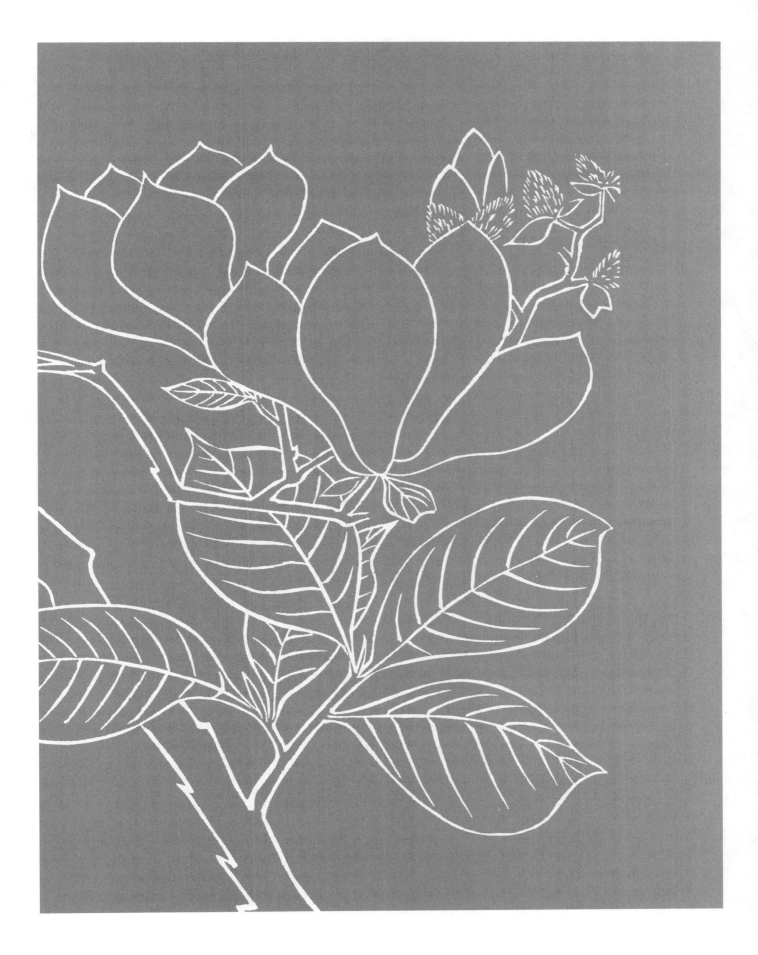

眼鼻喉用药

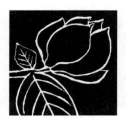

Remedies for the Nose, Throat and Eyes

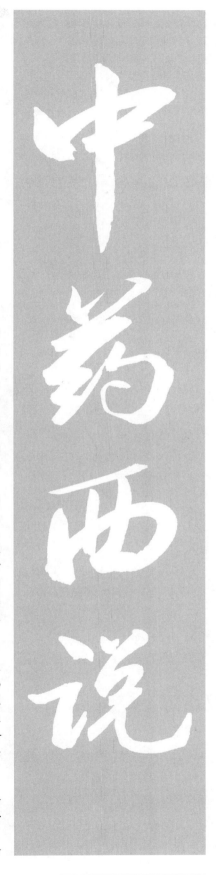

The most common disorders of the sense organs in the head are infections of the nose, throat and eyes (rather than the ear, nose and throat), therefore we consider these conditions in this section. Traditional Oriental herbal texts do not include a category for either upper respiratory infections or any of the sense organs. This is because their herb classifications are based on vitalistic treatment methods rather than anatomy and physiology. Nevertheless, we can find the majority of remedies for infections of the nose, throat and eyes in the section on "pungent herbs that release the exterior."

"Wind cold" and "wind heat" are the symptom patterns generated by upper respiratory infections, such as common cold, flu, sinusitis, rhinitis and laryngitis, as well as eye infections, such as conjunctivitis. "Wind" refers to the rapidly changing and painful nature of these conditions, while "cold" and "heat" refer to the absence or presence of any inflammatory or febrile response. Both these symptom pictures are considered external conditions because they affect surface tissues, not internal organs (See Holmes 1989 for a discussion of external conditions.)

Using the fourfold Western vitalistic herb classification as a basis, remedies for the nose, throat and eyes are divided into *restoratives, stimulants, relaxants* and *sedatives*. *Restoratives* and *stimulants* are taken from the traditional class of herbs "with pungent, warm qualities for releasing the exterior," while *relaxants* and *sedatives* are culled from the companion class of remedies "with pungent, cool qualities for releasing the exterior."

- **Restoratives** for the nose, throat and eyes treat deficiency conditions with chronic mucosal weakness, presenting clear nasal discharge.
- **Stimulants** for the nose, throat and eyes address deficiency

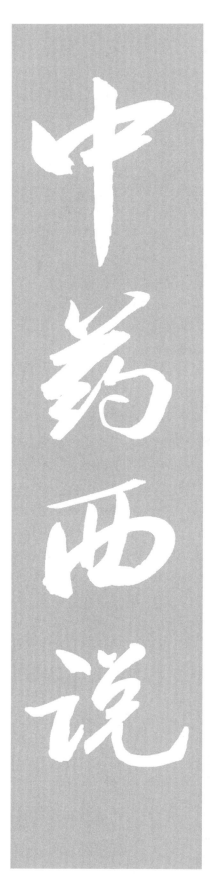

conditions with mucosal weakness, accompanied by nasal/sinus congestion and pain.

• **Relaxants** and **sedatives** for the nose, throat and eyes treat excess conditions with acute sinus, throat or eye inflammation, presenting pain, yellow purulent discharge and fever.

Because of the large overlap between *restoratives* and *stimulants* on one hand, and *relaxants* and *sedatives* on the other, these four herb types have been condensed into two categories: *restoratives/stimulants* and *relaxants/sedatives*.

The Remedies for the Nose, Throat and Eyes

Restoratives and Stimulants

At the onset of upper respiratory infections, the nose and sinuses display symptoms: nasal and sinus congestion, clear discharge, pain and frontal headache. Deficiency symptom patterns of the **external wind cold** type are generated, such as **head damp cold** and **lung wind cold.** These may include the viral conditions sinusitis, common cold (coryza), rhinitis and simple non-infectious catarrh caused by stress or allergy (allergic rhinitis).

The pungent, warm and dry effective qualities of the *restorative/stimulant* remedies in this section have a twofold action. First, they tone the mucus-lined nasal passages to stop catarrhal discharge and nasal drip by way of a *mucosal restorative* or *anticatarrhal* action. These *restoratives* include Magnolia Xin Yi Hua (the bud of various species of magnolia trees from the mountains of East and Central China) and Xanthium Cang Er Zi (Siberian cocklebur from Central and Northeast China), two botanicals frequently paired in herbal formulating.

Second, herbs in this section stimulate the sinuses to clear nasal congestion with a *nasal decongestant* action. This is the work of the *stimulants,* and includes Angelica Bai Zhi root (White angelica root, from the river valleys of coastal and Central China) and Perilla Zi Su Ye (Perilla leaf, a plant in the mint family found throughout Southeast Asia). Both the *anticatarrhal* and *decongestant* actions contribute to "dispelling wind cold."

The additional *anti-infective, antiseptic* and *analgesic* actions displayed in various degrees by these remedies reinforce their primary actions, making them effective and reliable for the infection and pain involved. Biochemically they are dominated by essential oils, which explains their tendency to be additionally somewhat *diaphoretic*—another property useful in helping resolve acute upper respiratory infections.

Relaxants and Sedatives

At an early stage of upper respiratory infections, the body's acute inflammatory response to bacterial proliferation may set in. This produces a yellow-green nasal discharge, and throat and eyes that become red, painful and swollen. These keynote signs characterize the syndromes **wind heat** and **lung wind heat,** which normally imply laryngitis, pharyngitis, tonsillitis, eye irritation, conjunctivitis or blepharitis.

Relaxant and *sedative* remedies for the nose, throat and eyes, such as Schizonepeta Jing Jie (the common Japanese catnip herb) and Chrysanthemum Ju Hua (the flower of the widely cultivated florist's chrysanthemum), bring relief through their *analgesic, anti-inflammatory, anti-infective* and *diaphoretic* properties. In this way they "dispel wind heat." Their therapeutic effects are mediated by their pungent, bitter and cool effective qualities on the vitalistic level and their high essential oil content on the biochemical level.

Another clinical way of dividing remedies in this section is to think of their primary tropism—nose/sinuses, throat or eyes. Some herbs are used predominantly because of their focus for treating sinus infections: Magnolia Xin Yi Hua (Yulan magnolia bud), Xanthium Cang Er Zi (Siberian cocklebur berry), Angelica Bai Zhi (White angelica root from Central China), Morus Sang Ye (the common mulberry leaf), Perilla Zi Su Ye (the Southeast Asian Perilla leaf) and Centipeda E Bu Shi Cao (the Southern Centipeda herb).

Then there are some remedies that excell at managing throat infections: Among them are Arctium Niu Bang Zi (the seed of the common burdock), Sterculia Pang Da Hai (Sterculia seed from Southeast Asia), Oroxylum Mu Hu Die (Oroxylum seed from Southeast Asia), Lasiosphaera Ma Bo (the common Puffball mushroom) and Chimonanthus La Mei Hua (Wintersweet flower).

Others, such as Chrysanthemum Ju Hua (Chrysanthemum flower), Celosia Qing Xiang Zi (the cultivated Silver quail-grass seed), Buddleia Mi Meng Hua (the cultivated Buddleia flower and bud), Equisetum Mu Zei (the common Horsetail herb), and Eriocaulon Gu Jing Cao (the marshland Pipewort herb) are used in particular for their *anti-inflammatory* and other actions in eye infections.

Many remedies in this section are frequently used in particular for children's eruptive fevers, such as measles, German measles and chickenpox. They help infection and resolve fever by causing sweating and bringing rashes to the surface, while at the same time relieving possible accompanying inflammation such as pharyngitis and conjunctivitis.

All remedies in the Nose, Throat and Eyes section are frequently combined with remedies that reduce infection, stimulate immunity, and reduce fever and inflammation in the Infection and Toxicosis section. The two remedy types are complementary when infection is severe and causes **fire toxins**—the stage of disease when symptoms present heat, redness, pain, swelling and purulence.

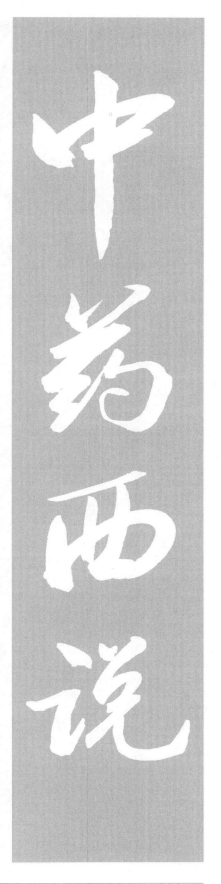

Nose, Throat and Eye Restoratives and Stimulants

REMEDIES TO RELIEVE NASAL CONGESTION AND PAIN, AND STOP DISCHARGE

➥ RELEASE THE EXTERIOR AND DISPEL WIND COLD WITH PUNGENT, WARM REMEDIES
Anticatarrhal nasal decongestants

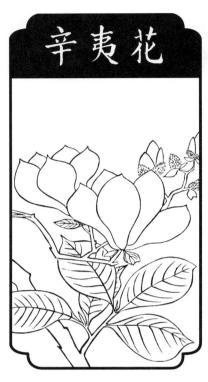

Magnolia Xin Yi Hua
Yulan Magnolia Bud

Botanical source: *Magnolia liliflora* Desrousseaux or *M. denudata* Desr. or *M. yulan* Desr. or *M. biondii* Pampanini (Magnoliaceae)
Pharmaceutical name: Gemma Magnoliae
Chinese names: Xin Yi Hua, Chun Hua, Yu Lan (Mand); San Yi Fa (Cant)
Other names: Lily flowered magnolia, "Pungent magnolia"; Shinika (Jap)
Habit: Large deciduous mountain shrub or small tree from Central and East China; aromatic, large, bell-shaped pink or white flowers open in summer.
Part used: the unopened flower bud

Therapeutic category: mild remedy with minimal chronic toxicity
Constituents: essential oil c. 3% (incl. pinene, camphene, limonene, linalol, cineol, terpineol, methylchavicol, citral, safrol, anethol, estragol), alkaloids, lignans (incl. eudesmin), flavonoids, magnolin, fargesin, vitamin A
Effective qualities: pungent, a bit astringent, a bit warm, neutral
  restoring, stimulating, astringing, relaxing
Tropism: upper respiratory, vascular, immune systems
  Lung, Stomach channels
  Air body

ACTIONS AND INDICATIONS
nasal/mucosal restorative and stimulant: mucostatic, decongestant, analgesic: mucosal deficiency with clear or purulent nasal discharge, sinus congestion and pain; sinusitis, rhinitis (incl. allergic), frontal headache
anti-infective (antiseptic, antiviral), anti-inflammatory: upper respiratory infections (acute and chronic, incl. common cold, influenza)
hypotensive: hypertension
uterine stimulant
antifungal: fungal skin conditions
immune regulator: immune stress with antibody-mediated cytotoxicity (incl. autoimmune disorders)

SYMPTOM PICTURE
head damp cold: stuffy or runny nose due to allergy or cold, sneezing, dizziness, frontal headache

PREPARATION
Use: The flower bud Magnolia Xin Yi Hua is decocted or may be used in tincture form.
Dosage: Decoction: 3-10 g
  Tincture: 2-4 ml
Caution: Prolonged use or overdosing of Yulan magnolia bud should be avoided, as it may cause some dizziness or eye inflammation. Being *uterine stimulant,* use this remedy very cautiously during pregnancy, and then only as small part of a large formula.

NOTES

In Chinese culture, the lily white satin flowers of this shrubby magnolia have been emblems of purity and sincerity for millenniums. The furry, unopened flower bud is an important remedy for acute and chronic sinusitis with discharge. High in essential oils, this pungent remedy acts as a *mucosal restorative* and *antiseptic* to the sinus and nasal passages, relieving catarrhal and congested, i.e., damp conditions. Yulan magnolia bud's *antifungal* action on skin conditions—presumably due to its essential oil content—is particularly strong.

In China's Daoist past, Yulan magnolia bud was one of many herbs famed for making the body light and the eyes shining, and for adding years to one's life span.

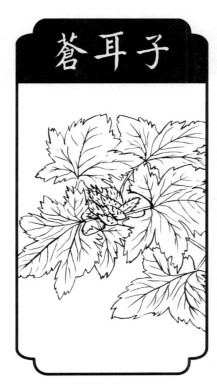

Xanthium Cang Er Zi
Siberian Cocklebur

Botanical source: *Xanthium sibiricum* Patrin or *X. strumarium* L. (Compositae)
Pharmaceutical name: Fructus Xanthii
Chinese names: Cang Er Zi, Er Dang, Cang Er, Xi Er (Mand); Chong Yi Ji (Cant)
Other names: Asian cocklebur; Burweed, "Green ear seed"; Sojishi (Jap)
Habit: Annual herb from the mountains of temperate Northeast Asia and Central China, growing especially on waste ground, along streams and villages; blooms in autumn with light green terminal or axillary flowerheads.
Part used: the fruit

Therapeutic category: medium-strength remedy with some chronic toxicity
Constituents: glycosides (incl. xanthostrumarin), fatty oil (incl. linoleic, oleic acid), xanthanol, hydroquinone, resin, alkaloids, organic acids, ceryl acohol, vitamin C
Effective qualities: sweet, a bit bitter and pungent, warm
   restoring, stimulating
Tropism: upper respiratory, musculoskeletal systems, pancreas
   Lung, Liver channels
   Warmth body

ACTION AND INDICATIONS

nasal/mucosal restorative/stimulant: mucostatic, decongestant, anti-inflammatory, antiallergic: chronic mucosal weakness with nasal discharge, sinus congestion and pain; chronic sinusitis, chronic allergic rhinitis
analgesic: headache, migratory myalgia (rheumatism), pain of paralysis, chronic low back pain
anti-infective: antibacterial, antifungal, interferon inducent
antipruritic: pruritus (from rashes, sores, urticaria, scabies, leprosy, etc.)
diuretic
hypoglycemiant, diuretic: diabetes

SYMPTOM PICTURES

head damp cold: stuffy nose and sinuses, sneezing, thick nasal discharge, frontal or other headache
wind damp obstruction: stiff painful joints, muscle aches and pains, skin itching

Preparation

Use: The berry Xanthium Cang Er Zi is decocted or used as tincture. External preparations are made for pruritic conditions.
Dosage: Decoction: 5-10 g
Tincture: 2-4 ml
Caution: Forbidden in rheumatic and other painful wind damp conditions due to Blood (metabolic) deficiency. An overdose or continuous longterm usage of this medium-strength remedy may result in nausea, vomiting, abdominal pain, low blood pressure and liver dysfunction.

Notes

Siberian cocklebur is the main remedy used in Chinese medicine for chronic paranasal sinusitis and allergic rhinitis, especially with headache present. The *analgesic* effect of this biochemically loaded botanical further extends to rheumatic and arthritic conditions, known in Chinese medicine as wind damp obstruction.

Although it also grows in North America and Europe, Cocklebur is hardly used in the West as a medicinal plant.

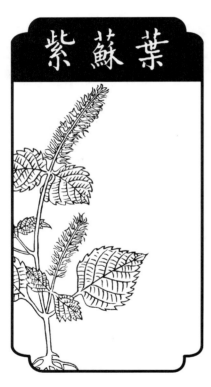

Perilla Zi Su Ye
Perilla Leaf

Botanical source: *Perilla frutescens* (L.) Britton var. *crispa* (Thunb.) Handel-Mazzetti or *P. fr.* var. *acuta* (Thunb.) Kudo (Labiatae)
Pharmaceutical name: Folium Perillae
Chinese names: Zi Su Ye, Jia Su Zi, Zi Su, Su Ye (Mand); So Yip (Cant)
Other names: Bushy perilla, Chiso, "Purple Su"; Shisoyo (Jap)
Habit: Pilose annual herb from Southeast Asia, Taiwan and Japan, growing in sunny, fertile areas near villages and roads; cultivated throughout China; racemes of minute white/purplish axillary/terminal flowers appear in summer.
Part used: the leaf

Therapeutic category: mild remedy with minimal chronic toxicity
Constituents: essential oil c.5% (incl. perillaldehyde, limonene, pinene, caryophyllene), perilla alcohol, cumic acid, arginine, flavonoids, anthocyanins, isoegomaketone
Effective qualities: pungent, warm, dry
stimulating, dispersing, relaxing
Tropism: respiratory, digestive systems
Lung, Large Intestine, Spleen channels
Air body

Actions and Indications

nasal stimulant: decongestant, stimulant diaphoretic, antibacterial: acute or chronic nasal/sinus congestion; sinusitis, common cold
antitussive: coughing, wheezing
gastric stimulant: gastric dyspepsia, acute gastroenteritis
antiemetic: vomiting, nausea (incl. morning sickness)
detoxicant: food poisoning (esp. from seafood); cholera
fetal relaxant: fetal unrest
interferon inducent

Symptom Pictures

lung wind cold and **head damp cold:** sneezing, stuffy nose, chills, feverishness, coughing

stomach Qi stagnation: painful distended abdomen, appetite loss, nausea, vomiting, flatulence, diarrhea

Preparation

Use: The leaf Perilla Zi Su Ye may be either infused or decocted, or used in tincture form.

Dosage: Infusion and decoction: 5-10 g
Tincture: 2-4 ml

Caution: Contraindicated in damp heat conditions of the digestive organs, and with heavy sweating during the onset of cold or flu.

Notes

A good, gentle pungent-warm *dispersing* remedy for the onset of colds, Perilla leaf is ideal when coughing and digestive upset (especially acute gastritis) join the overall symptom picture. This is clearly seen in the lung wind cold and stomach Qi stagnation syndromes above.

Because Perilla leaf contains a natural food preservative, it may also be used, to a limited extent, to prevent food from spoiling. The large leaves of the purple variety are also used for pickling vegetables, such as Japanese umeboshi plums, and should be eaten along with these.

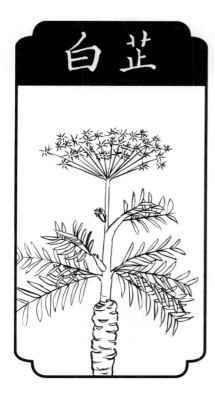

Angelica Bai Zhi
White Angelica Root *

Botanical source: *Angelica dahurica* (Fisch. ex Hoffm.) Bentham et Hooker f. or *A. anomala* Lallem. or *A. taiwaniana* Boissier (Umbelliferae)
Pharmaceutical name: Radix Angelicae dahuricae
Chinese names: Bai Zhi, Fang Xiang, Bai Zhi Xiang (Mand); Baak Ji (Cant)
Other names: Dahurian angelica; Byakushi (Jap)
Habit: Perennial herb from Central and North coastal China; grows in thickets in river valleys and marshes; also cultivated; blooms in summer with white-blossomed umbels.
Part used: the root

Therapeutic category: mild remedy with minimal chronic toxicity
Constituents: essential oil (incl. bergaptene, furocoumarins, incl. xanthotoxins marmesin, scopoletin, alloisoimperatorin, neobyakangelicol, byalangelicin, angelicol, oxypeucedanin, imperatorin, isoimperatorin, angelic acid, phellandrene), trace elements
Effective qualities: pungent, a bit sweet and bitter, warm, dry
stimulating, relaxing, dispersing
Tropism: upper respiratory, central nervous, urogenital systems
Lung, Stomach channels; Air body

Actions and Indications

nasal stimulant: decongestant, stimulant diaphoretic, anti-infective (antiviral, antibacterial): nasal/sinus congestion and pain; sinusitis, rhinitis, common cold, flu
nervous sedative, analgesic, anesthetic: headache (esp. at vertex), frontal sinus pain, toothache, stomachache, menstrual pain
uterine stimulant, emmenagogue: spasmodic dysmenorrhea, delayed menses
mucostatic: clear vaginal discharge (leucorrhea); gonorrhea
diuretic

maturant, detoxicant: beginning stage of boils, carbuncles, ulcers, etc., when red, painful and hot
interferon inducent
Miscellaneous: nasal polyp

SYMPTOM PICTURE
external wind cold: headache, stuffy nose and sinuses, nasal discharge, frontal pain, chills, sneezing

PREPARATION
Use: The root Angelica Bai Zhi is decocted or used as a tincture.
Dosage: Decoction: 3-10 g
Tincture: 2-4 ml
Caution: Contraindicated during pregnancy. Because of its rather drying nature, do not use in Blood (metabolic) or Yin deficiency. Avoid using with open boils and sores.

NOTES
With its aromatic, pungent, warm and dispersing qualities, White angelica root is the most *stimulating* and *drying* of herbs in this section. It is also one of the most versatile. White angelica excells at resolving painful congestion of the sinuses and nose, especially when accompanied by nasal discharge. Largely active in its broad *nasal decongestant, mucostatic, analgesic* and *anti-infective* effects is the high essential oil content, which includes significant coumarins. The remedy's excellent *analgesic* action is extended in formulas for relieving vertex headache of any kind.

Traditionally, White angelica root was considered more than a botanical for onsets of wind cold. It was also very much a woman's herb, commonly used for difficult, painful menses and white discharges, as well as for cosmetic purposes (Porter Smith 1881). This is not surprising, coming from an *Angelica,* and certainly is in keeping with the remedy's overal pharmacological and therapeutic profile.

The **Western Angelica root,** *Angelica archangelica,* is used for many of the above conditions (among others), and would present a fair substitute if necessary. Both plants contain a similar essential oil, and share identical and similar constituents such as phellandrene and angelic acid. However, of the two, White angelica is more *drying* and *analgesic.*

Note that in China's southwestern province Yunnan, the botanical source for the remedy Bai Zhi is frequently *Heracleum scabridum* Franchet—actually a species of cow parsnip.

Allium Cong Bai
Fresh Scallion Bulb

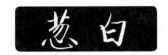

Botanical source: *Allium fistulosum* L. (Liliaceae)
Chinese names: Cong Bai (Mand); Chan Baak (Cant)
Category: mild remedy with minimal chronic toxicity
Constituents: essential oil, allicin, allyl sulfide, malic/palmitic/stearic/arachidic/oleic/linoleic acids, pectin, vitamins A, B1, B2, C
Effective qualities: pungent, warm, dry; stimulating, dispersing
Tropism: respiratory, digestive systems; Lung, Stomach channels

ACTIONS: *Diaphoretic, nasal decongestant, expectorant, antibacterial, antifungal, analgesic, digestant, diuretic*
INDICATIONS: The onset of upper respiratory infections of the wind cold type with nasal congestion; especially gram-positive bacterial and gram-negative bacillary infections; bronchitis, abdominal pain.
Dosage: Decoction: 2-5 fresh bulbs (or 3-10 g) in a short 5 minute decoction with the lid on, drunk hot.
Tincture: 2-4 ml.
Caution: None.

Centipeda E Bu Shi Cao
Centipeda Herb

Botanical source: *Centipeda minima* (L.) A. Brown and Ascherson (Compositae)
Chinese names: E Bu Shi Cao (Mand)
Category: mild remedy with minimal chronic toxicity
Constituents: alkaloid, glycoside, essential oil, saponin, bitter myriogynin
Effective qualities: pungent, warm; restoring, stimulating
Tropism: respiratory, digestive, musculoskelatal systems; Lung, Spleen channels

ACTIONS: *Nasal decongestant, anti-inflammatory, analgesic, detumescent, antitussive, antiemetic, antiparasitic*
INDICATIONS: Respiratory infections involving wind cold and lung wind cold, incl. rhinitis (all types), chronic bronchitis; abdominal pain, diarrhea, arthritis, vomiting, sore eyes; parasitic infestation (incl. roundworm, amoeba and malaria).

Topically for snake bite, boils, corns and neurogenic eczema.

Dosage: Short Decoction: 3-9 g
Tincture: 1-3 ml
Caution: None.

Nose, Throat and Eye Relaxants and Sedatives

REMEDIES TO REDUCE INFLAMMATION AND RELIEVE PAIN IN THE THROAT AND EYES
➤ RELEASE THE EXTERIOR AND DISPEL WIND HEAT WITH PUNGENT, COOL REMEDIES
Anti-inflammatories, analgesics, diaphoretics

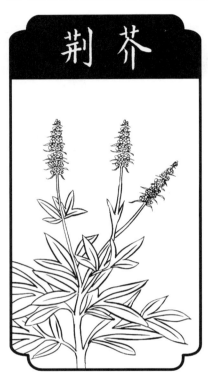

Schizonepeta Jing Jie
Japanese Catnip Herb

Botanical source: *Schizonepeta tenuifolia* Briquet (Labiatae)
Pharmaceutical name: Herba Schizonepetae
Chinese names: Jing Jie (Mand); Ging Gai (Cant)
Other names: Keigai (Jap)
Habit: Aromatic annual temperate Asian herb found on grassland and mountain slopes; mainly cutlivated in the provinces of Jiangsu, Zhejiang and Jiangxi; blooms in summer with terminal spikes of small pink flowers.
Part used: the herb

Therapeutic category: mild remedy with minimal chronic toxicity
Constituents: essential oil (incl. limonene, menthones)
Effective qualities: pungent, a bit warm, neutral
calming, relaxing, stimulating, dispersing
Tropism: upper respiratory, nervous systems
Lung, Liver channels
Warmth body

ACTIONS AND INDICATIONS
upper respiratory sedative: anti-inflammatory: upper respiratory infections with sore throat and irritability; pharyngitis, laryngitis
vasodilatant diaphoretic: common cold and flu with fever
rash-promoting, dermal resolvent: eruptive diseases (incl. measles); eczema, scabies, urticaria, boils, abscesses
nervous sedative, spasmolytic: unrest, headache, spasms, tremors, cramps, seizures
hemostatic: bleeding (mild), incl. blood in stool, nosebleed, uterine bleeding
anthelmintic: hookworm (ankylostomiasis)

SYMPTOM PICTURE
external wind cold/heat: sore throat, chills, sneezing, feverishness, headache, dizziness, unrest

PREPARATION
Use: The herb Schizonepeta Jing Jie is infused or used as a tincture. Charring brings out its *hemostatic* action.
Dosage: Infusion: 3-10 g
Tincture: 2-4 ml
Caution: Do not use this herb if sweating is already present in fevers or with fully erupted measles or sores. Liver wind conditions, i.e. those including spasms or tremors of the extremities, are also a contraindication.

NOTES
The pungent Japanese catnip has virtually identical uses to the Western variety, *Nepeta cataria*, except that it is also used to promote the eruption of rashes. This common remedy has essential

oils to show for both its *dispersing/stimulating* and its *relaxing/calming* effects. Both types of catnip may be used interchangeably for wind heat onset of infections with sore throat, chills, feverishness and irritability—their main indications.

Mentha Bo He
Asian Fieldmint Herb

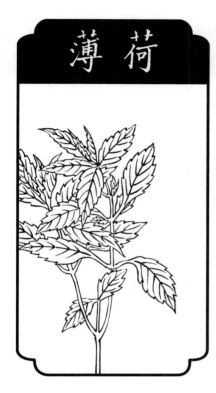

Botanical sourec: *Mentha arvensis* L. var. *haplocalyx* Briquet (Labiatae)
Pharmaceutical name: Herba Menthae arvensis
Chinese name: Bo He (Mand); Bok Hau, Bak Hau (Cant)
Other names: Cornmint; Hakka (Jap)
Habit: Hairy perennial temperate herb that prefers damp soil, such as river banks; cultivated in the coastal provinces Jiangsu, Jiangxi and Zhejiang; blooms in autumn in small lilac, pink or white axillary flower clusters.
Part used: the herb

Therapeutic category: mild remedy with minimal chronic toxicity
Constituents: essential oil c. 1.6% (incl. menthol 32-66%, menthone, camphene, limonene, pinene, pugelone, piperitone, azulene), tannins, resin, rosmarinic acid
Effective qualities: pungent, a bit sweet, cool
relaxing, calming, decongesting, dispersing
Tropism: upper respiratory, lymphatic, digestive systems
Lung, Liver channels
Warmth, Air bodies

ACTIONS AND INDICATIONS

upper respiratory sedative: anti-inflammatory, analgesic: acute upper respiratory infections with pain; pharyngitis, laryngitis, conjunctivitis, headache, earache, chest, rib and flank pain or pressure
vasodilatant diaphoretic: onset of common cold or flu with fever
rash-promoting: early stage of measles before eruptions
lymphatic decongestant: lymphadenitis from infection
choleretic, carminative: biliary dyspepsia, flatulence, nausea
antipruritic: pruritus
antitumoral: stomach cancer, local tumors
anesthetic, antiseptic

SYMPTOM PICTURE

external wind heat: headache, sore throat, swollen glands, itchy or red eyes, fever, some chills, no sweating

PREPARATION

Use: The herb Mentha Bo He should be infused or taken in tincture form. When part of a decoction it should be added at the end of cooking time and the decoction then left to infuse another 10 minutes.
Dosage: Infusion: 3-6 g
Tincture: 2-3 ml
Caution: Contraindicated if sweating has already begun (as in external deficiency conditions) and in Yin deficiency fevers.

NOTES

Asian fieldmint herb is commonly used to relax the pores and promote sweating at the onset of colds and flus. Its gentle *diaphoretic* effect also ensures full eruptions of rashes with measles, while the *analgesic* action relieves the pain of throat and eye infections. Being a mild *lymphatic stimulant* merely adds to Asian fieldmint's usefulness in these conditions traditionally classed as wind heat disorders.

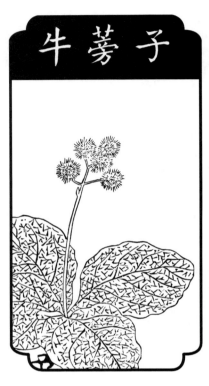

Arctium Niu Bang Zi
Burdock Seed

Botanical source: *Arctium lappa* L. (Compositae)
Pharmaceutical name: Fructus Arctii
Chinese names: Niu Bang Zi, Da Li Zi, Niu Zi, Shu Zhan Zi, Wu shi, Shu Nian (Mand); Ngau Gon Ji (Cant)
Other names: Great burdock, Cocklebur; Goboshi (Jap)
Habit: Wild and cultivated biennial herb growing on temperate grassy slopes, on roadsides and in gullies; lavender-colored flowers appear in summer as terminal corymb heads.
Part used: the fruit

Therapeutic category: mild remedy with minimal chronic toxicity
Constituents: arctiin, arctigenin, gobosterin, arachidic acid, essential oil, stearic/oleic/linoleic/palmitic acids, iodine, vitamins A, B1
Effective qualities: pungent, bitter, a bit sweet, cool, moist
  stimulating, dispersing, softening
Tropism: respiratory, digestive systems
  Lung, Stomach channels
  Warmth body

ACTIONS AND INDICATIONS

upper respiratory sedative: anti-inflammatory, demulcent: acute throat infections with pain and hoarseness; laryngitis, pharyngitis
diaphoretic, stimulant expectorant: common cold and flu with fever, productive cough
interferon inducent, antiviral, antibacterial, antifungal: miscellaneous infections (incl. HIV infection)
rash-promoting: incomplete rash formation in eruptive fevers (e.g. measles, chickenpox)
detoxicant: boils, carbuncle, ulcers
demulcent laxative: constipation from dryness
hypoglycemiant

SYMPTOM PICTURE

external wind heat and **lung wind heat:** fever, sore swollen throat, coughing with sputum, wheezing, dry stool

PREPARATION

Use: A short decoction is the best preparation for the crushed seed Arctium Niu Bang Zi. A tincture may also be used.
Dosage: Decoction: 5-10 g
  Tincture: 2-4 ml
Caution: Burdock seed should not be used in diarrhea or open purulent boils.

NOTES

A soothing *anti-inflammatory demulcent,* Burdock seed is one of the main remedies for red, swollen sore throat with onset of infection of the wind heat variety. Its *diaphoretic* and *anti-infective* actions are useful not only in upper respiratory infections but also in eruptive fevers.

In the Western herbal tradition, **Burdock root** is used for its *detoxicant diuretic* and *urinary restorative* properties.

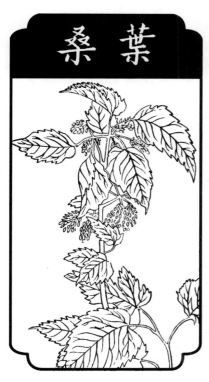

Morus Sang Ye
Mulberry Leaf

Botanical source: *Morus alba* L. (Moraceae)
Pharmaceutical name: Folium Mori
Chinese names: Sang Ye, Dong Sang Ye, Shuang Sang Ye (Mand); Song Yip (Cant)
Other names: White mulberry; Soyo (Jap)
Habit: Deciduous temperate East Asian tree, much cultivated for silkworm culture throughout China; flowers in May with stalked hanging catkins.
Part used: the leaf

Therapeutic category: mild remedy with minimal chronic toxicity
Constituents: organic acids, trace minerals, amino acids, phytoestrogens, flavonoids (incl. quercetin, isoquercetin, moracetin, rutin), sitosterol, campesterol, lupeol, myoinositol, inokosterone, ecdysterone, guaiacol, essential oil (incl. phenol, eugenol), fumaric/palmitic acids, amylase, sucrose, flucose, folic acid, choline, vitamins A, B1, B2
Effective qualities: sweet, a bit bitter, cool
calming, restoring, stimulating, dispersing
Tropism: respiratory tract, pancreas
Lung, Liver channels; Warmth body

ACTIONS AND INDICATIONS

upper respiratory sedative: anti-inflammatory, analgesic, antiseptic: acute upper respiratory infections with nasal congestion and pain; sinusitis, headache, pharyngitis, acute conjunctivitis
diaphoretic: onset of common cold and flu with fever
stimulant expectorant: acute bronchitis with coughing
hypoglycemiant: diabetes
vision restorative: poor vision, spots in vision
interferon inducent

SYMPTOM PICTURES

external wind heat: nasal congestion, painful sinuses, headache, fever

lung wind heat: feverishness, headache, dry cough, red, sore, tearing eyes, thirst

PREPARATION
Use: The leaf Morus Sang Ye is briefly decocted, infused or used in tincture form.
Dosage: Infusion and short decoction: 6-14 g
Tincture: 2-5 ml
Caution: None.

NOSE, THROAT AND EYE RELAXANTS/SEDATIVES

NOTES
The leaf of the East Asian Mulberry tree provides an excellent remedy for the symptom picture wind heat. Its *diaphoretic* and *expectorant* actions comprehensively resolve not only upper respiratory infections, but also fever and coughing. In the West, Elder flower is used in a similar way.

Chrysanthemum Ju Hua
Chrysanthemum Flower

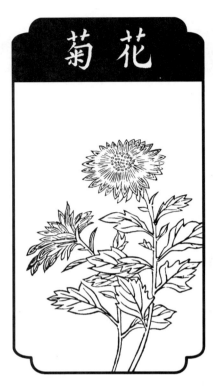

Botanical source: *Chrysanthemumx* x *morifolium* Ramatuelle (Compositae)
Pharmaceutical name: Flos Chrysanthemi
Chinese names: Ju Hua, Huang Ju Hua, Gan Ju Hua (Mand); Guk Fa (Cant)
Other names: Florist's chrysanthemum, Mum; Kikuka (Jap)
Habit: Widely distributed perennial East Asian herb; cultivated in Zhejiang, Anhui, Henan and Sichuan; white, yellow or pink flowers bloom in autumn.
Part used: the flowerhead

Therapeutic category: mild remedy with minimal chronic toxicity
Constituents: essential oil (incl. camphor, carvone, camphene, chrysanthenone, borneol, bornyl acetate), alkaloids, flavonoids (luteolin, cosmosiin, acacetinrhamnosyl), adenine, choline, stachydrine, chrysandiol, trimethylcyclohexene-carboxylic acid, amino acids, vitamins B1, E, trace minerals
Effective qualities: sweet, a bit bitter, cool
calming, relaxing
Tropism: respiratory, cardiovascular, nervous systems, eyes
Lung, Liver channels
Warmth, Air bodies

ACTIONS AND INDICATIONS
upper respiratory sedative: anti-inflammatory, anti-infective (antiviral, antibacterial, antifungal),
diaphoretic: early stage of acute infections (esp. upper and lower respiratory, esp. with fever, incl. sinusitis, tonsilitis, pharyngitis, bronchitis, conjunctivitis, trachoma)
resolvent detoxicant: boils, abscesses
nervous relaxant: headache, dizziness, tinnitus, vision problems
hypotensive coronary dilator: hypertension, coronary deficiency/disease with angina pectoris, arteriosclerosis
hair restorative: hair loss, early hair graying
antispirochetal

SYMPTOM PICTURES
external wind heat: fever, headache, dry red eyes, sore throat, irritability

heart Qi constraint (Liver Yang rising): dizziness, floaters in vision, headache, ringing in ears

heart blood and Qi stagnation: chest tightness and pain, palpitations, anxiety

PREPARATION
Use: The flower Chrysanthemum Ju Hua is either infused or used in tincture form. Chrysanthemum wine is traditionally drunk for longevity at the Chong Yang festival (the 9th day of the 9th month).
Dosage: Infusion: 10-20 g
Tincture: 2-5 ml
Caution: None.

Notes

In Chinese culture, the chrysanthemum is one of several plants elevated to the level of an emblem, inspiring more botanical writings through the ages than any other. This winter flower was described as a "virtuous recluse" by a Song philosopher, Zhou Dun-yi, because it prefers to flower alone in fall rather than in the "crowded market-place of spring." Chrysanthemum is generally associated with the wistful, romantic, withdrawn melancholy of that season—corresponding to the *aware* mood of the Japanese haiku poem.

There are actually two types of cultivated chrysanthemum, the white and the yellow (sweet) chrysanthemum. The white variety is better for treating problems with the eyes and vision. The yellow, being more dispersing by nature, is considered more effective in clearing wind heat syndromes that present symptoms of headache, red eyes and fever. A *cooling, anti-infective* and *diaphoretic* remedy for upper respiratory infections manifesting a fever and sore throat, Chrysanthemum flower is traditionally considered one of the best for wind heat conditions. Its *nervous-* and *vasorelaxant* properties were traditionally used to best advantage with local infections. Today, it also ranks, like the related Wild chrysanthemum, among China's top twelve remedies for systemic hypertension and coronary disease.

Camomile flower, in the same botanical family, is the closest Western herb with similar properties. Chrysanthemum flower is a more effective *antiseptic* and *hypertensive,* whereas Camomile (the German, Roman and Morroccan varieties) possesses superior *anti-inflammatory* and *analgesic* properties.

Chimonanthus La Mei Hua
Wintersweet Flower

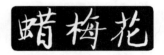

Botanical source: *Chimonanthus praecox* (L.) Link (Calycanthaceae)
Chinese names: La Mei Hua (Mand); Lat Mui Fa (C)

Category: mild remedy with minimal chronic toxicity
Effective qualities: pungent, bitter, neutral; calming
Tropism: respiratory, optic systems; Liver, Lung channels

ACTIONS: *Anti-inflammatory, analgesic, detoxicant*
INDICATIONS: Wind heat type infections, incl. tonsilitis, pharyngitis, difficulty in swallowing; red, irritated eyes; the recovery stage of measles; spider bites
Dosage: Decoction: 3-10 g
　　　　　Tincture: 2-4 ml
Caution: Forbidden during pregnancy as it is also a *uterine stimulant.*

Ilex Gang Mei
Rough Holly Leaf and Root *

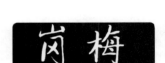

Botanical source: *Ilex asprella* (Hooker et Arn.) Champion ex Bentham (Aquifoliaceae)
Chinese names: Gang Mei (Mand); Gong Mui (Cant)
Category: mild remedy with minimal chronic toxicity

Effective qualities: pungent, bitter, cool; calming, astringing
Tropism: respiratory, digestive systems; Lung, Stomach channels

ACTIONS: *Anti-infective, anti-inflammatory, analgesic, astringent, detoxicant*
INDICATIONS: Wind heat onset of infections with fever, acute tonsilitis, pharyngitis, bronchitis; enteritis, hepatitis, mushroom poisoning.
Dosage: Decoction: 10-15 g
　　　　　Tincture: 2-4 ml
Caution: None.

NOSE, THROAT AND EYE RELAXANTS/SEDATIVES

Ilex Jiu Bi Ying
Round-Leaf Holly Leaf *

Botanical source: *Ilex rotunda* Thunberg (Aquifoliaceae)
Chinese names: Jiu Bi Ying (Mand); Gau Bit Ying
Category: mild remedy with minimal chronic toxicity

Effective qualities: pungent, bitter, cool; calming, astringing
Tropism: gastrointestinal, digestive, epidermal systems; Lung, Stomach channels

ACTIONS: *Anti-infective, anti-inflammatory, analgesic, astringent, hemostatic*
INDICATIONS: Onset of infections with wind heat, including colds, fever, tonsilitis, laryngitis; acute gastroenteritis, pancreatitis, peptic ulcer, rheumatic bone pain; externally for injuries, boils, burns, neurogenic dermatitis.
Dosage: Decoction: 10-15 g
    Tincture: 2-4 ml
Caution: None.

Tagetes Wan Shou Ju
African/French Marigold Flower

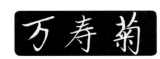

Botanical source: *Tagetes erecta* (Compositae)
Chinese names: Wan Shou Ju (Mand)
Category: mild remedy with minimal chronic toxicity
Constituents: essential oil (incl. syscaryophyllene, mycenol, cadinene, tagetenone)
Effective qualities: bitter, pungent, cool; calming, softening
Tropism: respiratory system; Lung meridian

ACTIONS: *Antiseptic, anti-inflammatory, analgesic, mucolytic expectorant*
INDICATIONS: Wind heat conditions such as upper respiratory infections, laryngitis, conjunctivitis; stomatitis, toothache, bronchitis; topically for mastitis and boils.
Dosage: Decoction: 10-15 g
    Tincture: 2-5 ml
    Essential oil: 2-4 drops in some water
Caution: None.
NOTES: The essential oil from various Tagetes species is distilled in parts of Africa, Australia, East Asia and the South of France; it is called Tagette or Tagetes essential oil.

Sterculia Pang Da Hai
Sterculia Seed

Botanical source: *Sterculia scaphigera* Wall. (Sterculiaceae)
Chinese names: Pang Da Hai, Tong Da Hai (Mand); Pan Dai Hoi (Cant)
Habitat: large tropical tree, Indo-Malayia and South China
Category: mild remedy with minimal chronic toxicity
Constituents: bassinose, arabinose, galactose
Effective qualities: sweet, cold; calming, astringing
Tropism: respiratory, digestive, cardiovascular systems; Lung, Large Intestine channels

ACTIONS: *Demulcent, anti-inflammatory, laxative, hypotensive, hemostatic*
INDICATIONS: Wind heat infections with sore throat, acute laryngitis, tonsilitis, hoarseness, cough due to acute bronchitis; dry stool, constipation, enteritis, nosebleeds, blood in stool, coughing blood; fever, sunstroke, toothache, intestinal parasites, hemorrhoids, fistula.

Dosage: Decoction or infusion: 4-10 g
Tincture: 1-3 ml
Topical applications are made to help the rashes of measles, etc. to surface.
Caution: None.

Oroxylum Mu Hu Die
Oroxylum Seed

Botanical source: *Oroxylum indicum* (L.) Ventenat (Bignoniaceae)
Chinese names: Mu Hu Die (Mand); Mok Fu Dai (Cant)
Habitat: Small (semi) tropical tree from India, south China and Malaysia
Part used: the winged disseminules (the flat seeds encased in a sheath the appearance of a silken pale yellow butterfly wing)
Category: mild remedy with minimal chronic toxicity
Constituents: oroxylin (incl. 3 flavonoids, baicalein, methylbaiclein, chrysin)
Effective qualities: a bit sweet, bitter; calming
Tropism: respiratory, digestive systems; Lung channels

ACTIONS: *Anti-inflammatory, analgesic, antitussive*
INDICATIONS: Wind heat infections with acute and chronic pharyngitis, hoarseness, acute bronchitis, whooping cough; epigastric pain.
Dosage: Decoction: 3-10 g
Tincture: 1-3 ml
Caution: None.

Lasiosphaera Ma Bo
Puffball Mushroom

Botanical source: *Lasiosphaera fenslii* Reich. or *L. nipponica* (Kawam.) Y. Kobayashi, or *Calvatia lilacina* (Lycoperdaceae)
Chinese names: Ma Bo (Mand); Ma Bot (Cant)
Category: mild remedy with minimal chronic toxicity
Constituents: gemmatein, tyrosine, urea, ergosterol, lipids, polysaccharide
Effective qualities: pungent, cool, dry; calming, astringing, thickening
Tropism: vascular, respiratory systems; Lung meridian

ACTIONS: *Anti-inflammatory, antibacterial, antiseptic, hemostatic, styptic, antitussive*
INDICATIONS: Acute throat inflammation (laryngitis, pharyngitis), hoarseness, cough; nosebleeds, bleeding from trauma, from lips, gums and mouth; surgical hemorrhage, frostbite. Topically in swabs, mouthwashes and gargles for painful throat, bleeding, etc.
Dosage: Decoction: 2-6 g
Tincture: 0.5-2 ml
Caution: Lasiosphaera Ma Bo is extremely dusty and should be handled with a mask over the mouth. The mushroom is cooked separately in a cheese cloth or filter paper nodulus. Contraindicated in voice loss from wind cold onset of infections.

Borax Peng Sha
Borax

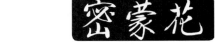

Geological name: *Borax*
Chinese names: Peng Sha, Zhong Peng Suan Na, Yue Shi (Mand); Paan Sha (Cant); "Peng granules"
Source: Western provinces Xizang (Tibet) and Qinghai
Category: mild remedy with minimal chronic toxicity

Constituents: hydrated sodium tetraborate
Effective qualities: sweet, salty, cool; calming, astringing, stimulating, dissolving
Tropism: respiratory, digestive systems; Lung Stomach channels

ACTIONS: *Anti-inflammatory, antibacterial, astringent, mucolytic expectorant, urinary litholytic*
INDICATIONS: Acute laryngitis, pharyngitis, tonsilitis and stomatitis with pain and swelling; mouth ulcers and sores; draining vaginal lesions; cough with hard sputum in acute bronchitis; urinary gravel and stones; toe blisters.
Dosage: Decoction: 3-6 g
Powder and pill: 1.5-3 g
Borax powder is also used for gargling and mouthwashes in tonsilitis, stuck bone in throat, and mouth and tongue sores. The powder may also be blown directly onto mouth and throat sores. A paste is prepared for external application in cases of skin ulcers.
Caution: Forbidden during pregnancy.
NOTES: Like the majority of other mineral remedies, borax was also used in metallurgy. Borax is collected on lake shores in arid western China, especially Tibet.

Buddleia Mi Meng Hua
Buddleia Flower and Bud

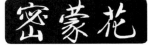

Botanical source: *Buddleia officinalis* Maximowicz (Loganiaceae)
Chinese names: Mi Meng Hua (Mand); Muk Mein Fa (Cant)

Category: mild remedy with minimal chronic toxicity
Constituents: buddleoglucoside, acacetin, buddlein
Effective qualities: sweet, cool; calming, restoring,
Tropism: optic, nervous systems; Liver channel

ACTIONS: *Anti-inflammatory, spasmolytic*
INDICATIONS: Eye inflammations with redness, swelling, pain; tearing, blood-shot eyes; cataract; irritability with ringing in ears, sleep loss, dizziness, fear of bright lights (photophobia).
Dosage: Decoction: 6-10 g
Tincture: 1-3 ml
Caution: None.

Celosia Qing Xiang Zi
Silver Quail-Grass Seed

Botanical source: *Celosia argentea* L. (Amaranthaceae)
Chinese names: Qing Xiang Zi (Mand); Ching Heung Ji (Cant)
Category: mild remedy with minimal chronic toxicity

Constituents: nicotinic acid, potassium nitrate
Effective qualities: bitter, cold; calming, astringing
Tropism: digestive, urinary, respiratory, optic systems; Liver channel

ACTIONS: *Anti-inflammatory, antipruritic, antiparasitic, antidiarrheal, vulnerary*
INDICATIONS: Wind heat or liver fire syndromes with red, painful swollen eyes; corneal opacity, superficial visual

obstructions, cataracts, eye inflammations, acute pruritus, leprosy; intestinal parasites; diarrhea, dysuria.
Topically for fractures.

Dosage: Decoction: 4-10 g
Tincture: 2-4 ml
External applications are made for skin and trauma conditions.

Caution: None.

Equisetum Mu Zei
Horsetail Herb

Botanical source: *Equisetum arvense* L. (Equisetaceae)
Chinese names: Mu Zei (Mand); Maan Chok (Cant)
Category: mild remedy with minimal chronic toxicity
Constituents: trace minerals, electrolytes, saponins, silicic acid, flavonoids, alkaloids, phytosterols
Effective qualities: sweet, bitter, astringent, cool; restoring, calming, astringing, stabilizing, solidifying
Tropism: optic, urinary, integumentary, digestive systems; Lung, Liver channels

ACTIONS: *Anti-inflammatory, draining/detoxicant diuretic, astringent, mucostatic, hemostatic, anhydrotic*
INDICATIONS: Wind heat syndrome producing eye inflammations with red, swollen, painful eyes; corneal opacity and other superficial visual obstructions (incl. pterygium); excessive tearing, blurred vision; damp heat infectious conditions (incl. dysentery, leucorrhea); hematuria, menorrhagia, uterine hemorrhage; edema, rectal prolapse, hemorrhoids, spontaneous sweating.
In the West, Horsetail herb is additionally used for other systemic conditions such as connective tissue weaknes, toxicosis and organic lung, kidney and bone disease.

Dosage: Long decoction: 3-10 g
Tincture: 1-4 ml

Caution: None.

Eriocaulon Gu Jing Cao
Pipewort Herb

Botanical source: *Eriocaulon buergerianum* Koernicke or *E. sieboldianum* Siebold et Zuccharini ex Steudel (Eriocaulaceae)
Chinese names: Gu Jing Cao (Mand); Guk Ging Chou (Cant)
Part used: the stalk and flowerhead, i.e. herb
Category: mild remedy with minimal chronic toxicity
Effective qualities: pungent, sweet, cool; calming
Tropism: optic, circulatory systems; Liver, Stomach channels

ACTIONS: *Anti-inflammatory, analgesic, vision restorative, antipyretic, anti-infective*
INDICATIONS: Corneal opacity, pterygium, painful eyes, night blindness, cataract; one-sided headache, sore throat, toothache, nosebleed, fever, infection from *Pseudomonas aeruginosa*.

Dosage: Decoction: 10-15 g
Tincture: 2-5 ml

Caution: Forbidden in metabolic deficiency. Contact with iron should be avoided.

Tamarix Xi He Liu
Chinese Tamarisk Tip

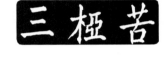

Botanical source: *Tamarix chinensis* Loureiro (Taxaceae)
Chinese names: Xi He Liu, Cheng Li (Mand); Sei Han Lao (Cant)
Part used: the tips or ends of the tree branches
Category: mild remedy with minimal chronic toxicity

Constituents: glycoside salicin
Effective qualities: sweet, salty, cool; stimulating, calming
Tropism: integumentary, musculoskeletal systems; Lung, Heart, Stomach channels

ACTIONS: *Diaphoretic, rash-promoting, anti-inflammatory, antipyretic, analgesic, diuretic, antiprutitic*
INDICATIONS: Wind heat type influenza, eruptive fevers (incl. measles and chickenpox); acute dermatitis, dermal pruritus; allergies, rheumatic myalgia, arthralgia.
Dosage: Decoction: 3-16 g
Tincture: 1-3 ml
Caution: None.

Evodia San Ya Ku
Bitter Evodia Root

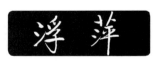

Botanical source: *Evodia lepta* (Spreng.) Merill (syn. *E. pteleaefolia* (Champ.) Merrill (Rutaceae)
Chinese names: San Ya Ku, San Cha Ku, San Jiao Bie, Bai Yun Xiang (Mand); Sam Ga Fu (Cant)

Category: mild remedy with minimal chronic toxicity
Constituents: unknown
Effective qualities: bitter, cold, calming
Tropism: respiratory, hepatic systems; Lung, Liver ch.

ACTIONS: *Anti-infective (antiviral), anti-inflammatory, detoxicant, refrigerant, antipyretic, analgesic, antipruritic*
INDICATIONS: Wind heat onsets of viral infections, incl. flu, cold, pneumonia, adenovirus, RSV, rubeola, varicella, CMV, meningitis, encephalitis; heatstroke, fever, tonsillitis, pharyngitis; viral hepatitis; rheumatoid arthritis, neuritis (incl. sciatica), lumbago; itch; poisoning by *Gelsmium elegans*.
 Topical applications are prepared for eczema, acute dermatitis, tissue trauma, infected wounds, abscesses.
Dosage: Decoction: 10-15 g. If the leaves are used, the dose is 10-30 g by short decoction.
Tincture: 2-5 ml
Caution: None.
NOTES: This remedy is an excellent prophylactic in the presence of viral epidemics such as the flu.

Spirodela Fu Ping
Duckweed Herb

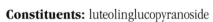

Botanical source: *Spirodela polyrrhiza* or *Lemna minor* L. (Lemnaceae)
Chinese names: Fu Ping (Mand); Fau Ping (Cant)
Category: mild remedy with minimal chronic toxicity

Constituents: luteolinglucopyranoside
Effective qualities: pungent, cool; decongesting
Tropism: urinary, epidermal, cardiovascular, systems; Lung channel

ACTIONS: *Diaphoretic, rash-promoting, diuretic*
INDICATIONS: Wind heat onsets of infections with headache, body aches, skin rashes, fever; oliguria; upper body edema.
Dosage: Short decoction: 10-20 g
Tincture: 2-4 ml
Caution: None.

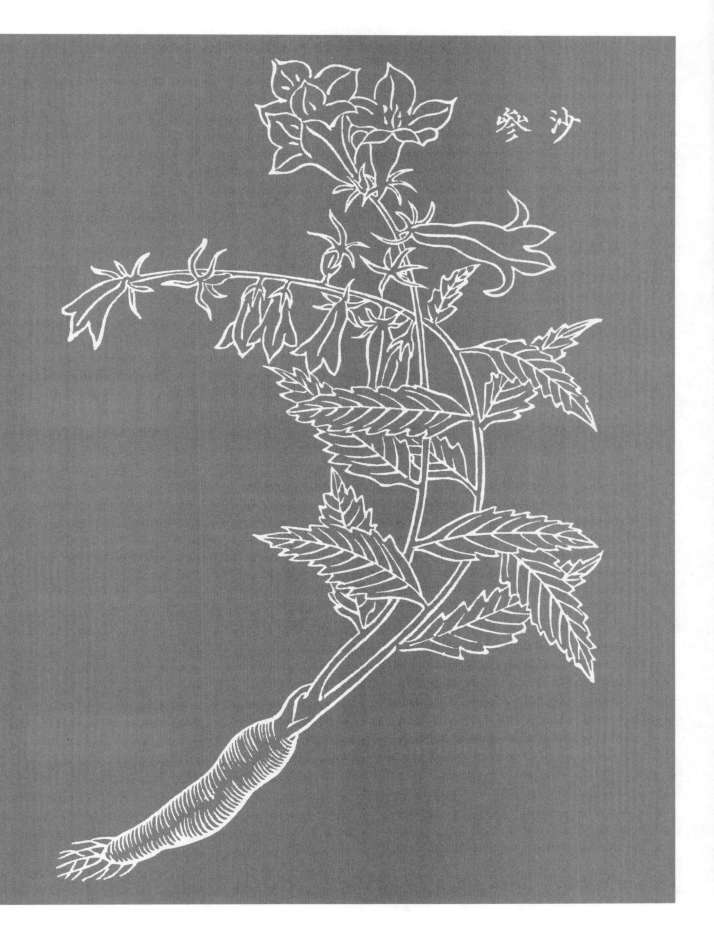

呼吸系统用药

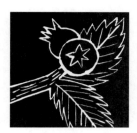

Remedies for the Respiratory System

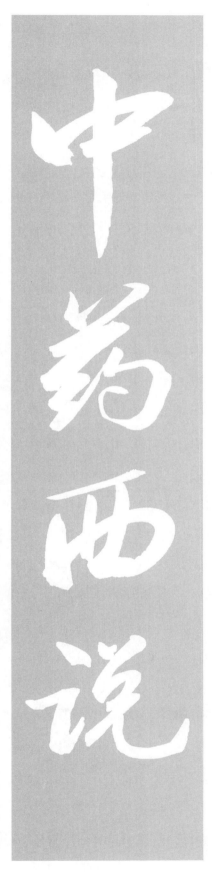

The Chinese pharmacy is particularly rich in remedies for respiratory ailments, not only because of the importance Oriental doctors have laid on treating acute pulmonary conditions, but also because of the constitutional factors inherent in Asians. Respiratory remedies include a wide variety of herb types ranging from *restorative cool demulcents,* such as Ophiopogon Mai Men Dong (Dwarf lilyturf root), to *cold astringents,* such as Lycium Di Gu Pi (Wolfberry root bark). Oriental herbal medicine is fully equipped to deal not only with infectious diseases but also—and especially, to our adavantage—various functional and preclinical pathologies.

Using the Western model of energetic herb actions, we may divide respiratory remedies into four types: *restoratives, stimulants, relaxants* and *sedatives.* These four correlate well with traditional Chinese herb categories for managing respiratory problems. However, the terms used in Chinese medicine differ somewhat from their Western counterparts.

Each remedy type addresses a particular type of bronchial condition, as follows:

- ***Respiratory restoratives*** treat two types of respiratory deficiencies:
    - deficiency conditions with dryness, irritation or inflammation (heat), presenting dry cough.
    - deficiencies accompanied by weak cough.
- ***Respiratory stimulants*** address deficiency and cold conditions with catarrhal congestion, presenting a productive cough.
- ***Respiratory relaxants*** treat excess conditions with bronchial spasm, presenting wheezing and uncontrollable cough.
- ***Respiratory sedatives*** treat excess conditions with infection and inflammation, displaying a productive cough.

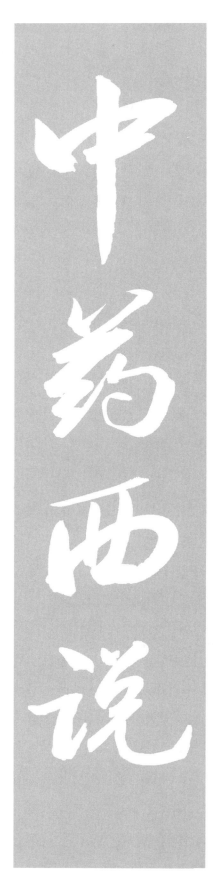

The Respiratory Remedies

Restoratives

The lungs are organs that, in terms of natural qualities, require coolness and moisture for optimum functioning. They dislike environmental heat and dryness, which cause problems involving irritation and inflammation. Such syndromes as **lung dryness** and **lung Yin deficiency** may arise, typically presenting dry, irritating cough and possibly blood-streaked sputum. If the whole system becomes dehydrated—whether due to climate, fever or constitution—signs of thirst; dry mouth and throat; hard, dry stool; hot spells and low-grade fever may join signs of the respiratory system.

In this case Oriental doctors speak of **Yin deficiency, Yin and fluids deficiency** and **deficiency heat** as the pathologies involved. The Yin, in this respect, represents the body's internal moisture and coolness. Such deficiency syndromes are found, for example, with chronic bronchitis, lung TB, croup, dehydration, heat exhaustion, diabetes, Sjögren's syndrome and low-grade remittent fevers.

Respiratory restorative herbs of the first type are sweet, cool and moist. They have a *demulcent* effect that soothes tissue irritation and reduce inflammation, and a *mucogenic* effect that promotes mucus secretion along the mucosa, thereby helping maintain moisture throughout the whole system. Their moisturizing and cooling action is not only a localized one, but a systemic one. This is why Chinese herbal texts discuss "nourishing the Yin, generating fluids, moistening dryness and clearing deficiency heat" with these *demulcents* and *mucogenics*.

Because *bronchial demulcents* renew bronchial sputum, they paradoxically often exert a secondary *mucolytic* action that softens and helps expectorate (cough up) dry, hard sputum. These *mucolytic expectorants* are therefore also frequently used for the syndrome **lung phlegm dryness,** characterized by difficult coughing with scanty, sticky sputum.

Six of the eleven *respiratory restoratives* presented here belong to the lily family, and most contain both saponins and mucilage as biochemical components of their therapeutic action. *Respiratory restoratives* include the commonly used root of the dwarf lilyturf from China, Korea and Japan (Ophiopogon Mai Men Dong); a highly-prized variety of fritillary from Sichuan province (Fritillaria Chuan Bei Mu); a bonnet bellflower variety from the sandy coastal provinces (Adenophora Nan Sha Shen; and two types of Solomon's seal (Polygonatum Huang Jing and Polygonatum Yu Zhu). No other pharmacy boasts such numbers in treating conditions of internal dryness and Yin deficiency, nor does anyone treat these conditions more effectively than the Chinese.

The second type of *respiratory restorative* addresses the Chinese subclinical syndrome **lung Qi deficiency,** characterized by shortness of breath, a feeble cough, fatigue, bouts of spontaneous sweating, hesitant, low voice and depression. This symptom complex often implies allergies, chronic bronchitis, lung tuberculosis and emphysema.

Respiratory restoratives of this type are said to "increase the Qi/energy." They include Astragalus Huang Qi (Astragalus root, a milkvetch type from the North China grasslands), Codonopsis Dang Shen (Downy bellflower root, a twining vine from the woods and gullies of the Northeast) and Panax Xi Yang Shen (American ginseng root from North America's Northeast). However, because these remedies are especially valuable for metabolic and hormonal deficiency conditions—essentially for systemically tonifying the body's Qi, of which lung Qi is a part—they are presented in the gastrointestinal and endocrine system sections.

Stimulants

Respiratory stimulants have a pungent, warm and dry nature that stimulates the bronchi, promoting a productive cough with expulsion of sputum. These remedies that "warm and transform phlegm cold" are called *stimulant expectorants*. They are appropriate in bronchial conditions of deficiency cold, such as **lung phlegm cold/damp.** This would be characterized by nasal and chest congestion, the coughing up of clear, white phlegm, and cold hands and feet. Bronchitis, bronchial asthma and emphysema are typical Western conditions that fall in this category.

The two remedies most widely used in classical formulations for these conditions are Pinellia Ban Xia (Prepared pinellia corm, a South Chinese alkaloidal plant in the arum family) and Platycodon Jie Geng (Ballonflower root, a saponin-rich type of bluebell common throughout Northeast Asia). The action of most *stimulant expectorants* is due largely to their essential oil content, through which they also disinfect the airways—although they variously also contain alkaloids, saponins and glycosides.

Several *stimulant expectorants,* such as the highly pungent Asarum Xi Xin (Asian wild ginger root and herb from North China and Japan) and Peucedanum Qian Hu (Asian masterwort root, an umbellifer from Mid and North China), also have a *diaphoretic* and *anti-infective* action. As a result, they are frequently used in **lung wind cold** syndromes. Some of these are already familiar to Westerners from related genuses growing in the United States and Europe. Among these are: *Asarum, Cynanchum, Sinapis* and *Peucedanum.*

Relaxants

Respiratory relaxants are used in symptom patterns of **lung Qi constraint,** such as in bronchial asthma and chronic bronchitis. Essentially, they are *bronchial dilators* that "circulate and lower lung Qi" or "ventilate the lungs," thereby relieving wheezing, chest tightness, difficult breathing and uncontrollable coughing.

Bronchodilators, also known as *antiasthmatics,* tend to be

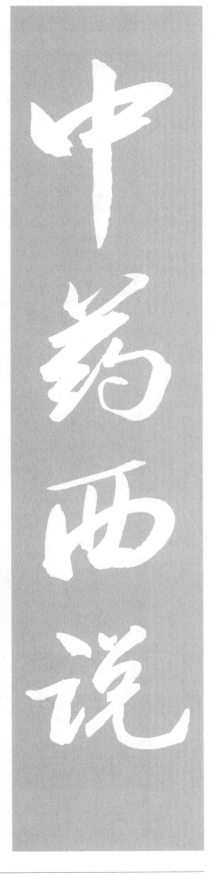

RESPIRATORY SYSTEM

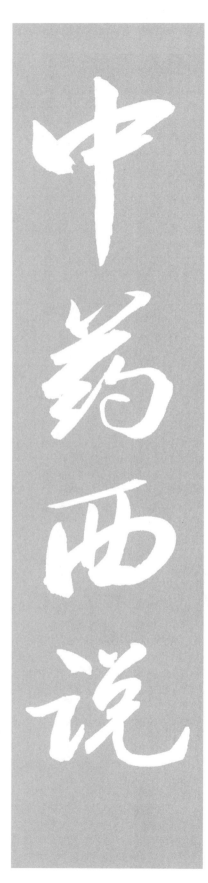

either pungent-warm or bitter-cold in nature. Chemically these remedies contain essential oils (e.g., in Perilla Zi Su Zi, the seed of the common and cultivated Perilla), alkaloids (e.g., ephedrine contained in Ephedra Ma Huang, the undershrub from Mongolia and North China), saponins and glycosides. These components account for their *relaxant* action on the bronchi and their frequent *anti-inflammatory* and *antitussive* (cough relieving) effect. Examples of true *antitussives* that treat uncontrollable coughing by neurologically reducing the cough reflex include Stemona Bai Bu (Stemona root from Central China and Taiwan), Aster Zi Wan (Tartary aster root from North Asia), Fritillaria Chuan Bei Mu (Sichuan fritillary bulb) and Fritillaria Zhe Bei Mu (Zhejiang fritillary bulb).

Interestingly, two mineral remedies are found among the wide selection of *antiasthmatics* in this section. The first is Hematite, a type of brown iron oxide from North China. The other is Stalactite tip, a spelunkine remedy collected throughout China that consists mainly of calcium carbonate.

A special type of *respiratory relaxant* or *antiasthmatic* owes its action to a tonification, in Chinese medical terms, of **Lung and Kidney Yang deficiency.** These remedies, which include Juglans Hu Tao Ren (Walnut meat) and Cordyceps Dong Chong Xia Cao (Caterpillar mushroom, an obscure fungus from East China and Tibet), relieve asthmatic breathing by restoring the underlying deficiency of the kidney-adrenal system. Their *adrenocortical restorative* action signals a systemic enhancement of metabolism. As a result, the three remedies in this category are also frequently used for systemic deficiency conditions presenting chronic tiredness and weakness, especially when also involving urogenital functions. Such functions fall under the umbrella of the Kidney Yang channel network in Chinese medicine.

Sedatives
Remedies in this category do not literally sedate respiratory functions; rather they sedate the heat and irritation of lung tissue brought on by infection. By reducing infection and inflammation, and by promoting expectoration, they are said to "cool and transform hot phlegm." *Respiratory sedatives* have *antiseptic, anti-inflammatory* and *astringent* properties in addition to *expectorant* ones. Their effective qualities are sweet-cool or bitter-cool, as seen, for instance, in the frequently used Houttuynia Yu Xing Cao (Fishwort herb from temperate East Asia) and Fritillaria Zhe Bei Mu (Zhejiang fritillary bulb from China's east coast).

The main symptom picture that *anti-inflammatory/antiseptic expectorants* address is **lung phlegm heat,** typified by coughing with expectoration of thick yellow or green phlegm, thirst and feverishness. When properly combined in a comprehensive formula, these remedies ensure adequate management of acute respiratory infections like bronchitis and bacterial pneumonia.

Respiratory Restoratives

REMEDIES TO PROVIDE MOISTURE, PROMOTE SECRETIONS AND RELIEVE RESPIRATORY DRYNESS

➥ NOURISH THE YIN, GENERATE FLUIDS AND MOISTEN DRYNESS
Bronchial demulcents, mucogenics, mucolytic expectorants

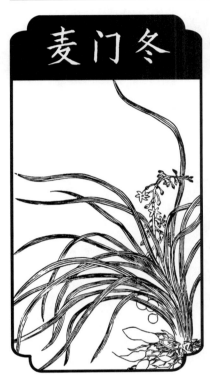

Ophiopogon Mai Men Dong
Dwarf Lilyturf Root

Botanical source: *Ophiopogon japonicus* (Thunb.) Ker-Gawler, syn. *Liriope spicata* Loureiro (Liliaceae)
Pharmaceutical name: Radix Ophiopogonis
Chinese names: Mai Men Dong, Mai Dong, Yang Jiu (Mand); Mek Mun Dung, Mek Dung (Cant)
Other names: Creeping lilyturf, Mondo grass, "Succulent winter wheat"; Bakumondo (Jap)
Habit: Evergreen perennial herb from Japan, Korea and temperate China, growing in mountain wilds or damp, shady spots in woods and forests; also cultivated; blooms in summer with racemes of small pale lilac to white flowers.
Part used: the root

Therapeutic category: mild remedy with minimal chronic toxicity
Constituents: steroidal saponins (ophiopogonins A, B, C, D) with aglycone ruscogenin, diosgenins, sterols (incl. beta-sitosterol and stigmasterol), ophioside, 5 homoiso flavanoids, glycosides, fructose, glucose, saccharose, saccharides, traces ess. oil (incl. longifoline, patchoulene, guaial, cyperene, humulene)
Effective qualities: sweet, a bit bitter and oily, cool, moist
  restoring, softening, thickening, calming
Tropism: respiratory, digestive, nervous systems
  Lung, Heart, Stomach channels; Warmth, Fluid bodies

ACTIONS AND INDICATIONS
respiratory restorative: bronchial demulcent, antitussive: dry respiratory conditions with dry cough; chronic bronchitis and pharyngitis, lung TB
mucolytic expectorant: cough with difficult expectoration
mucogenic, refrigerant: mucosal deficiency, dehydration with thirst; intermittent or low-grade fevers with dryness; hot spells, heat exhaustion, diabetes
hemostatic: coughing or vomiting of blood (hemoptysis, hematemesis)
demulcent laxative: constipation from dryness
nervous sedative: irritability, unrest
reproductive restorative, aphrodisiac: impotence, infertility
hypoglycemiant
antiseptic, leukocytogenic: infections, low WBC count

SYMPTOM PICTURES
lung phlegm dryness/Yin deficiency: dry throat and mouth, thirst, difficult dry cough, cough with blood-tinged or scanty, sticky sputum

Yin and fluids deficiency with **nerve excess:** hot spells or low-grade fever, thirst, dry mouth, lips and throat, irritability, sleep loss

stomach and intestines dryness: constipation, difficult dry stool, dry mouth/throat, dehydration, irritability

PREPARATION
Use: The root Ophiopogon Mai Men Dong is used in decoction or tincture form.
Dosage: Decoction: 6-14 g
Tincture: 2-4 ml
Caution: Being sweet, cool and moist by nature, this remedy should not be used for cough of the lung cold variety nor in digestive weakness with diarrhea.

NOTES
The small roots of the common East Asian ornamental, dwarf lilyturf, are a classic remedy for dry, Yin deficient conditions (with or without heat). Energetically cool, moistening and *restorative*, it contains saponins and exerts a *demulcent* and *mucus-generating* effect on the bronchial and digestive mucosa. Dwarf lilyturf can soften hard sputum, relieve dry coughs, lubricate dry constipation and relieve general symptoms of dehydration.

Dwarf lilyturf root is one of the few *Yin tonics* that is also considered a *reproductive tonic*. Since fairly recently it is also being applied to anginal heart conditions—no doubt because being an ingredient in Sheng Mai San, the Generate Pulse formula, which is used for these.

Asparagus Tian Men Dong
Shiny Asparagus Tuber

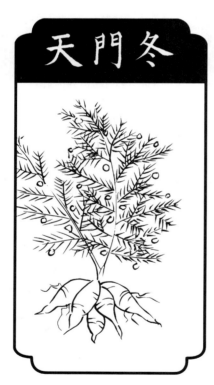

Botanical source: *Asparagus cochinensis* (Lour.) Merrill (Asparaginae)
Pharmaceutical name: Rhizoma Asparagi cochinensis
Chinese name: Tian Men Dong, Tian Dong, Tian Le, Wan Sui Teng (Mand); Tin Mun Dung, Tin Dung (Cant)
Other names: "Succulent winter aerial"; Tenmendo (Jap)
Habit: Perennial temperate East Asian climbing herb; grows in woods, thickets and on shaded, humid hillsides; small ivory flowers appear in summer.
Part used: the tuber

Therapeutic category: mild remedy with minimal chronic toxicity
Constituents: sitosterol, saponins (incl. asparagin and smilagenin), methoxymethylfufural, rhamnose, mucilage, sterols, oligosaccharide, glucose, starch, trace minerals (incl. iron, copper, zinc)
Effective qualities: sweet, bitter, oily, cool, moist
restoring, softening, decongesting
Tropism: respiratory, digestive, urogenital systems
Lung, Kidney, Stomach channels; Fluid, Warmth bodies

ACTIONS AND INDICATIONS
respiratory restorative: bronchial demulcent, antitussive: dry respiratory conditions with rasping cough; croup, whooping cough, lung TB, diphtheria
mucolytic expectorant: cough with difficult expectoration
mucogenic, antipyretic: mucosal deficiency, dehydration with dry sinuses, low-grade remittent fever, heat exhaustion, diabetes
demulcent laxative: constipation from dryness

draining/detoxicant diuretic: dysuria, edema, gout
reproductive restorative: impotence
antiseptic, antifungal, lymphocyte stimulant: infections, lung abscess, boils, snake bite
antitumoral, interferon inducent: leukemia, breast cancer

SYMPTOM PICTURES
lung phlegm dryness: harsh dry cough, dry sinuses, difficult scanty sticky expectoration, blood-tinged sputum

Yin and fluids deficiency: thirst, dehydration, hot spells, dry mouth and lips

stomach and intestines dryness: dry mouth and throat, constipation, difficult dry stool

PREPARATION
Use: The tuber Asparagus Tian Men Dong is decocted or used in tincture form. The tincture is less cooling than the decotion, although it enhances the herb's active side, such as its *expectorant* effects.

Dosage: Decoction: 5-15 g
  Tincture: 2-5 ml

Caution: Forbidden in diarrhea due to deficiency cold and cough due to wind cold.

NOTES
Respiratory conditions with dryness and Yin deficiency are the focus of Shiny asparagus root's action. However, its *moistening, restoring* effect extends to the whole system, beginning with the mucous membrane. This *cooling demulcent* relieves parchedness and dry constipation, and clears the empty heat of low fever or heat exhaustion.

There are more similarities between the Oriental and Western asparagus root than first meet the eye. The main difference is that while the Oriental variety is first and foremost a *respiratory restorative*, the Western asparagus is mainly a *nutritive, detoxicant* remedy. To some extent, these differences arise from different medical applications. Both asparagus types have shown *antitumoral* activity, for example.

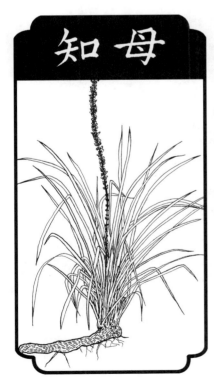

Anemarrhena Zhi Mu
Know Mother Root *

Botanical source: *Anemarrhena asphodeloides* Bunge (Liliaceae)
Pharmaceutical name: Radix Anemarrhenae
Chinese names: Zhi Mu, Ku Xin, Di Shen, Huo Mu (Mand); Ji Mou (Cant)
Other names: "Ant's eggs mother"; Chimo (Jap)
Habit: Perennial herb from north China (esp. Hebei, Shanxi) growing on exposed slopes and hillsides; elongated racemes of magenta speciform small flower clusters bloom in summer; the flowers open and release their fragrance with nightfall.
Part used: the root

Therapeutic category: mild remedy with minimal chronic toxicity
Constituents: steroidal saponins 6% (incl. timosaponin, sarsasapogenin, timosaponin, markogenin, asphonin, neogitogenin), timbiose, xanthone glycosides (mangiferin, isomangiferin, chimonin), tannin, mucilage, fatty oil, vitamins
Effective qualities: a bit sweet, bitter and oily, cool, moist
  restoring, calming, sinking
Tropism: respiratory, digestive, urogenital, endocrine systems
  Lung, Stomach, Kidney, Du channels; Fluid, Warmth bodies

RESPIRATORY RESTORATIVES

ACTIONS AND INDICATIONS
respiratory restorative: bronchial demulcent, antitussive: dry respiratory conditions with chronic dry cough; acute bronchitis, lung TB, pneumonia
mucogenic, refrigerant: mucosal deficiency with dryness; dehydration, heat exhaustion, diabetes, low-grade intermittent fevers (incl. scarlet fever, typhoid)
demulcent laxative: constipation from dryness
anti-inflammatory: mouth ulcers, stomatitis (incl. diabetic), receeding gums, dysuria
pituitary-adrenocortical restorative: adrenal cortex deficiency with weakness, fatigue, poor stamina; menopause
hypoglycemiant: hyperglycemia, diabetes mellitus
urogenital sedative: dysuria, oliguria; premature ejaculation, spermatorrhea, increased sex drive
antibacterial, antifungal: acute bronchitis, cystitis, fungal skin conditions

SYMPTOM PICTURES
lung (phlegm) heat dryness: dry cough, thirst, expectoration of thick yellow sputum, feverishness

Yin and fluids deficiency: night sweats, heat in palms, soles and sternum, dry lips, constipation, difficult urination

Kidney Yin deficiency: night sweats, nocturnal emissions, seminal incontinence, increased sexual drive

bladder damp heat: painful, difficult scanty urination, thirst, fever

PREPARATION
Use: The root Anemarrhena Zhi Mu is best prepared in decoction form; a glycerine extract and a tincture are the next best preparations.
Dosage: Decoction: 6-12 g
Tincture: 2-4 ml
Caution: Do not use with loose stool due to digestive deficiency because of its oily, cold demulcent quality.

NOTES
Anemarrhena is a singular night-blooming lily that includes *cooling (refrigerant), calming (urogenital sedative)* and *moistening (mucogenic secretory)* qualities. These qualities are effective in dry and hot (Yin-deficient) bronchial conditions with insufficient mucous and other secretions.

Classically, Know mother root is often combined with other remedies that clear heat and have a sinking energy, such as Fresh rehmannia root and Black figwort root. It teams up equally well with the other *respiratory demulcents* in this section. Besides fostering the Yin and generating fluids like other *Yin tonics*, Know mother provides the advantage of deeper, more systemic tonification through gentle stimulation of the pituitary/adrenal cortex axis. This action is due to the root's high content in steroidal saponins. In Chinese energetic terms, this action is related to the Extraordicary channel Du Mai. The remedy also goes some way to clear excess energy in the Du Mai, as can be seen by its ability to reduce sexual hyperstimulation and scanty, dripping or absent urination. Anemarrhena is a reliable *sexual sedative,* and is especially ideal when deficient heat from adrenocortical deficiency is present.

Ultimately, this botanical presents the gestalt of a widely applicable *restorative* of the most general and superior kind, especially useful for states of impending or actual adrenal burnout displaying signs of fatigue, stamina loss, dryness and heat. Its potential benefits for women in menopausal years are clear. There is no real therapeutic equivalent remedy in the West to Know mother root.

Trichosanthes Tian Hua Fen
Snakegourd Root

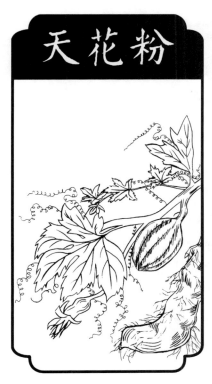

Botanical source: *Trichosanthes kirilowii* Maximowicz or *T. japonica* Regel or *T. uniflora* Hao (Cucurbitaceae)
Pharmaceutical name: Radix Trichosanthis
Chinese names: Tian Hua Fen, Gua Lou Gen, Hua Fen, Di Lou (Mand); Tin Fa Fun (Cant)
Other names: "Heavenly flower starch"; Tenkafun (Jap)
Habit: Perennial herbaceous climbing vine from Central and South China, Korea and Japan; grows on hillsides, along wood edges and in weed thickets in rich, moist soil; axillary white flowers bloom in summer and autumn.
Part used: the root

Therapeutic category: medium-strength remedy with some chronic toxicity
Constituents: saponins 1%, protein (incl. citrulline, arginine, glutamic acid, aspartic acid), tricosanthin, citrulline dihydrate, hydroxymethylserine, starch 25%, sterols sigmasterol and beta-sitosterol
Effective qualities: bitter, a bit sweet and sour, cool, moist
　　　　　　　　　　restoring, stimulating, calming
Tropism: respiratory, reproductive systems
　　　　　Lung, Stomach channels; Air, Warmth bodies

ACTIONS AND INDICATIONS

respiratory restorative: bronchial demulcent, antitussive, mucolytic expectorant: dry respiratory conditions with thirst, dry cough and difficult expectoration
mucogenic: mucosal deficiency, dehydration with thirst, heat exhaustion, diabetes
anti-inflammatory, antipyretic, antibacterial, antiviral: bronchitis, pneumonia, fever, laryngitis, HIV infection
antitumoral, interferon inducent: tumors, cancer (esp. mammary)
detumescent, detoxicant: swellings and non-suppurative sores, incl. abscesses (esp. breast abscess), boils, fistulas, carbuncles, hemorrhoids, mastitis
uterine stimulant: emmenagogue, oxytocic parturient, abortive: amenorrhea; prolonged pregnancy, stalled labor (uterine dystocia), miscarriage (incl. in second trimester)
hypoglycemiant: diabetes

SYMPTOM PICTURES

lung (phlegm) heat dryness: thirst, dry throat, dry or productive cough (with viscous or blood-streaked sputum)
Yin and fluids deficiency: unquenchable thirst, parched mouth, lips and throat, hot spells

PREPARATION

Use: The root Trichosanthes Tian Hua Fen is decocted or used in tincture form.
Dosage: Decoction: 8-16 g
　　　　　Tincture: 2-5 ml
Caution: Contraindicated in diarrhea due to digestive weakness and during pregnancy. Because of the protein tricosanthin, Snakegourd root has some cumulative toxicity, and should therefore not be used on its own for more than a month. In rare cases, idiosyncratic reactions may also be expected.

NOTES

The starchy root of this scrambling vine is valuable for generating respiratory moisture and coolness. Relieving signs of dry cough and dehydration, the remedy addresses conditions such as dry heat bronchitis, Yin deficiency fever and diabetes.

Snakegourd root's tropism for mammary conditions and toxic swellings of any kind is also noteworthy. Throughout history the root has also been used by decoction (today also trichosanthin by injection) to cause abortion at any time during gestation.

Today the root's compound tricosanthin is attracting much attention. It has become the active ingredient of GLQ223, an *antiviral* compound designed to counteract HIV infection, which acts by destroying infected macrophage cells. Here the remedy's *interferon-inducing* and *antitumoral* activities also engage.

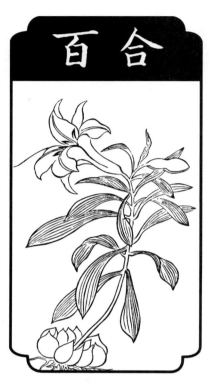

Lilium Bai He
Brown's Lily Bulb

Botanical source: *Lilium brownii* F.E. Brown var. *colchesteri* Wilson or *L. pumilum* De Candolle or *L. longiflorum* Thunberg (Liliaceae)
Pharmaceutical name: Bulbus Lilii
Chinese names: Bai He, Mo Lo (Mand); Baak Hap (Cant)
Other names: "Hundred meetings"; Byakugo (Jap)
Habit: Perennial central Chinese herb growing in loose fertile ground in grassland, sparse woodland and along forest edges; also cultivated; large, fragrant, cream solitary flowers appear in summer.
Part used: the bulb scales

Therapeutic category: mild remedy with minimal chronic toxicity
Constituents: alkaloids, starch, glucose, manna, iliosterin, anthocyanion, vit. C
Effective qualities: sweet, a bit bitter and oily, cool, moist
　　　　　　　　　　restoring, calming, sinking
Tropism: respiratory, cardiovascular, nervous systems
　　　　　Lung, Heart channels
　　　　　Fluid, Warmth bodies

ACTIONS AND INDICATIONS
respiratory restorative: bronchial demulcent, antitussive: dry respiratory conditions with constant dry cough; bronchitis, laryngitis, lung TB, hemoptysis, peptic ulcer
antiallergic: allergic asthma, spasmodic coughing
antipyretic, anti-inflammatory: low-grade fever, hot spells, heat exhaustion, laryngitis
neurocardiac sedative: unrest, irritability, palpitations, anxiety, apprehension; neurocardiac syndrome, neurosis, headache, visual disturbances
galactagogue: insufficient breast milk
diuretic

SYMPTOM PICTURES
lung heat dryness: chronic dry cough, scratchy sore throat, headache, feverishness, restlessness

Yin deficiency with **nerve excess:** irritability, anxiety, hot spells, sleep loss

heart Qi constraint with **nerve excess:** stress, anxiety, palpitations, sleeplessness, restlessness

PREPARATION
Use: The bulb Lilium Bai he is decocted or used in tincture form.
Dosage: Decoction: 10-30 g
　　　　　Tincture: 2-5 ml
Caution: Contraindicated in coughing found in wind cold or lung phlegm conditions, and in diarrhea.

NOTES

Frequently used for dry, hot and Yin deficiency conditions (simple or febrile), as in the above syndromes, Brown's lily bulb's primary tropism is for the chest. Here its *demulcent* effect wonderfully soothes harsh dry coughs, dry sore throats and allergic wheezing. The additional *neurocardiac sedative* action is a balm for any related worry, restlessness and headache. Combining as it does *sedative* and *galactagogue* actions, Brown's lily is also much used by postpartum mothers in Asia. Its use is perhaps even more appropriate in the West where the tendency is to cut short the puerperium because of social and work pressures.

Brown's lily root, Bai He Gen (Mand.) or **Baak Hap Gan** (Cant.), is preferred to the bulb for relieving apprehension and anxiety; it also treats dysuria and edema. Traditionally, drinking **lily flower** tea or eating the petals is said to help one overcome worry and sorrow, generally making it easier to get over unpleasant or unfortunate experiences.

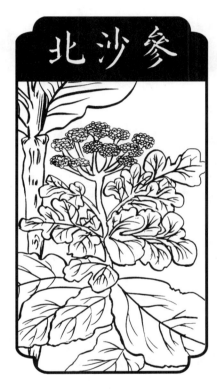

Glehnia Bei Sha Shen
Northern Sandroot *

Botanical source: *Glehnia littoralis* Fr. Schmidt ex Miquel (Umbelliferae)
Pharmaceutical name: Radix Glehniae
Chinese names: Bei Sha Shen, Bai (Sha) Shen (Mand); Bak Sa Sam (Cant)
Other names: Beech silver-top, "Sand ginseng"; Shajin, Hamabofu (Jap)
Habit: Perennial herb from the sea coasts of Mid and North China, Taiwan and Japan; also cultivated in soft, sandy soil; blooms in summer with short, terminal white-flowered umbels.
Part used: the root

Therapeutic category: mild remedy with minimal chronic toxicity
Constituents: alkaloids, stigmasterol, beta-sitosterol, phospholipids, essential oil, polysaccharides (glucosans), furanocoumarins (incl. imperatorin, isoimperatorin), mucilage
Effective qualities: a bit sweet and bitter, cool, moist
restoring, calming
Tropism: respiratory, digestive systems
Lung, Stomach channels
Warmth, Fluid bodies

ACTIONS AND INDICATIONS

respiratory restorative: bronchial demulcent, antitussive: dry respiratory conditions with thirst, dry cough, hoarseness; chronic bronchitis, pharyngitis, croup, lung TB

mucogenic, antipyretic: mucosal deficiency with dryness, dehydration, dermal pruritus worse in cold dry weather; low-grade intermittent fever, heat exhaustion

demulcent laxative: constipation from dryness

analgesic

SYMPTOM PICTURES

lung dryness: dry unproductive cough, dry throat and mouth, hoarseness, thirst

Yin and fluids deficiency: dry cough, thirst, dry lips and skin, hot spells

stomach dryness: dry mouth and throat, thirst, constipation, dry hard stool

PREPARATION
Use: The root Glehnia Bei Sha Shen should be decocted for best results, although a tincture can alternately be used.
Dosage: Decoction: 10-30 g
Tincture: 1-4 ml
Caution: Contraindicated in lung phlegm cold, stomach and intestines cold syndromes, and in wind cold coughing. Should never be combined with White bryony root.

NOTES
So-called because of its predilection for sandy maritime soil, Northern sandroot (*bei sha shen*) is unique for two reasons. First, it is the only remedy in this section dominated by liliaceaous plants that belongs to the parsley family: It is an umbellifer on the way to becoming a lily.

Second, Northern sandroot is the only umbellifer possessing sweet, moist, cooling qualities, rather than the usual pungent, dry, warming ones common to this family. Dry coughs with thirst, whether due to dry climes, city smog or low-grade fever, are its prime domain. With its systemic *moisturizing, mucus-generating* action, Northern sand root will relieve dehydration in general, with or without constipation.

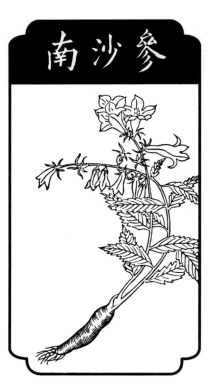

Adenophora Nan Sha Shen
Upright Ladybell Root *

Botanical source: *Adenophora stricta* Miquel or *A. tetraphylla* (Thunb.) Fischer or *A. capillaris* Hemslow (Campanulaceae)
Pharmaceutical name: Radix Adenophorae
Chinese names: Nan Sha Shen, Yu Ya Shen, Bao Ya Shen (Mand); Sa Sam (Cant)
Other names: Strict bellflower, "Southern sandroot"; Tsurigane ninjin (Jap)
Habitat: Perennial herb from temperate China growing on hillsides, in crevices or tussocks; in summer/autumn racemes of blue axillary flowers appear.
Part used: the root

Therapeutic category: mild remedy with minimal chronic toxicity
Constituents: *A. stricta*: saponins, phospholipids, sitosterol, taraxerone, octacasanoic acid, mucilage
A. tet.: essential oil, beta-sitosterol, alkaloid, stigmasterol, starch
Effective qualities: sweet, bitter, cool, moist
restoring, softening
Tropism: respiratory, digestive
Lung, Stomach channels
Fluid, Warmth bodies

ACTIONS AND INDICATIONS
respiratory restorative: bronchial demulcent, antitussive: dry respiratory conditions with thirst, dry cough, hoarseness; chronic bronchitis, croup, whooping cough, lung TB
mucolytic expectorant: dry cough with difficult expectoration
hemostatic: vomiting and coughing up of blood

Adenophora capillaris is additionally:
antitumoral: leukemia, cancer
aphrodisiac: impotence
antivenomous: insect and snake bites

Symptom Pictures

lung phlegm dryness: dry, difficult, unproductive coughing, expectoration of viscous sputum

lung Yin deficiency: dry cough, coughing up blood, low fever, thirst

Preparation

Use: The root Adenophora Nan Sha Shen is decocted or used in tincture form.
Dosage: Decoction: 10-18 g
Tincture: 2-4 ml
Caution: None.

Notes

The upright ladybell is only one of a thicket of bellflowers or bluebells used in fairly similar ways. Its root is considered one of the five *shen,* or ginseng, remedies—one for each of the Five Phases. *Sha shen,* meaning "sand root", treats Metal, the lungs. Nan Sha Shen, "Southern sandroot," is essentially a *bronchial demulcent* with chest-soothing and heat-clearing properties.

Three species of *Adenophora* are all known as **Nan Sha Shen.** The **Upright ladybell,** *A. stricta,* is particularly *secretion softening* as well as *expectorant;* the **Fourleaf bellflower,** *A. tetraphylla,* with its essential oil content, is also *antidotal* and *antipyretic;* the **Slim** or **Downy bellflower,** *A. capillaris,* is considered somewhat *aphrodisiac.* The **Remote bellflower** and **Common harebell,** *A. remotifolia* and *A. trachelioides,* are both called **Ji Ni.** This remedy is additionally an esteemed antidote to various poisons.

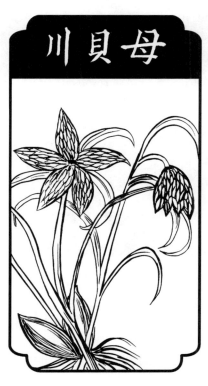

Fritillaria Chuan Bei Mu
Sichuan Fritillary Bulb

Botanical source: *Fritillaria cirrhosa* D. Don or *F. unibracteata* Hsio et K.C. Hsia or *F. przewalski* Maximowicz or *F. delavayi* Franchet (Liliaceae)
Pharmaceutical name: Bulbus Fritillariae cirrhosae
Chinese names: Chuan Bei Mu (Mand); Chyun Bui Mou (Cant)
Other names: Imperial/Crown/Tendrilled fritillary, "Sichuan shell mother"; Senbaimo (Jap)
Habit: Perennial temperate herb of the high Asian mountains, including west China, growing in grassy, damp areas near shrubs; viridian single terminal flower blooms in June.
Part used: the bulb

Therapeutic category: mild remedy with minimal chronic toxicity
Constituents: alkaloids (incl. fritimine, sipeimine, fritiminine, beilupeine, chinpeimine, verticine, fritillarine, verticinine), saponins
Effective qualities: sweet, bitter, a bit oily, cool, moist
restoring, softening, stimulating, calming
Tropism: respiratory, lymphatic systems
Lung, Heart channels; Warmth, Air bodies

Actions and Indications

respiratory restorative: bronchial demulcent, antitussive: dry respiratory conditions with difficult cough and chest constriction; acute or chronic bronchitis, lung TB; cough of any type
mucolytic expectorant: cough with difficult expectoration
antipyretic, anti-inflammatory: fever, laryngitis, acute mastitis, lymphangitis

resolvent, detumescent, lymphatic decongestant: nodules, swellings ; lymphadenitis, fibrocystic breast disorder, lymph gland TB; lung and breast abscess, scrofula, sores, goiter
antitumoral: lymphoma, Hodgkin's disease, cervical cancer, thyroid tumor
uterine stimulant, parturient: prolonged pregnancy, stalled labor (uterine dystocia)
galactagogue: insufficient lactation
diuretic: dysuria

Symptom Pictures
lung phlegm dryness/heat: difficult dry cough, chest tightness, production of scanty sputum

lung Yin deficiency: cough with scanty or blood-streaked sputum, thirst, tight chest, fever

Preparation
Use: The bulb Fritillaria Chuan Bei Mu is taken in decoction or tincture form.
Dosage: Decoction: 3-12 g
Tincture: 1-4 ml
Caution: Contraindicated in digestive weakness, especially with mucus present, and during pregnancy. Although this remedy is traditionally not to be used together with any kind of Aconite root, modern experiments have not found any incompatability between the two remedies.

Notes
Wildcrafted in the mountain ravines of China's western province, Sichuan, Chuan Bei Mu literally means "Sichuan shell mother." This is because its bulbs resemble a bunch of cowrie shells—like its relative, Zhe Bei Mu, from the eastern maritime province Zhejiang.

Sichuan fritillary can be labelled a specific for cough with expectoration of hard, viscous sputum. For symptom relief, it is a true *antitussive,* a cough reducer for any cough that becomes out of control. On the syndrome level, however, this prized remedy is a moist, cool *demulcent* for systemic treatment of dry, hot lung conditions. In this application it differs somwhat from its Zhejiang relative. Both fritillary types also exert an excellent *resolvent* action, especially on lymph gland swelling. Sichuan fritillary's *lymphatic decongestant* and *antitumoral* activities have been linked with its content in a long chain of alkaloids.

Heleocharis Bi Qi
Heleocharis Herb

Botanical source: *Heleocharis plantaginea* R. Br. (Cyperaceae), syn. *Eleocharis dulcis* Trin.
Chinese names: Bi Qi (Mand)
Habitat: Leafless sedge from tropical Asia
Category: mild remedy with minimal chronic toxicity

Effective qualities: sweet, cold, moist; restoring, softening
Tropism: respiratory, digestive systems; Lung, Stomach, Large Intestine channels

Actions: *Bronchial demulcent, mucogenic, mucolytic expectorant*
Indications: (Lung) Yin deficiency syndromes with dry cough and thirst; dry constipation, corneal opacity, benign surface swellings.
Dosage: Decoction: 30-90 g
Tincture: 2-5 ml
Caution: None.
Notes: The small starchy tubers found among the roots are edible and widely used in cooking.

Lycium Di Gu Pi
Wolfberry Root Bark

Botanical source: *Lycium chinense* Miller (Solanaceae)
Chinese names: Di Gu Pi (Mand); Dei Gwat Pei (Cant)
Category: mild remedy with minimal chronic toxicity
Constituents: betaine, cinnamic acid, sitosterol, linoleic acid, psyllic acid, tannin, saponin
Effective qualities: sweet, astringent, cold; restoring, astringing, solidifying, relaxing
Tropism: respiratory, vascular systems; Lung, Liver, Kidney channels

ACTIONS: *Antitussive, antipyretic, astringent, hemostatic, hypotensive, antilipemic, antipruritic, dermatropic, antiallergic, antibacterial*
INDICATIONS: Lung heat dryness and lung Yin deficiency syndromes with dry cough, wheezing, hemoptysis; Yin deficiency patterns with chronic low-grade and remittent fevers, night sweats; malaria; bleeding from nose, uterus; blood in urine, vomit or spittle, lung TB; hypertension, hypercholesterolemia; genital pruritus, allergic skin conditions (incl. contact dermatitis), chronic urticaria, erysipelas, eczema.
Dosage: Decoction: 6-14 g
Tincture: 2-5 ml
Caution: Forbidden in cold conditions of the digestive tract and in onset of infections, i.e. external conditions.
NOTES: Wolfberry root bark is therapeutically similar to the North American wild cherry bark.

Tremella Bai Mu Er
Silver Ear Mushroom

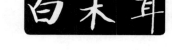

Botanical source: *Tremella fuciformis* Berk.
Chinese names: Bai Mu Er, Yin Mu Er (Mand); Baak Mou Ou (Cant)
Category: mild remedy with minimal chronic toxicity
Constituents: trace minerals (incl. calcium, potassium, magnesium, iron, sulfur), polysaccharides, vitamin B
Effective qualities: sweet, bland, moist, neutral; restoring, calming, nourishing
Tropism: respiratory, digestive systems; Lung, Stomach, Kidney channels

ACTIONS: *Demulcent, secretory, restorative, nutritive, radiation-protectant, immunostimulant*
INDICATIONS: Dry cough, coughing up blood in sputum with Lung/Kidney Yin and Fluids deficiency syndromes; dehydration, hot spells, emaciation, fatigue; radiation (incl. therapeutic), leukopenia; chronic or recurring infections
Dosage: Decoction: 3-10 g
Tincture: 1-3 ml
Soak up to 3 hours before using as vegetable in soups, stews. etc. Cook until tender.
Caution: None.

Respiratory Stimulants

REMEDIES TO PROMOTE EXPECTORATION AND RELIEVE COUGHING

➥ WARM AND TRANSFORM PHLEGM COLD

Stimulant expectorants

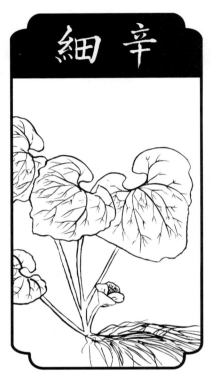

Asarum Xi Xin
Asian Wild Ginger Root and Herb

Pharmaceutical name: Radix et herba Asari
Botanical name: *Asarum sieboldii* Miqel or *A. heterotropoides* Fr. Schmidt var. *mandshuricum* (Maxim.) Kitag and spp. (Aristolochiaceae)
Chinese names: Xi Xin, Bei Xi Xin, Liao Xi Xin (Mand); Sai San (Cant)
Other names: "Fine pungent"; Saishin (Jap)
Habit: Cool, shade and moisture-loving perennial herb from North and Northeast China and Japan, preferring deep, loose fertile soil; purple-green solitary urceolate flowers arise from axils in May.
Part used: the entire plant

Therapeutic category: medium-strength remedy with some chronic toxicity
Constituents: essential oil 3% (incl. phenols, eucarvone, asarinin, elemicin, methyleugenol, isobutyldodecatatramine, demethylcoclaurine [hygenamine], palmitic acid, pinene safrole, ketone asaryl), resin
Effective qualities: pungent, a bit bitter, warm, very dry
    stimulating, relaxing, dispersing, eliminating
Tropism: upper and lower respiratory, nervous systems
    Lung, Kidney, Heart channels; Air, Warmth bodies

ACTIONS AND INDICATIONS
respiratory stimulant/relaxant: expectorant: catarrhal and spasmodic bronchial conditions with productive cough and wheezing; bronchitis, bronchial asthma
stimulant diaphoretic, anti-infective, diuretic: onset of flu and cold with pain, fever, upper and lower respiratory infections
nasal decongestant, anti-inflammatory: nasal and sinus congestion with pain; rhinitis, sinusitis, headache
uterine stimulant, parturient: amenorrhea, spasmodic dysmenorrhea, uterine dystocia
immune regulator: antiallergic: immune stress with immediate allergies (incl. rhinitis, nasal polyps); antibody-mediated cytotoxicity with allergies; immune complex disorders (incl. bronchial asthma, rheumatoid arthritis)
interferon inducent
nervous sedative, analgesic, antirheumatic: headache, aches and pains, arthritic neuralgia, rheumatic myalgia, chest pains, toothache
anesthetic: tooth extraction

SYMPTOM PICTURES
external wind cold: aches and pains, chills, sneezing, fatigue, no sweating, cold extremities
lung wind cold: coughing with watery white sputum, sneezing, congested nose and sinuses, headache, chills
lung phlegm cold: coughing with productive white watery sputum, wheezing, cold extremities
cold damp obstruction: joint and muscle pains, joint swelling and numbness

Preparation

Use: The root and herb Asarum Xi Xin is given a short decoction or else used in tincture form. The powder is used in insufflation (i.e., blown into the nose) for nasal polyp and for deafness.

Dosage: Decoction: 2-5 g
Tincture: 0.5-2 ml

Caution: Because of its warm, dry, stimulating qualities, Asarum Xi Xin is contraindicated in all hot and Yin deficient conditions, as well as in pregnancy. It is also nephrotoxic and should be avoided in those with renal deficiency. Asarum Xi Xin should not be used on its own for any length of time as it generates some cumulative toxicity.

Notes

Collected in northernmost China, Manchuria and Korea, Asian wild ginger root and herb is a strong, essential oil-laden remedy. It is a pungent *stimulant* to the arterial circulation and bronchi, generating warmth to chest and extremities, encouraging sweating, and opening and relaxing the chest. Hence, it is useful for cold, wind cold or phlegm cold syndromes affecting respiratory functions and surface structures. These conditions also benefit from Asian wild ginger's *antiallergic, immune regulating* and *analgesic* actions. Generally speaking, this remedy is interchangeable with both the European and American varieties of *Asarum*.

Hygenamine is thought to be the compound responsible for Asian wild ginger's *adrenergic* action, which includes the above effects (Chang and But 1987). Interestingly, the same constituent is also found in some other cold-clearing remedies, such as Evodia Wu Zhu Yu (Evodia berry) and Aconitum Fu Zi (Prepared Sichuan aconite root).

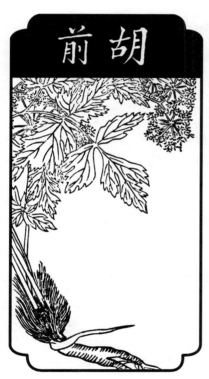

Peucedanum Qian Hu

Asian Masterwort Root *

Botanical source: *Peucedanum praeruptorum* Dunn or *P. decursivum* (Miq.) Maximowicz (Umbelliferae)
Pharmaceutical name: Radix Peucedani
Chinese names: Qian Hu, Yen Chuang Gong (Mand); Chin Wu (Cant)
Other names: "Before barbarian"; Zenko (Jap)
Habit: Perennial temperate East Asian herb growing on hillsides, shrubland and waste areas among damp thickets; blooms in autumn with umbels of terminal or axillary white blossoms.
Part used: the root

Therapeutic category: mild remedy with minimal chronic toxicity
Constituents: *P. praer.*: essential oil, peucedanins A, B, C, D, pyrano- and furanocoumarins (anomalin, peupraerin)
P. dec.: essential oil, glycosides (nodakenin, decursidin), umbelliferone, pyranocoumarins
Effective qualities: bitter, pungent, cool, dry
stimulating, relaxing, dispersing
Tropism: respiratory, digestive, reproductive systems
Lung, Spleen channels
Air, Fluid bodies

Actions and Indications

respiratory stimulant/relaxant: expectorant, bronchodilatant, antitussive: catarrhal and spasmodic bronchial disorders with productive/unproductive cough and wheezing; chronic and acute bronchitis

antibacterial, diaphoretic: all upper and lower respiratory infections
uterine stimulant, parturient: prolonged pregnancy, stalled labor, miscarriage, retained placenta
analgesic: pain in general
photosensitizer
antitumoral

SYMPTOM PICTURES
lung phlegm damp/heat: coughing with production of thick, copious or hard viscous sputum, tight chest
lung wind cold/heat: chills, feverishness, sneezing, coughing with production of sputum

PREPARATION
Use: The root Peucedanum Qian Hu is either decocted or taken in tincture form.
Dosage: Decoction: 4-10 g
Tincture: 2-4 ml
Caution: Forbidden during pregnancy.

NOTES
Containing a pungent, bitter essential oil, Asian masterwort root is a frequently used, versatile *respiratory stimulant/relaxant*. The root is used especially for the onset and early stages of respiratory infections with abundant sputum, wheezing and tight chest. According to Japanese research, its furanocoumarins have shown promising *antitumoral* and *platelet-inhibiting* activities.

This umbellifer is related to the **European masterwort,** *Peucedanum ostruthium*. Both masterwort varieties share the same or similar constituents, qualities, actions and traditional uses. Therapeutically they would easily be interchangeable.

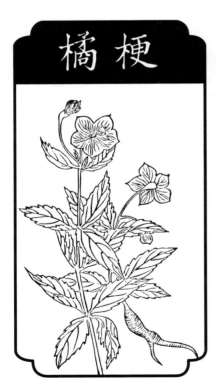

Platycodon Jie Geng
Balloonflower Root

Botanical source: *Platycodon grandiflorum* (Jacq.) De Candolle (Campanulaceae)
Pharmaceutical name: Radix Platycodonis
Chinese names: Jie Geng, Ku Jie Geng, Jin Geng (Mand); Gaat Gan (Cant)
Other names: Broad bluebell, Chinese bellflower; Kikyo (Jap)
Habit: Hardy erect perennial temperate herb from mid-coastal, north and northeast China, the Russian Far East, Korea and Japan, growing on waste ground and slopes; commonly cultivated; large bell-shaped purple, blue or white flowers appear singly at terminal styles or as racemes during summer.
Part used: the root

Therapeutic category: mild remedy with minimal chronic toxicity
Constituents: triterpenoid saponins (incl. platycodin, polygalacin), sterols (incl. stigmasterol and alpha-spinasterol), betulin, inulin, platycodonin, platycogenic acids
Effective qualities: sweet, a bit bitter and pungent, neutral, moist
stimulating, restoring
Tropism: respiratory, glandular systems
Lung, Stomach channels
Air, Fluid bodies

ACTIONS AND INDICATIONS
respiratory stimulant: expectorant, antitussive: catarrhal respiratory conditions with productive cough; chronic and acute bronchitis
respiratory demulcent, anti-inflammatory: throat infection with dry throat, voice loss; laryngitis, pharyngitis, pneumonia, tonsillitis
resolvent detoxicant: lung or throat abscess, vomiting of blood with pus, boils, carbuncles
hypoglycemiant: diabetes
antacid antisecretory: gastric ulcer due to hyperacidity, diarrhea; sloughing ulcers
nervous sedative (mild)
anticholinergic, antihistamine
antifungal: fungal skin conditions (dermatomycoses)

SYMPTOM PICTURE
lung wind cold/heat: coughing with production of clear sputum, chest pain, wheezing, voice loss, dry itchy throat

PREPARATION
Use: The root Platycodon Jie Geng is decocted or made into a tincture.
Dosage: Decoction: 3-10 g
Tincture: 2-4 ml
Caution: Contraindicated in coughing up of blood or hard dry sputum and in lung TB.

NOTES
Ballonflower root in the bluebell family is one of the most widely used and versatile respiratory remedies. Found in countless herbal formulas, this pectoral may be used in acute or chronic, hot or cold bronchial conditions, with or without sputum (the Chinese Coltsfoot). The lung wind cold or wind heat symptom picture above is therefore only one possible application. Fairly loaded with triterpenoid saponins and phytosterols, Ballonflower root also excels in treating a variety of simple and inflammatory throat conditions with its essentially sweet, *demulcent* qualities.

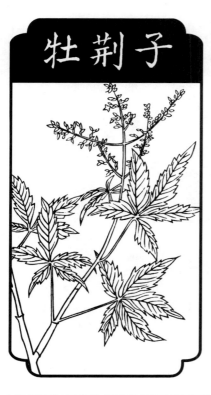

Vitex Mu Jing Zi
Five-Leaf Chastetree Berry

Botanical source: *Vitex negundo* L. var. *cannabifolia* (Sieb. et Zucc.) Handel-Mazzetti (Verbenaceae)
Pharmaceutical name: Fuctus Viticis negundis
Chinese names: Mu Jing Zi, Huang Jing Zi (Mand); Muk Ging Ji (Cant)
Other names: Taiwan Ninjin Boku (Jap)
Habit: Large shrub from temperate China commonly growing by roadsides and on sunny slopes; terminal violet flower panicles bloom during summer.
Part used: the fruit

Therapeutic category: mild remedy with minimal chronic toxicity
Constituents: flavonoid and cardiac glycosides, alkaloids, essential oil (incl. caryophyllene, elemene, pinene, sabinene, camphene, cineol, eugenol)
Effective qualities: bitter, a bit pungent, warm, dry
stimulating, relaxing, astringing, dispersing
Tropism: respiratory, digestive, urogenital systems
Lung, Spleen channels
Air, Warmth bodies

ACTIONS AND INDICATIONS
respiratory stimulant/relaxant: expectorant, bronchodilatant, antitussive: catarrhal bronchial conditions with productive cough and wheezing; chronic bronchitis, bronchial asthma
stimulant diaphoretic, antibacterial: common cold, flu, dysentery, malaria
arterial stimulant, antirheumatic: rheumatic myalgia, arthralgia; eczema
digestive stimulant, analgesic: dyspepsia, epigastric pain, diarrhea, chronic gastroenteritis, hernia
urogenital mucostatic: leucorrhea, gonorrhea
adrenocortical stimulant: general fatigue

SYMPTOM PICTURES
lung phlegm cold/damp: chronic coughing with expectoration of white sputum, wheezing, chills, poor appetite
lung wind cold: sneezing, coughing, chills, aches and pains, fatigue

PREPARATION
Use: The berry Vitex Mu Jing Zi is decocted or used in tincture form.
Dosage: Decoction: 6-12 g. Up to 60 g of the seed and root are used to prevent malarial attacks.
Tincture: 2-4 ml
Caution: None.

NOTES
On the Chinese mainland, Five-leaf chastetree berry is one of the outstanding popular remedies for congestive, catarrhal chest conditions. An herb only becomes popular because it works, and that alone should draw our attention to this *Vitex* variety—despite its relative obscurity in the West. Chronic bronchial conditions with cold, damp, rheumatic pains and poor appetite are the asterisk symptoms indicating the use of Five-leaf chasteberry.

Five-leaf chestetree root, Mu Jing Gen (Mand.) or **Muk Ging Gan** (Cant.), is used in a similar way to the berry.

The **berry** and **root** of *Vitex negundo* L., **Huang Jing,** are essentially used in the same way.

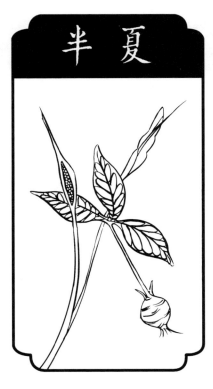

Pinellia Ban Xia
Prepared Pinellia Corm

Botanical source: *Pinellia ternata* (Thunb.) Breitung (Araceae)
Pharmaceutical name: Rhizoma Pinelliae preparatae
Chinese names: Ban Xia, Fa Ban Xia, Zhi Ban Xia (Mand); Bun Ha, Faat Bun Ha, Faat Ha (Cant)
Other names: "Midsummer ripe"; Hange (Jap)
Habit: Perennial herb from southern China, Korea and Japan; grows in shady and humid grass thickets by stream edges and on mountainsides; much cultivated; flowers in summer with a terminal spike of minute viridian flowers.
Part used: the prepared rhizomatous tuber

Therapeutic category: mild remedy with no chronic toxicity
Constituents: amino acids (incl. arginine, serine), alkaloids (ephedrine), polysaccharides, phytosterol, glucuronic acid, choline, fatty acid, glycoside, diglycosilic benzaldehyde, essential oil (incl. phenols), calcium oxalate, zinc
Effective qualities: pungent, a bit astringent, warm, dry
stimulating, restoring, softening
Tropism: stomach, intestines, lungs, lymphatic systems
Spleen, Stomach channels; Fluid, Air bodies

ACTIONS AND INDICATIONS

respiratory stimulant: expectorant, antitussive: catarrhal respiratory disorders with productive cough, chest distension and pain; acute and chronic bronchitis

mucosal restorative, mucostatic: excessive mucus production; chronic gastritis, leucorrhea, gonorrhea

lymphatic decongestant: lymphadenitis (incl. scrofula), lymph gland TB

resolvent detoxicant, antivenomous: deep-rooted boils, carbuncles, furuncles; snakebite, poisoning

antitumoral, interferon inducent: cervical, mammary, gastric cancer; lymphoma

immune regulator, antiallergic: immune stress with cell-mediated (delayed) allergies (incl. tubercular lesions, contact dermatitis, autoimmune disorders [incl. peptic ulcer])

antiemetic: nausea and vomiting in any condition (incl. pregnancy)

analgesic, hemostatic: pain in general; traumatic bleeding

Miscellaneous*:* otitis media, glaucoma (intraocular pressure), globus hystericus

SYMPTOM PICTURES

lung phlegm damp: coughing with production of copious sputum, tight painful chest

intestines mucous damp (Spleen damp): nausea, vomiting, abdominal distension with tenderness, headache, dizziness, heaviness of head and body

PREPARATION

Use: The prepared or processed corm Pinellia Ban Xia is decocted or used in tincture form. The raw corm is called **Sheng Ban Xia** (Mand.) or **Sang Bun Ha** or **So Bun Ha** (Cant.). Because in its raw state Pinellia corm is somewhat toxic, most commercially available Pinellia is already prepared in one way or another, and in pharmacy is called **Fa Ban Xia** (Mand.) or **Faat Bun Ha** (Cant.), "Prepared Ban Xia." Raw pinellia corm is processed by being first soaked in water and then boiled with alum (and sometimes with licorice root and calcium carbonate for a greater *stimulant expectorant* effect). Essentially, applying heat to the corm dissipates its acute toxicity.

When processed with alum and ginger juice, the remedy is called **Jiang Ban Xia** (Mand.) or **Geung Bun Ha** (Cant.) and is particularly effective for reducing vomiting.

Dosage: Decoction: 4-14 g
Tincture: 2-4 ml

Caution: Avoid combining this remedy with any type of Aconite root.

NOTES

Containing an interesting assortment of constituents (including amino acids, polysaccharides alkaloids and essential oil), the processed small, tuberous corm of the pinellia in the arum family is the most commonly used Chinese remedy for conditions involving sputum or mucus. This highly effective *expectorant* and *mucostatic* botanical is included in a large variety of standard prescriptions treating catarrhal respiratory and digestive disorders. In Chinese medicine, catarrhal conditions are described as injury through damp, and include manifestations of sputum, mucus and other impure fluids.

The significant *detoxicant, antitumoral* and *lymphatic decongestant* actions of Prepared pinellia corm have also found perennial use throughout East Asian medicine. Its *immune-regulating (antiallergic)* activities are fairly recent findings, however. They hold promise for type IV hypersensitivity responses, such as contact dermatitis and tubercular lesions, as well as autoimmune disorders in general (Kohda et al. 1982).

In South China the species *Typhonium flagelliforme* in the arum family is often used as botanical source for the remedy Ban Xia. This is the species usually exported to North America and so generally available. This remedy is properly known as **Shui Ban Xia** (Mand.) or **Seui Bun Ha** (Cant.) (Water Ban Xia) and is related to *Typhonium giganteum,* **Du Jiao Lan** (Giant typhonium root), with which it should also not be confused. It differs therapeutically from the true Ban Xia primarily in that it does not possess any *antiemetic* effect. Even so, more research is needed to ascertain the exact pharmacology and therapeutic actions of the distinct remedy Shui Ban Xia.

Gleditsia Zao Jiao
Honeylocust Pod

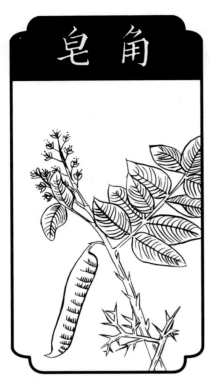

Botanical source: *Gleditsia sinensis* Lam. and *G. off.* Hems. (Leguminosae)
Pharmaceutical name: Fructus Gleditsiae
Chinese names: Zao Jiao, Zao Jia (Mand); Jou Gok (Cant)
Other names: Chinese locust, soap bean; Sokaku (Jap)
Habit: Deciduous temperate East Asian tree, growing along valley streams or in flatlands; blossoms in spring with racemes of fragrant yellowish or greenish white axillary flowers.
Part used: the fruit

Therapeutic category: mild remedy with minimal chronic toxicity
Constituents: triterpenoid saponins (incl. gledinin, gledigenin), gleditsia saponins B, C, D, E, G, stearic/palmitic/oleic/linolic/ linoleic, acid, ceryl alcohol, stigmasterol, sitosterol, tannins, nonacosane, heptacosane
Effective qualities: pungent, bitter, salty, warm, moist
   stimulating, softening
Tropism: respiratory, digestive, central nervous systems
   Lung, Large Intestine channels; Air, Fluid bodies

ACTIONS AND INDICATIONS

respiratory stimulant: expectorant: catarrhal bronchial conditions with productive cough; bronchitis
central nervous stimulant, analeptic: coma, stroke with facial paralysis, lockjaw, hemiplegia
uterine stimulant, parturient: stalled labor, placental retention
demulcent laxative: constipation from dryness
detoxicant, maturant, antibacterial, antifungal: boils, abscesses, sores, fungal infections
anthelmintic: roundworms
Miscellaneous: acute throat numbness, metal poisoning, dribbling saliva in children, tooth decay, rectal cancer

SYMPTOM PICTURE

lung phlegm damp: coughing, expectoration of copious white sputum

PREPARATION

Use: The bean pod Gleditsia Zao Jiao is used mainly powdered, made into pills, capsules, etc. For constipation and/or roundworms it is used as a suppository.
Dosage: Powder: 0.6-1.5 g
   Decoction: 2-5 g
   Tincture: 0.25-1.5 ml
Caution: Contraindicated during pregnancy.

NOTES

The thorny soap bean or honeylocust tree is common throughout China. Its pod is a popular remedy possessing a variety of uses derived from its *stimulant* nature. The various saponins it contains go some way to explaining this essential action. So do, however, the remedy's pungent, bitter and warm effective qualities—the time-tested, traditional explanation.

The sharp spines (thorns) of the honeylocust, called **Zao Jiao Ci** (Mand.) or **Jou Gok Chi** (Cant.), are used alone as a separate remedy. The remedy is used for treating fire toxin (purulent inflammatory) conditions such as tonsilitis, abscesses (e.g., lung) and boils, and retained placenta; topically for sores, ulcers, caked breasts, eczema and fungal infections. Dosage: 3-9 g. Contraindicated during pregnancy.

Cynanchum Bai Qian
Prime White Root *

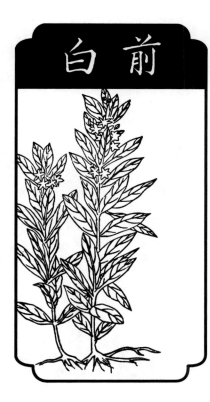

Botanical source: *Cynanchum stauntoni* (Decne.) Schltr. ex Leveillé or *C. glaucescens* (Decne.) Handel-Mazzetti (Asclepiadaceae)
Pharmaceutical name: Radix et rhizoma Cynanchi
Chinese names: Bai Qian, Sou Yao, Liu Xie Bai Qian, Shi Lan (Mand); Baak Chin, Bak Chin (Cant)
Other names: Byakuzen (Jap)
Habit: Pilose perennial herb from North China and Japan; grows in sandy soil in damp and shade along streams and rivers; cymes of small axillary purple flowers bloom in summer.
Part used: the root and rhizome

Therapeutic category: mild remedy with minimal chronic toxicity
Constituents: triterpenoid saponins, flavonoids, sucrose, amino acids, paenol, traces of alkaloids (incl. cynanchin)
Effective qualities: pungent, sweet, a bit salty, warm, dry
  stimulating, relaxing
Tropism: respiratory tract
  Lung channel
  Air body

ACTIONS AND INDICATIONS
respiratory stimulant: mucolytic expectorant, antitussive: catarrhal bronchial disorders with difficult, dry or productive cough; acute or chronic bronchitis
bronchial relaxant/dilator: bronchial asthma
immune regulator, antiallergic: immune stress with immediate allergies (incl. allergic rhinitis, dermatitis, urticaria)

SYMPTOM PICTURES
lung phlegm cold: coughing with clear white sputum, difficult expectoration, chest distension, gurgling in throat
lung Qi constraint: wheezing, tight chest, coughing

PREPARATION
Use: The root Cynanchum Bai Qian is either decocted or used in tincture form.
Dosage: Decoction: 4-10 g
  Tincture: 2-4 ml
Caution: Contraindicated in lung Qi deficiency or lung and Kidney Yang deficiency.

NOTES
Predominantly used in North China, First white root is a versatile traditional remedy for bronchial conditions, entailing both *stimulant* and *relaxant* effects. This means that both phlegm cold, or catarrhal, and Qi constraint, or spasmodic, bronchial conditions find relief through its use.

Today First white root is also proving very successsful in resolving stubborn outbreaks of hives as well as other type I allergic conditions.

Zingiber Sheng Jiang
Fresh Ginger Root

Botanical source: *Zingiber officinalis* (Willd.) Roscoe (Zingiberaceae)
Chinese names: Sheng Jiang, Sheng Jiang Pian (Mand); Sang Geung (Cant)
Category: mild remedy with minimal chronic toxicity
Constituents: essential oil
Effective qualities: pungent, hot; stimulating, dispersing
Habitat: Tropical plant from Asia and the Pacific Islands
Tropism: respiratory, digestive systems; Lung, Stomach channels

ACTIONS: *Stimulant expectorant, diaphoretic, gastric stimulant, antiemetic; helps detoxify other herbs in a formula.*
INDICATIONS: Coughing, chills and sneezing with lung wind cold syndrome; as adjunct in chronic bronchial conditions, or lung phlegm cold; deficiency cold gastrointestinal conditions.
Dosage: Decoction: 1-3 g
Tincture: 1-2 ml
Caution: Do not use in acute lung or stomach syndromes with heat.

Ardisia Zi Jin Niu
Marlberry Root and Herb

Botanical source: *Ardisia japonica* (Hornst.) Blume (Myrsinaceae)
Chinese names: Zi Jin Niu, Ai Di Cha (Mand); Ji Gam Ngau (Cant)
Habit: Small evergreen shrub from mid China, found in woodland shade and thickets; terminal small white or pink flowers open in summer.
Category: mild remedy with minimal chronic toxicity
Constituents: isocoumarin bergenin
Effective qualities: bitter, dry, neutral; stimulating, calming
Tropism: respiratory, digestive systems; Lung, Liver, Large Intestine channels

ACTIONS: *Stimulant expectorant, antitussive, anti-infective, vulnerary, anti-inflammatory, detoxicant, diuretic*
INDICATIONS: Chronic and acute bronchitis with cough (lung phlegm damp/cold syndrome), lung TB, pneumonia; traumatic injury; conjunctivitis, poisoning, influenza.
Dosage: Decoction: 16-30 g
Tincture: 2-5 ml
Caution: None.
NOTES: Marlberry root is a common, effective remedy for bronchial infections. The stem and leaf are used for treating cancer, especially of the liver. Various other *Ardisia* species are used in similar and other ways to Marlberry.

Respiratory Relaxants

REMEDIES TO RELAX THE BRONCHI AND RELIEVE WHEEZING

➥ CIRCULATE AND LOWER LUNG QI

Bronchodilatant antiasthmatics

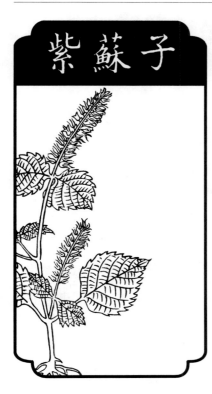

Perilla Zi Su Zi
Perilla Seed

Botanical source: *Perilla frutescens* (L.) var. *crispa* (Thunb.) Handel-Mazzetti or *P. frut.* var. *acuta* (Thunb.) Kudo (Labiatae)
Pharmaceutical name: Fructus Perillae
Chinese names: Zi Su Zi, Su Zi (Mand); So Ji (Cant)
Other names: Soshi (Jap)
Habit: Wild and cultivated pilose annual herb found throughout China, growing in sunny, fertile places, incl. roadsides and village borders; small white or purple axillary/terminal flowers on racemes appear in summer.
Part used: the fruit

Therapeutic category: mild remedy with minimal chronic toxicity
Constituents: perillaldehyde, essential oil (incl. limonene, pinene), perilla alcohol, cumic acid, arginine, vitamin B1
Effective qualities: pungent, warm, moist
relaxing, stimulating, softening
Tropism: respiratory, digestive systems
Lung, Large Intestine channels
Air body

ACTIONS AND INDICATIONS

respiratory relaxant: bronchodilator: spasmodic bronchial disorders with tight chest and wheezing; asthma (all types)
stimulant and mucolytic expectorant: catarrhal respiratory conditions with productive cough; chronic bronchitis
demulcent laxative: constipation from dryness

SYMPTOM PICTURES

lung Qi constraint: chest constriction, wheezing, coughing

lung phlegm damp/dryness: productive coughing with much liquid or viscous sputum, wheezing

PREPARATION

Use: The seed Perilla Zi Su Zi is either decocted or used in tincture form.
Dosage: Decoction: 4-10 g
Tincture: 2-4 ml
Caution: Forbidden in chronic diarrhea and asthma due to Qi deficiency.

NOTES

Being both *relaxant* and *stimulant,* the versatile respiratory remedy Perilla seed is mainly applied to the two asthmatic or bronchitic lung syndromes above.

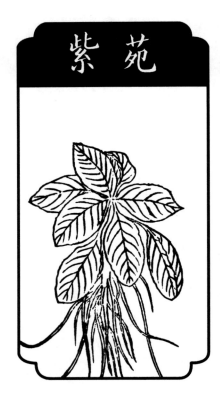

Aster Zi Wan
Tartary Aster Root *

Botanical source: *Aster tataricus* L. (Compositae)
Pharmaceutical name: Radix Asteris tatarici
Chinese names: Zi Wan, Zi Yuan, Qing Yuan (Mand); Ji Yan (Cant)
Other names: Purple aster, "Purple soft"; Shion (Jap)
Habit: Perennial herb from North Asia; grows in fields along streams and rivers in both mountains and lowlands; star-like flowerheads of green-lilac terminal flowers with yellow centers appear in spring.
Part used: the root

Therapeutic category: mild remedy with minimal chronic toxicity
Constituents: astersaponin, quercetin, oleic acid, lachnophyllol, anethole, epifriedelinol, friedelin, shionone, arabinose
Effective qualities: a bit bitter and pungent, warm, neutral
relaxing, stimulating, softening
Tropism: respiratory, urinary systems
Lung channel
Air body

ACTIONS AND INDICATIONS

respiratory relaxant: bronchodilator: spasmodic bronchial conditions with wheezing, spasmodic coughing; bronchial asthma
antitussive: coughing in general (incl. with expectoration of pus and blood)
mucolytic expectorant: acute and chronic bronchitis with difficult expectoration
antipyretic: fever (esp. summer fevers in children)
diuretic: dysuria, oliguria
hemostatic: hemorrhage (incl. puerperal)
nervous sedative: unrest, infantile crying
antibacterial, antifungal
antitumoral, interferon inducent: cancer (esp. ascitic cancer)

SYMPTOM PICTURES

lung Qi constraint: wheezing, tight chest, coughing made worse when lying down, restlessness
lung phlegm dryness: coughing, difficult expectoration, some production of dry viscous sputum

PREPARATION

Use: The root Aster Zi Wan is decocted or used in tincture form.
Dosage: Decoction: 3-10 g
Tincture: 2-4 ml
Caution: Use with caution in excess heat syndromes and coughs due to Yin deficiency with empty heat.

NOTES

Coughing in any condition, but especially with the above two symptom pictures, is relieved through Tartary aster root. Given equally for spasmodic and congestive catarrhal chest disorders, this *bronchial relaxant* excels at softening hard, viscous sputum.

None of the Aster varieties growing in North America seem to have been used for bronchial conditions, in spite of their overall *relaxing* and *stimulating* nature.

Prunus Xing Ren
Bitter Apricot Kernel

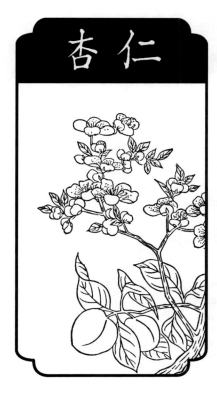

Botanical source: *Prunus armeniaca* L. or *P. arm.* var. *ansu* Maximowicz and spp. (Rosaceae)
Pharmaceutical name: Semen Pruni armeniacae
Chinese names: Xing Ren, Ku Xing Ren, Bei Xing Ren, Tian Mei (Mand); Baak Hang Yan (Cant)
Other names: Common apricot; Kyonin (Jap)
Habit: Deciduous tree from Mid and North China and Inner Mongolia, growing in plains and mountain valleys; also cultivated; blooms in spring with pink, then white, solitary flowers.
Part used: the seed

Therapeutic category: medium-strength remedy with some chronic toxicity
Constituents: glycoside amygdalin 3%, amino acids, emulsin, amygdalase, prunase, fatty oil, hydrocyanic acid, benzaldehyde
Effective qualities: bitter, warm, moist
    relaxing, restoring
Tropism: respiratory, digestive systems
    Lung, Large Intestine channels
    Air body

ACTIONS AND INDICATIONS
respiratory relaxant: bronchodilator, antitussive: spasmodic bronchial disorders with wheezing and spasmodic coughing; asthma, bronchitis
demulcent laxative: constipation due to dryness
antitumoral: tumors (incl. various cancers, leukemia, Hodgkin's disease)
immune regulator, antiallergic: immune stress with immediate allergies (incl. bronchial asthma, rhinitis, urticaria)
hemogenic: anemia

SYMPTOM PICTURES
lung Qi constraint with **dryness:** dry rasping cough, constant coughing, tight chest, wheezing

intestines dryness: constipation, difficult, hard dry stool

PREPARATION
Use: The kernel Prunus Xing Ren is crushed before use in decoction or tincture form.
Dosage: Decoction: 4-10 g
    Tincture: 2-4 ml
Caution: Forbidden in diarrhea. Do not take on its own continuously because of some slight toxicity, due to its hydrocyanic acid content.

NOTES
Current misidentifications to the contrary, the commonly used *respiratory relaxant* remedy Xing ren is the bitter apricot kernel, not the almond. The latter is called Ba Dan Xing. While the apricot is common and indigenous (originally from Shaanxi), the almond is fairly rare and was only imported from Persia via the Xinjiang town Kucha on the silk route during the seventh century Tang period.

Chinese success with Bitter apricot kernel in treating a variety of cancerous conditions is due to its laetrile content, which consists mainly of amygdalin. Its *blood-building* action with aplastic anemia is due to the hydrocyanic acid.

Bitter apricot flowers are traditionally included in cosmetic and fertility formulas.

There is a sweeter and moister variety of kernel from South China, called **Tian Xing Ren** (Mand.) or **Tim Hang Yan** (Cant.) ("sweet apricot kernel"), or **Nan Xing Ren** (Mand.) or **Naam Hang Yan** (Cant.) ("southern apricot kernel"). It is sometimes used instead of the regular kernel, especially with coughs of the dry or deficiency type.

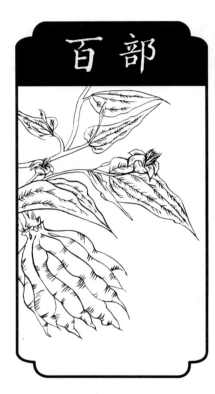

Stemona Bai Bu
Stemona Root

Botanical source: *Stemona japonia* (Blume) Miquel or *S. sessilifolia* (Miq.) Franchet et Savatier or *S. tuberosa* Loureiro (Stemonaceae)
Pharmaceutical name: Radix Stemonae
Chinese names: Bai Bu, Bai Bu Gen, Bo Bu (Mand); Baak Bou (Cant)
Other names: Wild asparagus, "Hundred parts"; Hyakubu (Jap)
Habit: Climbing herbaceous perennial vine from southern coastal provinces, central China and Taiwan, growing on sunny slopes in thickets; single lavender flowers on wiry peduncles open in spring.
Part used: the root

Therapeutic category: medium-strength remedy with some chronic toxicity
Constituents: alkaloids stemonine, stemonidine, isostemonidine, tuberostemonine, paipunine, acetic/citric/formic/malic/oxalic/cuccinic acids, calcium oxalate, resin, mucilage, saccharides
Effective qualities: sweet, bitter, warm, moist
                            relaxing, stimulating
Tropism: respiratory, digestive systems
               Lung channel; Air, Fluid bodies

ACTIONS AND INDICATIONS
respiratory relaxant/stimulant: bronchodilator, expectorant, antitussive: spasmodic and catarrhal bronchial disorders with acute or chronic cough; bronchitis, dry cough
bronchial demulcent: whooping cough, croup, lung TB
anthelmintic: intestinal parasites (esp. oxyuriasis, ancylostomiasis)
antiparasitic: lice (pediculus), ringworm, pinworm, trichomoniasis, schistosomiasis, giardiasis
pesticidal: insect infestation (e.g. maggots, mosquitoes, ticks, wiggler, aphids, cutworms, scabies, fleas, flies)
anti-infective: antibacterial, antifungal: bronchitis, cholera, dysentery, typhus, yeast/fungal infections

SYMPTOM PICTURE
lung Qi constraint with **dryness:** wheezing, chronic or constant dry coughing, chest constriction

PREPARATION
Use: The root Stemona Bai Bu is decocted or used in tincture form. Enemas and topical applications such as washes, compresses and vaginal sponges for parasitic/fungal/yeast conditions are also be prepared.
Dosage: Decoction: 4-12 g
                Tincture: 2-4 ml
                For intestinal parasites 30-60 g are taken daily for three or four days.
Caution: Not to be used at maximum dosage for several weeks continuously, as it has some cumulative toxicity. Possible side effects include dryness of the nose, mouth and throat, shortness of breath, chest discomfort, heartburn and dizziness. Contraindicated in weak digestion and diarrhea.

NOTES

Like several other botanical remedies in this section, Stemona root combines *relaxant* and *stimulant* actions on the bronchi. This bitter-sweet remedy is distinguished from the others, however, by a very useful secondary *demulcent* effect. Simple or infectious dry bronchial conditions with spasmodic coughing are best served by the *anti-infective* root. From the biochemical point of view, its efficacy relies heavily on a string of alkaloids.

Stemona root is also much used topically for treating parasites. The combination of *antiparasitic, antifungal* and *antibacterial* actions also make it desirable in managing vaginitis from yeast infection and trichomoniasis. Giardiasis is a condition for which it should work well.

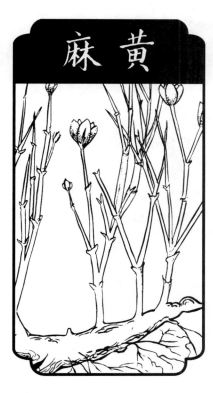

Ephedra Ma Huang
Ephedra Stem

Botanical source: *Ephedra sinica* Stapf (Ephedraceae)
Pharmaceutical name: Herba Ephedrae
Chinese names: Ma Huang, Long Sha, Bei Xiang (Mand); Ma Wong (Cant)
Other names: Chinese jointfir, Mormon tea (Am), "Numb yellow"; "Northern aromatic"; Mao (Jap)
Habit: Erect or prostate undershrub from Inner Mongolia and northern central China, growing on dry slopes and dry riverbeds; in summer, small pale orange terminal flowers appear.
Part used: the herb or stem

Therapeutic category: medium-strength remedy with some chronic toxicity
Constituents: alkaloids 1-2% (incl. 40-90% ephedrine, pseudoephedrine, norephedrine, pseudomethylephedrine, demethylpseudoephedrine, ephedine), essential oil, trace minerals (incl. chromium)
Effective qualities: a bit pungent, bitter and astringent, warm, very dry
relaxing, stimulating, dispersing, decongesting
Tropism: respiratory, urinary, sympathetic nervous systems
Lung, Bladder channels
Fluid body

ACTIONS AND INDICATIONS

respiratory relaxant: bronchodilator: spasmodic bronchial disorders with wheezing, coughing; bronchial asthma (all types), bronchitis
immune regulator, antiallergic: immune stress with immediate allergies (incl. bronchial asthma, urticaria, rhinitis); antibody-mediated cytotoxicity with autoimmune disorders
nasal decongestant: sinusitis, rhinitis
diaphoretic, antiviral, antibacterial: onset of flu and cold with no sweat; chronic bronchitis, rhinitis, tracheitis
draining diuretic: edema of middle and upper body, acute nephritis, oliguria
antienuretic: enuresis
sympathetic nervous stimulant, cardiac restorative, hypertensive: sympathetic nervous deficiency, low blood pressure; fatigue

SYMPTOM PICTURES

lung Qi constraint with **cold:** fatigue, wheezing, tight distended chest, coughing

external wind cold: chills, sneezing, headache, fatigue, body aches and pains, no sweating or urination

PREPARATION

Use: The stem Ephedra Ma Huang may be used in decoction or tincture form. The crude herb over one year old will lose potency because of the decrease of its essential oil content, which has proven crucial to its overall efficacy.

Dosage: Decoction: 2-8 g
Tincture: 1-3 ml

Caution: Because of its cumulative toxicity, do not take on its own at high doses or for extended periods. Side effects of this slight toxicity include raised blood pressure, unrest, tremors and heavy sweating. Use Ephedra Ma Huang with caution in deficiency conditions with sweating or wheezing, and never in high blood pressure, cardiac asthma, spontaneous sweating or insomnia.

NOTES

Ephedra stem is a classic component in formulas addressing spasmodic/asthmatic bronchitic conditions, both simple and allergic. Behind its effect of "circulating lung Qi" lies a *dilating* action on the bronchi, mediated by alkaloids and a characteristic fresh aromatic essential oil.

Being also a considerable *warming diaphoretic* and *diuretic,* Ephedra is traditionally much used for the onset of upper respiratory infections of the wind cold type with absence of sweating and urination. Its drying *nasal decongestant* action is clearly a good asset here with catarrh present.

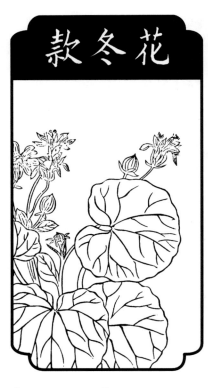

Tussilago Kuan Dong Hua
Coltsfoot Flower

Botanical source: *Tussilago farfara* L. (Compositae)
Pharmaceutical name: Flos Tussilaginis
Chinese names: Kuan Dong Hua, Ko Dong (Mand); Fong Dun Fa (Cant)
Other names: Coughwort, "Liking winter flower"; Kantoka (Jap)
Habit: Perennial temperate Eurasian herb preferring cool, moist climes and loose, fertile sandy soil; flowers in early spring with yellow capitate flowers.
Part used: the flower

Therapeutic category: medium-strength remedy with slight chronic toxicity
Constituents: sesquiterpenoid ester tussilagone, sesquiterpenoid farfaretin, bitter glycoside, inulin, triterpenoid saponins, pyrrolizidine alkaloids, ess. oil, sitosterol, rutin, taraxanthin, tussilaginyl methylbutyrates, gallic acid, palmitin, cholin, mucilage, tannins, calcium, trace minerals (incl. magnesium, zinc)
Effective qualities: pungent, sweet, neutral, moist
relaxing, stimulating, decongesting
Tropism: respiratory system; Lung meridian; Air, Warmth bodies
Lung channel; Air, Warmth bodies

ACTIONS AND INDICATIONS

repiratory relaxant: bronchodilator: spasmodic bronchial disorders with wheezing; bronchial asthma
stimulant expectorant, antitussive: catarrhal conditions with chronic and acute cough; bronchitis, emphysema, hemoptysis
anti-inflammatory, demulcent: laryngitis with pain, pleurisy, emphysema, lung TB; burns
detoxicant: lung abscess, boils

SYMPTOM PICTURES

lung Qi constraint: wheezing, tight chest, coughing

lung phlegm damp: coughing, expectoration of copious white sputum, with pus or blood

PREPARATION

Use: The flower Tussilago Kuan Dong Hua is briefly decocted, infused for 20 minutes or used in tincture form.
Dosage: Infusion/decoction: 5-10 g
Tincture: 2-4 ml
Caution: Tussilago Kuan Dong Hua should be avoided during pregnancy and breastfeeding. Do not take on its own continuously at maximum dosage for more than one month, as it contains alkaloids of slight cumulative toxicity.

NOTES

Identical in both Oriental and Western herbal medicine, Coltsfoot flower is mainly used as a gentle *relaxant/stimulant expectorant*. It is commonly combined with other herbs for different types of cough, bronchitis and asthma. **Coltsfoot leaf,** rather than the flower, is used for a *demulcent* effect in dry lung conditions.

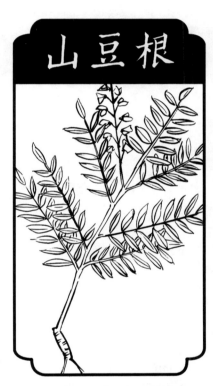

Sophora Shan Dou Gen
Pigeon-Pea Root

Botanical source: *Sophora subprostata* Chun et T. Chen (Leguminosae)
Pharmaceutical name: Radix Sophorae subprostatae
Chinese names: Shan Dou Gen, Guang Dou Gen (Mand); San Dau Gan (Cant)
Other names: "Mountain bean root"; Sanzukon (Jap)
Habit: Perennial woody shrub from South China (esp. Guangxi), growing in rocky cliffs; terminal racemes of pale yellow flowers open in early summer.
Part used: the root and rhizome

Therapeutic category: mild herb with minimal chronic toxicity
Constituents: alkaloids 0.93% (incl. 0.52% matrine, 0.35% oxymatrine, anagyrine, methylcytisine), flavonoids sophoranone, sophoranochromene, sophradin, sophoraponicin, pterorepine, trifolirhizin, genistein, maackian
Effective qualities: bitter, cold, dry
relaxing, stimulating, restoring
Tropism: respiratory, digestive, immune systems
Lung, Heart, Large Intestine channels
Warmth, Air bodies

ACTIONS AND INDICATIONS

respiratory relaxant: bronchodilator, mucolytic: spasmodic bronchial disorders with wheezing, coughing and difficult expectoration; allergic and bronchial asthma (acute and chronic), chronic bronchitis, emphysema
antipyretic, anti-inflammatory, analgesic: acute throat infections with difficult swallowing and swelling; pharyngitis, laryngitis, tonsillitis, lockjaw, gingivitis
antibacterial: acute infections (incl. enteritis, bacterial dysentery); reproductive infections, (incl. pelvic inflammatory disease, endometritis, cervicitis)
detoxicant, antivenomous, detumescent: boils, carbuncles, throat abscess, snakebite
cholagogue laxative: biliary dyspepsia, acute jaundice, constipation
antacid antisecretory: acid dyspepsia from hyperchlorhydria, gastric ulcer
antitumoral, immunostimulant, interferon inducent: tumors benign and cancerous (incl. cervical/laryngeal/lung/bladder cancer); leukemia
leukocytogenic: low WBC count due to chemo/radiotherapy (leukopenia)
vulnerary: head ulcers, injuries from all animal bites or stings, cervical erosion

Symptom Pictures

lung Qi constraint: wheezing, tight chest, coughing with difficult expectoration of scanty sticky sputum

lung heat dryness: swollen, painful sore throat, coughing, feverishness, thirst

intestines damp heat: urgent, painful bowel movement, loose stool, blood in stool

Preparation

Use: The root Sophora Shan Dou Gen is decocted or used as a tincture. For its *vulnerary* and *anti-inflammatory* effects, external swabs, compresses and douches are prepared.

Dosage: Decoction: 4-10 g
Tincture: 2-4 ml

Caution: Forbidden in diarrhea caused by poor digestive assimilation.

Notes

With its twin *relaxant/anti-inflammatory actions,* Pigeon-pea root is specific for relieving severe asthmatic conditions—as seen from the two lung syndromes above. Acute throat infections also benefit from these and *anti-infective* actions, signaled by bitter-cold-dry effective qualities.

The *anticancer* effect of Pigeon-pea root is thought to be due primarily to the alkaloids matrine and oxymatrine, and secondarily to the flavonoids. Enhancement of reticuloendothelial and phagocytic functions has been shown and, although good results have been achieved so far, more experimentation is needed to obtain a clearer pharmacological picture.

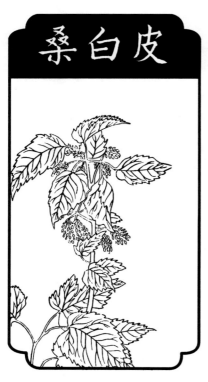

Morus Sang Bai Pi
Mulberry Root Bark

Botanical source: *Morus alba* L. (Moraceae)
Pharmaceutical name: Cortex radicis Mori albae
Chinese names: Sang Bai Pi (Mand); Song Baak Pei (Cant)
Other names: White mulberry; Sohakuhi (Jap)
Habitat: Small deciduous tree found throughout China, both wild and cultivated; flowers in May with stalked hanging catkins.
Part used: the root bark

Therapeutic category: mild remedy with minimal chronic toxicity
Constituents: flavone derivatives morusin, mulberrin, mulberrochromine, cyclomulberrin; betulinic acid, coumarins scopoletin and umbelliferone, amyrin, undecaprenol, dodecaprenol, mulberrofuran A, tannin, triterpenoid
Effective qualities: sweet, astringent, cold
relaxing, stimulating, decongesting, sinking
Tropism: respiratory, urinary, cardiovascular systems
Lung, Spleen channels
Air, Fluid bodies

Actions and Indications

respiratory relaxant: bronchodilator, antitussive: spasmodic bronchial conditions with wheezing, coughing; asthma, acute bronchitis

urinary sedative, draining diuretic: dysuria, strangury, edema, anuria; acute nephritis (Bright's disease)

hypotensive: hypertension

nervous sedative: irritability, unrest

interferon inducent

Symptom Pictures

lung Qi constraint: wheezing, chest constriction, coughing

lung heat: dry cough, coughing up blood, wheezing, thirst, unrest, irritability

fluid congestion with heat: water retention in face and extremites, thirst, fever, difficult/scanty urination

Preparation

Use: The root bark Morus Sang Bai Pi is decocted or used in tincture form. Stir-frying in honey changes its cooling effect into a warming one that is often used to treat chronic bronchitis.

Dosage: Decoction: 8-18 g
 Tincture: 2-4 ml

Caution: Contraindicated in lung Qi deficiency, coughing due to wind cold and excessive urination.

Notes

A good *respiratory relaxant* when the lung Qi fails to descend and constrains breathing, Mulberry root bark is most often used in hot or acute conditions. Thirst, fever and dry cough are here the key symptoms. Kidney edema and acute nephritis (including with hypertension) are other conditions calling for this *refrigerant, hypotensive diuretic* remedy.

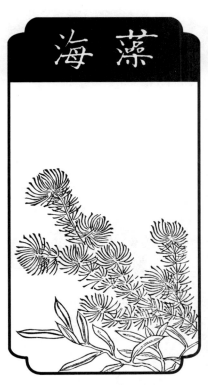

Sargassum Hai Zao
Sargassum Seaweed

Botanical source: *Sargassum fusiforme* (Harv.) Setch or *S. pallidum* (Turn.) C. Ag. (Sargassaceae)
Pharmaceutical name: Herba Sargassi
Chinese names: Hai Zao, Lou Shu(Mand); Hoi Chou (Cant)
Other names: Kaiso (Jap)
Part used: the whole thallus

Therapeutic category: mild remedy with minimal chronic toxicity
Constituents: mannitol, alginic acid, laminine, sargassan, polysaccharides, minerals and trace minerals (incl. iodine), glucose
Effective qualities: bitter, salty, cold, moist
 relaxing, softening, dissolving, diluting, decongesting
Tropism: respiratory, glandular, digestive, repoductive systems
 Stomach, Spleen, Liver, Kidney channels
 Fluid, Warmth bodies

Actions and Indications

respiratory relaxant: bronchodilator, expectorant: spasmodic bronchial disorders with wheezing; bronchial asthma, chronic bronchitis

detoxicant, dermatropic: metabolic toxicosis with arthritis, rheumatism, dermatitis, psoriasis

resolvent, dissolvent, lymphatic decongestant: lymphadenitis, lymphangitis, hypothyroid goiter, fibrocystic breasts

anticoagulant, antilipemic: thrombosis, hyperlipemia

antitumoral: tumors (incl. lymphoma, Hodgkin's disease, skin cancer)

radiation protective

analgesic, anti-inflammatory: groin pain, hernial pain, testicle inflammation, mumps
draining diuretic: edema
demulcent laxative: constipation
antifungal, antiviral: herpes simplex

PREPARATION
Use: The seaweed Sargassum Hai Zao is decocted or used in tincture form.
Dosage: Decoction: 10-16 g
Tincture: 2-4 ml
Caution: Forbidden in stomach and intestines cold, and not to be used continuously in hyperthyroid conditions.

NOTES
The extremely rich mineral and trace element content of this sea vegetable makes Sargassum beneficial in any respiratory condition presenting wheezing from constrained lung Qi. Likewise, it is very effective for most chronic swellings, especially swollen lymphatic glands. However, Sargassum's *dissolving, softening* and *diluting* actions—like that of all seaweeds—on tissues and fluids should be understood in context of its overall *resolvent detoxicant* effect.

Laminaria Kun Bu
Kelp Seaweed

Botanical source: *Laminaria* spp. (Laminariaceae)   **Chinese names:** Kun Bu (Mand)

NOTE: Kelp is very similar in nature, functions and uses to Sargassum Hai Zao (see previous page). The two remedies are interchangeable.
Dosage: Decoction: 3-10 g
Tincture: 0.5-2 ml
Caution: None.

Inula Xuan Fu Hua
Japanese Elecampane Flower

Botanical source: *Inula brittanica* L. or var. *chinensis* (Rupr.) Regel or *linariaefolia* Turczaninow or *japonica* Thunberg (Compositae)
Chinese names: Xuan Fu Hua, Fu Hua (Mand); Shuan Fuk Fa, Chuan Fuk Fa (Cant)
Other names: Senpukuka (Jap)
Habit: Perennial Northeast Asian herb growing on roadsides, field edges, damp lands and hillsides; terminal capitate yellow flowers bloom in autumn.

Category: mild remedy with minimal chronic toxicity
Constituents: flavonoids (quercetin, isoquercetin), inulin, taraxasterol, alkaloids, caffeic acid, chlorogenic acid, fatty oil, sesquiterpenes britanin and inulicin
Effective qualities: bitter, pungent, a bit warm, dry; relaxing, stimulating, decongesting
Tropism: respiratory, digestive, hepatic, urinary systems; Lung, Liver, Stomach, Spleen channels

ACTIONS: *Bronchodilator, antitussive, stimulant expectorant, digestive stimulant, antiemetic, draining diuretic, antibacterial*
INDICATIONS: Spasmodic bronchial conditions (lung Qi constraint syndrome) with wheezing, coughing; asthma, catarrhal conditions (lung phlegm damp) with productive cough; acute and chronic bronchitis; dyspepsia from stomach cold and intestines mucous damp (Spleen damp) syndromes; gastroenteritis; vomiting, belching, hiccup; edema.

Dosage: Infusion/decoction: 3-10 g
Tincture: 2-4 ml

When decocted, Inula Xuan Fu Hua should be first wrapped in filter paper, as the petals may cause gastric and bronchial irritation.

Caution: Avoid using in deficiency conditions, especially wind heat and dry respiratory conditions.

NOTES: It is interesting to note that while Elecampane root is being accepted as a good Qi tonic in the West, in the Orient it is the flower of this related elecampane, rather than the root, that has always been considered valuable—and then mainly as a *relaxant/stimulant expectorant*. This comes as no suprise, however, considering the presence in the Chinese pharmacopeia of other, more metabolism-oriented superior *Qi tonics* such as Astragalus root and Asian ginseng root.

If needed, the root of *Inula helenium,* Elecampane, would make a fairly good substitute for this remedy in both varieties of damp-related symptom pictures above.

Aristolochia Ma Dou Ling
Green Birthwort Capsule

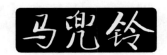

Botanical source: *Aristolochia contorta* Bunge or *A. debilis* Siebold et Zuccarini (Aristolochaceae)
Chinese names: Ma Dou Ling (Mand); Ma Dau Ling (Cant)
Habit: Perennial spreading vine from North China
Category: medium-strength remedy with chronic toxicity

Constituents: alkaloids aristolochine and magnoflorine, aristolochic and aristolochinic acid
Effective qualities: bitter, cold, neutral, dry; relaxing, decongesting
Tropism: respiratory, cardiovascular, hepatobiliary systems; Lung channel

ACTIONS: *Bronchodilator, antitussive, anti-inflammatory, hypotensive, draining diuretic, detumescent, immunostimulant, antitumoral, antibacterial, antifungal*

INDICATIONS: Lung Qi constraint syndrome with acute asthma, acute bronchitis; dry cough, wheezing; hemoptysis; hypertension, edema, ascites; various infections (incl. chronic abscess, tonsilitis, hepatitis, liver cirrhosis, lung TB, pneumonia); painful swollen hemorrhoids and fistulas; tumors, cancer.

Dosage: Decoction: 3-10 g
Tincture: 1-3 ml

Toasting Aristolochia Ma Dou Ling in honey first can prevent the possible side-effects of nausea and vomiting.

Caution: The fruit capsule and root of this plant possess some cumulative toxicity due to aristolochic acid: They should not be used continuously. For the same reason, the tincture of this remedy can cause idiosyncratic reactions. These include nausea, gastric discomfort and mild diarrhea. This remedy is contraindicated in diarrhea due to stomach and intestines cold, in coughing or wheezing due to deficiency cold, and during pregnancy.

NOTES: Green birthwort capsule is a reliable *relaxant* for acute asthmatic conditions, i.e., when the Qi constrains the lungs, with dry coughing. The *hypotensive* effect of both fruit and root is mild but consistent. The *antitumoral* and *anti-infective* actions of Green birthwort capsule are due to its content in aristolochic acid.

Caragana Jin Ji Er
Caragana Root

Botanical source: *Caragana sinica* (Buchol) Rehder and spp. (Leguminosae)
Chinese names: Jin Ji Er, Tu Huang Qi (Mand)
Category: mild remedy with minimal chronic toxicity
Constituents: alakaloids, flavonoids, coumarin lactones, phytosterols
Effective qualities: sweet, neutral, dry; relaxing, decongesting, astringing
Tropism: respiratory, cardiovascular, urinary systems, immune; Lung, Spleen, Heart channels

Actions: *Bronchodilator, hypotensive, restorative, draining diuretic, anti-inflammatory, antiseptic, mucostatic, antirheumatic, immunosuppressant*
Indications: Wheezing from bronchial asthma and bronchitis; palpitations, with hypertension; edema, leucorrhea, rheumatism, lupus erythematosus.
Dosage: Decoction: 10-40 g
Tincture: 2-5 ml
Caution: Caragana Jin Ji Er may very rarely cause allergic reactions in some people, such as skin itching or skin rashes, as well as dizziness, drowsiness or nausea.
Notes: Caragana root is called **Tu Huang Qi** or "local Huang Qi" because it is popularly used in the same way as Huang Qi, Astragalus root, namely as a *Qi/energy tonic*. **Caragana flower, Jin Que Hua** or **Yang Que Hua**, is a popular remedy for dizziness and vertigo.

Haematitum Dai Zhe Shi
Hematite

Geological source: Haematitum
Chinese name: Dai Zhe Shi (Mand); Doi Ji Sek (Cant)
Source: The mineral ore is obtained in North China. It is also known as red orchre or brown iron oxide.
Category: medium-strength remedy with some chronic toxicity
Constituents: diferric trioxide, calcium/aluminum/silicon oxide, clay, iron, trace minerals (incl. aluminum, silicon, magnesium, tin, arsenic, manganese)
Effective qualities: bitter, cold, dry; relaxing, sinking, astringing
Tropism: respiratory, digestive, central nervous, cardiovascular systems; Liver, Stomach, Pericardium channels

Actions: *Bronchodilator, nervous sedative, antiemetic, hemostatic, hemogenic*
Indications: Wheezing, asthma from constrained lung Qi; tinnitus, vertigo, headache, pressure behind eyes, sudden deafness, vomiting, belching, hiccups; uterine bleeding, vomiting blood, nosebleed; anemia, spleen deficiency.
Dosage: Decoction: 10-30 g. The mineral Hematite is decocted 30 minutes before the remainder of a formula is added to the decoction.
Caution: Contraindicated in pregnancy and for continuous use at regular doses due to slight cumulative toxicity.
Notes: An adjunct remedy in formulas for acute conditions such as acute asthma or vomiting, Hematite also excells at relieving the neurological symptoms of rising energy, such as ringing in the ears, sudden deafness, vertigo and headache.

Stalactitum E Guan Shi
Stalactite Tip

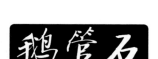

Geological source: *Stalactitum* or *Balanophylla* spp.
Chinese names: E Guan Shi, Shi Zhong Ru, Zhong Ru She (Mand)
Source: Caves throughout China
Category: mild remedy with minimal chronic toxicity
Constituents: calcium carbonate, trace minerals
Effective qualities: sweet, warm; relaxing, stimulating
Tropism: respiratory, endocrine systems; Lung channel

Actions: *Stimulant expectorant, antitussive, galactagogue*
Indications: Productive coughing and wheezing with lung Qi constraint syndrome with deficiency and cold; insufficient breast milk.
Dosage: Decoction: 10-16 g. Decoct alone for 30 minutes before adding any other herbs.
Caution: Do not use excessively, as it may cause indigestion. Forbidden with coughing up of blood.
Notes: **E Guan Shi** and **Zhong Ru** are both the tips of tubular stalactites. E Guan Shi is small and slender and has a radiated internal structure, whereas Zhong Ru is thicker and coarser, and usually shows a hollow center.

Iphigenia Shan Ci Gu
Iphigenia Bulb

Botanical source: *Iphigenia indica* A. Gray (Liliaceae)
Chinese names: Shan Ci Gu, Cao Bei Mu, Tu Bei Mu, Yi Bi Jian (Mand); San Chi Gu (Cant)
Category: strong remedy with acute toxicity

Constituents: alkaloids colchinine 0.12%, isocolchinine, lumicolchinine, cornigerine, N-formyl-N-deacetylcolchinine
Effective qualities: bitter, warm; relaxing, calming
Tropism: respiratory, nervous systems; Lung channel

ACTIONS: *Bronchodilator, analgesic, antitumoral*
INDICATIONS: Asthma, bronchitis from constrained lung Qi; gout, nasopharyngeal and salivary gland tumors (incl. cancerous); adenoma, hepatoma, lymphosarcoma, breast cancer.
Dosage: Decoction: 0.1-0.5 g
Tincture: 1-3 drops
Caution: This very toxic remedy is only to be used under supervision. Side-effects include vomiting, diarrhea, abdominal pain, stupor, chills and exhaustion.
NOTES: In the People's Republic the *antitumoral* compound colchincinamide is also synthesized.

There are several other botanical sources for the remedy Shan Ci Gu: the bulb of *Tulipa edulis* Bak. (also in the lily family, and also known as **Guang Zi Gu**); the corm of *Cremastra variabilis* (Blume) Nakai (Orchidaceae) (especially used for lung tumors and gastric cancer); the corm of *Pleione bulbocodioides* (Frenchet) Rolfe (Orchidaceae). All contain similar and identical alkaloids to *Iphigenia indica,* and are considered sweet, a bit pungent and cold in effect. They are additionally used to treat furuncles, insect and snake bites, and lymphadenitis.

REMEDIES TO RESTORE THE ADRENAL CORTEX AND RELIEVE WHEEZING

➥ TONIFY LUNG AND KIDNEY YANG, AND ARREST WHEEZING

Adrenocortical restorative antiasthmatics

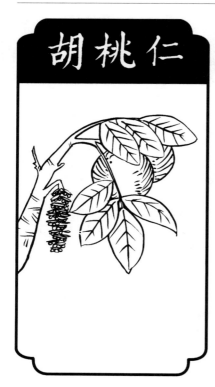

Juglans Hu Tao Ren
Walnut Meat

Botanical source: *Juglans regia* L. (Juglandaceae)
Pharmaceutical name: Semen Juglandis
Chinese names: Hu Tao Ren, Hu Tao Rou, Fen Xin Mu (Mand); Hap Tou Yan (Cant)
Other names: English/Persian walnut, "Persian peach"; Koto (Jap)
Habit: Deciduous pantemperate tree cultivated on flatlands; blooms in summer with drooping flower spikes.
Part used: the seed

Therapeutic category: mild remedy with minimal chronic toxicity
Constituents: linoleic/oleic/linolenic/lauric/myristic/arachic acid, juglone, betulin, carotene, proteins, trace minerals, calcium, iron, phosphorus, tannins, phytin, inositol, phytosterols, oxydase, vitamins A, B2, C, E
Effective qualities: sweet, warm, moist
 restoring, relaxing, nourishing, thickening, solidifying
Tropism: respiratory, urogenital, digestive, musculoskeletal systems
 Lung, Kidney, Large Intestine, Yang Qiao channels; Air, Fluid bod-

ACTIONS AND INDICATIONS

respiratory relaxant: bronchodilator: spasmodic bronchial conditions with wheezing, chronic cough; chronic asthma, lung TB, pneumonia
adrenocortical restorative, cholinergic: weak lungs, chronic fatigue and weakness; adrenal cortex deficiency, menopause, tinnitus
urogenital restorative, antienuretic: incontinence with enuresis, pollakiuria, spermatorrhea
musculoskeletal restorative: weak lumbars, knees and legs; lumbago, degenerative bone conditions (incl. osteomalacia); weight loss
resolvent detoxicant, dermatropic: chronic skin conditions (incl. dermatitis, eczema, herpes)
antilithic, lithagogue: kidney and bladder stones
antacid antisecretory: acid dyspepsia from hyperchlorhydria; gastric and duodenal ulcer
intestinal demulcent: constipation, dry hard stool, colic
Miscellaneous: premature hair graying

SYMPTOM PICTURES

adrenocortical deficiency (Lung and Kidney Yang deficiency): chronic cough, wheezing, fatigue, weakness
genitourinary cold and **musculoskeletal deficiency (Kidney Yang deficiency):** frequent urination, seminal incontinence, loss of sexual desire, weak back and knees, cold extremities

PREPARATION

Use: The seed Juglans Hu Tao Ren is decocted or used in tincture form.
Dosage: Decoction: 10-30 g
 Tincture: 2-4 ml
Caution: Contraindicated in lung phlegm heat, coughing due to heat, Yin deficiency with empty heat, watery stool.

NOTES

Chinese medicine uses the seed, i.e., the meat, of this "Persian peach" (Hu Tao), whereas Western herbal medicine uses its fruit rind (hull) and leaf. Their uses are somewhat different, although they overlap in that they both treat acute and chronic skin conditions, weakness from skeletal deficiency, degenerative bone disease and constipation due to internal dryness.

The main therapeutic value of Walnut meat lies in its tonifying action on the adrenal cortex and its resultant *restorative* and *relaxant* effects on the bronchi. These successive actions rank Walnut meat a Kidney Yang remedy in Chinese medicine, that is, a remedy for the syndrome that includes adrenal, urinary and genital as well as respiratory deficiency.

While Walnut meat is also used for its *astringent* action on urogenital functions and Walnut hull/leaf on the intestinal tract and capillaries, all three parts are effective in treating urinary and seminal incontinence.

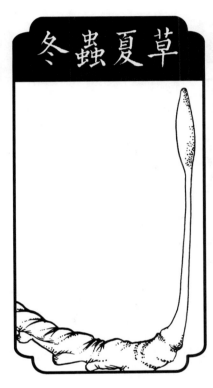

Cordyceps Dong Chong Xia Cao
Chinese Caterpillar Mushroom

Botanical source: *Cordyceps sinensis* (Berk.) Saccardo and spp. (Clavicipitaceae) and host larvae *Hepialus armoricanus* Oberthur and spp. or *Holotrichia koraiensis* (Hepialidae)
Pharmaceutical name: Sclerotium Cordycepsis
Chinese names: Dong Chong Xia Cao, Dong Cao, Chong Cao (Mand)
Other names: Tochukaso (Jap); Aweto (Tib); Dong Chong Ha Chou (Cant)
Habit: Grows in the cool, forested hills and mountains of East China and Tibet; prefers loose, fertile leafy soil; in autumn, the mushroom grows underground from the anterior end of previously infected host larvae and eventually surfaces during the following summer.
Part used: the fruiting body or the cultured mycelia

Therapeutic category: mild remedy with minimal chronic toxicity
Constituents: proteins 25-32%, mannitol, cordycepic acid, cordycepin, polysaccharides, nucleosides (uracil, uridine, adenine, adenosine), lipids, 18 amino acids, ergosterol, cellulose, saturated and unsaturated acids, vitamin B 12, trace elements (incl. phosphorus, cobalt, iron, copper, zinc, magnesium)
Effective qualities: sweet, neutral, dry
                      restoring, relaxing, astringing, calming
Tropism: respiratory, endocrine, immune, reproductive, musculokeletal, digestive, systems
                Lung, Kidney, Yang Qiao channels; Air, Fluid bodies

ACTIONS AND INDICATIONS

respiratory relaxant: bronchodilator, antitussive: spasmodic bronchial disorders with wheezing; infantile cough, asthma, chronic bronchitis, emphysema
adrenocortical and respiratory restorative, cholinergic: lung weakness, lung TB; fatigue, weakness, backache, impotence; convalescence, menopause, premature aging, renal failure
hemostatic: hemoptysis
genital astringent, anhydrotic: seminal incontinence with spermatorrhea, excessive day or night sweats
neurocardiac sedative, hypotensive: neurocardiac syndrome with irritability, anxiety; hypertension, arrhythmia
antilipemic: hyperlipemia
immunostimulant, antibacterial: infections in general; chronic lung TB, streptococcal pneumonia

antitumoral: cancer (incl. lung and nasopharyngeal cancer)

SYMPTOM PICTURES

adrenocortical deficiency (Lung and Kidney Yang deficiency): wheezing, fatigue, loss of stamina

lung Yin deficiency: coughing with blood-tinged sputum, fatigue, dreaminess

genitourinary cold with **Yin deficiency (Kidney Yin and Yang deficiency/Kidney Essence deficiency):** fatigue, weak legs and back, night sweats, seminal incontinence, impotence

PREPARATION

Use: The fungus Cordyceps Dong Chong Xia Cao is decocted or used in tincture form. Preparing the mushroom for consumption with duck is said to enhance its benefits.

Dosage: Decoction: 6-14 g
Tincture: 2-4 ml

Caution: Use with care in external conditions, i.e., with the onset of infections.

NOTES

Chinese caterpillar mushroom is an unusual remedy that originates in Sichuan and southern Tibet and now grows in other provinces, such as Shaanxi and Yunnan. Consisting of a fungus and its larval host, it develops largely in the dark of the soil before surfacing (see Habit for details).

The Caterpillar mushroom is traditionally compared to Oriental ginseng for its life-extending abilities. The mushroom's action is almost totally *restorative,* applying to the bronchi, on the one hand, and the whole system through *adrenocortical* and *immune stimulation,* on the other. The remedy's primary tropicity for respiratory functions is evinced in its *bronchial relaxant, antitussive, hemostatic* and *antiseptic* actions. This clearly spells out usage for symptom patterns entailing fatigue, shallow breathing, coughing, wheezing—in Chinese medicine defined as a deficiency of both Lung and Kidney Yang. Consumptive, Yin-deficient lung conditions are the other important indication that calls for Caterpillar mushroom.

The cultured mycelia have been shown to be equally as effective therapeutically as the natural mushroom (Zhang Shu-lan et al. 1985), and have been undergoing extensive clinical trials.

Gecko Ge Jie
Toad-Headed Lizard

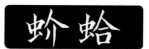

Zoological source: *Gecko gecko* L. or *G. verticilatus* Laurentii (Geckonidae)
Chinese names: Ge Jie (Mand); Gap Gwai (Cant)
Habit: Small nocturnal lizard from (sub)tropical Asia (different from the gecko lizard)
Part used: the whole animal

Category: mild remedy with minimal chronic toxicity
Constituents: amino acids, lipids
Effective qualities: salty, neutral; relaxing, restoring, astringing
Tropism: respiratory, endocrine urinary, reproductive systems; Lung, Kidney, Chong, Ren channels

ACTIONS: *Bronchodilator, antitussive, adrenocortical and respiratory restorative, cholinergic, urogenital restorative, estrogenic*

INDICATIONS: Chronic spasmodic bronchial conditions with cough, wheezing, fatigue; emphysema, asthma, tracheitis; lung Qi constraint with Lung and Kidney Yang deficiency syndrome; fatigue, low stamina; lung TB with coughing up blood; Kidney Yang deficiency syndrome with enuresis/pollakiuria, loss of sexual interest, impotence.

Dosage: Powder: 3-6 g
Decoction: 10-18 g

Gecko Ge Jie is usually used in powder form, but may also be decocted.

Caution: Contraindicated in wheezing due to external wind cold, and in external heat conditions.

NOTES: Toad-headed lizard's *cholinergic* action on the adrenal cortex causes the pronounced *bronchial relaxant* effect. Chronic asthma with systemic deficiency is here the main indication.

Respiratory Sedatives

REMEDIES TO PROMOTE EXPECTORATION AND REDUCE BRONCHIAL INFECTION

➧ COOL AND TRANSFORM PHLEGM HEAT

Anti-inflammatory antiseptic expectorants

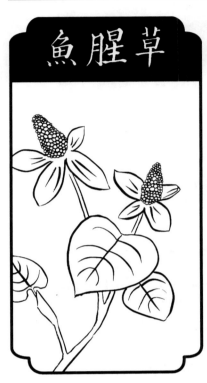

魚腥草

Houttuynia Yu Xing Cao
Fishwort Herb *

Botanical source: *Houttuynia cordata* Thunberg (Saururaceae)
Pharmaceutical name: Herba Houttuyniae
Chinese names: Yu Xing Cao, Ju Cai, Ji Cai (Mand); Yu Chin Chou (Cant)
Other names: "Fish smelling herb"; Gyoseiso (Jap)
Habit: Perennial creeping herb with fishy scent from temperate East Asia and subtropical Himalayas; grows in shady, dank places by streams, ponds, swamps and ditches; blooms in summer with spikelets of white terminal flowers.
Part used: the herb or leaf, sometimes the whole plant (herb and root)

Therapeutic category: mild herb with minimal chronic toxicity
Constituents: essential oil (incl. decanoyl acetaldehyde, methylnonylketone, capric aldehyde, ketodecanal, methyllauryl sulfide, pinene, camphene, myrcene, linalool, bornyl acetate), capric acid, calcium sulfate/chloride, flavonoids, (incl. quercitrin, isoquercitrin, quercetin, reynoutrin, rutin, cordarine, hyperin)
Effective qualities: pungent, cold, dry
   calming, stimulating, astringing, decongesting
Tropism: respiratory, digestive, urinary systems
   Lung, Liver channels
   Warmth, Fluid bodies

Actions and Indications

respiratory sedative: anti-infective (antiviral, antibacterial, antifungal, immunostimulant),
antitussive: acute respiratory, epidermal, intestinal and urinary tract infections; bronchitis, acute and chronic pneumonia, influenza, emphysema, TB; psoriasis, dermatitis, tinea, enteritis, dysentery, cystitis; esp. *Staphylococcus*, *Streptococcus*, gram-negative bacilli, *Mycobacterium tuberculosis*
detoxicant, anti-inflammatory: lung abscess, chronic suppurative otitis media, laryngitis, mastitis, cellulitis, acute dermatitis; hemorrhoids, boils, carbuncles, swellings, insect bites
anticatarrhal: diarrhea; acute enteritis, dysentery, leucorrhea; rectal prolapse
draining diuretic: chronic nephritis, edema, cystitis, dysuria
interferon inducent

Symptom Pictures

lung phlegm heat: coughing, expectoration of thick green sputum, feverishness, thirst

intestines damp heat: diarrhea, painful bowel movement, abdominal pain, thirst

bladder damp heat: painful, burning difficult urination, thirst

Preparation

Use: The herb Houttuynia Yu Xing Cao is infused, briefly decocted or used in tincture form. The fresh herb is more effective than the dried and, like it, may be applied topically for urticaria and fungal skin infections.

Dosage: Infusion or decoction: 10-30 g
Tincture: 2-4 ml
Caution: Forbidden in deficiency cold syndromes.

NOTES

High in essential oils, Fishwort herb is a good broad-based *anti-infective (antiviral, antibacterial, antifungal)* remedy for the respiratory, urinary and intestinal organs. The herb addresses both damp heat (i.e., catarrhal) infections, and those of the fire toxin (i.e., pyogenic/febrile) type.

With bronchial infections presenting productive coughing and fever, this *expectorant* really shines. Like the similar *mucostatic* remedy Plantain leaf, Fishwort acts here as a true *sedative* to reduce inflammation, resolve sputum, detoxify and relieve coughing. As a reliable *anti-inflammatory* (note the significant flavonoids present in the plant), a variety of simple, suppurative (and possibly allergic?) inflammatory disorders are also treated with it. Lung abscess with hemoptysis is here one of the main traditional indications.

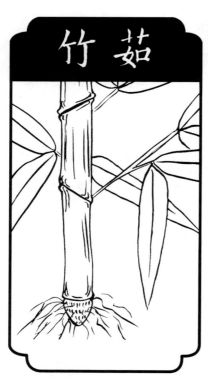

Phyllostachys Zhu Ru
Black Bamboo Shaving

Botanical source: *Phyllostachys nigra* (Lodd.) Munro var. *henonis* (Mitf.) Stapf ex Rendle and spp (Gramineae)
Pharmaceutical name: Caulis Phyllostachis in taeniis
Chinese names: Zhu Ru (Mand); Jok Yu (Cant)
Other names: Black/Purple/Henon bamboo, Partridge cane; Chikujo (Jap)
Habit: Tall evergreen (sub)tropical Chinese bush growing on moist, fertile ground by streamsides and in remote hills; long cultivated in Japan.
Part used: the culm shaving without the green skin

Therapeutic category: mild remedy with minimal chronic toxicity
Constituents: fentosan, lignan, triterpene, cellulose
Effective qualities: sweet, cool, dry
calming, relaxing, astringing
Tropism: respiratory, central nervous, vascular, digestive systems
Lung, Stomach, Gallbladder channels
Warmth, Air bodies

ACTIONS AND INDICATIONS

respiratory sedative: anti-infective, antibacterial: acute respiratory infections; acute bronchitis with tight chest and coughing
antipyretic: fevers, heat stroke
antiemetic gastric relaxant: vomiting, nausea, morning sickness; chronic gastritis
hemostatic: coughing or vomiting blood, nosebleed, menorrhagia
nervous relaxant, anticonvulsant: agitation, infantile seizures, epilepsy
fetal relaxant: fetal unrest
interferon inducent

SYMPTOM PICTURES

lung phlegm heat: expectoration of thick yellow sputum, tight chest, coughing up blood, irritability
stomach heat: sour or bitter regurgitation, bad breath, intolerance of heat

PREPARATION
Use: The shaving Phyllostachis Zhu Ru is decocted or used in tincture form; the latter is less cool than the decoction.
Dosage: Decoction: 4-10 g
Tincture: 2-4 ml
Caution: Contraindicated in nausea or vomiting due to cold in the stomach.

NOTES
A graceful, thin-walled yet strong native of South China, the black bamboo was introduced to Europe in 1829 and to the U.S. in 1909. The culm shaving is a specific remedy for acute lung infections with fever. Its *relaxant* nature is especially useful during pregnancy, to relieve morning sickness and fetal unrest.

Black bamboo leaf, Zhu Ye (Mand.) or **Jok Yip** (Cant.), is sweet and cold in quality. Its *refrigerant, antipyretic, secretory, nervous relaxant, diuretic* and *antiemetic* properties are given in fever with thirst and irritability, convulsions in children, vomiting and nosebleeds.
Dose: 6-12 g. Forbidden with diarrhea present.

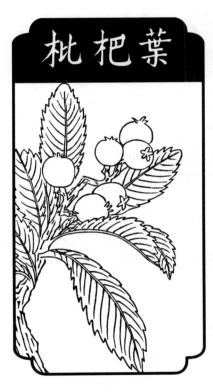

Eriobotrya Pi Pa Ye
Loquat Leaf

Botanical source: *Eriobotrya japonica* (Thunb.) Lindley (Rosaceae)
Pharmaceutical name: Folium Eriobotryae
Chinese names: Pi Pa Ye, Pa Ye (Mand); Pei Pai Yip (Cant)
Other names: Japanese medlar; Biwayo (Jap)
Habit: Small evergreen shrub or tree growing in Central China's uplands; also cultivated on the southwest coast; dense terminal white blossom panicles appear in autumn and early winter.
Part used: the leaf

Therapeutic category: mild remedy with minimal chronic toxicity
Constituents: essential oil (incl. nerolidol, farnesol), amygdalin, tannin, saponin, organic acid, glucose, vitamins B and C
Effective qualities: bitter, cool, dry
calming, stimulating, relaxing, astringing
Tropism: respiratory, digestive systems
Lung, Stomach channels
Air, Warmth bodies

ACTIONS AND INDICATIONS
respiratory sedative: antitussive, expectorant: bronchial infections with productive cough; acute and chronic bronchitis
gastric sedative, antiemetic: nausea, vomiting, hiccups, belching; gastritis
urinary sedative: dysuria, fever
hemostatic, vulnerary: nosebleed; coughing up blood; chaps, sores, ulcers
antibacterial, antiviral

SYMPTOM PICTURES
lung phlegm heat: coughing with expectoration of thick yellow or dry sputum, wheezing, thirst
stomach fire with **Qi reflux:** belching, hiccups, nausea, vomiting, thirst

PREPARATION
Use: The leaf Eriobotrya Pi Pa Ye is briefly decocted or used in tincture form. *Astringent, antiseptic* topical applications can be prepared for sores, etc.
Dosage: Decoction: 6-16 g
  Tincture: 2-5 ml
Caution: Contraindicated in coughing due to lung wind cold and in vomiting from stomach cold.

NOTES
Loquat leaf can be used in various lung symptom pictures with coughing and thirst as main symptoms. Like most other remedies, it is rarely used on its own, but usually combined.

The sweet tasting **Loquat fruit** is used as a cooling medicinal food for cough, thirst, dry throat and nausea, but should not be eaten in excessive quantities.

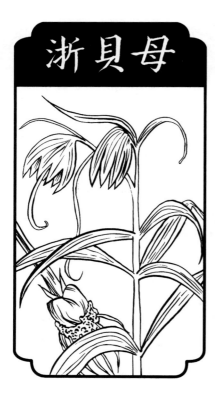

Fritillaria Zhe Bei Mu
Zhejiang Fritillary Bulb *

Botanical source: *Fritillaria thunbergii* Miquel, syn. *F. verticillata* Willdenow var. *thunbergii* Baker (Liliaceae)
Pharmaceutical name: Bulbus Fritillariae
Chinese names: Zhe Bei Mu, Xiang Bei, Zhe Bei (Mand); Chit Bui Mou (Cant)
Other names: "Zhejiang shell mother"; Setsubaimo (Jap)
Habit: Perennial temperate herb at home in the sandy soil of China's mild coastal climates, especially Zhejiang; partial to humid warmth and sunlight; also cultivated; terminal umbels of solitary yellow flowers appear in spring.
Part used: the bulb

Therapeutic category: mild remedy with minimal chronic toxicity
Constituents: alkaloids (incl. peimine, peiminine, peimidine, peimiphine, peimisine, peimitidine), steroid propeimine, glucoalkaloid peiminoside
Effective qualities: bitter, cool, moist
  calming, stimulating, softening
Tropism: respiratory, lymphatic systems
  Lung, Triple Heater, Liver, Stomach channels
  Air, Warmth bodies

ACTIONS AND INDICATIONS
respiratory sedative: antitussive, antiseptic: acute or chronic respiratory infections with constant coughing; bronchitis, pneumonia
mucolytic expectorant: cough with difficult expectoration
anti-inflammatory: laryngitis, acute mastitis
resolvent, detumescent, lymphatic decongestant: nodules, swellings, lymphadenitis (esp. in neck), fibrocystic breast disorder, lung or breast abscess, scrofula, sores
antitumoral: tumors (incl. lymphoma, Hodgkin's disease, breast cancer)
uterine stimulant
hypotensive: hypertension

SYMPTOM PICTURE
lung phlegm heat/dryness: coughing, difficult expectoration of gluey yellow purulent sputum, tight chest, fever

PREPARATION

Use: The bulb Fritillaria Zhe Bei Mu is decocted or used in tincture form.
Dosage: Decoction: 3-12 g
Tincture: 1-4 ml
Caution: Contraindicated in gastric deficiency and during pregnancy. Although this remedy is traditionally forbidden with any kind of Aconite root, modern experiments have not found any incompatability between the two remedies.

NOTES

The Zhejiang fritillary is a liliaceous plant noted for its *heat-clearing* and *mucolytic expectorant* effects on the bronchi. The bulb is much used in acute bronchitis with difficult expectoration. Because it will reduce cough of any origin or type (the alkaloids peimine and peiminine have proven active here), this *antitussive respiratory sedative* remedy is often combined with *respiratory stimulants* and *relaxants,* depending on the overall symptom picture presenting.

Zhejiang fritillary bulb is also a noted *softening resolvent* remedy that can reduce swellings and lumps of many kinds, including lymphatic swelling, fibrocystic breasts and tumors.

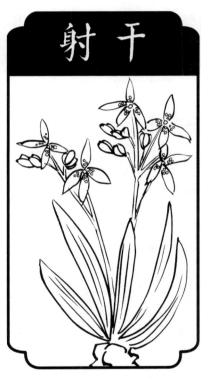

Belamcanda She Gan
Leopard Flower Root

Botanical source: *Belamcanda chinensis* (L.) De Candolle (Iridaceae)
Pharmaceutical name: Rhizoma Belamcandae
Chinese names: She Gan, Pian Ju, Wu Shan (Mand); Sei Gon, Sei Gam (Cant)
Other names: Blackberry lily, "Lance"; Yakan, Karasu ogi (Jap)
Habit: Perennial herb from mideastern China, Japan, the Russian Far East and Indonesia, growing in rich, damp grassland and slopy mountain ground; also cultivated; terminal racemes of red-spotted orange flowers appear in summer.
Part used: the rhizome

Therapeutic category: medium-strength remedy with some chronic toxicity
Constituents: belamcandin, iridin, tectoridin, tectorigenin, mangiferin
Effective qualities: bitter, cold, moist
relaxing, calming, stimulating, softening
Tropism: respiratory, digestive, reproductive, urinary systems
Lung, Liver channels
Warmth, Air bodies

ACTIONS AND INDICATIONS

respiratory sedative/relaxant: antitussive, antiviral, antibacterial: respiratory infections with coughing and wheezing (esp. in children); acute bronchitis, pneumonia, emphysema
mucolytic expectorant: cough with difficult expectoration
anti-inflammatory, detumescent: acute laryngitis, pharyngitis, tonsillitis with pain and swelling; boils, swellings
uterine stimulant, emmenagogue: amenorrhea, dysmenorrhea
hepatic stimulant: liver congestion, hepatitis, splenomegaly
draining diuretic: edema (incl. of the glottis)
stimulant laxative: constipation
antitumoral: breast cancer, throat tumors
antifungal, antivenomous: skin and throat infections; rabid dog bites, snakebites

Symptom Pictures
lung phlegm heat: wheezing, coughing, expectoration of thick yellow sputum

lung heat dryness and **lung phlegm dryness:** dry cough, painful swollen red throat, swallowing difficulty, hoarseness, constipation

Preparation
Use: The root Belamcanda She Gan is decocted or used as a tincture.
Dosage: Decoction: 3-9 g
Tincture: 1-3 ml
Caution: Because it has some cumulative toxicity, do not use on its own continuously, and do not exceed dosages. Belamcanda She Gan is forbidden during pregnancy and breastfeeding, and in diarrhea from intestinal deficiency.

Notes
Leopard flower root's multi-pronged *sedative, relaxant* and *stimulant* actions on the bronchi soften and dissolve hard old sputum, promote expectoration, and relieve coughing and wheezing. In bacteriological terms, Leopard flower is active in reversing viral and bacterial respiratory infections. From the therapeutic perspective, however, the asterisk signs for this *anti-inflammatory* remedy are a dry cough and an inflamed, swollen sore throat. Its bitter, cold and moist qualities are especially effective when heat and/or dryness constrain lung Qi, causing coughing and wheezing.

Leopard flower root's ability to relieve swelling—of the throat, liver or spleen—marks another of its therapeutic themes.

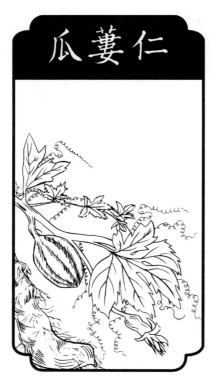

Tricosanthes Gua Lou Ren
Snakegourd Seed

Botanical source: *Trichosanthes kirilowii* Maximowicz and spp. (Cucurbitaceae)
Pharmaceutical name: Fructus Trichosanthis
Chinese names: Gua Lou Ren, Gua Lou Zi, Lou Ren/Shi, Di Lou (Mand); Gwa Lok Yan, Gwa Lok Ji (Cant)
Other names: Karonin (Jap)
Habit: Perennial herbaceous climbing vine from Central and South China and Vietnam; grows on hillsides, along wood edges and in weed thickets; axillary white flowers bloom in summer and autumn.
Part used: the fruit, i.e. the seed and pericarp

Therapeutic category: mild remedy with minimal chronic toxicity
Constituents: trichosanic acids, resins, fatty oil, tricosanthine
Effective qualities: sweet, bitter, sour, cool, moist
calming, stimulating, relaxing, dissolving, softening
Tropism: respiratory, cardiovascular, digestive systems
Lung, Stomach, Large Intestine channels; Warmth, Air bodies

Actions and Indications
respiratory sedative/relaxant: spasmodic bronchial infection with chest constriction and pain; bronchitis, pneumonia, pleurisy, emphysema

bronchial demulcent, expectorant: dry, harsh or difficult cough, cough with bloody sputum

demulcent laxative: constipation from dryness

coronary dilator: angina pectoris
stimulant diuretic: anuria
resolvent detoxicant: mastitis, nonsuppurative sores, breast abscess and swelling, eczema
antitumoral: tumors, cancer (incl. granuloma, hepatoma)
antibacterial: infections (esp. with *Escherichia coli, Shigella, Pseudomonas, Vibrio*)

Symptom Picture
lung phlegm heat: chest pain, production of thick yellow sputum, difficult expectoration, feverishness, thirst

Preparation
Use: The seed Trichosanthes Gua Lou Ren should be decocted or used in tincture form. Briefly stir-fried or toasted, the seeds become wearmer by nature and are then used to treat chronic bronchitis.
Dosage: Decoction: 10-14 g
Tincture: 2-5 ml
Caution: Contraindicated in diarrhea due to intestines cold. Do not combine with Ginger root, White oxknee root or Aconite root.

Notes
The seed of a scrambling vine, the snakegourd, uniquely combines sweet, bitter and sour taste qualities. As a result, its action on the bronchi is *demulcent, relaxant, mucolytic* and *stimulant* all at the same time. Snakegourd seed is a comprehensive remedy for acute, spasmodic phlegm heat conditions arising from infection, with keynote symptoms of harsh, dry cough, painful expectoration and chest constriction.

Tricosanthes Gua Lou
Snakegourd Fruit

Botanical source: *Tricosanthes kriliowii* Maximowicz (Cucurbitaceae)
Chinese names: Gua Lou (Mand); Gwa Lok (Cant)

Constituents: triterpenoid saponins, organic acids, resin, saccharides

Notes: The nature, functions, uses and dosages of this herb are the same as Trichosanthes Gua Lou Ren, Snakegourd seed, above, but somewhat less strong and without the *demulcent laxative* action.

Tricosanthes Gua Lou Pi
Snakegourd Rind

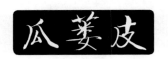

Botanical source: *Tricosanthes kriliowii* Maximowicz (Cucurbitaceae)

Chinese names: Gua Lou Pi (Mand); Gwa Lok Pei (Cant)

Notes: The nature, functions, uses and dosages of Snakegourd fruit rind are generally the same as Snakegourd seed (above). However, the fruit rind possesses the respiratory actions only, and is less strong. On the other hand, of the whole plant it has shown the best *antitumoral* and *cancer-inhibiting* action.

Benincasa Dong Gua Ren
Waxgourd Seed

Botanical source: *Benincasa hispida* (Thunb.) Cogniaux (Cucurbitaceae)
Chinese names: Dong Gua Ren, Dong Gua Zi (Mand); Dong Gwa Yan, Dong Gwa Ji (Cant)
Other names: Wintermelon, Ash/Whitegourd, Tunka; Tokanin (Jap)
Habit: Perennial Asian herb found throughout China; in early summer, single flowers arise from leaf axils.

Category: mild remedy with minimal chronic toxicity
Constituents: urease, fixed oil (incl. palmitic/stearic/linoleic acid), saponins, guanidine, adenine, histidine, citrulline
Effective qualities: sweet, cold, moist; stimulating, softening, decongesting
Tropism: respiratory, digestive, urinary systems; Lung, Large Intestine, Small Intestine, Stomach channels

ACTIONS: *Mucolytic expectorant, anti-inflammatory, resolvent detoxicant, draining diuretic, urinary demulcent, demulcent laxative, interferon inducent*
INDICATIONS: Bronchial infection with dry cough and scanty sputum (lung phlegm heat/dryness syndrome); acute bronchitis, lung and intestinal abscess, enteritis; hemorrhoids, infectious leucorrhea, edema (esp. of legs); ascites, urinary irritation (dysuria), constipation, abdominal distension.
Dosage: Decoction: 10-20 g
Tincture: 2-4 ml
Caution: Use cautiously with deficiency cold conditions, with diarrhea and with edema caused by malnutrition.
NOTES: The *stimulating, softening, decongesting* qualities of Waxgourd seed, when applied to the two main areas of its tropism, the lungs and urinary tract, produce good results with acute bronchitic conditions and lung abscess. Renal edema and infectious leucorrhea likewise benefit from these effects. In vitalistic terms, phlegm damp and damp heat are the conditions resolved.

Waxgourd rind, Dong Gua Pi (Mand.) or **Dong Gwa Pei** (Cant.), is used for treating edema, scanty urination and thirst in hot weather. Dose: 15-30 g.

Phragmites Lu Gen
Water-Reed Root

Botanical source: *Phragmites communis* (L.) Trinius (Gramineae)
Chinese names: Lu Gen, Wei Jing, Wei Gen (Mand); Lou Gan (Cant)
Other names: Common reed, Reed grass; Rokon (Jap)
Habit: Tall perennial pancontinental temperate and tropical marsh grass found at pond and stream borders, as well as in swamps.

Category: mild remedy with minimal chronic toxicity
Constituents: coixol, tricin, asparamide, xylose, arabinose, glucose, galactose, fat, starch, vitamin B1 and 2, C
Effective qualities: sweet, cold, moist; calming, sinking, dissolving
Tropism: respiratory, digestive, urinary systems; Lung, Stomach channels

ACTIONS: *Expectorant, anti-inflammatory, antiseptic, detoxicant, antiemetic, diuretic, antilithic, antipyretic, rash-promoting*
INDICATIONS: Acute bronchitis with thick yellow sputum, lung abscess; acute gastritis with vomiting; urinary tract infections, hematuria, urinary stones; spiking fever; eruptive fever (e.g. measles, chickenpox).
Dosage: Decoction: 15-30 g. Up to 60 g may be used when promoting rashes in eruptive fevers.
Tincture: 2-5 ml
Caution: Forbidden in stomach cold syndromes.

NOTES: Appropriately a *refrigerant sedative* remedy for acute respiratory, gastric and urinary tract infections, Water reed root addresses lung phlegm heat and bladder damp heat syndromes equally well. Blood in the urine, scanty urination (also found in eruptive fevers) and dangerous spiking fever are its special indications.

Water reed twig, Phragmites Wei Jing (Mand.) or **Lou Ging** (Cant.), is used in the same way as the root.

Momordica Luo Han Guo
Arhat Fruit

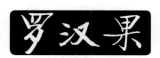

Botanical source: *Momordica grosvenori* Swingle (Cucurbitaceae)
Chinese names: Luo Han Guo (Mand); Lok Haan Gok (Cant)
Category: mild remedy with minimal chronic toxicity

Constituents: glucose
Effective qualities: sweet, neutral; restoring, calming, softening
Tropism: respiratory systems; Lung, Spleen channels

ACTIONS: *Demulcent, anti-inflammatory, antitussive*
INDICATIONS: Hot and Yin deficient bronchial conditions, especially with dry cough; lymph gland swelling.
Dosage: Decoction: 10-16 g, or 1/2 to 2 fruits
Tincture: 2-4 ml
Caution: None.

Phyllostachys Zhu Li
Black Bamboo Sap

Botanical source: *Phyllostachys nigra* (Lodd.) Munro var. *henonis* (Mitf.) Stapf ex Rendle and spp (Gramineae)
Chinese names: Zhu Li (Mand); Jok Lai (Cant)

Category: mild remedy with minimal chronic toxicity
Effective qualities: sweet, very cold; relaxing, calming
Tropism: respiratory, nervous systems; Stomach,

ACTIONS: *Anti-infective, anti-inflammatory, antiemetic, astringent, hemostatic, antipyretic, analeptic, nervous relaxant, anticonvulsant*
INDICATIONS: Acute bronchitis in lung phlegm heat syndromes with coughing and tight chest; coughing up blood, nosebleed; fever, coma, stroke with paralysis of hands and feet, hemiplegia, seizures, epilepsy; wind phlegm syndromes.
Dosage: Decoction: 10-60 g in decoction. For acute bronchitis: 10-18 g
Tincture: 2-5 ml
Caution: Forbidden in coughing due to cold conditions and diarrhea due to small intestine deficiency. Often mixed with ginger juice to mitigate its very cold quality.

Phyllostachys Zi Zhu Gen
Black Bamboo Root

Botanical source: *Phyllostachys nigra* (Lodd.) Munro var. *henonis* (Mitf.) Stapf ex Rendle and spp

(Gramineae)
Chinese names: Zi Zhu Gen (Mand); Ji Jok Gan

Notes: Phyllostachys Zi Zhu Gen is identical in nature, functions and uses to Phyllostachys Zhu Li (see above). In addition, it is a *nervous sedative, diuretic* and *astringent* used for anxiety and unrest, especially nocturnal restlessness.

Dosage: Decoction: 4-15 g
Tincture: 1-3 ml

Caution: None.

Plantago Che Qian Cao
Plantain Leaf

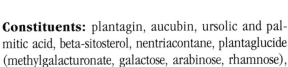

Botanical source: *Plantago asiatica* L. or *P. major* De Candolle or *P. depressa* Willdenov (Plantaginaceae)
Chinese names: Che Qian Cao (Mand); Che Chin Chou (Cant)
Habit: Perennial herb found worldwide by roadsides, villages and wild areas.
Therapeutic category: mild remedy with minimal chronic toxicity

Constituents: plantagin, aucubin, ursolic and palmitic acid, beta-sitosterol, nentriacontane, plantaglucide (methylgalacturonate, galactose, arabinose, rhamnose), vitamins B1, C
Effective qualities: sweet, cold, moist; calming, sinking decongesting
Tropism: respiratory, digestive, urinary, reproductive systems; Lung, Liver, Spleen channels

Actions: *Anti-infective (antiseptic, antibacterial), expectorant, detoxicant, anti-inflammatory, antipyretic, antitumoral, draining diuretic, mucostatic, optitropic*
Indications: Acute bronchial infection (lung [phlegm] heat syndrome); acute urinary tract infection, blood in urine, prostatitis (bladder damp heat syndrome); boils, abscesses, carbuncles, acute enteritis, dysentery, gonorrhea; jaundice, hepatitis, nephritic edema, pyelonephritis, urinary tract stones, dysuria; leucorrhea, poor vision.
Dosage: Decoction: 15-30 g
Tincture: 2-5 ml
The crushed fresh leaves are applied topically for boils and such like.
Caution: Do not use with spermatorrhea present.

Pumus Fu Hai Shi
Pumice

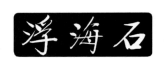

Geological source: Pumus
Chinese names: Fu Hai Shi, Hai Fu Shi, Shui Shi (Mand); Faan Hoi Sek (Cant)
Category: mild remedy with minimal chronic toxicity
Constituents: silicates of potassium, calcium, sodium and aluminum; silicon dioxide
Effective qualities: salty, cool, moist, calming, softening, dissolving
Tropism: respiratory, urinary, lymphatic systems; Lung, Kidney channels

Actions: *Mucolytic expectorant, antiseptic, hemostatic, diuretic, detumescent, resolvent detoxicant*
Indications: Acute bronchitis (lung phlegm heat syndrome) with coughing, difficult expectoration, coughing up blood (hemoptysis); acute urinary tract infections (bladder damp heat syndrome); swellings (incl. lymphadenitis).
Dosage: Decoction and powder: 6-10 g. For acute urinary infections the remedy is powdered and taken directly (e.g. in capsules).
Caution: Contraindicated in coughing due to deficiency cold.
Notes: Pumice is a mineral produced by volcanic eruptions. The bones of *Costazia aculeata* Canu et Bassler or *C. costazii* Audouin are sometimes substituted for the mineral.

Cyclina Hai Ge Ke
Clam Shell

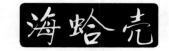

Zoological source: *Cyclina sinensis* Gmelin (Veneridae)
Chinese names: Hai Ge Ke, Hai Ke, Ge Li (Mand); Hoi Gap Hok (Cant)
Source: China's coastal provinces
Therapeutic category: mild remedy with minimal chronic toxicity

Constituents: calcium carbonate, iron, chitin, trace minerals (incl. iodine), vitamins
Effective qualities: salty, bitter, neutral, dry; stimulating, softening, decongesting
Tropism: respiratory, urinary, digestive systems; Lung, Kidney, Heart channels

ACTIONS: *Stimulant expectorant, antitussive, anti-inflammatory, analgesic, detumescent, diuretic, mucostatic, antacid antisecretory*

INDICATIONS: Acute bronchitis (lung phlegm heat syndrome) with couging and wheezing, difficult expectoration and chest/rib pain; urinary irritation/pain, lumbar pain, incontinence with enuresis/leucorrhea/spermatorrhea; goiter, lymphadenitis (incl. scrofula); edema (incl. with anuria).

The calcined powder is used internally for gastric pain, gastric hyperacidity with acid regurgitation, and internally for burns.

Dosage: Decoction of the raw or roasted/calcined shell pieces or powder: 6-16 g
Powder or pill: 1-3 g
If using Clam shell powder in a formula, place in a cheesecloth bag before adding to the decoction.

Caution: Forbidden in Qi deficient and cold syndromes.

NOTES: Wen Ge, Asian Venus clam shell, *Meretrix meretrix* Lamarck, is similar in qualities, constituents, tropism, actions and indications as Clam shell. The two clam shell types are used interchangeably. Dose: 2-6 g of the crushed shell.

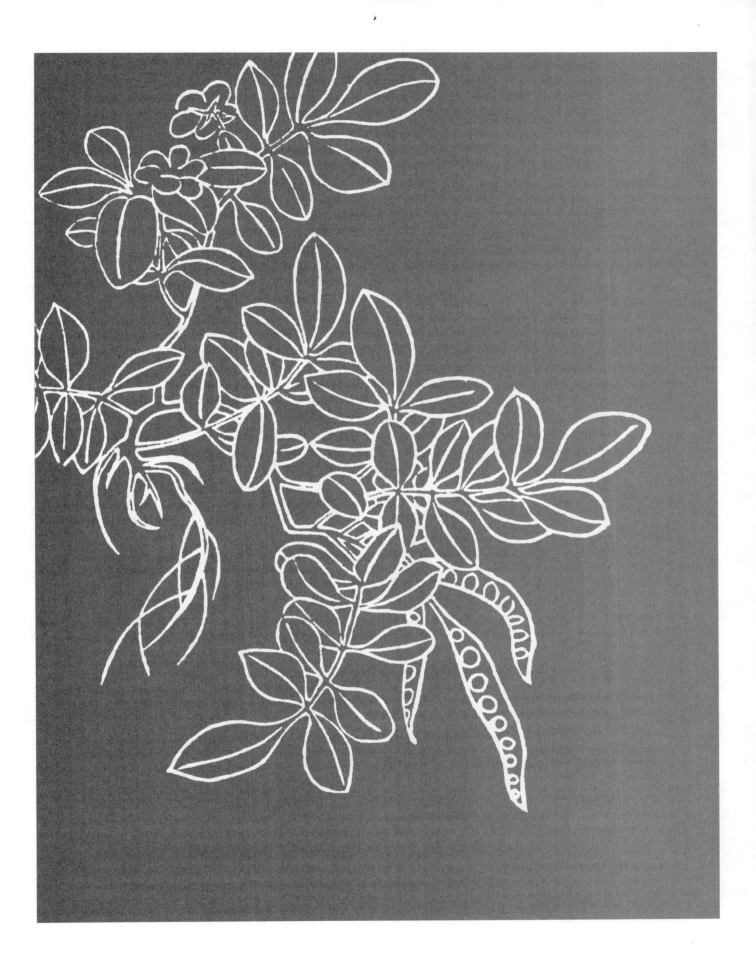

心血管系统用药

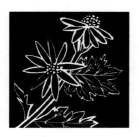

Remedies for the Cardiovascular System

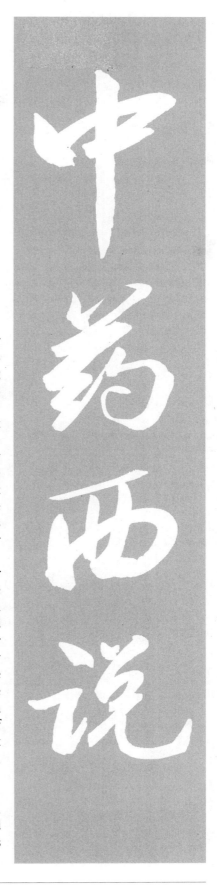

The Oriental pharmacopeia has always possessed remedies for various cardiovascular problems, but it is only in recent years that researchers in the People's Republic of China began putting much time and effort into investigating them. The impetus behind new research involves a problem in terminology: Traditional therapeutic classifications of herbal remedies do not describe cardiac or vascular conditions as such, because these herb classes define vitalistic treatment methods rather than body systems. Cardiovascular remedies are found primarily in the classes that "vitalize the Blood and disperse Blood stasis," that "warm the interior and clear cold," that "settle and calm the spirit" and that "nourish the heart and calm the spirit." Yet it is evident from the modern point of view that it is cardiovascular conditions that are being referred to in these earlier descriptions.

From the perspective of any vitalistic medicine—whether Chinese, Greek or Ayurvedic—the heart organ is thought to be intimately involved with affective and spiritual faculties (*shen* in Chinese medicine). Many disorders manifesting emotional and mental symptoms are an expression of heart/cardiovascular imbalance on an energetic or vitalistic level. Even though every organ serves as a physical substrate for spiritual faculties of some kind, it is in cardiac pathology that the connection between the physiologic and spiritual/energetic is most obvious and, in clinical practice, unavoidable. An especially good example of this connection is in tense and excess conditions of the heart accompanied by anxiety, panicky feelings and inner unrest, where *cardiac relaxants* and *sedatives* are given.

Using the fourfold rubric of Western herbal energetics, Oriental herbal remedies for cardiovascular problems are classed as *restoratives, stimulants, relaxants* and *sedatives*. Each type is used to address a particular condition, as follows:

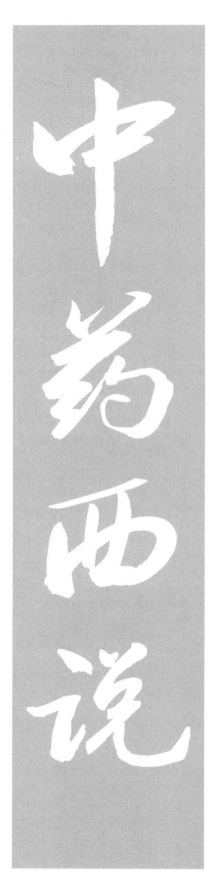

- ***Cardiovascular restoratives*** treat three types of cardiovascular deficiency:
  - simple functional deficiency.
  - coronary circulation deficiency with anginal chest pain.
  - vascular deficiency presenting bleeding.
- ***Cardiovascular stimulants*** address deficiency conditions with poor arterial circulation, displaying cold extremities.
- ***Cardiovascular relaxants*** treat excess conditions with spasms and high blood pressure, presenting irritability.
- ***Cardiovascular sedatives*** treat excess conditions with neurocardiac hyperactivity, accompanied by emotional and mental disturbance, such as anxiety.

The above classification scheme serves not only to make the highly effective Oriental cardiovascular botanicals more accessible to the practitioner, but further allows for organization of various cardiovascular disorders within a logical therapeutic framework.

The Cardiovascular Remedies

Restoratives

Restorative remedies for the cardiovascular system are divided into three kinds:
- *cardiac restoratives* that enhance heart functioning and relieve palpitations.
- *coronary restoratives* that promote coronary circulation and relieve chest pain.
- *hemostatics* and *styptics* that stop bleeding.

Simple *cardiac restoratives* address the symptom pattern **heart Qi deficiency** that implies chronic cardiac insufficiency. These remedies are so varied and used for so many other purposes, however, that they are not presented separately in this text. Instead, they are to be found throughout this and other sections of the Materia Medica. Examples of highly effective *cardiac restoratives* are Crataegus Shan Zha (the berry of two species of Asian hawthorn found throughout China) and Rehmannia Shu Di Huang (Prepared rehmannia root, a type of figwort from China's eastern coast).

The second type of *restorative* is specifically *coronary restorative*. By improving coronary circulation it relieves conditions arising from coronary deficiency, such as angina pectoris, coronary artery disease and coronary thrombosis. This type has a *resolvent* action as part of its overall *restorative* effect, which includes *antilipemic* and *anticoagulant* actions: *Coronary restoratives* can prevent and treat hyperlipidemia, atherosclerosis and thrombosis. The majority are also systemic *vasodilators* and therefore treat peripheral arterial deficiency. In traditional

Chinese medical terms, these remedies are described as "vitalizing the Blood and dispersing Blood stasis in the heart."

The syndrome summarizing this condition is **heart blood and Qi stagnation.** Its prominent symptoms are chest tightness, chest pains that extend down the left arm, shortness of breath, palpitations, fatigue and feelings of anxiety and panic. Note that the preventive role of *coronary restoratives* in these anginal conditions is no less important than their use as remedies for curing.

Of the many herbal agents currently used for the coronary circulation in Chinese clinics, the most prominent are chosen. These include the much-researched remedies Ginkgo Yin Xing Ye (the leaf of the East Asian ginkgo tree) and Crataegus Shan Zha (the common Asian hawthorn berry), as well as the frequently used Ligusticum Chuan Xiong (the root of a montane lovage species from Sichuan and Central China) and Carthamus Hong Hua (safflower, a dye plant cultivated throughout Asia). From the biochemical point of view, the most active constituents of these botanicals are glycosides and essential oils.

The third type of *restorative* works by astricting the capillaries, bringing about a *hemostatic* effect. *Hemostatics* are used to stop bleeding of almost every kind, whether acute or chronic, local or systemic. The majority also have a *coagulant* action that speeds up clotting time. Note that hemorrhage in Oriental medicine is treated not only with *hemostatics* from this section, but also with remedies that address the underlying condition that gave rise to it. The most common patterns that predispose to bleeding of endogenous origin are Spleen Qi deficiency, Blood heat and Yin deficiency with rising Yang. *Hemostatics* in this section may also be combined with *vulnerary* remedies in the Tissue Trauma section in case of bleeding due to injury. *Vulneraries* treat the pain, inflammation and swelling caused by tissue trauma, not any bleeding present.

Except for their *astringent* and *coagulant* actions, these remedies are not alike in either their effective qualities, including taste, or their chemical constituents. They include such unusual agents as the common Cattail pollen (Typha Pu Huang) and an herb common to both Oriental and Western herbal medicine, Great burnet root, Sanguisorba Di Yu.

Stimulants

Cardiovascular stimulants can be specified as *cardiac* and *arterial stimulants* that promote outward blood circulation, enhance metabolic activities and relieve cold. Because warmth, metabolism and energy production are considered essential aspects of the body's Yang energies in Oriental medicine, these types of remedies are said to "tonify the Yang, warm the interior and dispel cold." They are further described as "warming the channels and collaterals." As such, they treat deficiency of the body's Yang energies, found, for example, in the syndrome **Heart and Kidney Yang deficiency.**

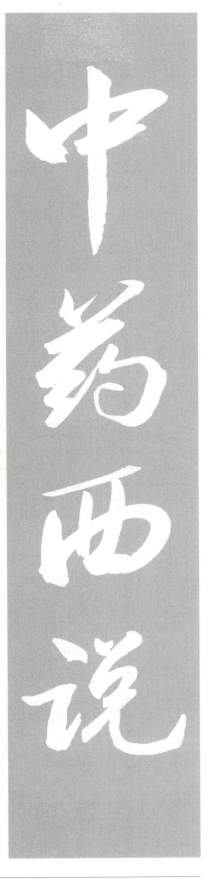

CARDIOVASCULAR SYSTEM

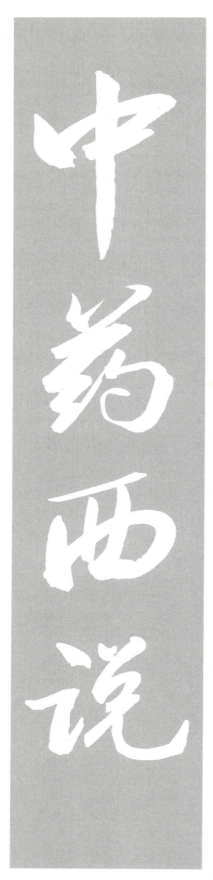

As expected from their pungent, hot, dry nature, *cardiovascular stimulants* are used specifically for symptom patterns of internal cold. These include **stomach and intestines cold, genitourinary cold, uterus cold** and even **wind/damp/cold obstruction.** All these conditions have a Yang deficiency at their root. They involve poor arterial supply to the organ, systems or tissues involved, and invariably display cold hands and feet, proneness to chills, cold skin and lethargy.

The syndrome **Devastated Yang** is the most severe and acute of all Yang deficiency conditions. It entails circulatory collapse with fainting and coma, and may arise, for example, from shock or congestive heart failure. Remedies that address this syndrome "rescue devastated Yang" with their immediate *stimulant* action on adrenergic and cardiovascular functions.

Chinese *cardiovascular stimulants,* like those used in the West, contain essential oil as an important constituent. The exceptions are Aconitum Fu Zi (Prepared Sichuan aconite root from Mid and North China) and Bufo Chan Su (Toad venom)—both alkaloidal remedies.

A word of caution. There are many professional and popular herb books in English that describe Chinese remedies as promoting blood circulation, when what they really mean is that the herbs "vitalize the Blood" (*huo xue*) in the traditional Oriental medical sense. The two concepts are not equivalent at all (see the *restoratives* above, the introductions to the Reproductive System and Tissue Trauma remedies, as well as p. 74). The tradition of misinterpreting Chinese medical terms goes back to such early compilers as Bernard E. Read and unfortunately today is still alive and well. We can be on the lookout for such misinterpretations (well-intentioned though they may be) simply by questioning any purported action on the circulation as we know it in the West.

Relaxants

Cardiovascular relaxants generally have *vasodilatory* and *hypotensive* actions that make them useful for tense or spasmic conditions of the coronary, cerebral or systemic circulation. Such conditions include arterial spasms, high blood pressure and essential hypertension, causing symptoms of irritability, headache, dizziness, ringing in ears, rapid heart beat and palpitations. The syndrome most descriptive of this condition is **heart Qi constraint,** which is said to arise from a stagnation of the Qi in the chest. This syndrome may also involve **Liver Yang rising** (the Yang functions of the energetic Liver channel, not the liver organ itself; see p. 37 for a discussion of differences between Western organs and Chinese channel networks).

In vitalistic terms, *cardiovascular relaxants* are said to "circulate heart Qi," thereby releasing constrained or stagnant Qi in the hub of the cardiovascular system, cardiac and coronary functioning. Some of these remedies are also able, where neccessary, to "subdue Liver Yang." They include very effective *hypotensives* like Ilex Mao Dong Qing (the root of the furry holly, a temperate evergreen shrub), Prunella Xia Ku Cao (Selfheal spike, an herb also used in the West) and Catharanthus Chang Chun Hua (the root and herb of the Madagascar periwinkle, also an important *anticancer* remedy). These remedies share few energetic qualities or chemical constituents.

Sedatives

When autonomic nervous and cardiac functions become excessively stressed, anxiety, unrest, agitation and sleep loss result. These symptoms are summed up in the syndromes **Heart Yin deficiency** with **nerve excess,** and **Heart fire.** They may result from a variety of conditions, including stress, anxiety states, phobias, panic attacks and posttraumatic stress disorder. By calming nervous and cardiac overactivity, *cardiovascular sedatives* gently relax the heart and calm mental, emotional and behavioral excess.

Traditional and modern Chinese texts divide these *neurocardiac sedatives* into two groups. The first group consists of "heavy remedies that settle and calm the spirit," including Stegodon Long Gu (Dragon bone—actually the fossilized remains of prehistoric reptiles) and Ostrea Mu Li (Oyster shell). These mineral substances sedate mainly through their high calcium and magnesium content, and are said, energetically speaking, to possess strong *sinking* and *stabilizing* effects.

The second group comprises "light remedies that nourish the heart and calm the spirit," such as the botanicals Polygala Yuan Zhi (Thin-leaf milkwort root from Mongolia and North China), Scrophularia Xuan Shen (Black figwort root from dank North Chinese lowlands) and Zizyphus Suan Zao Ren (the seed of the sour or wild jujube, a subtropical shrub). Most of these act through a variety of glycosides.

These *neurocardiac sedatives* are similar to the *nervous sedatives* in the section for the nervous system, in that they calm the spirit and relieve unrest and agitation. Unlike the latter, however, they emphatically possess a neurocardiac action. As such they primarily reduce emotional anxiety and distress, rather than relieve pain.

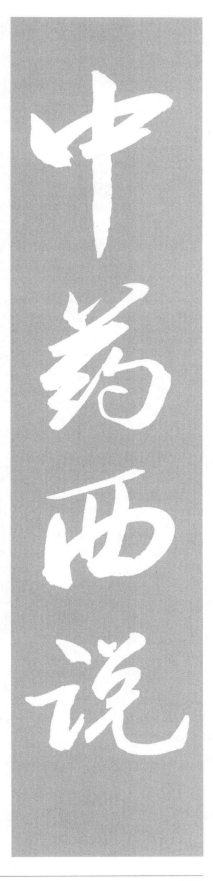

Cardiovascular Restoratives

REMEDIES TO RESTORE CORONARY CIRCULATION AND RELIEVE CHEST PAIN

➥ VITALIZE THE BLOOD AND DISPERSE BLOOD STASIS IN THE HEART

Coronary restoratives

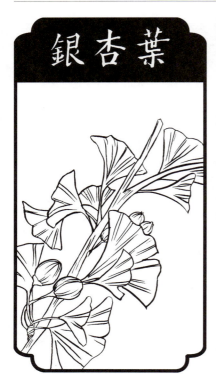

Ginkgo Yin Xing Ye
Ginkgo Leaf

Botanical source: *Ginkgo biloba* L. (Ginkgoaceae)
Pharmaceutical name: Folium Ginkgoidis
Chinese names: Yin Xing Ye, Bai Guo Ye (M); Gan Hang Yip, Baak Gwat Yip (C)
Other names: Maidenhair tree
Habit: Large, hardy deciduous East Asian tree fond of deep, rich sandy soil; much cultivated in Central and South China, Korea and Japan.
Part used: the leaf of the tree

Therapeutic category: medium-strength remedy with some chronic toxicity
Constituents: flavonoid glycosides up to 24% (incl. heterosides quercetin, kaempferol, isorhamnetin; coumarin esters, proanthocyanidins, catechins), terpenoids (incl. bilobalide, ginkgolides, sciadopitysin, ginkgetin, bilobetin), organic acids (incl. vit. C), rutin, SOD, sterols, carotenoids
Effective qualities: sweet, bitter, astringent, neutral, dry
  decongesting, relaxing, raising, restoring, diluting, astringing
Tropism: cardiovascular, respiratory, urogenital systems
  Heart, Lung, Kidney, Du channels
  Fluid, Air bodies

ACTIONS AND INDICATIONS

cardiovascular/coronary restorative: systemic vasodilator: coronary deficiency with angina pectoris; coronary disease, peripheral arterial deficiency with pain or paresthesia of the extremities, cerebral ischema and occlusion with concentration and memory loss, vascular headaches; cerebrovascular accident, trauma to the head, arteritis of the lower limbs, diabetic vasoconstriction

circulatory resolvent: antilipemic, anticoagulant: atherosclerosis, hypercholesterolemia, thrombosis (incl. cerebral, coronary)

venous/vascular/capillary restorative, venous decongestant: varicose veins, hemorrhoids, leg ulcers, phlebitis, edema, purpura, capillaritis

nervous restorative: cerebral insuffficiency with depression, tinnitus, vertigo, memory loss, senility; Alzheimer's, Parkinson's disease, CFS

antioxidant (free radical inhibitor): premature aging, toxicosis, poor vision, retinal (macular) degeneration

bronchial relaxant: asthma (incl. allergic), spasmodic coughing; chronic bronchitis

intestinal relaxant, spasmolytic: abdominal pain, colic

antiemetic: nausea, vomiting

urogenital astringent: leucorrhea

anti-inflammatory, vulnerary: wounds with bruising, bleeding

antifungal

Symptom Pictures

heart blood and Qi stagnation: chest tightness or pain, shortness of breath, palpitations, fatigue

venous blood stagnation: varicose veins, phlebitis, thrombosis

nerve and brain deficiency (Kidney Essence deficiency): absentmindedness, forgetfulness, depression, dizziness, premature senility

lung Qi constraint: spasmodic coughing, tight chest, wheezing

Preparation

Use: The leaf Ginkgo Yin Xing Ye may be briefly decocted or infused for 15-20 minutes. The tincture extract is also excellent.

Dosage: Decoction: 6-12 g
Tincture: 2-4 ml

Caution: Prolonged use of Ginkgo leaf may cause mild side effects such as dizziness, headache, fatigue, gastric or chest discomfort, loss of appetite, constipation or diarrhea. The remedy belongs to the medium-strength category because it has shown some cumulative toxicity (Chang & But 1987), and should therefore not be used continuously on its own over a two- or three-month period.

Notes

The ginkgo tree is the oldest species of tree extant. In China, where it survived the last ice age, this auspicious tree was planted (appropriately enough) in geomantically powerful sites connected with ancestor worship, especially around temples and tombs. To the 18th-century European mind, the delicate, fan-shaped leaf of this "silver apricot" *(yin xing)* resembled the maidenhair fern.

It is fascinating to observe how a relatively minor herbal remedy, once relegated to modern research labs, can yield such a variety of properties. Ginkgo leaf exerts a general *restoring* effect on the circulation. This effect results from two component actions: a *restorative/relaxant* action on the coronary arteries and capillaries, and a *decongestant* action on the systemic veins. Deficient microcirculation from any cause and at any site, therefore, is Ginkgo leaf's most telling indication. Peripheral and cerebral, as well as coronary vascular disorders will benefit from its use in this connection. Signs of stasis of the venous circulation, such as varicose veins, are also helped.

Less is known about Ginkgo leaf's *restorative* action on the nervous system, but the various brain centers are clearly the main benefactors. In the vitalistic language of Oriental medicine, Kidney Essence is tonified as symptoms such as loss of mental focus, poor memory, dizziness and depression—often associated with premature senility—are relieved.

German research also indicates a two-fold protective action from free-radical damage. First, in preventing premature aging (with attendant symptoms), and second, in decreasing the damage caused by environmental toxins (especially chemical pollutants). Ginkgo leaf is just one of several remedies used in ancient times that, because of current health needs, is currently experiencing a welcome rebirth.

Ginkgo nut, Bai Guo or Yin Guo (Mand.) or **Baak Gwat** or **Gan Gwat** (Cant.) is the seed of the ginkgo tree. It is sweet, bitter, astringent and neutral in qualities. Its *stimulant expectorant, bronchodilatant, antitussive,* and *urogenital mucostatic* actions address bronchitis presenting lung phlegm damp with coughing, expectoration of copious sputum, wheezing (asthma), leucorrhea, spermatorrhea, urinary incontinence and discharges in the urine. Dose: 3-10 g.

Caution: Ginkgo seed's status is medium-strength with considerable cumulative toxicity, and should therefore not be used on its own continuously or overdosed. Negative effects are the same as for Ginkgo leaf (see Caution above). The remedy is also a *uterine stimulant* that is forbidden during pregnancy.

Crataegus Shan Zha
Asian Hawthorn Berry

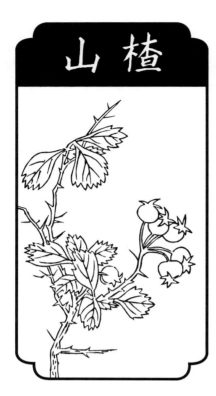

Botanical source: *Crataegus pinnatifida* Bunge var. *major* N.E. Bremek or *C. cuneata* Siebold et Zuccarini and spp. (Rosaceae)
Pharmaceutical name: Fructus Crataegi
Chinese names: Shan Zha, Ye Shan Zha, Shan Li Hong (Mand); San Jiau (Cant)
Other names: Mountain hawthorn; Sansa (Jap)
Habit: Deciduous shrub growing in sunny, wild upland regions throughout temperate China; small corymbs of terminal white flowers appear in summer.
Part used: the fruit

Therapeutic category: mild remedy with minimal chronic toxicity
Constituents: triterpenoids (incl. amygdalin, quercetin), ursolic/crategolic/citric/tartaric/caffeic/stearic/chlorogenic acids, phlobaphene, choline, epicatechol, flavonoids, nonacosane, oleanolic acid, daucosterol, stigmasterol, vanillin, fumaric and succinic acid, digestive enzymes, trace elements, vitamin C
Effective qualities: a bit sour, astringent and sweet, neutral, dry
    relaxing, restoring, calming, diluting, softening, dissolving,
        diluting, astringing
Tropism: cardiovascular, nervous, digestive, reproductive systems
    Heart, Pericardium, Liver, Spleen, Stomach, Yin Wei channels
    Air, Fluid bodies

ACTIONS AND INDICATIONS

cardiovascular/coronary restorative: systemic vasodilator: coronary deficiency with angina; coronary disease, peripheral arterial deficiency
circulatory and systemic resolvent: anticoagulant, antilipemic, antilithic: atherosclerosis, thrombosis, hyperlipidemia, arteriosclerosis, urinary or biliary stones
cardiac restorative: cardiac deficiency with palpitations, dyspnea
cardiovascular relaxant, hypotensive: high blood pressure, essential hypertension, neurocardiac disorder, coronary artery spasm
nervous sedative, sympathetic inhibitor: unrest, anxiety, hot flushes; menopausal syndrome, cardiac and postpartum pain
uterine restorative: amenorrhea, delayed menses, postpartum lochial retention with pain
enzymatic digestant: dyspepsia with heartburn (esp. from fat and protein), intestinal fermentation
secretory: dry mouth, thirst
astringent, mucostatic: diarrhea, leucorrhea
antibacterial, vermifuge: enteritis, bacillary dysentery

SYMPTOM PICTURES

heart blood and Qi stagnation: chest tightness or pain, shortness of breath, fatigue

heart Qi constraint: palpitations, headache, dizziness, feeling stressed

heart Blood and Qi deficiency: fatigue, labored breathing, palpitations, poor sleep

heart and Kidney Yin deficiency with **nerve excess:** sleep loss, unrest, anxiety, low fever, hot spells, dry mouth

food stagnation: painful distended abdomen and epigastrium, flatulence, diarrhea

Preparation

Use: The berry Crataegus Shan Zha is decocted or used in tincture form.
Dosage: Decoction: 8-16 g
Tincture: 2-4 ml
Caution: Use cautiously in digestive weakness without food stagnation present, and also in acid regurgitation.

Notes

The Asian hawthorn berry, no less than the Western, is a superlative remedy for the heart and blood vessels, both functionally and substantially. The sheer depth of its *restorative, relaxant* and *resolvent* action on this system is unequaled, confirming application for heart Qi, Blood and Yin deficiency syndromes, as well as for coronary deficiency itself. Hawthorn berry may be seen as a true "heart governor" or "heart protector" operating through the Yin Wei extra channel.

Traditional prescriptions also make frequent use of the sweet-sour "mountain hawthorn" for indigestion of fats and proteins resulting from enzyme deficiency.

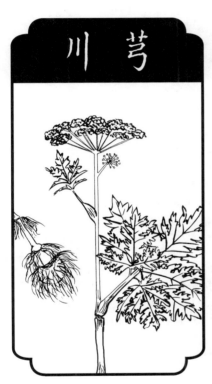

Ligusticum Chuan Xiong
Sichuan Lovage Root

Botanical source: *Ligusticum wallichii* Franchet (Umbelliferae)
Pharmaceutical name: Radix Ligustici wallichii
Chinese names: Chuan Xiong, Xiong Qiong, Hu Qiong, Xiang Guo (Mand); Chyun Gung (Cant)
Other names: Senkyu (Jap)
Habit: Perennial herb from temperate mountane China, especially Sichuan; also cultivated; blooms in summer with small white blossoms on compound terminal umbels.
Part used: the root

Therapeutic category: mild remedy with minimal chronic toxicity
Constituents: essential oil (over 180 components, incl. ligustilide 58%, sabinene, butylidine phthalide, terpinolene, terpinene, terpineol), alkaloids (incl. tetramethylpyrazine [chuanxionqin]), phenolic compounds, organic acids, ferulic acid, amino acids, trace minerals
Effective qualities: pungent, a bit bitter and sweet, warm, dry
restoring, dissolving, diluting, raising, stimulating, relaxing, calming
Tropism: cardiovascular, reproductive, nervous, digestive systems
Pericardium, Liver, Gallbladder, Chong, Yin Wei, Ren channels
Air, Fluid, Warmth bodies

Actions and Indications

cardiovascular/coronary restorative: systemic vasodilator: coronary deficiency with angina pectoris, coronary disease, myocardial infarct; cerebrovascular occlusion/ischemia/embolism, vascular headaches
circulatory resolvent: antilipemic, anticoagulant: hyperlipemia, atherosclerosis, thrombosis
arterial and capillary stimulant: peripheral arterial deficiency with pain, cold or paresthesia
cardiovascular relaxant/restorative, hypotensive: palpitations, anxiety, vertigo, leg cramps; stress, neurocardiac disorder, hypertension, coronary artery spasm with angina
uterine relaxant, spasmolytic, estrogenic: spasmodic dysmenorrhea
uterine stimulant, emmenagogue, parturient: delayed menses, amenorrhea, irregular menstruation; prolonged pregnancy, stalled labor, placental retention; infertility

nervous sedative, analgesic: PMS, unrest, headache (all types), abdomen, subcostal and joint pain, vertigo, myalgia, neurodermatitis, toothache
radiation-protective: radiation sickness (e.g. radiation therapy)
antibacterial, lymphocyte stimulant: bacterial infections
interferon inducent

Symptom Pictures

heart blood and Qi stagnation with **Qi constraint:** feeling stressed, anxiety spells, unrest, palpitations, chest tightness or pain, dizziness

uterus Qi constraint and Blood congealed: difficult or irregular painful menses with clots, palpitations, restlessness

Qi constraint with **nerve excess:** feeling stressed, unrest, irritability, chest, epigastric and abdominal pain, flank soreness, cold extremities

Preparation

Use: The root Ligusticum Chuan Xiong should be decocted in the standard way or used in tincture form. Its pain and spasm-relieving properties are more pronounced in the tincture.

Dosage: Decoction: 3-10 g
  Tincture: 1-3 ml

Caution: Being a *uterine stimulant,* Sichuan lovage root is contraindicated during pregnancy. It should also not be used in heavy menstrual bleeding, Yin deficiency with empty heat, Qi deficiency conditions, and headaches due to Liver Yang rising. Overdosing may bring on vomiting and dizziness.

Notes

Traditional Chinese medicine ascribes to this fragrant species of lovage from the Western province, Sichuan, an important Blood-enlivening effect. Today, this perennially reliable action has been scientifically vindicated: Its influence is seen to extend deep into cardiovascular dynamics, involving *vasodilatant* and *arterial stimulant* actions combined. With its rich biochemical coverage of essential oils and alkaloids, Sichuan lovage root stands out as a highly versatile *cardiovascular restorative, relaxant* and *stimulant* all in one. Consequently, the remedy is one of the most frequently used for coronary blood deficiency and spasms—whether induced by nervous stress, fatty deposits or high blood pressure.

In the past, Sichuan lovage root was put to use first and foremost in gynecological conditions. It was considered fully the equal of its botanical cousin, Dong quai root, in *stimulating* and *relaxing* menstrual functions. Today we can also see an *estrogenic* hormonal action at work that supports traditional usage for amenorrhea and spasmodic dysmenorrhea. In energetic terms the remedy's combined indications for menstrual, pregnancy-related and neurocardiac conditions points to a definite action on the Chong and Yin Wei extra meridians. Taking Sichuan lovage's gentle *sedative* and *analgesic* actions into account, its success with various types of PMS should also now be clear. Likewise, the remedy's status as a versatile agent for various forms of pain is evident. Its additional *capillary stimulant* and *vasodilatant* actions are further proof that the traditional usage of Sichuan lovage for relieving many types of headache—as for most types of coronary obstruction today—was and still is entirely justified.

Salvia Dan Shen
Cinnabar Sage Root *

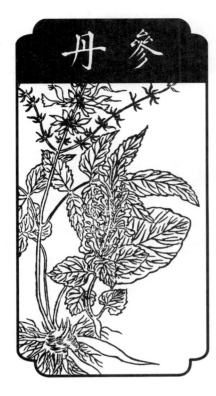

Botanical source: *Salvia miltiorrhiza* Bunge, *S. trijuga* or *S. przewalskii* (Labiatae)
Pharmaceutical name: Radix Salviae miltiorrhizae
Chinese names: Dan Shen, Zi (Dan) Shen (Mand); Daan Sam (Cant)
Other names: Red-root sage, Purple sage, "Scarlet root"; Tanjin (Jap)
Habit: Perennial hairy herb from Northeast and coastal China, growing on sunny slopes, roadsides, streamsides and forest outskirts; prefers moist, sandy soil; in summer racemes of small scarlet/crimson terminal flowers open.
Part used: the root

Therapeutic category: mild remedy with minimal chronic toxicity
Constituents: naphtoquinones (incl. tanshinones I and II, isotanshinones I and II, cryptotanshinones, salvilenone), tanshinol, diterpenoid phenol salviol, aldehydic and catechuic acids, phenyllactic and phenolic acids (danshensu A and B), crystalline miltirone, teraxeryl acetate, friedelin, butylallophanate, inulin, feruginol, Ro–060980, 17 amino acids, 14 trace minerals (incl. zinc, selenium, molybdanum, manganese, iron, copper), vitamin E
Effective qualities: sweet, a bit bitter and astringent, cool, dry
 restoring, stimulating, diluting, dissolving, relaxing, calming, sinking
Tropism: cardiovascular, reproductive, hepatic, nervous systems
 Liver, Heart, Pericardium, Chong, Yin Wei channels; Air, Fluid bodies

ACTIONS AND INDICATIONS

cardiovascular/coronary restorative: vasodilator, capillary stimulant: coronary deficiency with angina; coronary disease, myocardial infarct, peripheral arterial deficiency, arrhythmia
circulatory resolvent: antilipemic, anticoagulant, fibrinolytic: hyperlipemia, atherosclerosis, thrombosis, menstrual clots, postpartum hematoma
detoxicant, dermatropic, diuretic: metabolic toxicosis with eczema, psoriasis, liver or spleen enlargment, arthritis, acne, skin ulcers, boils
liver restorative/protective, protein anabolism stimulant: liver cirrhosis, hepatitis, toxicosis
leukocytogenic: low WBC count (leukopenia)
antitumoral, immunostimulant, lymphocyte stimulant: gynecological tumors, endometriosis; infections in general
nervous sedative: PMS, insomnia, unrest, palpitations; stress, neurosis, neurocardiac syndrome
uterine relaxant, spasmolytic: spasmodic dysmenorrhea, abdominal lumps, intestinal cramps
uterine stimulant, emmenagogue, parturient: amenorrhea, retained placenta, miscarriage
antioxidant (free radical inhibitor): premature aging, toxicosis
anticontusion, vulnerary, antiseptic: sprains, strains, fractures, wounds

SYMPTOM PICTURES

heart blood and Qi stagnation with **Qi constraint:** chest tightness, chest pains, palpitations, shortness of breath, worry, anguish

uterus Qi constraint and Blood congealed: painful, difficult menses, clots with flow, irritability

Qi constraint with **nerve excess:** chest, epigastric or abdominal pain, unrest, irritability, feeling stressed

metabolic toxicosis with **skin damp heat:** skin rashes, malaise, joint and muscle pains, fetid urine, tender flanks, headaches

Nutritive level heat: sleeplessness, palpitations, irritability, unrest

PREPARATION
Use: The root Salvia Dan Shen is decocted or used in tincture form.
Dosage: Decoction: 6-16 g
Tincture: 2-5 ml
Caution: Use with care during pregnancy. Avoid before childbirth and before or after surgery. Large doses should not be used when there is bleeding.

NOTES
In the days of Daoist shamanism the cinnabar red-colored root of this sage suggested a relation to the blood and acquired the status of the type of *shen* (ginseng) associated with the element Fire, and therefore the heart. Although highly valued in the distant past, in the traditional Oriental repertoire this botanical is not considered a major remedy.

Today, that is changing. Because of current health concerns, Cinnabar sage has re-emerged in the People's Republic as an important, routinely used remedy for deficient and obstructive coronary heart conditions. Happily for traditionalists, it literally does increase circulation through the coronary arteries, clean up blood sludge and break up congealed blood. A major aspect of its cardiocirculatory effects involves deep-acting *resolvent* and *detoxicant* actions. Cinnabar sage root addresses a wide spectrum of toxicosis conditions in general—conditions nicely summed up in the traditional Greek medical concept "fluids dyskrasia." In tandem with this, it has more recently proven to be a liver's best friend—enhancing many of its functions, such as its microcirculation and cellular regeneration, thereby preventing fibrosis.

Nor should this remedy be forgotten as a versatile woman's ally with both *uterine relaxant* and *stimulant* actions. As a first-aid remedy, it has shown activity in speeding up fracture healing. Cinnabar sage, the Fire ginseng, is clearly arising once again, Phoenix-like, to stake its ancient claim on our loyalties.

Salvia Shi Jian Chuan is the root or herb of **Chinese sage,** *Salvia chinensis.* This remedy is used primarily for its *detoxicant, analgesic, anti-inflammatory* and *detumescent* properties for ostealgia, toxicosis presenting boils or abscesses, and various forms of cancer. Dose: 10-20 g.

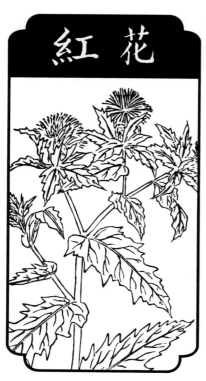

Carthamus Hong Hua
Safflower

Botanical source: *Carthamus tinctorius* L. (Compositae)
Pharmaceutical name: Flos Carthami
Chinese names: Hong Hua, Huang Lan Hua, Yao hua, Chuan Hong Hua (Mand); Hong Fa (Cant)
Other names: Dyer's saffron, "Red flower"; Koka (Jap)
Habit: Annual or biennial temperate herb cultivated throughout Asia; orange-carmine, tubular terminal blossoms appear in summer.
Part used: the flower

Therapeutic category: mild remedy with minimal chronic toxicity
Constituents: palmitic/stearic/arachic/oleic/linoleic/linolenic acids, dipalmitin, sitosterol glucoside, dihydroflavanones (carthamin, carthamone, neocarthamin), polyacetylenes, polysaccharide, safflor yellow, lignans, fatty oil
Effective qualities: a bit pungent and bitter, warm
restoring, stimulating, relaxing, diluting, dissolving
Tropism: reproductive, vascular, digestive, epidermal systems
Heart, Liver, Chong channels; Fluid, Air bodies

ACTIONS AND INDICATIONS

cardiovascular/coronary restorative: vasodilator: coronary deficiency with angina; coronary disease
circulatory resolvent: antilipemic, anticoagulant: atherosclerosis, hyperlipemia, thrombosis, cerebral ischemia
hypotensive: chronic hypertension
spasmolytic, analgesic: coronary artery spasm with angina; spasmodic dysmenorrhea with menstrual cramps, abdominal lumps and pain, pain from blood clots (incl. menstrual, postpartum and traumatic); arthralgia
uterine stimulant, emmenagogue, parturient, abortive: amenorrhea, prolonged pregnancy, stalled labor (uterine dystocia), placental retention (lochioschesis), miscarriage
anticontusion, vulnerary, detumescent: tissue injuries, fractures, strains, sprains, nonsuppurative boils, sores, carbuncles, purple erythema, spleen and liver enlargement
diuretic: chronic nephritis
rash-promoting diaphoretic: measles, scarlet fever
immunostimulant anti-infective: antibacterial, antifungal: miscellaneous infections (incl. candidiasis)
interferon inducent

SYMPTOM PICTURES

heart blood and Qi stagnation: chest tightness and pain, palpitations, fatigue

uterus Qi stagnation with **blood congealed:** absent, delayed or difficult menses, painful clotted flow

PREPARATION

Use: The flower Carthamus Hong Hua is infused or briefly decocted; it may also be used in tincture form.
Dosage: Decoction: 4-12 g
Tincture: 2-4 ml
Caution: Forbidden during pregnancy and in menorrhagia because it stimulates the uterus.

NOTES

Used in Chinese, Ayurvedic and Greek medicine alike, the Safflower is said to originate in Tibet. The highest quality safflower by reputation is certainly Tibetan. While this plant's scarlet flowers have traditionally been used for making dyes and cosmetic rouge, medicinally it is a versatile cardiovascular, gynecological and obstetrical remedy.

Like several other remedies in this section, Safflower today is commonly used to improve the coronary and cerebral microcirculation. On the coronary arteries the remedy specifically exerts a *restorative* effect through *vasodilatory, antilipemic* and *anticoagulant* actions on one hand, and a *relaxant* effect through its *spasmolytic* and *analgesic* actions on the other. As a result, Safflower provides comprehensive protection from both deficiency (hyperlipemic) and spasmodic forms of coronary disease and angina. Cerebral ischemia, atherosclerosis and hypertension are also addressed as a result of its comprehensive *resolvent* effect on the blood vessels. Collectively, these vascular actions are happily viewed by traditionalists as modern manifestations of the remedy's "Blood-vitalizing" effect. This effect traditionally refers to its ability to reduce pain, swelling and ecchymosis in the case of tissue injury such as sprains, strains and fractures—which explains its inclusion in numerous decoctions, compresses and plasters for the treatnment of soft tissue trauma.

Safflower's combined *stimulant* and *relaxant* action on the uterus have been used since prehistory for a variety of menstrual and pregnancy-related conditions. In energetic terms, both Qi stagnation and congealed Blood in the uterine area are addressed, thereby providing pain relief from uterine atonicity, spasms or blood clots. One interesting application of these actions is the remedy's traditional use—similar to Sichuan lovage root's—for cleansing the uterus and strengthening the mother about two weeks into the postpartum.

The polyacetylenes in this plant have proven *antiseptic* and *antifungal* in a variety of infectious conditions.

Pueraria Ge Gen
Kudzu Root

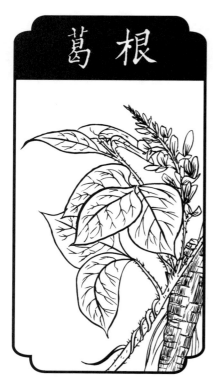

Botanical source: *Pueraria lobata* (Willd.) Ohwi or *P. omeiensis* Wang et Tang or *P. thomsanii* Bentham or *P. hirsuta* (Thunb.) Schneider (Leguminosae)
Pharmaceutical name: Radix Puerariae
Chinese names: Ge Gen, Ge Teng, Gan Ge (Mand); Gwaat Gan (Cant)
Other names: Kudzu vine; Kakkon (Jap)
Habit: Hairy, twining perennial vine from Central China, Korea and Japan, growing in moist, shaded areas on hillsides, roadsides and in thickets; also cultivated; in summer and autumn, racemes of pink/magenta flowers develop.
Part used: the root

Therapeutic category: mild remedy with minimal chronic toxicity
Constituents: isoflavonoids (incl. puerarin, daidzenin, daizin), allantoin, sitosterol, daucosterol, dehydroxyisoflavone, methylhydantoin, arachidic acid, mucilage
Effective qualities: sweet, pungent, neutral, moist
   restoring, raising, relaxing, softening
Tropism: cardiovascular, digestive systems
   Spleen, Stomach, Heart channels
   Fluid, Air bodies

ACTIONS AND INDICATIONS

cardiovascular/coronary restorative: systemic vasodilator: coronary deficiency with angina; coronary disease, myocardial and cerebral ischemia, vascular headache (incl. migraine), peripheral arterial deficiency; early acute deafness
cardiovascular relaxant, hypotensive: hypertension (esp. with stiff neck and dizzness)
mucogenic: dehydration with thirst, dry mouth; diabetes, heat exhaustion
demulcent, spasmolytic: diarrhea; acute gastroenteritis, intestinal colic, dysentery
rash-promoting antipyretic: fevers, eruptive fevers (e.g. measles, chickenpox)
hypoglycemiant: hyperglycemia
antiemetic: vomiting
antivenomous: insect and snakebites

SYMPTOM PICTURES

heart blood and Qi stagnation: chest tightness/pain, dizziness, shortness of breath
heart Qi constraint (Liver Yang rising): headache, dizziness, stiff neck, ringing in ears
external wind heat: feverishness, thirst, stiff neck, shoulders and upper back, loose stool
stomach fire: thirst, dry mouth and throat, great appetite

PREPARATIONS

Use: The root Pueraria Ge Gen is best decocted or used in tincture form. *Emollient* poultices may also be prepared.
Dosage: Decoction: 5-20 g
   Tincture: 2-4 ml
Caution: None.

NOTES

A whole new dimension has been added to this sweet, starchy *demulcent* remedy, traditionally used for fevers of the wind heat type with thirst, stiff neck and dizziness, as well as for diarrheal conditions. Recent studies have shown Kudzu root to possess *restorative* and *relaxant* actions on cardiac and coronary functions, evincing remarkable success with tense deficiency conditions such as angina, hypertension and migraine (Chang and But 1987). Translated back into vitalistic physiology, these actions indicate application to the preclinical syndromes coronary blood deficiency, heart blood stasis and Qi contraint, and Liver Yang rising.

Kudzu root's extracted cardiac glycoside puerarin is used for other circulatory conditions, such as central retinal arterial occlusion, as well as for the disorders mentioned.

Kudzu flower, Ge Gen Hua or **Gwat Fa** (Cant.), relieves thirst, hemorrhoidal bleeding and drunkenness. Dose: 4-10 g.

Kudzu leaf, Ge Gen Ye (**Gwat Yip**), treats bleeding wounds and snakebites. Dose: 15-60 g.

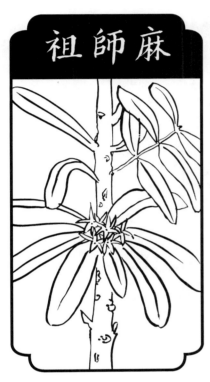

Daphne Zu Shi Ma
Giraldi's Daphne Bark *

Botanical source: *Daphne giraldii* Nitsche or *D. retusa* Hemslow or *D. tangutica* Maximowicz (Thymelaceae)
Pharmaceutical name: Cortex seu cortex radicis Daphne giraldii
Chinese names: Zu Shi Ma (Mand)
Habit: Small deciduous shrub found in the mountainous wooded regions of temperate central China; flowers in June with clusters of three to eight capitulate flowers.
Part used: the bark or root bark

Therapeutic category: medium-strength remedy with some chronic toxicity
Constituents: diterpenes (incl. daphnetin, daphnin, syringin), coumarins, saponin, daphnetoxin
Effective qualities: bitter, pungent, warm, dry
    restoring, dissolving, diluting, calming
Tropism: cardiovascular, nervous systems
    Heart, Pericardium channels
    Fluid, Air bodies

ACTIONS AND INDICATIONS
cardiovascular/coronary restorative, systemic vasodilator: coronary deficiency with angina; coronary disease, peripheral arterial deficiency with leg pain
anticoagulant, antilipemic: thrombosis, thrombangiitis obliterans, hyperlipidemia
nervous sedative, analgesic: acute myalgia, arthralgia, lumbar and leg pain, epigastric pain
anti-inflammatory, vulnerary, hemostatic: wounds, injuries (incl. with bleeding)
antibacterial

SYMPTOM PICTURES
heart blood and Qi stagnation: chest pains and tightness, anxiety, rapid breathing
wind/damp/cold obstruction: numbness, pain and redness in joints or muscles

PREPARATIONS
Use: The bark Daphne Zu Shi Ma is preferably used in tincture form. It also may be decocted.
Dosage: Decoction: 3-12 g
    Tincture: 2-4 ml
Caution: Being of cumulative low toxicity, continuous use of this remedy is contraindicated.

NOTES

A traditional *vulnerary* remedy from the Western provinces for traumatic injury, Giraldi's daphne bark has now found a modern niche as a very reliable *analgesic*. When coupled with its *coronary restorative* effect, this botanical has achieved high success rates in both anginal/thrombotic coronary conditions and arthritis.

Like the majority of other Chinese remedies, in clinical practice Giraldi's daphne bark is now usually combined with other herbs into a comprehensive formula, which itself is often used alongside acupuncture treatment.

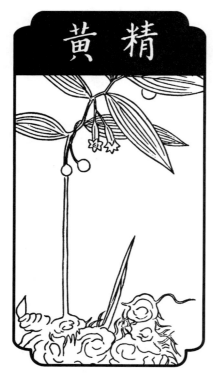

Polygonatum Huang Jing
Siberian Solomon's-Seal Root

Botanical source: *Polygonatum sibiricum* Redoute or *P. cyrtonema* Hua or *P. kingianum* Collett et Hemsley (Liliaceae)
Pharmaceutical name: Rhizoma Polygonati sibirici
Chinese names: Huang Jing, Tu Zhu, Xien Ren Yu Liang (Mand); Wong Jing (Cant)
Other names: "Yellow essence"; Osei (Jap)
Habit: Perennial herb from the mountains of North and Central China; also cultivated; axillary spikes of greenish white flowers develop during summer.
Part used: the rhizome

Therapeutic category: mild remedy with minimal chronic toxicity
Constituents: *P. cyrt.*: mucilage, aspartic acid, carboxylic acid, homserine, diaminobutyric acid, cardiac glycoside, anthraquinones, alkaloid
Effective qualities: sweet, neutral, moist
    restoring, relaxing, dissolving
Tropism: cardiovascular, respiratory, urinary systems
    Lung, Spleen, Heart channels
    Fluid, Air bodies

ACTIONS AND INDICATIONS

cardiac/coronary restorative: coronary deficiency/disease with angina; cardiac deficiency, myocardial ischemia
cardiac relaxant, hypotensive: palpitations, hypertension
circulatory resolvent, antilipemic: atherosclerosis, hyperlipidemia, hepatic fatty infiltration
antioxidant (free radical inhibitor): toxicosis, premature aging
demulcent respiratory restorative: dry respiratory conditions with dry cough; chronic bronchitis, lung TB
mucogenic: mucosal deficiency with thirst; dehydration, heat exhaustion, diabetes
adrenocortical restorative: fatigue, weakness, convalescence, menopause
hypoglycemiant: hyperglycemia, diabetes
diuretic: chronic glomerulonephritis
antibacterial, antifungal, lymphocyte stimulant

SYMPTOM PICTURES

heart blood and Qi stagnation: chest pain and tightness, wheezing, fatigue
Yin and fluids deficiency: hot spells, fatigue, thirst, dry mouth and throat
lung Qi deficiency: fatigue, weakness, shortness of breath, palpitations
lung dryness: dry cough with scanty sputum, dry throat, thirst

PREPARATION
Use: The root Polygonatum Huang Jing is decocted or used in tincture form.
Dosage: Decoction: 9-30 g
Tincture: 2-4 ml
Caution: Forbidden with intestinal damp, poor digestion and diarrhea.

NOTES

Two plant sources for the remedy Huang Jing are commonly used: *Polygonatum sibiricum* and *P. cyrtonema*, Chinese Solomon's-seal. Both are generally considered *restorative* and *moistening*, and are commonly given in convalescence after chronic illness, as well as for the two respiratory symptom complexes above.

This *antioxidant* botanical is found in many a life-extension formula, such Shi Jin-mo's Antiaging Formula. Steamed and eaten, the rhizome was understandably considered by Daoists to be "extra ration of the immortals." Today, Siberian Solomon's-seal root is routinely included in prescriptions for cardiac, coronary and other circulatory disorders because of its outstanding *restoring* and *relaxing* effects on the whole circulation. Its role as a *Qi tonic* derives partly from these effects and partly from its toning action on the adrenal cortex.

Ilex Si Ji Qing
Wintergreen Holly Leaf

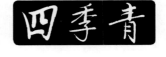

Botanical source: *Ilex chinensis* (Aquifoliaceae)
Chinese names: Si Ji Qing, Dong Qing Ye, Gong Lao Ye (Mand); (Cant)
Therapeutic category: mild remedy with minimal chronic toxicity

Constituents: glycosides
Effective qualities: bitter, pungent, dry, cool; calming, astringing, decongesting, dissolving
Tropism: cardiovascular, respiratory, urinary, systems; Lung, Stomach, Bladder channels

ACTIONS: *Coronary restorative, anti-infective, anti-inflammatory, astringent, antitumoral*
INDICATIONS: Coronary deficiency with angina, coronary disease; acute, hot bronchial infections, pneumonia, upper respiratory infections; gastrointestinal, urinary and reproductive infections with damp heat; ulcers, burns.
Dosage: Decoction: 10-15 g
Tincture: 2-5 ml
Caution: None.

REMEDIES TO PROMOTE ASTRICTION AND STOP BLEEDING

➥ STOP BLEEDING
Astringent hemostatics, styptics

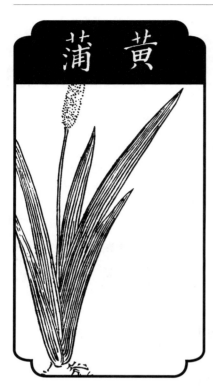

Typha Pu Huang
Cattail Pollen

Botanical source: *Typha latifolia* L. or *T. angustifolia* L. or *T. angustata* Bory et Chaub and spp. (Typhaceae)
Pharmaceutical name: Pollen Typhae
Chinese names: Pu Huang, Xiang Pu, Gan Pu (Mand); Pu Wong (Cant)
Other names: Reed mace, Kossack asparagus, "Yellow/fragrant Pu"; Hoo (Jap)
Habit: Perennial aquatic herb from temperate Asia, Europe and North America; grows in and around swamps, pools and ponds.
Part used: the pollen

Therapeutic category: mild remedy with minimal chronic toxicity
Constituents: fatty oil (incl. sitosterol stearic acid, sitosterol glucoside, palmitic acid, triacontanol, pentacosane), essential oil, flavonoids (incl. typhaneoside, kaempferolrutinoside, 2 neohesperidosides, rhamnosyl-glucoside), typhasterol, alkaloids, leucine, valine, aminopurine
Effective qualities: sweet, pungent, neutral
  astringing, thickening, stimulating, relaxing, dissolving
Tropism: cardiovascular, digestive, reproductive systems
  Liver, Spleen, Heart channels
  Fluid, Air bodies

ACTIONS AND INDICATIONS
hemostatic, coagulant, styptic: passive uterine bleeding (metrorrhagia), bleeding wounds or injuries, blood in stool, urine or sputum, subcutaneous bleeding
astringent, antipruritic: leucorrhea, genital pruritus
capillary stimulant, vasodilator, hypotensive: angina pectoris, coronary disease, peripheral arterial deficiency, hypertension
antilipemic: hyperlipemia, atherosclerosis
uterine stimulant, parturient, abortive: amenorrhea, miscarriage, retained placenta
analgesic: postpartum pain and blood retention, dysmenorrhea, chest and abdominal pain, sprains, strains
anti-inflammatory: burns, scalds, dermatitis, mouth ulcers

SYMPTOM PICTURE
heart blood and Qi stagnation: anxiety, irritability, chest pains, headaches

PREPARATION
Use: The pollen Typha Pu Huang is decocted or used in tincture form. The raw remedy is used to disperse congealed Blood, while toasted it is considered better for arresting bleeding. The powdered remedy is used for skin conditions and sores. External applications can also be made for skin and genital conditions.
Dosage: Decoction: 4-12 g
  Tincture: 1-4 ml
Caution: This *uterine stimulant* is contraindicated during pregnancy.

NOTES

In addition to its more traditional *hemostatic* and *analgesic* uses for stopping hemorrhage, the pollen of cattail cobs is an important modern Chinese remedy for treating hypercholesterolemia with angina pectoris or hypertension.

Like the similar remedy Rubia Qian Cao Gen, Cattail pollen also has a gynecological emphasis, relieving uterine pain due to congealed Blood (in this case literally clots) in menstruation and postpartum. As a *uterine stimulant,* it also hastens expulsion of the afterbirth.

Rehmannia Sheng Di Huang
Fresh Rehmannia Root

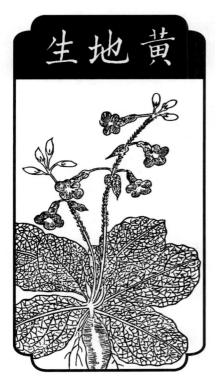

Botanical source: *Rehmannia glutinosa* (Gaertner) Liboschitz *f. hueichingensis* (Chao et Schih) Hsiao (Scrophulariaceae)
Pharmaceutical name: Radix Rehmanniae
Chinese names: Sheng Di Huang, Sheng Di, Gan Di Huang (Mand); Sang Dei (Wong) (Cant)
Other names: Chinese foxglove, "Earth yellow"; Shojio (Jap)
Habit: Hairy perennial herb from coastal and North China; grows in loamy, humid soil on sunny hillsides, roadside wasteground and in marshes; also widely cultivated; terminal maroon-purple or cream flowers emerge in spring.
Part used: the fresh root

Therapeutic category: mild remedy with minimal chronic toxicity
Constituents: alcohols (incl. mannitol, stigmasterol), sitosterol, campesterol, saccharides, arginine, rehmannin, iridoid glycosides catalpol and aucubin, nelittoside, amino acid, stachyose, iron, vitamin A
Effective qualities: sweet, a bit bitter, cold, moist
  restoring, relaxing, sinking, dissolving
Tropism: cardiovascular, digestive, glandular (endocrine and exocrine) systems
  Heart, Liver, Kidney channels
  Warmth, Fluid bodies

ACTIONS AND INDICATIONS

hemostatic, coagulant: blood in stool/urine/spittle, nosebleed, intermenstrual bleeding (metrorrhagia)
cardiotonic: cardiac deficiency
hypotensive, antilipemic: hypertension, hyperlipidemia; unrest, insomnia
antipyretic, mucogenic: fevers in general, dehydration, heat exhaustion; mouth and tongue sores
pituitary-adrenocortical restorative: fatigue, poor stamina from adrenocortical deficiency; menopause
hypoglycemiant: hypoglycemia, diabetes with thirst and heat
detoxicant, diuretic: chronic rheumatoid and arthritic conditions; skin cysts
liver protective: infectious hepatitis
antiallergic
leukocytogenic: low WBC count (leukopenia)

SYMPTOM PICTURES

Blood and Nutritive level heat: blood in stool, urine or spittle, heavy menstrual flow, fever, thirst

Yin and fluids deficiency: hot spells, esp. in soles, palms and sternum; dry mouth and lips, thirst, palpitations, fatigue

Heart fire: irritability, sleep loss, low-grade fever, mouth and tongue sores

Preparation

Use: For best results, Rehmannia root should be used absolutely fresh, which is termed **Sheng Di Huang** (Mand.) or **Sang Dei Wong** (Cant.). Second best is **Gan Di Huang** (Mand.) or **Gaan Dei Wong** (Cant.), the sun-dried root. Both fresh and sun-dried roots are decocted or used in tincture form.

Dosage: Decoction: 9-30 g
Tincture: 2-4 ml

Caution: Fresh rehmannia root is contraindicated in the following conditions: bronchial sputum, intestinal mucus (lung phlegm damp and intestines mucous damp syndromes), and in Yang deficiency. The remedy is also forbidden during pregnancy accompanied by Blood/metabolic deficiency or digestive weakness.

Notes

The *hemostatic* properties of the fresh or sun-dried Rehmannia root only come fully into play in febrile conditions; in vitro research has yielded confusing results concerning its *hemostatic* action. This highlights the significant difference between the theoretical potential actions of a botanical in the lab and its practical, empirically tested clinical applications.

In distinction to the wine-cured root (Rehmannia Shu Di Huang), the fresh root is reserved for conditions presenting fever, dryness or hemorrhage. In Chinese medical terms, the remedy is applied to conditions displaying heat at the Blood and Nutritive levels, and to Yin and fluids deficiency presenting symptoms of deficiency heat and dryness.

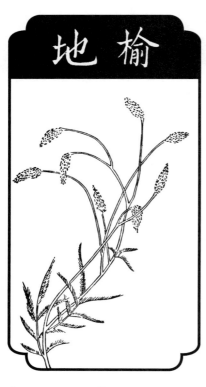

Sanguisorba Di Yu
Great Burnet Root

Botanical source: *Sanguisorba officinalis* L. (Rosaceae)
Pharmaceutical name: Radix Sanguisorbae
Chinese names: Di Yu, Hong Di Yu, Suan Zhe (Mand); Dei Yu (Cant)
Other names: Garden burnet, Bloodwort; Jiyu (Jap)
Habit: Perennial pantemperate herb growing on upland slopes and plains throughout China; in autumn, dark purple obovate flower spikes appear.
Part used: the root and rhizome

Therapeutic category: mild remedy with minimal chronic toxicity
Constituents: diyu glycosides, saponins sanguisorbins, carboxyl steroids, tannin, tannic/gallic acids, glucose, ziyuglycosides, vitamin A
Effective qualities: bitter, sour, astringent, cool, dry
astringing, solidifying, thickening
Tropism: vascular, reproductive systems
Liver, Large Intestine, Stomach channels
Fluid, Warmth bodies

Actions and Indications

hemostatic, coagulant: bleeding hemorrhoids, blood in stool, gastric and intestinal hemorrhage, functional menorrhagia, nosebleed, coughing up blood; any type of bleeding
astringent: diarrhea; chronic gastroenteritis, bacillary dysentery, leucorrhea
anti-inflammatory, vulnerary, styptic: scalds, burns, injuries with bleeding, ulcers
detoxicant, antibacterial, antifungal: furunculosis, eczema
antiemetic: nausea, vomiting

Preparation

Use: The root Sanguisorba Di Yu is decocted or used in tincture form. External preparations are applied to bleeding wounds, infantile eczema, burns, etc.
Dosage: Decoction: 8-16 g
Tincture: 2-5 ml
Caution: Do not use in deficiency cold conditions.

Notes

In Chinese medicine as in traditional Western medicine, Great burnet root is used for its outstanding *hemostatic* and *anti-inflammatory* effects.

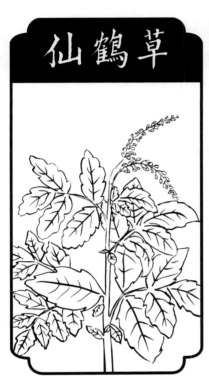

Agrimonia Xian He Cao
Furry Agrimony Herb *

Botanical source: *Agrimonia pilosa* Ledebour var. *japonica* (Miq.) Nakai (Rosaceae)
Pharmaceutical name: Herba Agrimoniae pilosae
Chinese names: Xian He Cao, Mao Jiao Ying (Mand); Sin Hok Chou (Cant)
Other names: Senkakuso (Jap)
Habit: Perennial ubiquitous herb growing on hillsides, by roadsides, grassy thickets and in grasslands; flowers in autumn with terminal or axillary yellow flowers forming long terminal racemes.
Part used: the herb

Therapeutic category: mild remedy with minimal chronic toxicity
Constituents: condensed tannin (phlobaphene), agrimonin, flavonoids (luteolin, apigenin), palmitic acid, daucosterol, glucopyranoside, essential oil, phloroglucinol derivatives, pimic acid, tannin, vitamin K
Effective qualities: bitter, pungent, astringent, neutral
astringing, thickening, solidifying, restoring
Tropism: cardiovascular, digestive, respiratory systems
Lung, Liver, Spleen channels; Fluid body

Actions and Indications

hemostatic, coagulant: coughing or vomiting blood, blood in urine or stool, nosebleed
astringent, anti-inflammatory, antibacterial: enteritis, bacterial dysentery, conjunctivitis, laryngitis; enuresis, diarrhea; heatstroke
antiparasitic: vermifuge, antiprotozoal, antimalarial: infection and infestation (incl. vaginal trichomoniasis, malaria, tapeworm)
detoxicant: boils, carbuncles
analgesic: abdominal pain, headache
cardiotonic: cardiac deficiency

Preparation

Use: The herb Agrimonia Xian He Cao is decocted or used in tincture form. Suppositories can be prepared for diarrhea and tapeworm. Eye and mouth washes, douches and vaginal sponges are also used.
Dosage: Decoction: 8-16 g
Tincture: 2-4 ml
Caution: This remedy may occasionally cause nausea, palpitations or flushing of the face; avoid using in excess heat conditions.

NOTES

Modern Chinese research on the *hemostatic* properties of this herb comes to varied and indefinite conclusions. As Furry agrimony herb was traditionally combined with one or more other *hemostatic* agents, depending on the type of hemorrhage being treated, it's safe to conclude that this remedy is best used in conjunction with another *hemostatic* for maximum results.

Both the Chinese and Western type of Agrimony are used to stop bleeding, but the latter is preferably used for its *anti-inflammatory* and *mucostatic* properties.

Cirsium Da Ji
Japanese Thistle Herb

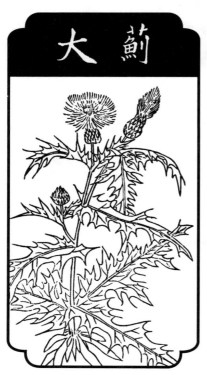

Botanical source: *Cirsium japonicum* De Candolle (Compositae)
Pharmaceutical name: Herba seu radix Cirsii japonici
Chinese names: Da Ji (Mand); Daai Gei (Cant)
Other names: "Great thistle"; Taikei (Jap)
Habit: Perennial herb from temperate East Asia, growing on sunny slopes and roadsides; blooms in summer with racemes of pale magenta flowers.
Part used: the herb or root

Therapeutic category: mild remedy with minimal chronic toxicity
Constituents: stigmasterol, beta-sitosterol, taraxasteryl acetate, amyrin, essential oil, bitter
Effective qualities: sweet, astringent, cool
astringing, thickening, relaxing
Tropism: vascular, reproductive systems
Liver, Spleen, Heart channels
Fluid body

ACTIONS AND INDICATIONS

hemostatic: coughing and vomiting blood, functional uterine bleeding, blood in stool and urine, nosebleed, traumatic bleeding
detumescent, vulnerary: injuries with swelling; abscesses, carbuncles, furunculosis, non-suppurating sores, skin swellings
anti-inflammatory: nephritis, hepatitis, mastitis, acute appendicitis
hypotensive: hypertension
diuretic

PREPARATION

Use: The herb Cirsium Da Ji is decocted or used in tincture form; external applications are used for sores, swellings, etc.
Dosage: Decoction: 8-20 g (up to 60 g for the fresh herb)
Tincture: 1-4 ml
Caution: Forbidden in stomach and intestines cold.

NOTES

Japanese thistle is a simple *hemostatic* used especially for coughing or vomiting blood.

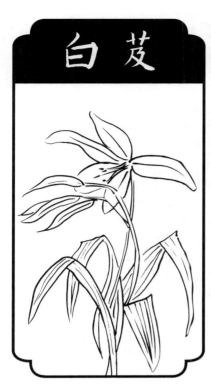

Bletilla Bai Ji
Amethyst Orchid Root *

Botanical source: *Bletilla striata* (Thunb.) Reichenbach f. (Orchidaceae)
Pharmaceutical name: Rhizoma Bletillae
Chinese names: Bai Ji (Mand); Baak Kap, Baak Gei (Cant)
Other names: Common bletilla, "White spreading"; Byakukyu (Jap)
Habit: Perennial herb from Central, South and East China and Japan; grows on mountainsides in moist, rich sandy soil, shrubland and fields; slender, pale purple, magenta or pink flowerheads open in late spring.
Part used: the rhizome

Therapeutic category: mild remedy with minimal chronic toxicity
Constituents: mucilage (bletilla glucomannan), starch, glucose, essential oil
Effective qualities: bitter, sweet, cool, moist
　　　　　　　　　　astringing, thickening, solidifying
Tropism: vascular, respiratory, digestive systems
　　　　　　Lung, Stomach, Liver channels
　　　　　　Fluid, Warmth bodies

ACTIONS AND INDICATIONS

hemostatic, coagulant: coughing or vomiting of blood, nosebleed, blood in urine or stool
vulnerary, styptic, demulcent: wounds with bleeding, burns, chronic ulcers (incl. malignant ulcers); gastric and duodenal ulcer with dyspepsia or bleeding, enteritis, chronic dry cough, lung TB, bronchiectasis, silicosis, hemorrhoids, suppurative infections
emollient: chapped or dry skin on hands and feet, scalds
detumescent: chronic nonsuppurative sores, chillblains, abscesses
antibacterial, antifungal: lung TB (incl. with hemoptysis), gram-positive bacilli

PREPARATION

Use: The root Bletilla Bai Ji is decocted or used in tincture form. Highly efficacious external applications are also made for bleeding wounds, ulcers, sores, chapped skin, burns, etc.
Dosage: Decoction: 5-16 g
　　　　　　Tincture: 1-4 ml
Caution: Contraindicated in hemoptysis with onset of infections, in the early stage of lung abscess and in stomach or lung heat.

NOTES

Among gardening and houseplant pundits in both East Asia and the U.S., bletilla is known as a hardy ground orchid that takes little time investment to produce violet to pink blooms—even in winter. Among Chinese doctors and pharmacists, the rhizome of the amethyst orchid furnishes a good *coagulant hemostatic* remedy for various forms of passive bleeding. Its *demulcent* effect, on the other hand, is put to use with dry, irritated conditions of the mucosa: peptic ulcer, bronchial dryness with dry cough and such like are here the prime beneficiaries. This sweet and moist remedy operates primarily because of its mucilage content—but then again, we note that it also contains a bitter essential oil of unknown composition.

Amethyst orchid root is often used topically for its *emollient* and *resolvent* actions, especially for the above surface conditions. It would certainly also be an excellent ingredient in a cosmetic face or hand lotion.

Cynanchum Bai Wei
Swallow-Wort Root

Botanical source: *Cynanchum atratum* Bunge or *C. versicolor* Bunge (Asclepiadaceae)
Chinese names: Bai Wei (Mand); Baak Mai (Cant)
Category: mild remedy with minimal chronic toxicity
Constituents: essential oil, cynanchol, cardiotonic glycosides
Effective qualities: bitter, salty, astringent, cold; astringing, calming, solidifying
Tropism: cardiovascular, urinary, respiratory systems; Liver, Stomach, Kidney channels

ACTIONS: *Hemostatic, refrigerant, antipyretic, diuretic, detoxicant, antitussive*
INDICATIONS: Blood in urine, fevers, especially low-grade, remittent fevers with Yin deficiency (e.g. postpartum, CFS); cardiac deficiency, urinary tract infection, enuresis, laryngitis, abscess, snake bites; cough.
Dosage: Decoction: 4-10 g
    Tincture: 2-4 ml
Caution: Forbidden in diarrhea.

Stellaria Yin Chai Hu
Stellaria Root

Botanical source: *Stellaria dichotoma* L. var. *lanceolata* Bunge (Caryophyllaceae)
Chinese names: Yin Chai Hu, Cha Qi Fan Lu (Mand)
Category: mild remedy with minimal chronic toxicity
Constituents: gypsogenin
Effective qualities: sweet, cool, dry; restoring, astringing
Tropism: vascular systems; Liver, Kidney, Gallbladder, Stomach channels

ACTIONS: *Hemostatic, antipyretic, antilipemic*
INDICATIONS: Uterine bleeding, blood in urine, coughing up blood, nosebleeds; low-grade fever with Yin deficiency, night sweats; infantile nutritional impairment, malaria.
Dosage: Decoction: 3-10 g
    Tincture: 1-3 ml
Caution: Forbidden in fever with metabolic deficiencies and in wind cold onset of infections.

Dioscorea Shu Liang
Dyer's Yam Root

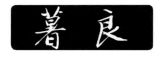

Botanical source: *Dioscorea cirrhosa* Loureiro (Dioscoreaceae)
Chinese names: Shu Liang (Mand)
Category: mild remedy with minimal chronic toxicity
Constituents: tannins
Effective qualities: sweet, astringent, cool; astringing, restoring, calming
Tropism: vascular system; Liver, Lung channels

ACTIONS: *Hemostatic, astringent, analgesic, diuretic, antipyretic*
INDICATIONS: Uterine, urinary and rectal bleeding, vomiting blood; arthralgia, paresthesia; typhoid.
    Topically for injuries, burns, boils.
Dosage: Decoction: 10-15 g
    Tincture: 2-5 ml
Caution: None.

Cephalanoplos Xiao Ji
Field Thistle Herb and Root

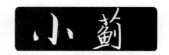

Botanical source: *Cephalanoplos segetum* (Bunge) Kitamura (Compositae)
Chinese names: Xiao Ji (Mand), Siu Gei (Mand)
Category: mild remedy with minimal chronic toxicity
Constituents: saponins, alkaloids

Effective qualities: sweet, astringent, cool; astringing, solidifying, relaxing, calming
Tropism: vascular, digestive, urogenital systems; Heart, Liver, Spleen channels

ACTIONS: *Hemostatic, coagulant, mucostatic, vulnerary, detoxicant, diuretic, nervous sedative, hypotensive, antilipemic, anti-infective*
INDICATIONS: Functional bleeding of many kinds, incl. blood in urine and stool, uterine bleeding, coughing up blood, nosebleed, traumatic bleeding; stress, agitation; boils, abscesses, wounds; nephritis, hepatitis, hypertension; diptherial and streptococcal infections.
Dosage: Decoction: 10-20 g
Tincture: 2-5 ml
Caution: Use only with signs of stasis present; forbidden during pregnancy as it is a *uterine stimulant*.

Callicarpa Zi Shu
Callicarpa Leaf

Botanical source: *Callicarpa pedunculata* R. Brown and spp. (Verbenaceae)
Chinese names: Zi Zhu, Zi Zhu Cao (Mand)
Category: mild remedy with minimal chronic toxicity
Constituents: condensed tannins, resin, flavonoids, carbohydrates, hydroxyl compounds, calcium, magnesium, iron salts
Effective qualities: bitter, neutral, dry; astringing, solidifying
Tropism: vascular systems; Liver, Spleen channels

ACTIONS: *Hemostatic, coagulant, anti-inflammatory, anti-infective*
INDICATIONS: Coughing and vomiting blood, nosebleed, blood in stool and urine, uterine bleeding, gastric bleeding traumatic, surgical and dental bleeding; hemorrhoids (with or without bleeding); burns.
Dosage: Decoction: 6-20 g
Tincture: 2-5 ml
The crushed or powdered leaf is applied topically onto bleeding wounds.
Caution: None.

Sonchus Ku Cai
Annual Sowthistle Herb

Botanical source: *Sonchus oleraceus* L. (Asteraceae)
Chinese names: Ku Cai (Mand)
Category: mild remedy with minimal chronic toxicity
Effective qualities: bitter, astringent, cold, dry; astringing, solidifying, calming, sinking
Tropism: vascular, respiratory, digestive, urinary systems; Lung, Spleen channels

ACTIONS: *Hemostatic, astringent, anti-inflammatory, anti-infective, antitumoral*
INDICATIONS: Functional uterine bleeding, coughing, vomiting of blood, blood in the stool and urine, nosebleed; acute enteritis, appendicitis, mastitis, stomatitis, pharyngitis, tonsilitis, infectious hepatitis, cirrhosis; breast, skin, stomach and liver cancer.

Dosage: Decoction: 15-30 g
Tincture: 2-5 ml
Caution: None.
Note: This remedy is one of the best for functional uterine bleeding.

Dioscorea Huang Yao Zi
Potato Yam Tuber

Botanical source: *Dioscorea bulbifera* L. (Dioscoreaceae)
Chinese names: Huang Yao Zi (M); Wong San Ji (C)
Category: medium-strength remedy with some chronic toxicity
Constituents: terpenoid/steroidal saponins (incl. diosbulbins A, B, C, D, diosgenin, phenanthrenes), tannins, iodine, vitamins
Effective qualities: bitter, astringent, neutral; restoring, solidifying
Tropism: vascular, respiratory, endocrine systems; Heart, Liver channels

Actions: *Hemostatic, detumescent, detoxicant, antitumoral, antibacterial, antitussive, demulcent*
Indications: Bleeding (incl. uterine and pulmonary); hypothyroid goiter, hyperthyroidism, lymphadenitis, tubercular lymphadenitis; laryngitis, gonorrhea, syphilis, food poisoning, insect/snake bites, carbuncles, simple sores; gastrointestinal, esophageal, uterine and thyroid tumors (incl. cancer); dry cough, asthma, whooping cough.
Topically for animal bites (incl. dog and snake bites).
Dosage: Decoction: 3-12 g.
Tincture: 1-4 ml
Up to 30 g in decoction are used for treating cancer.
Caution: Avoid continuous and longterm use which may lead to liver damage or jaundice; watch for signs such as nausea, vomiting. Forbidden with ulcerated abscess present.

Nelumbo Lian Fang
Lotus Receptacle

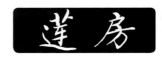

Botanical source: *Nelumbo nucifera* Gaertner (Nymphaeaceae)
Chinese names: Lian Fang (Mand); Ling Fong (Mand)
Part used: the receptacle or peduncle
Category: mild remedy with minimal chronic toxicity
Constituents: nelumbine, nicotinic acid, thiamine, proteins, starch, carotene, riboflavin, vitamin C
Effective qualities: bitter, astringent, warm, dry; astringing, solidifying, relaxing
Tropism: vascular, urigenital systems; Liver, Spleen, Kidney channels

Actions: *Hemostatic, astringent, fetal relaxant, antitumoral*
Indications: Uterine bleeding, menorrhagia, blood in urine; infantile diarrhea from food poisoning; fetal unrest, threatened miscarriage; cervical cancer; lochial retention; pemphigus.
Dosage: Decoction: 3-10 g
Tincture: 1-3 ml
Caution: None. The *fresh* remedy should be used when treating diarrhea from food poisoning in children.

Celosia Ji Guan Hua
Cock'scomb Herb

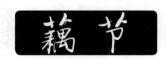

Botanical source: *Celosia cristata* L. (Amaranthaceae)
Chinese names: Ji Guan Hua (Mand); Gai Gun Fa (Cant)
Category: mild remedy with minimal chronic toxicity

Effective qualities: sweet, astringent, cool; astringing, solidifying
Tropism: vascular, digestive, urinary systems; Bladder, Liver, Large Intestine channels

Actions: *Hemostatic, atringent, mucostatic, anti-inflammatory, antiparasitic*
Indications: Many types of bleeding, including uterine, hemmorrhoidal, blood in stool; dysentery, leucorrhea, urinary tract infection, eye inflammation; trichomoniasis.
Dosage: Decoction: 10-15 g
Tincture: 2-5 ml
Caution: None.

Nelumbo Ou Jie
Lotus Root Node

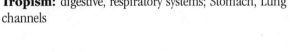

Botanical source: *Nelumbo nucifera* Gaertner (Nymphaeaceae)
Chinese names: Ou Jie (Mand); Ngao Jit (Cant)
Category: mild remedy with minimal chronic toxicity

Effective qualities: sweet, astringent, neutral; astringing
Tropism: digestive, respiratory systems; Stomach, Lung channels

Actions: *Hemostatic, astringent*
Indications: Bleeding (incl. nosebleeds), coughing and vomiting of blood, uterine bleeding.
Dosage: Decoction: 10-30 g
Tincture: 2-4 ml
Caution: None.
Note: The charred remedy, known as **Ou Jie Tan** (Mand.) or **Ngao Jit Taan** (Cant.), is said to have a superior *hemostatic* action.

Homo Xue Yu Tan
Charred Human Hair

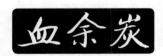

Zoological source: *Homo sapiens* L. (Hominidae)
Chinese names: Xue Yu Tan, Luan Fa Shuang (Mand)
Category: mild remedy with minimal chronic toxicity
Constituents: eukeratin, sulfur

Effective qualities: bitter, astringent, neutral, dry; astringing, calming
Tropism: vascular, urogenital systems; Heart, Liver, Kidney channels

Actions: *Hemostatic, urinary sedative, diuretic*
Indications: Bleeding in general (esp. nosebleeds, uterine bleeding); urinary irritation, blood in urine.
Dosage: Powder: 4-10 g
Caution: None.

Cardiovascular Stimulants

REMEDIES TO PROMOTE CIRCULATION AND RELIEVE COLD

➺ TONIFY THE YANG, WARM THE INTERIOR AND DISPEL COLD;
RESCUE DEVASTATED YANG

Arterial circulatory stimulants

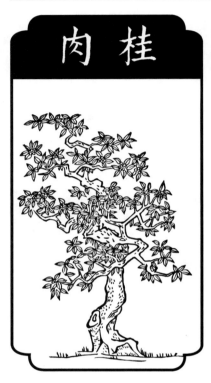

Cinnamomum Rou Gui
Cassia Cinnamon Bark

Botanical source: *Cinnamomum cassia* Blume (Lauraceae)
Pharmaceutical name: Cortex Cinnamomi cassiae
Chinese names: Rou Gui, Yu Gui, Guan Gui, Gui Xin (Mand); Yok Gwai (Cant)
Other names: Saigon cinnamon; Nikkei (Jap)
Habit: Evergreen cultivated subtropical tree from Guangxi, Guandong, Hainan, Taiwan, Vietnam and Java; flowers in early summer with cymose panicles of yellow-white flowers.
Part used: the inner bark

Therapeutic category: mild remedy with minimal chronic toxicity
Constituents: essential oil 1-2% (incl. cinnamic aldehyde/acid/acetate, eugenol, phellandrene, phenylpropyl acetate), mucilage, starch, tannin, sucrose
Effective qualities: pungent, sweet, astringent, hot, dry
  stimulating, decongesting, astringing
Tropism: cardiovascular, reproductive, digestive, respiratory systems
  Liver, Kidney, Spleen, Bladder, Dai channels
  Warmth, Air bodies

ACTIONS AND INDICATIONS

cardiovascular/arterial circulatory stimulant: arterial deficiency with cold skin and extremities, fatigue; hypothermia
spasmolytic, analgesic: spasm and pain in general (incl. abdominal pain); hernia, intestinal colic, spasmodic dysmenorrhea, lumbar pain, rheumatic myalgia, headache
uterine stimulant: amenorrhea
astringent, mucostatic: urogenital discharges, chronic diarrhea
draining diuretic: edema, jaundice, oliguria
leukocytogenic: low WBC count (leukopenia)
antibacterial, antifungal, antiviral
antiallergic

SYMPTOM PICTURES

Heart and Kidney Yang deficiency (Yang deficiency): palpitations, exhaustion, dizziness, cold skin and estremities

genitourinary cold (Kidney Yang deficiency): fatigue, lumbar pain, sore knees, urinary and seminal incontinence, cold extremities and skin

uterus cold: menstrual cramps, delayed or absent menses, easily chilled

stomach and intestines cold (Spleen Yang deficiency): epigastric or abdominal pain, nausea, fatigue, loose stool, cold extremities

Preparation

Use: The bark Cinnamomum Rou Gui may be decocted or taken in tincture form; the latter brings out its warming and stimulating qualities. An essential oil is made from the bark and the leaf of this East Asian cinnamon variety (also called Saigon cinnamon), but both types are not suited for internal use, as they are highly irritating unless given in a gelatin capsule (2 drops) with some olive oil (see Holmes 1989).

Dosage: Decoction: 2-5 g
Tincture: 0.25-2 ml

Caution: Contraindicated in pregnancy and Yin deficiency syndromes with empty heat.

Notes

The bark of the Sumatran and South Chinese Cassia cinnamon tree is essentially an *arterial circulatory stimulant* with pungent, sweet and very warming qualities. Add to this excellent pain and spasm relieving properties, and the result is a superlative, perennial remedy for treating internal deficiency cold conditions. The keynote symptoms here are pain and coldness caused by spasms and insufficient arterial circulation. Urogenital, digestive and cardiovascular deficiencies, seen in the Yang deficiency syndromes above, stand to benefit the most.

Cassia cinnamon bark is additionally a good *astringent* and *mucostatic* for damp cold discharges and, because of its high essential oil content, is considerably *antimicrobial* in conditions involving chronic or hidden infection, especially with fungal terrain present.

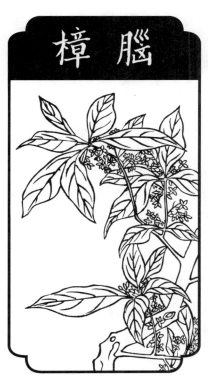

Cinnamomum Zhang Nao
Camphor Flake

Botanical source: *Cinnamomum camphora* (L.) Siebold (Lauraceae)
Pharmaceutical name: Camphora
Chinese names: Zhang Nao, Chao Nao, Hu Nao, Xiang Zhang (Mand)
Other names: Laurel camphor, Gum camphor; Shono (Jap)
Habit: Evergreen (sub)tropical Asian tree growing in plains, low hills, on slopes and in damp soil along rivers and roadsides; blooms in spring and summer with panicles of small pale yellow or green flowers.
Part used: the stearopten flakes prepared from the tree and root bark

Therapeutic category: medium-strength remedy with some chronic toxicity
Constituents: essential oil (incl. geraniol, carvacrol, cynol, limonenes, phellandrenes, azulene, bisabolene, camphene), flavonoid quercetin
Effective qualities: pungent, a bit bitter, warm with cooling potential, dry
stimulating, dispersing, restoring, raising, relaxing, calming
Tropism: cardiovascular, nervous, respiratory, digestive, reproductive, urinary systems
Heart, Spleen, Lung, Kidney, Liver, Large Intestine, Bladder, Du, Yang Qiao, Dai, Yang Wei channels; Warmth, Air, Fluid bodies

Actions and Indications

cardiovascular/arterial circulatory stimulant, hypertensive: cardiac and circulatory deficiency; hypothermia, circulatory collapse, congestive cardiac failure, low blood pressure, peripheral arterial deficiency, heatstroke
central nervous stimulant, psychogenic, analeptic: shock, collapse or coma with cold extremities; cerebral contusion
stimulant diaphoretic, nasal decongestant: onset of cold or flu, acute or chronic sinusitis, rhinitis
antipyretic: remittent and intermittent fevers

antidepressant nervous restorative: cerebral deficiency with exhaustion, depression, stupor, poor memory and concentration; neurasthenia, schizophrenia

nervous sedative/relaxant, spasmolytic, analgesic: nervous unrest, anxiety, insomnia, spasms, pain, mania, delirium; myalgia, neuralgia, gout, occipital headache, dysmenorrhea, dysuria, toothache, trauma pain

urogenital relaxant, mucostatic, diuretic: strangury, pollakiuria, dysuria, dysmenorrhea, leucorrhea, spermatorrhea

bronchial relaxant: asthma, whooping cough

intestinal relaxant: diarrhea, abdominal pain (incl. from parasites), cholera

aphrodisiac/anaphrodisiac: sexual disinterest/overexcitement

antiemetic: nausea, vomiting

anti-inflammatory: ear, nose, throat, joint, skin inflammations (esp. with discharge); acute mastitis

vulnerary, detumescent: chronic sores; wounds, injuries, contusions, fractures, swellings, ulcers

antifungal, antiseptic, dermal, antipruritic: fungal skin conditions, scabies, ringworm, pruritus, coldsores

anti-infective, antidotal, antivenomous: lung TB, infections in general; herb, food and chemical poisoning, centipede bite

Symptom Pictures

Heart and Kidney Yang deficiency (Yang deficiency): mental stupor, exhaustion, cold weak limbs, palpitations, pale or blue face

devastated Yang: chills, cold extremities, diarrhea with undigested food, prostration, fainting

nerve and brain deficiency (phlegm damp Heart obstruction): exhaustion, depression, confusion, unrest, sleep loss, disorientation

external wind cold with **head damp cold:** congested painful nose and sinuses, nasal dripping, sneezing, chills, fear of cold and draughts, aches and pains, unrest

lung phlegm cold with **Qi constraint:** coughing, production of sputum, wheezing, tight chest

bladder Qi constraint: urgent, difficult, frequent urination, bladder fullness

intestines mucous damp (Spleen damp): fatigue, nausea, loose mucousy stool, cold extremities

Preparation

Use: The flakes or granules of Cinnamomum Zhang Nao are usually taken in pill form, but may also be tinctured. The camphor tree root bark itself may also be used, and the leaves and branches especially are used externally. Excellent washes, compresses and liniments are prepared for topical use.

Dosage: Pill of flake: 0.25-1 g

Tincture of flake: 0.25-0.5 ml (6-12 drops)

Decoction of wood or root bark: 15-30 g

Essential oil: 1-2 drops in warm water

Small doses are generally more *stimulating,* large ones more *relaxing/sedating*.

Caution: Camphor flake is forbidden during pregnancy, in Qi deficiency and Yang excess conditions with heat, or in those prone to epilepsy. It should never be used continuously by itself due to slight cumulative toxicity.

Notes

The camphor tree is indignous to China, Taiwan and Japan. The massive, ancient tree, with its dense, aromatic, insect proof wood, has been valued in furniture making, incense making, perfumery and medicine since time immemorial. The icy white flakes used in Chinese medicine, the result of a lengthy boiling and sublimation process, is one way of preparing the wood (extracting the essential oil is another).

Although deservedly much applied to external conditions with pain, inflammation, swelling and infection, Camphor flake is also valued for its *cardiovascular* and *nervous stimulant* action. In energetic terms, it is defined as a systemically *Yang-tonifying* remedy that treats Yang deficiency conditions presenting exhaustion, depression and cold. Paradoxically, built into this primary systemic stimulation (or warming tonification) is an equally powerful *relaxant* and *sedative* effect that relieves spasmodic, painful and low-grade febrile states. Clearly, it is by engaging the circulation that Camphor is useful in such a variety of conditions, balancing quite opposite states with its adaptive, mercurial energy.

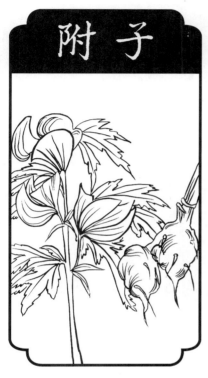

Aconitum Fu Zi
Prepared Sichuan Aconite Root

Botanical source: *Aconitum carmichaeli* Debeaux (Ranunculaceae)
Pharmaceutical name: Radix lateralis Aconiti carmichaeli praeparatae
Chinese names: Fu Zi, Shou Fu Zi, (Shu) Fu Pian (Mand); Fu Ji (Cant)
Other names: Sichuan wolfsbane; Bushi (Jap)
Habit: Perennial herb from Central and North China, especially Sichuan, preferring sunlit and mildly warm, moist conditions; also cultivated; in summer, small purple flower racemes appear.
Part used: the processed lateral root tuber

Therapeutic category: mild remedy with minimal chronic toxicity
Constituents: alkaloids 0.5-1% (incl. aconitine, hypaconitine, mesaconitine, jesaconitine, atisine), hygenamine, coryneine, polysaccharides
Effective qualities: pungent, a bit sweet, hot, neutral, dry
    stimulating, relaxing, restoring, decongesting
Tropism: cardiovascular, digestive, nervous systems
    Heart, Spleen, Kidney, Du, Yang Qiao channels
    Warmth, Air bodies

ACTIONS AND INDICATIONS

cardiovascular/arterial circulatory stimulant, hypertensive: cardiac deficiency and circulatory failure; hypotension, hypothermia, heatstroke; bradycardia, congestive heart failure, sick sinus syndrome with arrhythmia
central nervous stimulant, analeptic: shock, collapse or coma with profuse sweating, cold extremities, prostration
pituitary-adrenocortical stimulant/restorative: loss of stamina, fatigue; meopausal syndrome
analgesic, anti-inflammatory, spasmolytic, lymphocyte stimulant: acute abdominal pain, diarrhea, dysentery, cholera, neuralgia, myalgia (muscular rheumatism), arthritis
hypotensive, coronary dilator: hypertension
hypoglycemiant
antipyretic: fevers
draining diuretic: edema

SYMPTOM PICTURES

Heart and Kidney Yang deficiency (Yang deficiency): fear of cold, exhaustion, shallow breathing, cold skin and extremities

devastated Yang: chills, fainting, cold limbs, diarrhea with undigested food, prostration

genitourinary cold (Kidney Yang deficiency): cold back and knees, infertility, impotence, copious urination, water retention, mental stupor

intestines cold (Spleen and Kidney Yang deficiency): early morning diarrhea, abdominal pain, fatigue

cold damp obstruction: nerve, muscle and joint pains worse in cold or damp weather

PREPARATION

Use: Aconite root can be used only when processed properly to nullify its extremely toxic nature. The prepared lateral root tuber of Sichuan aconite, Aconitum Fu Zi (Shou Fu Zi) is decocted or used in tincture form.

Dosage: Decoction: 5-10 g. When used as a reinforcement for tonifying remedies, the dosage range is 1.5-5 g.
 Tincture: 2-4 ml
 For shock and coma, up to 20 g decoction or 8 ml tincture may be given.

Caution: Contraindicated during pregnancy and breastfeeding, and in Yin deficiency with false cold and true heat.

NOTES

Prepared Sichuan aconite root is *the* time-hallowed remedy for Yang deficiency conditions with systemic arterial deficiency. In acute shock and coma, with severe heart weakness and congestive heart failure, and in chronic cold and Yang deficient conditions of the digestive, urinary and reproductive systems, this medicinal is a foremost *cardiovascular stimulant*. Aconitine, atisine and other alkaloid types, as well as the cardiotonic hygenamine, are here active.

The well-known *analgesic* properties of Prepared Sichuan aconite root apply to both arthritic and rheumatic conditions, as they can involve an element of cold. Recently, the polysaccharides have shown *hypoglycemiant* activity (Yamada and Kiyohara 1989). Clearly, although the actions of this remedy are few, its practical syndrome applications are many.

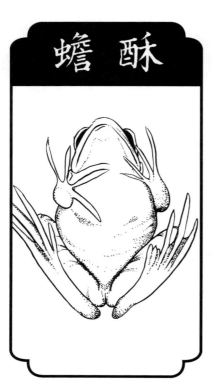

Bufo Chan Su
Toad Venom

Zoological source: *Bufo bufo gargarizans* Cantor or *B. melanostictus* Schneider (Bufonidae)
Pharmaceutical name: Secretio Bufonis
Chinese names: Chan Su (Mand)
Other names: Senso (Jap)
Part used: the dried venomous secretion of the toad skin glands

Therapeutic category: medium-strength remedy with some chronic toxicity
Constituents: cardiotonic glycosides (bufotoxins) with aglycones (sterols) bufogenins and bufotoxins (incl. bufagin, bufotalin, cinobufagin, cinobufotalin, telocinbufagin, bufalin, gamabufalin, resibufogenin, cinobufotalidin, arenobufagin, bufarenogen, desacetylcinobufagin, bufotalidin, hellebriganin, resibufagin, cinobufotoxin), epinephrine, indole derivative bufotenine, bufotenidine and serotonin, sitosterol, campesterol, bufosteroids, serotonine, bufothionine, tryptamine, adrenaline, dehydrobufoteinine, suberic acid, trace elements (incl. copper)
Effective qualities: sweet, pungent, warm, dry
 stimulating, decongesting, raising, relaxing
Tropism: cardiovascular, central nervous, respiratory, glandular systems
 Heart, Kidney, Lung, Stomach, Du, Yang Qiao channels
 Air, Warmth bodies

ACTIONS AND INDICATIONS

cardiovascular/arterial circulatory and adrenal medulla stimulant: hypertensive, adrenergic: cardiac deficiency and circulatory failure; congestive heart failure, sick sinus syndrome, hypotensio, hypothermia, shock, neonatal asphyxia, toxic pneumonia, respiratory failure, pulmonary heart disease, surgical bleeding, heatstroke, carbon monoxide poisoning, poisoning of hypnotics and anesthetics

central nervous stimulant, psychogenic, analeptic: shock, collapse or coma with profuse sweating, prostration, cold extremities
bronchial stimulant/relaxant: expectorant, antitussive, antiasthmatic: bronchitis, bronchial asthma
uterine stimulant
antitumoral (mild), *immunostimulant:* tumors, cancer
radiation-protective: radiation sickness
leukocytogenic: leukopenia, leukocytosis
resolvent detoxicant, detumescent, diuretic: eczema, boils, carbuncles/furuncles (esp. on back), cankers, sores, swellings, ulcers; food poisoning, acute pyogenic infections
anti-inflammatory, analgesic: acute laryngitis, acute tonsilitis, stomatitis, chronic ostemyelitis, toothache, fibromyositis
anesthetic (slow onset but long-lasting)
antibacterial
anticoagulant

SYMPTOM PICTURES

Heart and Kidney Yang deficiency (Yang deficiency): cold skin and extremities, fear of cold, exhaustion, stupor

devastated Yang: chills, fainting, cold limbs, diarrhea with undigested food, prostration

heart/lung fluid congestion: coughing, difficult breathing from exertion or lying down, sweating, chills, fatigue, irritability

lung Qi constraint with **phlegm cold:** coughing, production of white sputum, tight chest, wheezing, cold extremities

PREPARATION

Use: The toad secretion Bufo Chan Su is usually decocted. External applications for skin tumors and other conditions above are also prepared.

Dosage: Decoction: 0.015-0.03 g
Tincture: 0.05-0.1 ml or up to 3 drops

Caution: Use only under professional supervision, especially as regards dosage. Contraindicated during pregnancy breastfeeding and nursing because of its medium-strength status. For the same reason Bufo Chan Su is not to be used continuously at maximum dosage. Signs of accumulated toxicity from Bufo Chan Su include malaise, unrest, nausea, numbness of the mouth, lips and extremities, dizziness and chest discomfort.

NOTES

The mainstream traditional use of Toad venom is as a *resolvent detoxicant* and *analgesic* remedy for topical use. Painful swollen carbuncles and furuncles, and painful conditions as toothache, sores, painful throat and myalgia were the primary conditions treated with it.

Now that Toad venom has been validated by extensive Chinese research, it has become a commonly used modern medicinal. Its reliable *stimulant* action on the body's Yang (including cardiovascular, sympathetic nervous and adrenal medullar functions) reflect deep neuroendocrine activity on the Du Mai, Yang Qiao and to some extent Yang Wei extra channels. In this sense, Toad venom is a specific remedy that treats a large variety of conditions entailing circulatory failure. This remedy's particular action on the heart muscle is like digitalis, but more rapid and short-lived, and without any cumulative effect (Chang and But 1987).

The successful application in the People's Republic of Toad venom for radiation sickness also merits note.

Thevetia Huang Hua Jia Zhu Tao
Peruvian Thevetia Leaf and Seed

Botanical source: *Thevetia peruviana* (pers.) K. Schuman (Apocynceae)
Chinese names: Huang Hua Jia Zhu Tao (Mand); Wong Fa Gaap Juk Tou (Cant)
Therapeutic category: strong remedy with acute chronic toxicity

Constituents: cardiac glycosides (incl. thevetin A and B, peruvoside, neriifolin, ruvoside, perusitin, cerberin), bornesitol, vertiaflavone
Effective qualities: pungent, bitter, warm; stimulating
Tropism: cardiovascular, urinary, digestive systems; Heart, Spleen channels

ACTIONS: *Cardiovascular stimulant, diuretic, detumescent, anthelmintic*
INDICATIONS: Congestive heart failure, paropxysmal supraventricular tachycardia, atrial fibrillation; coronary disease; intestinal parasites.
Dosage: Decoction: 1-3 g
Tincture: 0.25-1 ml
Caution: Use only under clinical supervision. Doses for this strong status remedy must be respected. Signs of intoxications include vomiting, salivation, apetite loss, tiredness and shortness of breath.
NOTES: The extracted glycosides, rather than the leaf and seed itself, are most commonly used in China today.

Cardiovascular Relaxants

REMEDIES TO RELAX THE BLOOD VESSELS AND RELIEVE IRRITABILITY

➥ CIRCULATE HEART QI, RELEASE CONSTRAINT AND SUBDUE LIVER YANG

Hypotensive vasodilators

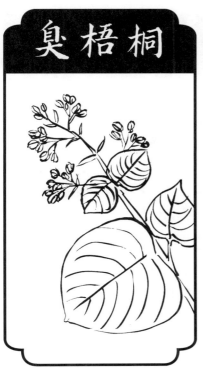

Clerodendrum Chou Wu Tong
Forked Glorybower Leaf

Botanical source: *Clerodendrum trichotomum* Thunberg (Verbenaceae)
Pharmaceutical name: Folium Clerodendri
Chinese names: Chou Wu Tong, Ba Jia Wu Tong (Mand)
Other names: Mayflower/Harlequin glorybower, Clerondendron, "Stinking parasol tree"; Kusagi (Jap)
Habit: Deciduous shrub or small subtropical Asian tree growing on uplands; also cultivated; blooms in autumn with fragrant cymes of white flowers.
Part used: the young leaf (usually with twig)

Therapeutic category: mild remedy with minimal chronic toxicity
Constituents: alkaloids, glycosides (clerodendrins A, B), bitters, inositol, glucu-ronide, clerodendronin A and B, acacetin, organic acids
Effective qualities: bitter, sweet, neutral
          relaxing, calming
Tropism: cardiovascular, nervous, musculoskeletal, respiratory systems
       Heart, Liver, Lung, Yin Wei channels
       Air body

ACTIONS AND INDICATIONS

cardiovascular relaxant: hypotensive: tense/spasmodic cardiovascular disorders with dizziness; essential hypertension, neurocardiac syndrome, peripheral arterial deficiency with pain
nervous sedative, analgesic, anti-inflammatory: stress, unrest, migraine, severe intermittent headache; hemiplegia, myalgia, arthralgia, rheumatoid arthritis
bronchial relaxant: asthma, bronchitis
antimalarial, anthelmintic: malaria, intestinal parasites
dermatropic, antipruritic: boils, eczema, neurodermatitis, tinea manuum
diuretic

SYMPTOM PICTURE

heart Qi constraint and **heart Yin deficiency** with **nerve excess (Liver Yang rising):** throbbing headache, dizziness, unrest, sleep loss, irritability

PREPARATION

Use: The leaf Clerodendrum Chou Wu Tong is decocted or used in tincture form. When part of a decoction formula, it should be added 10 minutes before the end of cooking time to preserve its *hypotensive* action. External applications have been useful with dermatitis. Only very large doses are effective for asthmatic conditions.
Dosage: Decoction: 10-15 g
          Tincture: 2-4 ml
Caution: None.

NOTES

Forked glorybower leaf is a straightforward *neurocardiac relaxant* and *sedative,* best applied to heart Qi constraint (also known as excess Liver Yang) conditions with high blood pressure. The leaf's *hypotensive* effect, due to the component clerodendrin, has proven superior to Eucommia bark, but inferior to Rauwolfia root. Excellent *analgesic* and *anti-inflammatory* activity has also been shown by the remedy.

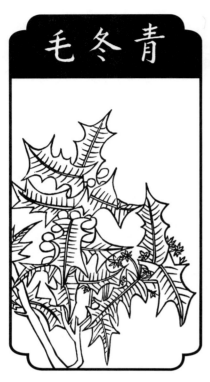

Ilex Mao Dong Qing
Furry Holly Root *

Botanical source: *Ilex pubescens* Hooker et Arnold (Aquifoliaceae)
Pharmaceutical name: Radix seu folium Ilicis pubescentis
Chinese names: Mao Dong Qing, Mao Pi Shu (Mand); Mou Dung Ching (Cant)
Other names: Downy holly, "Winter green"
Habit: Evergreen shrub from temperate China, growing among shrubs in grassland and mountains; pinkish flowers bloom in fascicles in early summer.
Part used: the root or leaf

Therapeutic category: mild remedy with minimal chronic toxicity
Constituents: flavonoids, phenolic compounds, sterols, triterpenoid saponins, ilexsaponin A, tannin, amino acids, saccharides, oleanolic/ursolic acid
Effective qualities: pungent, bitter, cool, dry
    relaxing, calming, stimulating
Tropism: cardiovascular, nervous, respiratory systems
    Heart, Lung, Liver channels
    Air, Warmth bodies

ACTIONS AND INDICATIONS

cardiovascular relaxant: coronary dilator, hypotensive: tense/spasmodic cardiovascular disorders with dizziness; essential hypertension, myocardial infarct, cerebral thrombosis, phlebitis, neurocardiac syndrome
coronary restorative: coronary deficiency/disease, angina pectoris
bronchodilator, antitussive, expectorant: asthma, cough; bronchitis
analgesic: chest pains, pain in general
antipyretic, anti-inflammatory, antibacterial: febrile infections, tonsillitis, laryngitis, retinitis, vasculitis, uveitis; burns, erysipelas; suppurative skin eruptions

SYMPTOM PICTURES

heart Qi constraint (Liver Yang rising): headache, dizziness, irritability

heart blood and Qi stagnation: chest tightness or pain, shortness of breath, anxiety

external wind heat and **lung wind heat:** fever, shivers, sore throat, aches and pains, coughing, wheezing

PREPARATION

Use: The root Ilex Mao Dong Qing is used in decoction, tincture or extract (flavanoid glycosides) form. Externally it is frequently applied to burns and scalds to reduce inflammation and pain.
Dosage: Decoction: 20-90 g
    Tincture: 2-5 ml
   High doses are needed for cardiovascular conditions and phlebitis.
Caution: Contraindicated in people with tendency to bleeding. Idiosyncratic reactions such as headache, dizziness, nausea, constipation, etc., are occasionally possible with this remedy.

NOTES

The root or leaf of the Furry holly provides another trusty *relaxant* wind heat remedy that is finding renewed application for modern disorders. Both *vasodilatant* and *spasmolytic*, its main relevant applications today are essential hypertension and coronary disease with angina.

Dong Qing (Mand). or **Dung Ching** (Cant.) is the generic name for a variety of *Ilex* species growing in southern China, all used in similar, but distinct ways for their *anti-inflammatory, analgesic, detumescent* and *astringent* properties.

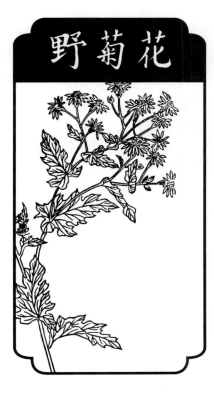

Chrysanthemum Ye Ju Hua
Wild Chrysanthemum Flower

Botanical source: *Chrysanthemum indicum* L. (Compositae)
Pharmaceutical name: Flos Chrysanthemi indici
Chinese names: Ye Ju Hua, Ye Huang Zhu (Mand); Gam Guk Fa (Cant)
Other names: Nogikuka (Jap)
Habit: Ubiquitous perennial herb from China and Japan, found on slopes and roadsides; corymbose racemes of terminal/axillary yellow flowers appear during late autumn and winter.
Part used: the flower

Therapeutic category: mild remedy with minimal chronic toxicity
Constituents: glycosides (luteolin, chrysanthemin, stachydrin and cholin), daucosterol, essential oil (incl. thujone, camphor, yejuhua lactone), acacetin, cumambrin A, coumarins, polysaccharides, monobehenate, palmitic acid, chrysanthemol, tannin, vitamins A, B1
Effective qualities: bitter, pungent, cold
　　　　　　　　　　　relaxing, sinking, decongesting
Tropism: cardiovascular, central nervous systems
　　　　　Lung, Liver channels; Air, Warmth bodies

ACTIONS AND INDICATIONS

cardiovascular relaxant: peripheral vasodilator, hypotensive: tense/spasmodic cardiovascular disorders with dizziness; essential hypertension, peripheral arterial deficiency, headache
anti-infective: antibacterial, antiviral: common cold, flu, hepatitis, dysentery, encephalitis
resolvent detoxicant, anti-inflammatory, dermatropic, antipruritic: deep-rooted boils, carbuncles, inflamed ulcers, conjunctivitis, mastitis, scrofula, pruritus
lymphatic decongestant: lymphadenitis, lymphangitis, tonsilitis

SYMPTOM PICTURES

heart Qi constraint (Liver Yang rising/Liver fire): dizziness, ringing in ears, headache

external wind heat: feverishness, sore throat, swollen glands

PREPARATION

Use: The flower Chrysanthemum Ye Ju Hua should be used both internally and externally for the above conditions. For external washes and compresses, the fresh herb should be used by preference. It is either infused in the normal way or used as a tincture.
Dosage: Infusion: 10-20 g
　　　　　Tincture: 2-5 ml
Caution: None.

CARDIOVASCULAR RELAXANTS

NOTES
Its excellent *anti-infective* and *detoxicant* actions notwithstanding, the Wild chrysanthemum flower from northern China is especially used these days to treat essential hypertension. In practice, its *relaxant* effect on the whole circulation is often complemented with other *vasodilators, coronary restoratives* and *resolvents* from this and other sections.

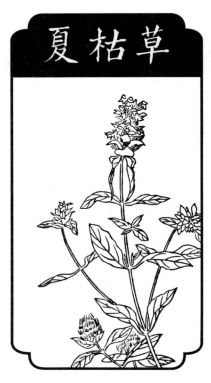

Prunella Xia Ku Cao
Selfheal Spike

Botanical source: *Prunella vulgaris* L. (Labiatae)
Pharmaceutical name: Spica Prunellae
Chinese names: Xia Ku Cao (Mand); Ha Gu Chou, Ha Bu Chou (Cant)
Other names: Chinese healall, "Summer withering"; Kagoso (Jap)
Habit: Sprawling perennial temperate Eurasian herb, growing on roadsides, hillsides and forest edges; the flower spike blooms in summer with small white or violet terminal blossoms.
Part used: the flower spike or herb

Therapeutic category: mild remedy with minimal chronic toxicity
Constituents: oleanolic/ursolic/caffeic acids, rutin, tannins 5%, hyperoside, essential oil (incl. camphor, cineol, pinene, linalool, myrcene, phellandrene), fenchone, triterpenoid saponins, cyanidin, delphinidin, alkaloids, soluble salts (incl. 68% potassium chloride), resin, jiangtangsu, vitamins A, B1, C, K, trace minerals (incl. zinc)
Effective qualities: a bit sweet, pungent, bitter and astringent, cold, dry
 relaxing, dissolving, sinking, astringing
Tropism: cardiovascular, digestive, lymphatic systems
 Liver, Gallbladder, Lung channels
 Air, Warmth bodies

ACTIONS AND INDICATIONS
cardiovascular relaxant: vasodilator, hypotensive: tense/spasmodic cardiovascular disorders with dizziness; hypertension, tinnitus, headache, eyeball pain, photophobia
antipyretic: high fever, heat exhaustion, heat cramps
resolvent detoxicant, detumescent: toxicosis (esp. metabolic [incl. rheumatism, gout], heavy metal [incl. sulfur, mercury]); swollen glands (esp. in neck), lipoma, goiter, boils, abscesses
lymphatic decongestant: lymphadenitis, lymphangitis, cervical lymph gland TB
broad-spectrum anti-infective: antiviral, antibacterial, anti-inflammatory, phagocyte stimulant: acute conjunctivitis, keratitis, mastitis, stomatitis; HIV infection, herpes simplex
leukocytogenic: leukopenia
draining diuretic: edema
hypoglycemiant
astringent, vulnerary: wounds, sores, ulcers, contusions
hemostatic: bleeding, menorrhagia

SYMPTOM PICTURES
heart Qi constraint (Liver Yang rising/Liver fire): headache, dizziness, irritability, red, painful, swollen eyes

metabolic/heavy metal toxicosis: malaise, aches and pains, dizziness, concentration loss

Preparation

Use: The flower spike Prunella Xia Ku Cao should be infused for best results; the decoction or tincture are also good.
Dosage: Infusion: 8-18 g
Tincture: 2-5 ml
Caution: Avoid using in digestive deficiency.

Notes

The same plant as used in the West, Selfheal spike is a good example of a remedy with *relaxant, heat-clearing, detoxicant* and *anti-inflammatory* properties that are well documented in both traditional Chinese and Greek texts.

Today, its excellent *hypotensive* action has generated much research in China. Relieving neurological symptoms in the head—especially from heavy metal poisoning, for example—is another of Selfheal's specialties. The remedy's *detoxicant* action is evident in the areas of metabolic toxicosis (e.g., rheumatic disorders) and heavy metal toxicosis.

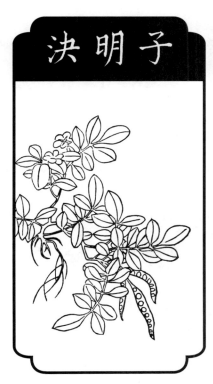

Cassia Jue Ming Zi
Sickle Senna Seed

Botanical source: *Cassia tora* L. or *C. obtusifolia* L. (Leguminosae)
Pharmaceutical name: Semen Cassiae torae
Chinese names: Jue Ming Zi, Cao Jue Ming (Mand); Chou Kit Ming (Cant)
Other names: Sicklepod, Fetid cassia, Coffee weed, "Determining brightness"; Ketsumeishi (Jap)
Habit: Annual Southeast Asian herb; grows in sunny situations on waste ground and roadsides and near villages; cultivated throughout China; showy pale yellow flowers open in late summer, singly or in twos, on leaf axils.
Part used: the seed

Therapeutic category: mild remedy with minimal chronic toxicity
Constituents: chrysophanol, aloe-emodin, emodin, rhein, physcion, glucoside obtusin, rubrofusarin, torachryson, toralactone, fatty oil, mucilage, proteins, vitamin A
Effective qualities: bitter, sweet, salty, cool, moist
relaxing, restoring, softening
Tropism: cardiovascular, digestive systems
Liver, Gallbladder, Large Intestine channels
Air, Warmth body

Actions and Indications

cardiovascular relaxant: hypotensive, antilipemic: tense/spasmodic cardiovascular disorders; hypertension, hyperlipemia
demulcent, anti-inflammatory: itchy/red/swollen/painful/bloodshot/tearing eyes; acute conjunctivitis, retinitis, corneal ulcer, boils, furunculoid sores
demulcent laxative: constipation, dry stool
hepatic, diuretic: hepatitis, liver cirrhosis, ascites
vision restorative, optitrophic: poor eyesight; photophobia, night blindness, glaucoma, retinal degeneration
antibacterial
Miscellaneous: infantile malabsoption and malnutrition

Symptom Pictures
heart Qi constraint (Liver Yang rising): headache, red painful eyes, light oversensitivity, blurred vision

intestines dryness: chronic constipation, difficult bowel movement, hard dry stool

Preparation
Use: The seed Cassia Jue Ming Zi may be decocted or used in tincture form.
Dosage: Decoction: 10-15 g
Tincture: 2-4 ml
Caution: Do not combine with Cannabis seed for a *demulcent laxative* effect.

Notes
Oriental herbalists have traditionally made most use of Sickle senna seed for irritated, inflamed or tearing eyes as well as a variety of vision disorders. Little is still known about its dynamics in this area—except that it works.

Nowadays practitioners also take into account Sickle senna seed's good *hypotensive* and *diuretic* effects when prescribing. The *relaxant* action reverses symptoms of constrained Qi in the heart, and is especially indicated when high blood cholesterol, etc., is part of overall findings.

Rauvolfia Luo Fu Mu
Rauvolfia Root

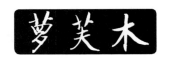

Botanical source: *Rauvolfia verticillata* (Lour.) Baillon or *R. yunnanensis* Tsiang var. *angustifolia* Wu or *R. latifrons* Tsiang or *R. serpentina* Bentham (Apocynaceae)
Chinese names: Luo Fu Mu, Bai Hua Lian, Shan Ma Di (Mand); Lou Fuk Muk (Cant)
Habit: Evergreen East Asian shrub; flowers throughout summer with corymbs of small white flowers.
Category: medium-strength remedy with some chronic toxicity

Constituents: alkaloids 1-3%: basic quaternary ammonium alkaloids (incl. serpentine, serpentinine, sarpagine, samatine), tertiary amine derivatives (incl. yohimbine, ajmaline, ajmalicine, tetraphylline, tetraphyllicine), weakly basic secondary amines (incl. reserpine 0.002-0.16%, rescinnamine, deserpidine, raunesine, canescine)
Effective qualities: bitter, dry, cold; calming, relaxing, sinking
Tropism: cardiovascular, nervous, hepatobiliary systems; Heart, Liver, Bladder, Yin Wei channels

Actions: *Hypotensive, nervous sedative (hypnotic, sympathetic inhibitor), analgesic, hypnotic, antipyretic, anti-inflammatory, hepatic decongestant, dermatropic, detumescent, detoxicant, antivenomous*
Indications: Hypertension with headache and dizziness (Liver Yang rising syndrome); insomnia, unrest; mania, anxiety states, phobias, obsessive-compulsive disorder, chronic manic psychosis, chronic schizophrenia, hyperthyroid conditions with sympathetic nervous excess, malnutrition; Yang excess conditions; abdominal pain of acute infections, vomiting; obstinate high fever, malaria; acute hepatitis with jaundice, cholecystitis (liver damp heat); laryngitis with painful throat; urticaria, neurogenic eczema with pruritus, contact and seborrheic dermatitis; boils, furunculosis, snake and scorpion bite; traumatic injury with pain, swelling and discoloration.
Dosage: Decoction: 10-14 g
Tincture: 1-3 ml
Topical applications are also made for tissue trauma and venomous bites.
Caution: Contraindicated in depressive states, parasympathetic hypertonia and excess gastric hydrochloric acid or peptic ulcer. Rauwolfia Luo Fu Mu possesses mild cumulative toxicity. If taken continuously over 2 months, signs of mild intoxication may appear, including dizziness, somnolence, sleeploss, diarrhea and tiredness.
Notes: Rauvolfia root is more than just a reliable remedy for tense cardiovascular conditions. With its *sinking* and *heat-clearing* qualities, this *sedative/relaxant* botanical has proven highly effective in chronic psychotic and schizoid conditions, as well as excess Yang states such as mania and high fever. Hives and other forms of eczema have also cleared up dramatically under its application.

Catharanthus Chang Chun Hua
Madagascar Periwinkle Root and Herb

Botanical source: *Catharanthus roseus* (L.) G. Don (Apocynaceae)
Chinese names: Chang Chun Hua (M); Cheung Cheun Fa
Category: medium-strength remedy w. chronic toxicity
Constituents: over 70 alkaloids, incl. 28 bi-indole alkaloids (incl. vinblastine, vincristine, leurosine, vincadioline, leurosidine, perivine, catharanthine)
Effective qualities: bitter, cool; relaxing, calming
Tropism: cardiovascular, urinary, endocrine systems; Liver, Pericardium channels

ACTIONS: *hypotensive, antitumoral, hypoglycemiant, hypnotic, diuretic, astringent, emmenagogue*
INDICATIONS: Hypertension; heart Qi constraint and heart Yin deficiency with nerve excess (Liver Yang rising) syndromes; many types of tumors (incl. cancerous, esp. lung, lymphatic); acute lymphocytic leukemia, diabetes mellitus, amenorrhea, insomnia.
Dosage: Decoction: 9-15 g
Tincture: 1-3 ml
Caution: Forbidden during pregnancy and lactation, and not to be used on its own continuously because of its medium-strength status.
NOTES: This remedy and its extracted alkaloids has become important in the treatment of many types of cancer.

Apocynum Luo Bu Ma
Lance-Leaf Dogbane Root and Herb

Botanical source: *Apocynum lancifolium* Russam or *A. venetum* L. or *A. hendersonii* Hooker (Apocynaceae)
Chinese names: Luo Bu Ma, Ze Qi Ma (M); Lo Bou Ma (C)
Category: strong remedy with some acute toxicity
Constituents: cardiotonic glycosides (incl. cymarin, strophanthidin, acetyl compound), alpha-amyrin lupeol, hydroxyacetophenone, catechin, rutin, neoisorutin
Effective qualities: bitter, dry, cold; sinking, relaxing
Tropism: cardiovascular, nervous systems; Heart, Spleen channels

ACTIONS: *Hypotensive, cardiotonic, draining diuretic*
INDICATIONS: Hypertension, cardiac deficiency, heart disease; edema, hepatitis, nephritis.
Dosage: Decoction: 3-9 g; Tincture: 0.25-1 ml
The herb is also rolled into a cigarette and used as a smoke in chronic bronchitis with cough and wheezing.
Caution: Do not exceed these dosages! Not for continuous use because of its strong status. Signs of intoxication include diarrhea, nausea, vomiting and slow heart beat.

Salsola Zhu Mao Cai
Salsola Root and Herb

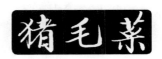

Botanical source: *Salsola collina* Pallas or *S. ruthenica* Iljin or *S. richteri* Iljin (Chenopodiaceae)
Chinese names: Zhu Mao Cai, Ci Peng, Zha Peng Ke (Mand)
Category: mild remedy with minimal chronic toxicity
Constituents: *S. ruthenica*: succinic acid, betaine, polysaccharides
Effective qualities: sweet, bland, cool; relaxing
Tropism: cardiovascular, nervous systems; Heart, Bladder channels

ACTIONS: *Hypotensive, analgesic, hypnotic* (mild)
INDICATIONS: Hypertension, headache, restlessness.
Dosage: Decoction: 10-30 g
Tincture: 2-5 ml
Caution: None.

Cardiovascular Sedatives

REMEDIES TO CALM THE HEART, SEDATE THE NERVES AND RELIEVE ANXIETY

➥ SETTLE AND CALM THE SPIRIT WITH HEAVY REMEDIES

Neurocardiac sedatives

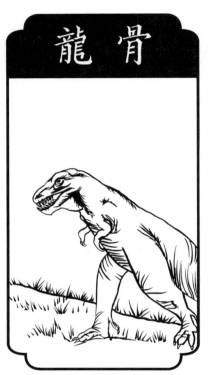

Stegodon Long Gu
Dragon Bone

Zoological source: *Stegodon orientalis* Owen or *S. rhinocerus sinensis* Owen or *Hipparion* spp. (Saurischia, Ornithischia, Artiodactyla)
Pharmaceutical name: Os Stegodontis
Chinese names: Long Gu (Mand); Lung Gwat (Cant)
Other names: Mammal bone; Ryokotsu (Jap)
Source: The skeleton fossils are found in Inner Mongolia, and Shanxi, Shaanxi, Gansu and Hebi provinces.
Part used: the fossilized vertebrate bone

Therapeutic category: mild remedy with minimal chronic toxicity
Constituents: calcium carbonate (up to 82%) and phosphate, iron, potassium, sulfates, silicon dioxide, ferric/aluminum/manganese/calcium oxide, hydroxy apatite, organic acids (incl. acetic/isobutyric/valeric/propionic acids)
Effective qualities: sweet, astringent, neutral, dry
  calming, sinking, astringing, solidifying, stabilizing
Tropism: cardiac, nervous, reproductive systems
  Heart, Liver, Kidney, Large Intestine, Yin Wei, Yang Wei, Dai channels

ACTIONS AND INDICATIONS
neurocardiac sedative: hypnotic: cardiac hyperfunctioning with palpitations, anxiety; acute neurocardiac syndrome, anxiety states, phobias; nightmares
nervous sedative, hypotensive: insomnia, unrest, paranoia, fright seizures; essential hypertension
sexual sedative: sexual overstimulation in both sexes (nymphomania, satyriasis), premature ejaculation
mucostatic, hemostatic, anhydrotic: incontinence with leucorrhea, spermatorrhea, diarrhea; uterine bleeding, spontaneous sweating
vulnerary: chronic ulcers and sores, scrotal/vaginal pruritus, chronic wet eczema

SYMPTOM PICTURES
Spirit Instability with **nerve excess:** emotional distress, anxiety, palpitations, unrest, sleep loss
Liver and Kidney Yin deficiency with **nerve excess (Liver Yang rising/Floating Yang):** irritability, unrest, sleep loss, dizziness, night sweats, seminal discharges

PREPARATION
Use: The bone Stegodon Long Gu is decocted or used in powder form. When decocted, it should be cooked alone for 20-30 minutes before any other herbs are added. The calcined remedy, known as **Duan Long Gu** (Mand.) or **Taan Lung Gwat** (Cant.), is better at restraining fluids, stopping uterine bleeding and night sweats and healing chronic sores.

Powdered Dragon bone is used topically for its *astringent* and *vulnerary* action on rectal prolapse, sores, itching due to damp, nosebleed, etc.
Dosage: Decoction: 15-30 g

Caution: Contraindicated in damp heat and excess external conditions.

NOTES

Dragon bone, a literal translation of Long Gui, is the fossilized remnants of large prehistoric mammalian vertebrate reptiles such as the dinosaur. Because these remnants were traditionally believed actually to come from the mythological animal, the dragon, spiritual ruler of the East, the remedy was associated with various magic practices in its collection, preparation and administration.

Today it is clear that Dragon bone's high mineral content ensures a safe, general, medium-strength *sedative* action on the nerves, heart and genital organs. Dragon bone's *stabilizing* and *solidifying* energies also provide a good *astringent* effect for treating various discharges.

Fossilized **Dragon tooth, Long Chi** (Mand.) or **Lung Ji** (Cant.), has the same uses as the bone, but is considered a stronger *neurocardiac sedative* for palpitations, anxiety, insomnia, nightmares, delirium and convulsions. Dragon tooth is also used to treat arthritis, osteomyelitis and gastralgia. It is decocted in the same way as Dragon bone and used at a dosage of 10-16 g.

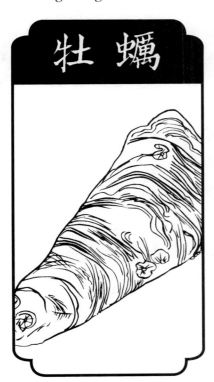

Ostrea Mu Li
Oyster Shell

Zoological source: *Ostrea gigas* Thunberg or *O. rivularis* Gould or *O. talienwahensis* Crosse (Ostreidae/Pterioidae)
Pharmaceutical name: Concha Ostreae
Chinese names: Mu Li, Sheng Mu Li (Mand); Mao Lai (Cant)
Source: China's coastal provinces
Other names: Borei (Jap)
Part used: the shell

Therapeutic category: mild remedy with minimal chronic toxicity
Constituents: calcium tricarbonate (80-95%)/phosphate/sulfate, potassium, magnesium, ferric oxide, silicon dioxide, iodine, zinc, aluminum, amino acids, trimethyl-amine, succinic acid, vitamins A, B1, B2, D, F, sterols, lipids, betaine, glycogen, taurin, glutathione, keratin, oburidine, adenine, glycolipids
Effective qualities: salty, astringent, cool, dry
calming, sinking, softening, astringing, solidifying, stabilizing
Tropism: nervous, cardiac, reproductive, digestive systems
Heart, Liver, Kidney, Gallbladder, Yin Wei, Yang Wei, Dai channels

ACTIONS AND INDICATIONS

neurocardiac sedative: hypnotic: cardiac hyperfunctioning with palpitations, anxiety; acute neurocardiac syndrome, anxiety states, phobias
nervous sedative/relaxant, spasmolytic, anticonvulsant: insomnia, unrest, tinnitus, blurred vision, spasms, seizures; epilepsy, neurosis, hypocalcemia
hypotensive: hypertensive with headache, dizziness
sexual sedative: sexual overstimulation in both sexes (nymphomania, satyriasis), premature ejaculation
astringent, antacid antisecretory: dyspepsia from gastric hyperacidity, peptic ulcer, diarrhea
mucostatic, hemostatic, anhydrotic: leucorrhea, menorrhagia, intermenstrual bleeding, night/day sweats
antienuretic: incontinence with enuresis, pollakiuria, nocturnal spermatorrhea
hypoglycemiant: hyperglycemia, diabetes
antipyretic: low-grade fevers
dissolvent, detumescent: scrofula, goiter, lymphadenitis, spleenomegaly
Miscellaneous: tuberculosis

Symptom Pictures

Spirit Instability with **nerve excess:** anxiety, restlessness, palpitations, sleep loss

Yin deficiency with **nerve excess (Liver Yang rising/Floating Yang):** irritability, dizziness, sleep loss, hot spells or low fever, spasms

stomach Qi constraint: painful heavy stomach, sour eructations, appetite loss, sweating, anxiety

Preparation

Use: Ostrea Mu Li, the crushed oyster shell, is decocted. For best results with fluids leakage and gastric hyperacidity, it should first be calcined or roasted. This is called **Duan Mu Li** (Mand.) or **Taan Mao Lai** (Cant.).

Dosage: Decoction: 10-30 g

Caution: Contraindicated in high fever without sweating and not to be combined with Ephedra Ma Huang, Cornus Wu Zhu Yu or Asarum Xi Xin.

Notes

The mineral rich shell of the oyster for millenniums has provided Oriental practitioners with a reliable *sedative* remedy adapted to the nerves, heart and sexual organs. Just as the dense shell sinks to the ocean floor, so its heavy minerals are seen to exert a *sinking, calming* effect on the whole system. Yin deficiency conditions involving autonomic nervous imbalance presenting anxiety, hot flushes, sleep loss and spasms were found here to be the best indications.

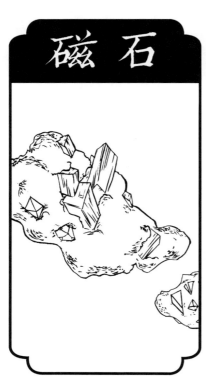

Magnetitum Ci Shi
Magnetite

Geological source: *Magnetitum*
Pharmaceutical name: Magnetitum
Chinese names: Ci Shi, Huo Ci Shi, Xuan Shi (Mand); Chi Sek (Cant)
Other names: Lodestone, Loadstone, Magnetic iron oxide; Jiseki (Jap)
Source: China's northeast coastal provinces, Guangdong
Part used: the mineral

Therapeutic category: mild remedy with minimal chronic toxicity
Constituents: black iron oxide (incl. triferric tetroxide 69%, ferric/ferrous 31%/magnesium/aluminum/silicon oxides), calcium, manganese
Effective qualities: pungent, salty, cold
          calming, sinking, relaxing, restoring
Tropism: cardiovascular, nervous, respiratory systems
          Heart, Kidney, Liver, Lung, Yin Wei channels
          Air body

Actions and Indications

neurocardiac sedative: hypnotic: cardiac hyperfunctioning with palpitations, anxiety; acute neurocardiac syndrome, anxiety states

nervous sedative/relaxant, spasmolytic, anticonvulsant: unrest, insomnia, infantile tremors or fright seizures, dizziness, vertigo, tinnitus; hypocalcemia

respiratory relaxant: chronic asthma, tracheitis

hemogenic: anemia

auditory and optic restorative: poor hearing, deafness; blurred vision

Symptom Pictures

Spirit Instability with **nerve excess:** palpitations, anxiety, restlessness, sleep loss

Liver and Kidney Yin deficiency with **nerve excess (Liver Yang rising):** dizziness, blurred vision, ringing in ears, irritability, flushed face

Lung and Kidney Yang deficiency: chronic wheezing, fatigue

Preparation

Use: The mineral Magnetitum Ci Shi is first prepared by being fired, dipped in vinegar and pulverized. It is then decocted. When decocting, first cook it alone for 20-30 minutes before adding other herbs.
Dosage: Decoction: 10-30 g
Caution: None.

Notes

A cold, *sedative* mineral remedy to both the neural and cardiac functions, Magnetite is most often used in formulas for clearing empty heat and hyperactivity. The remedy's heavy, mineral qualities are traditionally seen as pacifying the Liver's rising Yang energy with their *sinking, downward-moving* energies. Magnetite's *refrigerant* effect is ideal for treating severe Yin–deficient conditions with constrained Qi in the heart, as the symptom pictures indicate. The remedy's built-in *relaxant* action on neuromuscular functions are made use of in peripheral spasms and infantile seizures.

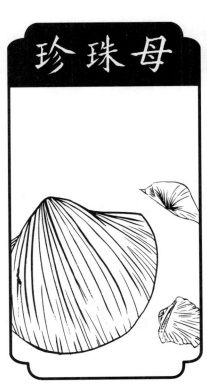

Pteria Zhen Zhu Mu
Mother of Pearl Shell

Zoological source: *Pteria margaritifera* L. or *P. martensii* Dunker (Pteridae) and *Hyriopsis cumingii* Lea and *Cristaria plicata* Leach (Unionidae)
Pharmaceutical name: Concha Pteriae
Chinese names: Zhen Zhu Mu (Mand); Jen Ju Mou (Cant)
Other names: Nacre; Chinju (Jap)
Source: China's coastal provinces
Part used: the shell

Therapeutic category: mild remedy with minimal chronic toxicity
Constituents: calcium carbonate, minerals and trace minerals
Effective qualities: sweet, salty, cold, dry
    calming, sinking, relaxing
Tropism: cardiovascular, nervous
    Heart, Liver, Yin Wei channels
    Air body

Actions and Indications

neurocardiac sedative: hypnotic: cardiac hyperfunctioning with palpitations, anxiety; acute neurocardiac disorder, anxiety states

nervous sedative/relaxant: spasmolytic, anticonvulsant: unrest, tinnitus, spasms, dizziness, insomnia; mania, hysteria, hypocalcemia; seizures

analgesic: headache

vision restorative: night-blindness, bloodshot eyes, cataract, pterygium

Symptom Picture
Spirit Instability with **nerve excess (Liver Yang rising/Floating Yang):** unrest, dizziness, headache, ringing in ears, spasms, sleep loss

Preparation
Use: The shell Pteria Zhen Zhu Mu is powdered and taken directly, or decocted first.
Dosage: Powder and decoction: 10-30 g
Caution: Forbidden in a cold abdomen.

Notes
Relying heavily (no pun intended) on its mineral and trace element content, the maritime remedy Mother of pearl is found in formulas treating excess conditions of the autonomic nervous system affecting the heart. In Chinese medicine these conditions are encapsulated in the traditional symptom pictures Liver Yang Rising or Floating Yang.

Pteria Zhen Zhu
Pearl

Zoological source: *Pteria margaritifera* L. or *P. martensii* Dunker (Pterioidae)
Chinese names: Zhen Zhu (Mand); Jen Ju (Cant)
Category: mild remedy with minimal chronic toxicity
Constituents: calcium/magnesium carbonate 93%, calcium phosphate, ferric oxide, 6 amino acids
Effective qualities: sweet, salty, cold, dry; calming, relaxing, restoring
Tropism: cardiac, nervous, digestive systems; Heart, Liver, Yin Wei channels

Actions: *Hypnotic, depressant, anticonvulsant, antipyretic, vision restorative, vulnerary, amtacid anti-secretory*
Indications: Acute neurocardiac syndrome (Spirit Instability with nerve excess [Liver Yang rising] syndromes) with palpitations, anxiety, fright; anxiety states, agitation, childhood seizures, epilepsy; fevers with thirst in Heart Fire syndromes; blurred vision from pterygium, corneal opacity and other superficial visual obstructions; chronic sores and ulcers (incl. mouth ulcers), throat numbness; gastric hyperacidity, peptic ulcer.
Dosage: Powder and pill: 0.3-1 g. Use Pearl powder topically for skin blemishes and roughness, pimples, blackheads, swollen lymph glands and superficial visual obstructions (prepare eyedrops for these).
Caution: Use cautiously during pregnancy.

Calcitum Han Shui Shi
Calcite

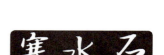

Geological source: *Calcitum* or *Gypsum rubrum*
Chinese names: Han Shui Shi (Mand); Haan Soi Sek (Cant)
Category: mild remedy with minimal chronic toxicity
Constituents: calcium carbonate, magnesium sulfate
Effective qualities: pungent, salty, cold; calming
Tropism: nervous, cardiac systems; Heart, Stomach, Kidney channels

Actions: *Hypnotic, depressant, antipyretic, anti-inflammatory, draining diuretic*
Indications: Irritability, agitation, (esp. from high fever, hypocalcemia); conjunctivitis; vomiting; edema; burns.
Dosage: Decoction: 10-20 g
   Topically Calcite is only used for for scalds and burns.
Caution: Forbidden in cold deficient conditions of the stomach and intestines.

Fluoritum Zi Shi Ying
Purple Fluorite

Geological source: *Fluoritum*
Chinese names: Zi Shi Ying (Mand); Fluor-spar
Category: mild remedy with minimal chronic toxicity
Source: the southern province Guangdong
Constituents: calcium fluorite, silicon dioxide
Effective qualities: sweet, warm; relaxing, solidifying
Tropism: nervous, cardiac, respiratory, reproductive systems; Heart, Liver, Yin Wei channels

ACTIONS: *Hypnotic, depressant, bronchodilator, hemostatic*
INDICATIONS: Neurocardiac syndrome, anxiety states; fright, palpitations, mental stupor with Spirit Instability syndrome; wheezing and coughing with lung Qi constraint; menorrhagia, uterine bleeding, infertility; fatigue.
Dosage: Decoction: 6-16 g. Simmer separately for 30 minutes first, if adding other ingredients.
Caution: None.

Pinus Hu Po
Amber Resin

Botanical source: *Pinus succinifera* Conv. (Pinaceae)
Chinese names: Hu Po, Xue Po (Mand); Fu Pa (Cant)
Source: China's Southwest
Part used: the fossilized underground pine resin
Category: mild remedy with minimal chronic toxicity
Constituents: succoxyabietic/succinoabietinolic/succinosilvic/succinic acids; succinoabietol, succinore-sinol, benzine, resin
Effective qualities: sweet, neutral; calming, relaxing, dissolving
Tropism: nervous, cardiovascular, reproductive systems; Heart, Liver, Bladder, Small Intestine, Yin Wei channels

ACTIONS: *Hypnotic, spasmolytic, anticonvulsant, analgesic, urogenital relaxant/stimulant, hemostatic, detoxicant, detumescent, vulnerary*
INDICATIONS: Neurocardiac syndrome with anxiety, palpitations, forgetfulness, nightmares (Spirit Instability with nerve excess syndrome); anxiety states; infantile and epileptic seizures; dysuria, strangury, oliguria (incl. from urinary stone); amenorrhea, dysmenorrhea with lower abdominal lumps, anuria, scrotal and penile pain and swelling; postpartum pain; sores, menorrhagia, hematuria; skin ulcers, carbuncles; coronary disease.
Dosage: Powder, pill: 1-3 g internally and topically.
Caution: Forbidden in Yin deficiency with empty heat.

Cinnabarum Zhu Sha
Cinnabar

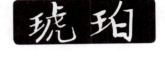

Geological source: *Cinnabarum*
Chinese names: Zhu Sha, Tan Sha (Mand); Ju Sa (Cant)
Source: The mineral ore is mined in the provinces of Yunnan, Guizhou, Hunan and Sichuan.
Category: medium-strength remedy with chronic toxicity
Constituents: red mercuric sulfide c. 99%, phosphates, magnesium and ferric oxide
Effective qualities: sweet, cool; calming
Tropism: cardiovascular, nervous systems; Heart, Yin Wei channels

ACTIONS: *Hypnotic, depressant, spasmolytic, anticonvulsant, anti-inflammatory, expectorant, antivenomous, antiputrefactive, topical antibacterial/antiparasitic/antifungal*
INDICATIONS: Neurocardiac syndrome (Spirit Instability with nerve excess) with insomnia, anxiety, unrest; anxiety states, nightmares, seizures, sore throat, acute bronchitis; topically for boils, furuncles, snakebite, parasitic and fungal skin infections.
Dosage: Powder: 0.3-1 g internally and topically.
Caution: Use Cinnabarum Zhu Sha only under professional supervision! Never to be taken continuously for more than a few days, and never to be heated, to prevent mercury poisoning. Only use internally in full heat conditions.

CARDIOVASCULAR SEDATIVES

➤ NOURISH THE HEART AND CALM THE SPIRIT WITH LIGHT REMEDIES
Neurocardiac sedatives

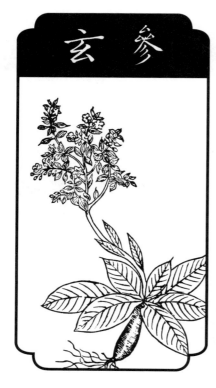

Scrophularia Xuan Shen
Black Figwort Root *

Botanical source: *Scrophularia ningpoensis* Hemsley or *S. buergeriana* Miquel (Scrophulariaceae)
Pharmaceutical name: Radix Scrophulariae ningpoensis
Chinese names: Xuan Shen, Yuan Shen, Hei Shen, Zhong Tai (Mand); Yin Sam, Yan Sam (Cant)
Other names: Ningpo figwort, "Black ginseng"; Gen Jin (Jap)
Habit: Perennial moisture-loving herb from North China's lowlands, Zhejiang and Sichuan; grows in tussocks and thickets, along streams, gullies and other boggy places; autumn sees emerging panicles of dark purple terminal or axillary flowers.
Part used: the root

Therapeutic category: mild remedy with minimal chronic toxicity
Constituents: scrophularin, iridoids, harpagosides (70%), stachyose, essential oil (incl. monoterpenes), alkaloids, fatty acid, phystosterol, asparagine, oleic/stearic/linoleic acids, carotene, dextrose
Effective qualities: sweet, a bit salty and bitter, cold, moist
  calming, sinking, relaxing, restoring, dissolving, softening
Tropism: cardiovascular, nervous, urinary, glandular systems
  Heart, Pericardium, Kidney, Lung, Stomach, Yin Wei channels
  Warmth, Air bodies

ACTIONS AND INDICATIONS

neurocardiac sedative: hypnotic: neurocardiac hyperfunctioning with anxiety, insomnia; stress, neurocardiac syndrome, anxiety states, phobias, sleep disorder, menopausal syndrome
cardiovascular relaxant/restorative, vasodilator, hypotensive: hypertension, hot spells
pituitary-adrenocortical restorative: adrenal cortex deficiency with fatigue, loss of stamina; menopause
anti-inflammatory, antipyretic: acute painful pharyngitis, laryngitis, tonsilitis, gingivitis, lymphadenitis, conjunctivitis; diphtheria, scarlet fever, typhoid
resolvent detoxicant, diuretic: metabolic toxicosis, carbuncles, goiter, erysipelas
lymphatic decongestant, detumescent: lymphadenitis, scrofula
mucogenic: dehydration (esp. of fever or heat exhaustion); dry cough
demulcent laxative: dry hard stool, constipation
diuretic
interferon inducent, antibacterial, antifungal

SYMPTOM PICTURES

heart Yin deficiency with **nerve excess:** anxiety, unrest, palpitations, sleeplessness, irritability
Yin and fluids deficiency with **nerve excess:** hot spells, irritability, thirst, dry mouth, constipation
Blood and Nutritive level heat: sleep loss, irritability, fever

PREPARATION

Use: The root Scrophularia Xuan Shen is decocted or used in tincture form.

Dosage: Decoction: 9-30 g
Tincture: 2-4 ml
Caution: Use cautiously in diarrhea due to digestive deficiency or damp.

NOTES

Because of its *neurocardiac sedative* and systemic *heat-clearing* effects, the sweet, cold natured Black figwort root is classed as a *sedative* more than a *relaxant* remedy. Its main target is the cardiovascular system. The remedy is mainly applied for chronic neurogenic stress conditions of the heart (with or without hypertension), presenting mental and emotional, as well as physical symptoms, dominated by anxiety, insomnia and palpitations. Through deep adrenocortical support, Black figwort replenishes the underlying deficiency (the Kidney/adrenal Yin) usually found in these longstanding conditions that often also present chronic tiredness and hot spells.

Like its cousin the Western figwort, *Scrophularia nodosa*, Black figwort root has significant *anti-inflammatory* and *antipyretic* actions (harpagosides at work). These classically address Yin and fluids-deficient conditions with heat, dehydration and nervous irritation. Like the Western variety, Black figwort is also a *detoxicant, lymphatic decongestant* and *diuretic*—although here their similarities end.

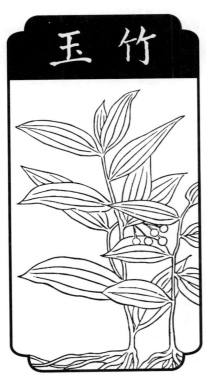

Polygonatum Yu Zhu
Fragrant Solomon's Seal Root

Botanical source: *Polygonatum odoratum* (Miller) Druce var. *pluriflorum* (Miq.) Ohwi or *P. plurifolium* Allioni (Liliaceae)
Pharmaceutical name: Rhizoma Polygonati odorati
Chinese names: Yu Zhu, Wei Shen, Wei Zhui, Nu Wei (Mand); Yak Jok, Yak Chok, Yak Jak (Cant)
Other names: "Jade bamboo"; Gyokuchiku (Jap)
Habit: Perennial herb from China and Japan's temperate mountain regions; grows on hillsides in damp, shady grass thickets and beneath trees and shrubs; much cultivated; small, light green bell-shaped axillary flowers open in summer.
Part used: the rhizome

Therapeutic category: mild remedy with minimal chronic toxicity
Constituents: cardioactive glycosides (incl. convallamarin, convallarin), glycosides quercitol and kaempferol, chelidonic acid, starch, mucilage, vit. A
Effective qualities: sweet, neutral with warming/cooling potential, moist
calming, sinking, relaxing, restoring, stimulating, dissolving
Tropism: cardiovascular, respiratory, digestive, nervous, muscular systems
Heart, Lung, Stomach, Liver, Yin Wei channels

ACTIONS AND INDICATIONS

neurocardiac sedative: hypnotic, spasmolytic: neurocardiac hyperfunctioning with tension, insomnia; neurocardiac syndrome, stress, anxiety states, phobias
cardiovascular relaxant, spasmolytic: spasms (incl. arterial, coronary); spasms and cramps of hands, legs and sinews; heat cramps
cardiovascular stimulant: cardiac deficiency, arrhythmia, congestive heart failure, stroke, hypothermia, angina pectoris, heat exhaustion
antilipemic, resolvent: hyperlipemia, atherosclerosis, cysts
respiratory demulcent restorative, antitussive: dry bronchial conditions with dry cough, scratchy throat

mucogenic, antipyretic: mucosal deficiency, dehydration with dry mouth; low remittent fever, diabetes, heat syndrome
demulcent laxative: dry constipation
diuretic, dermatropic: poor complexion, freckles
interferon inducent

Symptom Pictures

heart Yin deficiency with **nerve excess** and **internal wind:** palpitations, agitation, anxiety, dizziness, spasms and cramps of sinews and limbs

heart Yang deficiency: pale complexion, palpitations, chilliness, mental confusion or depression, dizziness

Yin and fluids deficiency with **nerve excess (Liver Yang rising/Floating Yang):** hot spells, thirst, unrest, sleep loss, palpitations

lung and stomach heat dryness: dry cough, dry throat and mouth, irritability, increased hunger, constipation

Preparation

Use: The root Polygonatum Yu Zhu is decocted or used in tincture form.
Dosage: Decoction: 8-30 g
Tincture: 1-4 ml
Caution: Contraindicated in stomach cold; use cautiously in high blood pressure and tachycardia.

Notes

Fragrant Solomon's seal root from the mountains of North China is emerging as a superlative cardiovascular remedy. With its alkaloid content, this liliaceous remedy is essentially *sedative* and *relaxant* to both nervous and cardiovascular systems. In traditional Chinese energetics it can be said to work on the Yin Wei extra meridian—like the majority of *neurocardiac sedative* remedies in this section. Any Qi constraint and Yin deficient condition entailing nervous, cardiac and coronary stress, and leading to palpitations, unrest and tremors, calls for its *sinking, calming* energies. The botanical also "clears internal wind," reducing arterial and coronary spasms. As Fragrant Solomon's seal contains cardioactive glycosides, it may also be given in heart Yang deficiency patterns seen in heart failure and heat exhaustion, for example.

The more traditional gestalt of Fragrant Solomon's seal root is a remedy that enriches the Yin fluids. As such, it promotes mucosal secretions and moisture in dry respiratory and intestinal conditions (including acute infections) with dry mouth, throat or chest. Like other *respiratory restoratives,* this remedy should be a prime choice when Yin deficiency conditions involve stress, emotional disturbances or spasms of the limbs.

Fragrant Solomon seal's *dissolvent* or *resolvent* effect is seen in its evident success in reducing excessive blood lipids. More traditionally, it has a special reputation for resolving cysts, especially when combined with Rehmannia Shu Di Huang or Rehmannia Sheng Di Huang (Suk Dei, Sang Dei in Cantonese).

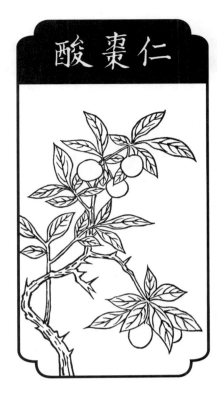

Zizyphus Suan Zao Ren
Sour Jujube Seed

Botanical source: *Zizyphus spinosa* Hu, syn. *Z. jujuba* Miller var. *spinosus* Bunge (Rhamnaceae)
Pharmaceutical name: Semen Zizyphi spinosae
Chinese names: Suan Zao Ren, Jin Zao Ren, Shan Zao (Mand); San Jou Wan, Jou Wan (Cant)
Other names: Wild/Spiny jujube, "Mountain jujube"; Sansonin (Jap)
Habit: Spiny, tall deciduous shrub from subtropical Asia, also found in North China's dry slopes and hills, and by roadsides; etiolated yellow flowers bloom in autumn in axillary cymes.
Part used: the seed

Therapeutic category: mild remedy with minimal chronic toxicity
Constituents: triterpenoid saponins (jujubosides A and B, rutin), flavonoids spinosin and zyvulgarin, triterpenes (betulin, betulininc acid, ceanothic acid, alphitolic acid), ebelinlactone, ferulic and ursolic acids, fatty oil 31%, sterols, vitamin C, manganese
Effective qualities: sweet, a bit sour, cool, moist
  calming, sinking, relaxing, stabilizing
Tropism: cardiovascular, autonomic nervous, digestive systems
  Heart, Spleen, Liver, Gallbladder, Yin Wei channels; Air, Fluid bodies

ACTIONS AND INDICATIONS

neurocardiac sedative: hypnotic, analgesic: neurocardiac hyperfunctioning with anxiety, alarm, insomnia; stress, neurocardiac syndrome, sleep disorder, anxiety states, neurosis, phobias; pain in general
cardiac relaxant, hypotensive: palpitations, hypertension
anticonvulsant: seizures (esp. with hot spells)
anhydrotic: spontaneous sweating, night sweats
demulcent laxative: dry stool or constipation
oxygenator, anti-altitude sickness: high altitude reactions (incl. fatigue, vomiting)
immunostimulant

SYMPTOM PICTURES

heart Yin deficiency with **nerve excess (Liver Yang rising/Floating Yang):** unrest, irritability, anxiety, unrest, apprehension, palpitations, sleep loss, night sweats, hot spells

PREPARATION

Use: The seed Zizyphus Suan Zao Ren is decocted or used in tincture form. When toasted first, it becomes more warming and sedative. The toasted (quick-fried) seed is called Chao Suan Zao Ren (Suk Jou Wan in Cantonese).
Dosage: Decoction: 10-18 g
  Tincture: 2-4 ml
Caution: Use carefully in full heat conditions and severe diarrhea.

NOTES

The kernel of the sour or wild jujube fruit is a sweet, cool *sedative* remedy with a specific tropism for neurocardiac functions. In relieving mental and emotional states such as apprehension, anxiety and worry with hot spells, as well as physiological ones such as high blood pressure, Sour jujube seed adresses Qi constraint and Yin deficient syndromes of the heart.

More recently, Sour jujube has shown tissue oxygenating properties in both laboratory and live experiments (Wan Jia-zhen 1986); it is now often combined with Schisandra Wu Wei Zi (Schisandra berry) for treating high altitude reactions.

Cimicifuga Sheng Ma
Rising Hemp Root *

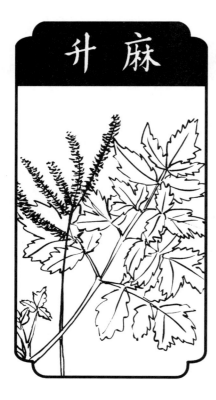

Botanical source: *Cimicifuga foetida* L. or *C. heracleifolia* Komarov or *C. dahurica* (Turcz.) Maximowicz (Ranunculaceae)
Pharmaceutical name: Radix Cimicifugae foetidae
Chinese names: Sheng Ma, Jou Ma (Mand); Jing Ma, Song Ma (Cant)
Other names: Fetid black cohosh, Chinese/Stinking bugbane; Shoma (Jap)
Habit: Pubescent perennial herb from Northeast Asia (including Russia's Far East), growing in mountain valleys and grasslands; in summer, minuscule white flowers appear on terminal panicles.
Part used: the root

Therapeutic category: mild remedy with minimal chronic toxicity
Constituents: triterpenoids (incl. dahurinol, cimicifugenol, cimisinol), glycosides cimicifugenol and methylcimicifugoside, furochromones (cimifugin, visaminol, norvisnagin, visnanin), cinnamic acid derivatives (ferulic/isoferulic/caffeic acids), phenocarboxylic acids, steroids sitostrol and stigmasterol, cimitin, tannins, resin cimicifugin (macrotin)
Effective qualities: sweet, pungent, a bit bitter, cool, dry
  calming, relaxing, restoring, stabilizing
Tropism: nervous, cardiovascular, respiratory, digestive, reproductive systems
  Liver, Heart, Lung, Stomach, Yin Wei channels
  Air, Warmth bodies

ACTIONS AND INDICATIONS
neurocardiac sedative: hypnotic, analgesic: neurocardiac hyperfunctioning with anxiety, irritability; neurocardiac syndrome, stress, anxiety states, sleep disorder; headache, colic, myalgia, neuralgia, dysmenorrhea
cardiac relaxant, hypotensive: palpitations, hypertension
anti-inflammatory, antipyretic, antibacterial, antiviral: laryngitis, gingivitis, stomatitis, tonsilitis, bronchitis, enteritis, erysipelas, typhoid, malaria, shingles (herpes zoster)
diaphoretic, rash-promoting: measles, smallpox, scarlet fever
astringent: chronic diarrhea, canker sores, mouth ulcers
uterine decongestant: menorrhagia, congestive dysmenorrhea
estrogenic
antiprolapse: gastroptosis, uterine prolapse, rectal prolapse, rectocele
antitumoral

Cimicifuga heracleifolia is additionally:
interferon inducent, antioxidant

SYMPTOM PICTURES
heart Yin deficiency with **nerve excess (Liver Yang rising):** anxiety, palpitations, sleep loss, irritability, restlessness

external wind heat: headache, aches and pains, sore throat, irritability, anxiety, feverishness

Preparation

Use: The root Cimicifuga Sheng Ma is either decocted or used in tincture form. Excellent mouthwashes and gargles may be prepared for mouth and throat inflammations.

Dosage: Decoction: 3-6 g
Tincture: 2-3 ml

Caution: Contraindicated in Yin deficiency heat, dyspnea or asthma and in fully erupted eruptions. Doses should not be exceeded, as this herb can cause gastric irritation.

Notes

There are more similarities between this Asian and the American variety of *Cimicifuga* (Black cohosh root) than at first suspected. If these similarities are not clear on first viewing, the reason probably lies in Rising hemp root not being considered an herb of major importance: It has only recently been given some scientific attention and certainly could bear wider usage.

The truth is that both *Cimicifugas* types are *neurocardiac sedatives/relaxants* that are applied to a variety of tense cardiovascular states, such as neurocardiac disorder and hypertension. Both will resolve external/lung wind heat conditions with bronchitis, shingles or eruptive fever. Both types are *antipyretic, anti-inflammatory, analgesic* and *estrogenic*.

Here is a good example of how the bias of health care needs can completely dominate a remedy's therapeutic image, to the exclusion of its intrinsic nature.

In South China and the U.S through export, the species *Serratula chinensis* is the source of the remedy Sheng Ma. This remedy is properly known as **Guang Dong Sheng Ma.** Although similar in most functions to Cimicifuga Sheng Ma, Serratula Sheng Ma does not possess the other remedy's *antiprolapse* effect. Serratula Sheng Ma is used mainly for promoting the eruption of measles (*diaphoertic, dermatropic*) and for reseving fire toxin (*anti-inflammatory, detoxicant, antimicrobial*). Empirically, it also seems to exert a *sedative* action on the nervous system.

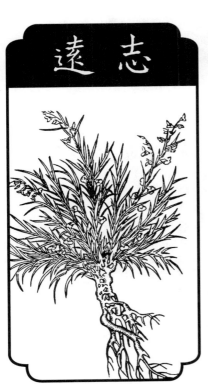

Polygala Yuan Zhi
Thin-Leaf Milkwort Root *

Botanical source: *Polygala tenuifolia* Willdenow (Polygalaceae)
Pharmaceutical name: Radix Polygalae
Chinese names: Yuan Zhi, Xiao Cao, Xi Xie Yuan Zhi (Mand); Yuen Ji, Yan Ji (Cant)
Other names: Chinese seneca root; Onji (Jap)
Habit: Perennial herb from north and northeast China growing on hillsides, roadsides and in meadows; blossoms in summer with racemes of purple axillary or terminal flowers.
Part used: the root

Therapeutic category: mild remedy with minimal chronic toxicity
Constituents: triterpensoid saponins (tenuigenin A and B), resin, glycosides, fatty acids, polygalitol, tenuidine, tenuifolin, onsitin, amyrin, xanthones
Effective qualities: a bit sweet, sour, pungent and salty, neutral, dry
calming, relaxing, raising, stimulating, softening
Tropism: cardiovascular, nervous, respiratory systems
Heart, Lung, Liver, Yin Wei, Du channels
Air, Fluid bodies

ACTIONS AND INDICATIONS

neurocardiac sedative: hypnotic: neurocardiac hyperfunctioning with anxiety, insomnia; neurocardiac syndrome, stress, anxiety states, sleep disorder, agitation, mental disorientation, nightmares, menopausal syndrome
anticonvulsant: seizures (incl. in children)
cardiac relaxant, hypotensive: hypertension
nervous restorative: cerebral deficiency, memory loss, weakness, mental fatigue, stress; Alzheimer's, concussion
mucolytic/stimulant expectorant: chronic bronchitis, bronchiectasis; cough with viscous sputum
uterine stimulant: emmenagogue, oxytocic parturient: delayed, scanty or absent menses, prolonged pregnancy, stalled labor
hepatic stimulant: jaundice, liver congestion, appetite loss
resolvent detoxicant: boils, carbuncles, breast abscess, acute mastitis; toxicosis
interferon inducent, antibacterial: miscellaneous infections

SYMPTOM PICTURES

heart Yin deficiency with **nerve excess (Liver Yang rising):** anxiety, palpitations, apprehension, nervous tension, sleep loss

nerve and brain deficiency: fatigue, absent-mindedness, forgetfulness, mental stupor

lung phlegm damp: coughing, wheezing, difficult expectoration with production of viscous sputum

PREPARATION

Use: The root Polygala Yuan Zhi is either decocted or used in tincture form.
Dosage: Decoction: 4-12 g
Tincture: 2-4 ml
Caution: Do not use in Yin deficiency conditions with empty heat, gastritis, peptic ulcer and during pregnancy.

NOTES

In tense neurocardiac and neurocirculatory conditions, Thin-leaf milkwort root mainly addresses mental and emotional imbalances. Not only are high anxiety and stress states relieved, but mental powers are also increased. This botanical's *restorative* action on the brain enhances such faculties as concentration, understanding and memory—findings that go back to Shamanistic times. Because of this, Thin-leaf milkwort is currently given by some practitioners in Altzheimer's disease. Clearly, however, other conditions involving cerebral insufficiency, such as myalgic encephalitis (ME), will also benefit.

The famed root has also been believed traditionally to promote willpower, "strength of character" (Porter Smith 1871) and dream intensity—reasonable possibilities if we also consider its *stimulant* action on the liver, signaled by the sour taste quality.

Thin-leaf milkwort is one of several milkworts used in herbal medicine worldwide. To resolve lung phlegm damp syndromes, its *stimulant expectorant* action is considered stronger than that of Balloonflower root (Platycodon Jie Geng). Both its constituents and clinical uses vicariously mirror **Seneca root** (*Polygala senega*) in North America and **Bitter milkwort** (*Polygala amara*) in Europe. Bronchial disorders presenting old, hard sputum that is difficult to cough up are those most benefitted by Thin-leaf milkwort. Its pungent, sour effective qualities are evidence here of its energetic action.

If necessary, the Thin-leaf milkwort can be replaced by **Siberian milkwort**, *Polygala sibirica*, known as **Tian Yuan Zhi** (Mand.) or **Tin Yan Ji** (Cant.).

Nardostachys Gan Song
Indian Spikenard Root

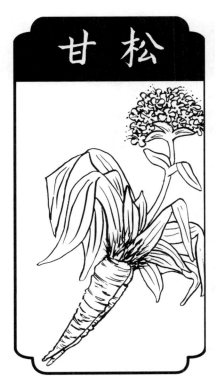

Botanical source: *Nardostachys jatamansi* De Candolle or *N. chinensis* Batalin (Valerianaceae)
Pharmaceutical name: Radix Nardostachis
Chinese names: Gan Song, Ku Mi Zhi, Gan Song Xiang (Mand)
Other names: Indian/Himalayan nard, Syrian nard
Habit: Perennial temperate herb growing in the rocky soil of the Himalayan high alpine meadows; also cultivated; blooms in summer with several small terminal panicles of pale pink flowers.
Part used: the root

Therapeutic category: medium-strength remedy with some chronic toxicity
Constituents: *Nard. jat.*: essential oil 1-2%, (incl. sesquiterpenones [valeranone 5-20%], sesquiterpenes [incl. dihydroazulenes], sesquiterpenols, sesquiterpenals, cineol, methylcarvacylester, jatamansinic acid, coumarins)
Nard. chin.: essential oil (incl. nardosinone, aristolenon, sesquiterpenones [incl. valeranone, nardostachone], acids [incl. aristoleen])
Effective qualities: bitter, pungent, sweet, neutral, dry
    calming, relaxing, stimulating, restoring, raising
Tropism: cardiovascular, nervous, respiratory, digestive, reproductive systems
    Heart, Liver, Spleen, Lung, Yin Wei, Du channels; Air, Fluid bodies

ACTIONS AND INDICATIONS
neurocardiac sedative: hypnotic: neurocardiac hyperfunctioning with palpitations, anxiety, insomnia; stress, neurocardiac syndrome, tachycardia, anxiety states, hysteria, neurosis, sleep disorder, angina pectoris
hypotensive: hypertension, cardiac arrhythmia
anticonvulsant: seizures, epilepsy
stimulant expectorant: bronchitis, cough
intestinal relaxant: spasmolytic, carminative: dyspepsia, intestinal colic, IBS
uterine stimulant, emmenagogue: amenorrhea, dysmenorrhea
nervous restorative: cerebral deficiency with depression
hair restorative: hair loss, early hair graying
venous decongestant: varicose veins, hemorrhoids
antibacterial, antifungal, antimalarial: miscellaneous infections (incl. sore throat; *Staphylococcus*); malaria
detoxicant, dermatropic: ulcers, boils, skin disorders (incl. psoriasis)

SYMPTOM PICTURES
heart Yin deficiency with **nerve excess (Liver Yang rising):** anxiety, palpitations, sleep loss

lung phlegm damp: coughing, expectoration of white sputum, unrest

intestines Qi constraint (Liver/Spleen disharmony): indigestion worse under stress, abdominal pains and lumps

PREPARATION
Use: The root Nardostachys Gan Song is decocted or used in tincture form. Its extracted essential oil is also used for skin care, aromatherapy and perfumery.
Dosage: Decoction: 3-5 g
    Tincture: 1-2 ml
    Essential oil: 1-2 drops in a gel capsule

Caution: Do not use on its own continuously due to its low cumulative toxicity. Avoid in Qi deficiency and Blood heat conditions, as well as during pregnancy.

NOTES

Originating in the Himalayas, Indian spikenard root was brought back to the Central Kingdom during the Tang dynasty by homeward-bound Buddhist monks, who called it Ku Mi Zhi. While its earthy, mossy, spicy scent was used as a perfume and deodorant, in internal medicine the root found favor as a general *sedative, relaxant* and *stimulant*. The result of these opposing actions ultimately gives Indian spikenard a balancing, regulating character useful in both deficiency and excess conditions of cardiac, uterine and digestive functions. The remedy is especially indicated for arrhythmia and tachycardia.

The plant's essential oil content largely contributes to its therapeutic effects, and is also used in extracted form. It too is a very valuable *cardiovascular relaxant* remedy. Sesquiterpenes and several variants thereof make up most of its fractions—but note the presence of *anticoagulant, sedative* and *spasmolytic* coumarins that also support use in coronary disorders.

Indian spikenard root should not be confused with the North American *Aralia* species of spikenards.

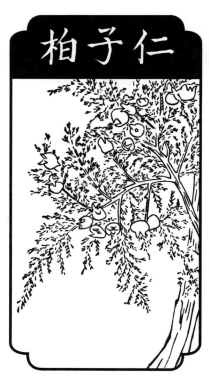

Biota Bai Zi Ren
Oriental Arborvitae Berry

Botanical source: *Biota orientalis* (L.) Endicher, syn. *Thuja orientalis* L. (Cupressaceae)
Pharmaceutical name: Semen Biotae orientalis
Chinese names: Bai Zi Ren, Bo Zi Ren (Mand); Ji Yan, Baak Ji Yan (Cant)
Other names: Hakushinin (Jap)
Habit: Aromatic evergreen tree or pyramidal shrub from Northeast China and Korea, found on dry slopes; also cultivated; flowers in spring with catkins.
Part used: the seed

Therapeutic category: mild remedy with minimal chronic toxicity
Constituents: saponins, benzene, essential oil (incl. monoterpenes [pinene, caryophyllene], thujone), fixed oil, fatty acids, bitter pinipicrin, resin, tannin
Effective qualities: sweet, pungent, neutral, moist
    calming, relaxing, astringing, softening, stabilizing
Tropism: cardiovascular, nervous, glandular systems
    Heart, Liver, Kidney, Large Intestine channels
    Air, Fluid bodies

ACTIONS AND INDICATIONS

neurocardiac sedative: hypnotic: neurocardiac hyperfunctioning with insomnia, anxiety; stress, neurocardiac syndrome, anxiety states, hysteria
analgesic (mild): headache
astringent, anhydrotic: furtive sweating, seminal incontinence
demulcent laxative: constipation due to dryness, postpartum and senile constipation

SYMPTOM PICTURES

heart Yin deficiency with **nerve excess (Liver Yang rising):** anxiety, unrest, palpitations, sleep loss, forgetfulness, headache

intestines dryness: constipation, difficult dry stool, general dryness

PREPARATION
   Use: The seed Biota Bai Zi Ren is decocted or used in tincture form.
   Dosage: Decoction: 8-18 g
            Tincture: 1-4 ml
   Caution: Contraindicated in loose stool or catarrhal conditions in general.

NOTES
   Oriental arborvitae berry finds its main application in worry, apprehension, etc., that results from constrained heart Qi—in Western terms from excess autonomic nervous influence on the heart. The added *intestinal demulcent* action makes this botanical appropriate for postpartum unrest with constipation from loss of blood or fluids.

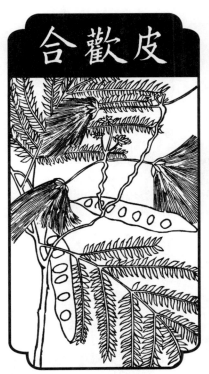

Albizzia He Huan Pi
Mimosa Bark

Botanical source: *Albizzia julibrissin* Durazzini or *A. lebbek* Bentham (Leguminosae)
Pharmaceutical name: Cortex Albizziae
Chinese names: He Huan Pi (Mand); Hap Fun Pei (Cant)
Other names: Silk tree, Pink siris, "Meeting happiness"; Gokanhi (Jap)
Habit: Widespread large deciduous tree from subtropical Asia, esp. Central China's mountain valleys and forest borders; cultivated in North and South China; in summer, pink flowers appear in short terminal racemes of up to three flowers.
Part used: the tree bark

Therapeutic category: mild remedy with minimal chronic toxicity
Constituents: saponins, tannins, albizzin, albiotocin
Effective qualities: sweet, astringent, neutral, dry
              calming, relaxing
Tropism: cardiac, central nervous systems
         Heart, Spleen Lung, Liver, channels; Air, Fluid bodies

ACTIONS AND INDICATIONS
   neurocardiac sedative: hypnotic: neurocardiac hyperfunctioning with anxiety, apprehension, emotional distress; stress, neurocardiac disorder, anxiety states, phobias, paranoid disorders, insomnia, sleep disorder
   resolvent detoxicant: boils, abscesses, carbuncles (incl. lung abscess with vomiting of pus)
   vulnerary, analgesic: traumatic pain and swelling (incl. fractures); chronic pain of joint and muscles of extremities
   oxytocic, diuretic, vermifuge

SYMPTOM PICTURE
   heart Yin deficiency with **nerve excess (Liver Yang rising):** anxiety, irritability, restlessness, sleep loss, chest tightness

PREPARATION
   Use: The bark Albizzia He Huan Pi is decocted or used in tincture form. External applications for trauma are also prepared.
   Dosage: Decoction: 10-16 g
            Tincture: 2-4 ml
   Caution: Do not use without presence of heart Qi constraint.

NOTES

Found from Iran through to Japan, the auspicious mimosa tree blossoms yearly with short-lived but suave-scented pompons of pink flowers. To the delight of Confucianists, it is known in the East to promote family affection and harmony. The remedy He huan pi literally translates as "common happiness bark." Certainly, Mimosa bark has seen long use as a medicinal for chronic emotional or nervous stress affecting the heart on every level: an herb for worry and for broken hearts due to deficient heart Yin. Because of its combination of *sedative* and *vulnerary* actions, Mimosa bark is also a good trauma herb.

Mimosa flower, He Huan Hua (Mand.) or **Hap Fun Fa** (Cant.) is used for the same heart syndrome as the bark. Like the bark, it will relieve abdominal pain and spasmodic lumps due to Liver channel stagnation caused by emotions. Mimosa flower is also said to improve memory and promote sleep.

Nelumbo Lian Zi Xin
Lotus Plumule

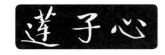

Botanical source: *Nelumbo nucifera* Gaertner (Nymphaeaceae)
Chinese names: Lian Zi Xin, Lian Xin, Lian Zi Rui (Mand); Ling Ji Sam (Cant)
Habit: Perennial water plant mainly cultivated in ponds; flowers in summer with large pink-white terminal capitate flowers.
Part used: the plumule and radicle
Category: mild remedy with minimal chronic toxicity
Constituents: alkaloid neferine
Effective qualities: sweet, neutral; calming, relaxing
Tropism: cardiovascular, nervous systems; Heart chan.

ACTIONS: *Hypnotic, antipyretic, hypotensive, hemostatic*
INDICATIONS: Unrest, irritability, delirium, insomnia, palpitations (esp. during fever and with heart fire syndrome); hypertension, coughing up blood.
Dosage: Infusion and decoction: 2-6 g
  Tincture: 0.5-2 ml
Caution: Contraindicated in abdominal lumps and constipation.

Polygonum Ye Jiao Teng
Flowery Knotweed Stem

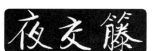

Botanical source: *Polygonum multiflorum* Thunberg (Polygonaceae)
Chinese names: Ye Jiao Teng, Shou Wu Teng (Mand); Ye Gou Tong, Gam Gou Tong (Cant)
Category: mild remedy with minimal chronic toxicity
Constituents: anthraquinones (incl. emodin, chrysophanic acid, chrysophanol, emodin monomethyl ether)
Effective qualities: sweet, a bit bitter and astringent, neutral, dry; calming, astringing, stabilizing
Tropism: cardiac, nervous, muscular, digetive systems; Heart, Liver channels

ACTIONS: *Hypnotic, analgesic, anhydrotic, dermatropic, antifungal*
INDICATIONS: Insomnia, stress, nightmares, anxiety, irritability; neurocardiac syndrome, anxiety states, heart Yin deficiency syndrome; generalized muscular soreness, pain or paresthesia; excessive daytime sweating; pruritus, eczema, urticaria, scabies, fungal infections.
Dosage: Decoction: 10-26 g
  Tincture: 2-4 ml
  Washes and such like are prepared for external use in the skin conditions above.
Caution: Use cautiously with diarrhea present.

Triticum Fu Xiao Mai
Wheat Berry

Botanical source: *Triticum aestivum* L. (Gramineae)
Chinese names: Fu Xiao Mai (Mand); Fau Siu Maak, Fou Siu Maak, Fu Siu Maak (Cant)
Category: mild remedy with minimal chronic toxicity
Constituents: calcium, phosphorus, iron, potassium, niacin, arginine, thiamine, riboflavin
Effective qualities: sweet, a bit salty, cool; calming, restoring
Tropism: cardiovascular, nervous, urinary systems;

ACTIONS: *Hypnotic* (mild), *anhydrotic, urinary restorative*
INDICATIONS: Palpitations, insomnia, irritability, emotional instability, mental confusion; heart Yin deficiency syndrome; excessive daytime or night-time sweating; bedwetting in children (enuresis).
Dosage: Decoction: 10-16 g
Tincture: 2-4 ml
Caution: None.

Glycine Dan Dou Chi
Fermented Soybean

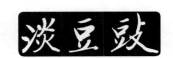

Botanical source: *Glycine max* L. Merr. (Leguminosae)
Chinese names: Dan Dou Chi (Mand); Tam Dou Sai (Cant)
Category: mild remedy with minimal chronic toxicity
Constituents: lipids, sitosterol, stigmasterol, lecithin
Effective qualities: sweet, somewhat bitter, neutral
Tropism: nervous system; Lung, Spleen channels

ACTIONS: *Hypnotic* (mild), *diaphoretic* (mild)
INDICATIONS: Insomnia, unrest and irritability (especially after illness); onset of colds with unrest, especially with Yin deficiency.
Dosage: Decoction: 10-18 g
Tincture: 2-4 ml
Caution: None.

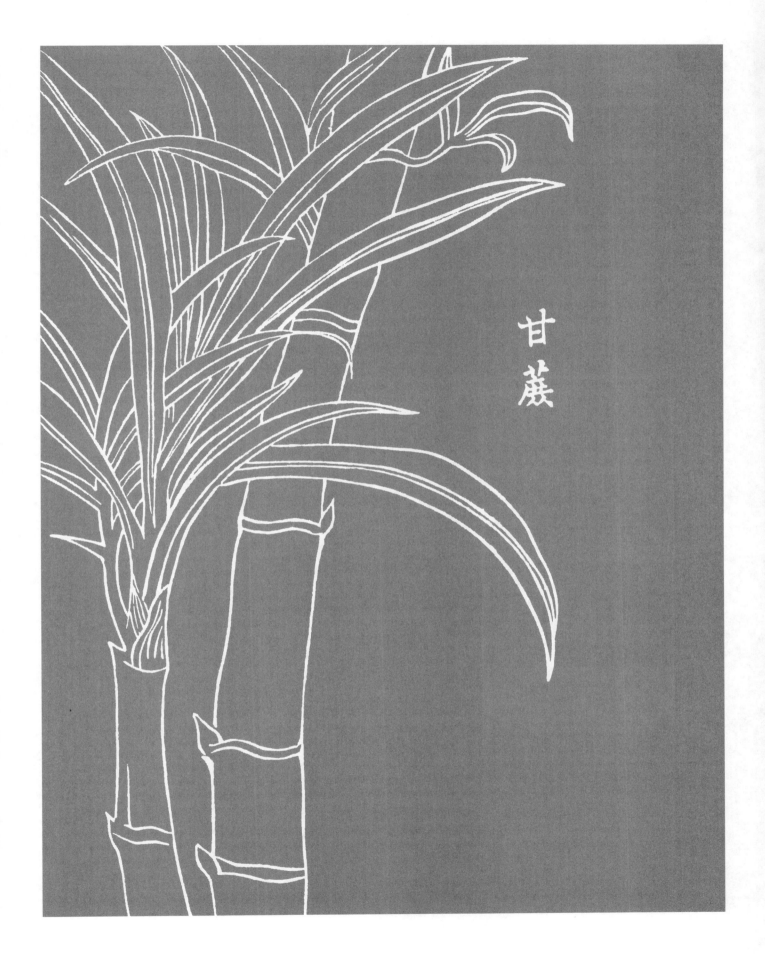

胃腸道用藥

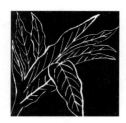

Remedies for the Gastrointestinal System

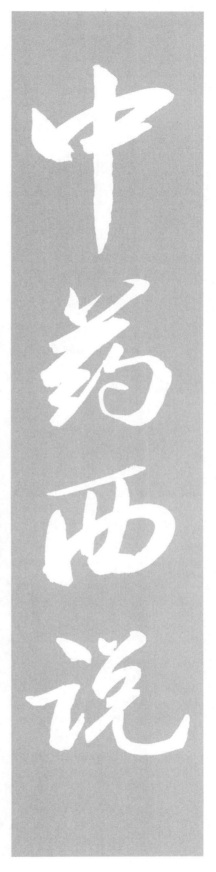

It has not been a secret to Asian practitioners that nutrition and energy largely depend on digestive functions. Similarly, they have long understood that problems involving digestive organs demand specific treatment protocols, and so have developed more herb categories for the gastrointestinal than for any other body system.

From the practical point of view, the sheer number of Chinese remedies addressing digestive disorders necessitates making an initial separation between those for the gastrointestinal system and those for the hepatobiliary system. Next, the numerous gastrointestinal remedies themselves can be clarified and better defined for us in the West by applying the fourfold Western energetic differentiation of herbs according to *restoring, relaxing, stimulating* and *sedating* principles of treatment. This primary differentiation allows us to organize the gastrointestinal remedies into a logical and coherent therapeutic framework, affording a clear and manageable overview of both herb categories and the pathologies they address.

- ***Gastrointestinal restoratives*** treat deficiency conditions of the digestive tract involving either:
  - functional deficiency with poor absorption of nutrients, presenting fatigue.
  - deficiency and dryness with mucosal or fluid deficiency, accompanied by constipation.
  - deficiency and damp with deficient fluid resorption, presenting diarrhea.
- ***Gastrointestinal stimulants*** address deficiency conditions compounded by various factors:
  - deficiency with insufficient digestive secretions, displaying appetite loss and fatigue.
  - deficiency and cold with spasms, presenting abdominal pain.

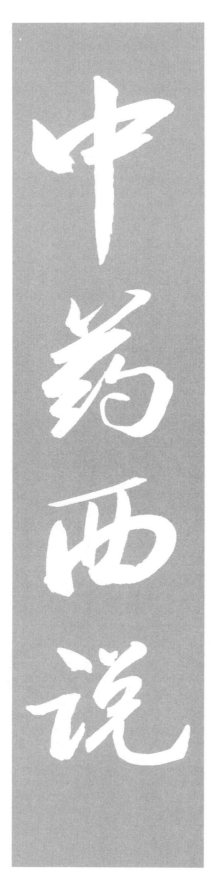

- deficiency and damp with excess mucus, accompanied by abdominal fullness.
- deficiency and food stagnation with digestive enzyme deficiency, presenting abdominal fullness.
- large intestine deficiency with accumulations, accompanied by constipation.

• *Gastrointestinal relaxants* address excess conditions with tension, displaying spasms and abdominal pain.

• *Gastrointestinal sedatives* address excess conditions with acute infection, presenting diarrhea and purulent discharge.

The Gastrointestinal Remedies

Restoratives

Restorative herbs for the digestive tract are separated into three types:

- *sweet digestants* that restore digestive functions, increase nutrient absorption and relieve fatigue.
- *moist demulcents* that moisten the stomach and intestines, relieve mucosal dryness and relieve constipation.
- *dry astringents* that promote astriction and stop diarrhea.

Gastrointestinal restoratives of the first type are dominated by the sweet taste. When taken over a period of time, they regulate and enhance the digestive functions of the stomach, duodenum and small intestine, and gradually build physical strength. Their actions include regulating digestive secretions (including pancreatic enzymes), both locally and through hormonal control. They also gradually regulate the intestinal flora, increase nutrient absorption and may increase small intestine blood cell produc-tion (if Nikishima's theory on hemopoesis is correct [Nikishima 1962]). In addition, these *restoratives* supply actual nutrients to the system, notably amino acids. Because they enhance anabolic processes, they may also be qualified as *anastative nutritives*. Their action is summed up in the phrase "benefit the Spleen and tonify the Qi"—the spleen denoting the sum total of these anabolic gastrointestinal functions.

The subclinical condition or syndrome treated by the *sweet digestants* is **stomach and small intestine Qi deficiency** (in Chinese medicine usually known as **Spleen Qi deficiency).** This condition is defined by a symptom complex that includes loss of appetite, stuffiness in the abdomen, epigastrium or chest, loose stool, diarrhea, belching, fatigue and weight loss. Clearly, these *restoratives* should also be used in formulations for chronic disorders like metabolic acidosis, celiac disease, Crohn's disease, peptic ulcers and ulcerative colitis, as well as for more short-term conditions like enteritis.

Chinese medicine has historically placed particular emphasis on "strengthening the Spleen" (i.e., enhancing digestion and absorption) with these particular *sweet digestants*. Indeed, a whole medical lineage, initiated by Li Dong-yuan, evolved on the basis of this one therapeutic strategy. While in the West digestive herbs are dominated by *bitter digestants,* in Asia they are primarily represented by these *sweet digestants.*

Sweet digestants include widely known and frequently used herbs such as Atractylodes Bai Zhu (White atractylodes root, a type of North Asian thistle), Panax Xi Yang Shen (American ginseng root from northeast North America) as well as the roots of several bellflowers. They invariably contain triterpenoid saponins which may act in a way analogous to adrenocortical and other hormones, thus explaining their systemic *restorative* effect on gastric and intestinal digestive functions.

Because nutrient uptake by the small intestine and liver are so interdependant, it comes as no surprise to see considerable overlap between this type of *gastrointestinal restorative* and *liver restoratives* that enrich liver Yin functions. An herb rich in saponins and amino acids such as Codonopsis Dang Shen (the root of the Downy bellflower, a lovely twining vine from the mountain woods of Northeast China) would comfortably fit either category.

The second type of *gastrointestinal restorative* is *demulcent* and *laxative* because of its moist nature. Dendrobium Shi Hu (Stonebushel herb in the lily family), for example, provides moisture to the stomach, thus relieving conditions of gastric mucosal deficiency. A simple *gastric demulcent,* it treats the syndrome **stomach dryness** while also hydrating the entire system. The symptomatology of **stomach dryness** (also known as **stomach Yin deficiency)** includes indigestion, epigastric discomfort, distension and a sensation of lumps, dry heaving, hunger without appetite and anxious agitation. After the preclinical stage there may appear conditions such as chronic gastritis, diabetes mellitus, neurogenic gastric conditions including peptic ulcers, and the end stage of fevers.

The remaining remedies in this section are specifically *demulcent laxatives,* addressing **intestines dryness** and relieving hard, dry stool and constipation. They are said to "moisten the intestines and unblock the bowels." Two of them are seeds containing large amounts of lipids, accounting for their *lubricant laxative* action. Many fruit kernels, such as those of the apricot, peach, plum and prune, have moist qualities signaling a *demulcent laxative* effect.

The third type of *restorative* to the digestive tract is of a dry, astringent and either neutral or warm quality. The effect of *astringent restoratives* on the gut is astricting and toning, thereby promoting adequate fluid resorption in the colon and relieving diarrhea. In traditional terms they "promote astriction and restrain leakage from the intestines." They are used to speed up the resolution of acute intestinal deficiency conditions, such as colitis (including food poisoning and *Staphylococci* infection),

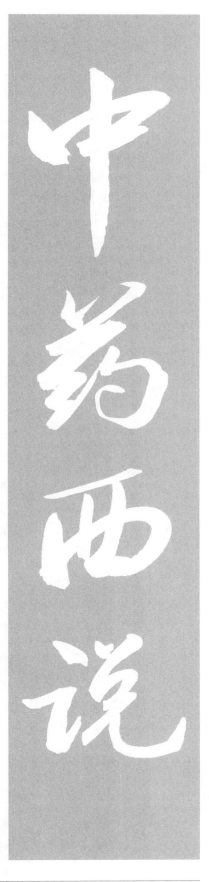

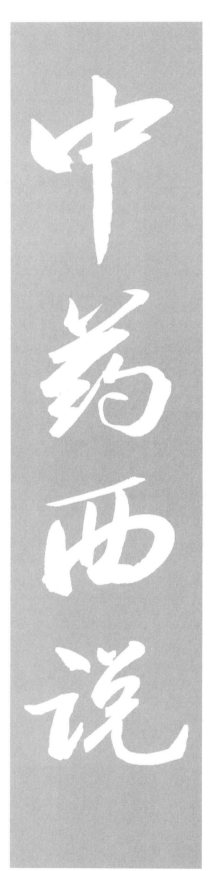

food allergies and antibiotics reactions, as well as chronic disorders such as (gastro)enteritis, dysentery, ulcerative colitis, celiac disease and Crohn's disease. In addition, many of these remedies are secondarily effective in astricting genital discharges such as leucorrhea, spermatorrhea and menorrhagia.

The syndrome **intestines damp cold** aptly sums up the specific symptomatology for *antidiarrheal* remedies. Its key symptoms are loss of appetite, chronic diarrhea with undigested food, abdominal pain, tiredness, mental fatigue and cold extremities. The Chinese syndrome **summer heat,** consisting of the above symptom picture plus fever, is also treated by some of these *astringents*. Because it is prevalent in warmer weather, it suggests catarrhal enteritis caused by food poisoning.

Astringent antidiarrheals include important cosmopolitan remedies like Myrobalan fruit from India (Terminalia He Zi), Opium poppy husk originally from the Middle East (Papaver Ying Su Ke) and Black plum from China (Prunus Wu Mei). Cuttlefish bone (Sepia Hai Piao Xiao) is unique not only because it is an animal remedy also used in homeopathy, but also because it promotes astriction without itself being dry, has an additional *hemostatic* action and is currently much used to reduce gastric hyperacidity and ulcers.

The minerals Red kaolin (Halloysitum Chi Shi Zhi, from Central and East China) and Clay ironstone (Limonitum Yu Liang Shi, from Guangdong in the South) are two highly effective *antidiarrheal* and *hemostatic* remedies in this section.

Stimulants

Because digestion can malfunction in a variety of ways where stimulation is required as a treatment strategy, botanical remedies for these disorders must be chosen according to the specific presenting condition. Consequently, *gastrointestinal stimulants* are divided into five types:
• *bitter, cool digestants* that promote digestion, stimulate secretions and relieve appetite loss and fatigue.
• *pungent, hot, analgesic digestants* that promote digestion, reduce colic and relieve abdominal pain.
• *pungent, warm, dry digestants* that promote digestion, resolve mucus and relieve abdominal fullness.
• *enzymatic digestants* that promote digestion, stimulate enzyme secretions, remove food stagnation and relieve adominal fullness
• *stimulant laxatives* that promote bowel movement and relieve constipation.

The first type of *gastrointestinal stimulant* has a strong, clean bitter taste because of its bitter compounds. Bitterness stimulates gastric, pancreatic, biliary and intestinal secretions, thereby awakening appetite, promoting digestion and ultimately generating strength and lightness. *Bitter digestants* are given for **stomach and intestines Qi stagnation** conditions presenting appetite loss, indigestion, fatigue, infrequent bowel movement and malaise. Acute and chronic gastritis, simple intestinal atony and atonic constipation (inactive colon) also respond well to *bitter digestants.*

A prime example of a currently used Chinese *bitter digestant* is Swertia Dang Yao (Chinese green gentian root). Although the Asian pharmacy, like the Western, has several intensely bitter remedies, the majority are rarely used for this purpose in actual practice; hence, they are found in categories other than this.

Containing generous quantities of essential oils, the second type of *gastrointestinal stimulant* is generally very pungent, hot and dry in character. Its stimulating effect on digestive functions is reflected in the cold, deficient symptom patterns it is prescribed for: **stomach cold** and **intestines cold.** These syndromes correlate in Chinese medicine with a deficiency of Spleen Yang—also known as "the middle"—and in Greek and Ayurvedic systems with weak digestive fire. Indigestion or colic with epigastric or abdominal pain, cold limbs and extremities, nausea, appetite loss, diarrhea and a bright white complexion are the keynotes of both symptom complexes. These symptoms are seen in chronic disorders such as chronic gastritis, chronic enteritis and ulcerative colitis.

Numerous *pungent digestants,* such as the tropical remedies Clove bud (Eugenia Ding Xiang) and Dried ginger root (Zingiber Gan Jiang), are also *relaxant* and *analgesic* by nature (relieving spasm and pain). Their primary function, however, is still stimulation and warming in digestive conditions characterizes by cold and deficiency; they are said to "warm the middle and dispel cold." The same cannot be said of true *intestinal relaxants* that work more systemically through autonomic nervous relaxation.

The third type of *gastrointestinal stimulant* also contains essential oils manifesting pungent, warm and dry qualities. With its *carminative, mucolytic* and *antiseptic* actions, this type effectively resolves dampness due to excessive intestinal mucus and microbial toxins. Overproduction of mucus and microbial toxicosis can create symptoms such as indigestion; loss of appetite; heaviness in the abdomen and body; lethargy, abdominal distension and gurgling; nausea; a sticky, sweet taste in the mouth; a feeling of tightness in the head; and alternating constipation and diarrhea with reduced assimilation. These symptoms typify the syndrome **intestines mucous damp** (classically known as **Spleen damp)** often found along with conditions such as intestinal dysbiosis, gastritis, enteritis and diverticulitis.

Ubiquitous in Chinese herbal formulas are Atractylodes Cang Zhu (Black atractylodes root, a thistle type from China's northeast mountains) and Agastache Huo Xiang (Rugose giant hyssop herb from subtropical East Asia), both *dry digestants* that "transform Spleen damp" with their aromatic quality.

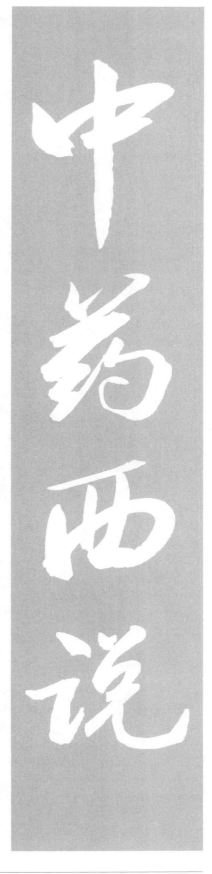

GASTROINTESTINAL SYSTEM

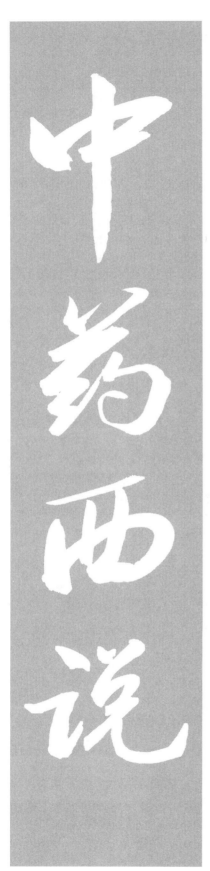

The fourth type of *gastrointestinal stimulant* is sweet and/or pungent by nature. It provides enzymes that facilitate digestion and stimulate enzyme release in the pancreas. *Enzymatic digestants* treat enzymatic insufficiency and imbalance of the intestinal microflora, also known as intestinal dysbiosis. An imbalanced gut flora can cause intestinal fermentation, microbial toxicosis, candidiasis and many other conditions as it progresses. The basis of these conditions is aptly expressed in the symptom picture **food stagnation,** the keynote symptoms of which are indigestion, regurgitation and epigastric and abdominal bloating, fullness and dull pain.

Enzymatic digestants that "dissolve food stagnation and transform accumulation" include fermented sprouting grains such as barley and rice (Hordeum Mai Ya and Oryza Gu Ya), and the enzyme-rich gizzard lining of chicken (Gallus Ji Nei Jin).

The fifth type of *gastrointestinal stimulant* works by irritating the colon wall, thereby causing bowel movement. Its action is described as a *stimulant laxative* or "downward draining" one and is not determined by any single biochemical constituent. Because of its habit-forming effect, this type of *laxative* is for occasional use in acute recalcitrant constipation rather than for regular use. This holds true whether *stimulant laxatives* are used singly or as part of a formula. The most commonly used *laxative* of this type, in both Oriental and Western herbal medicine, is Senna Fan Xie Ye, otherwise known as Senna leaf.

Relaxants
When stress and nervous and emotional tension affect digestion over a long period of time, the resultant syndrome is called **intestines Qi constraint.** Its keynote symptoms are abdominal pain or colic, nausea, vomiting, appetite loss, irregular bowel movement and variable consistency of the stool. This symptom complex may be subclinical and may occur in other conditions, including those unrelated to stress. Instances of these are irritable bowel syndrome (mucous colitis), spastic colon (intestinal colic), diverticulitis, colitis and enteritis.

Because *gastrointestinal relaxants* exert a *relaxant* action on the smooth muscles of the digestive tract, relieving pain and spasm, they are also called *intestinal analgesics* and *spasmolytics.* In Chinese terms they "circulate the Qi in the middle and release constraint." On the whole they posess pungent, bitter and warm qualities, and their dominating constituents are essential oils and glycosides. Magnolia Hou Po (the bark of several species of large magnolia trees from Central China) and Lindera Wu Yao (the root of a shrub from montane Central and South China, and Taiwan) are among the most commonly used *relaxants* in this section. Because they operate by relaxing autonomic nervous functions, the *intestinal spasmolytics* also relax other smooth muscles, such as the uterus and bronchi.

It should be emphasized that the sources of abdominal pain are many. Although these *intestinal spasmolytics* may help with pain relief, they may not treat the source of a disorder in the face of insufficient diagnosis.

Sedatives

Gastrointestinal sedatives are applied for acute inflammatory, infective and diarrheal conditions, as summed up by the vitalistic symptom pattern **intestines damp heat.** The symptomatology of this syndrome includes abdominal pain, urgent burning stool, chronically loose fetid stool (usually with blood and pus), fever and thirst. It clearly denotes such conditions as acute gastroenteritis, bacillary and amoebic dysentery, Crohn's disease, acute ulcerative colitis and enterocolitis.

Remedies in this section are bitter, astringent and cold in character, and have strong *anti-infective, antiseptic* and *anti-inflammatory* actions. They are said in Oriental medicine to "clear damp heat from the large intestine." Only six botanicals of this type are presented in this section because other remedies used for acute intestinal infections generally treat a whole variety of infections. These others therefore appear in the section of remedies for infection and toxicosis.

Classic *gastrointestinal sedatives* include Pulsatilla Bai Tou Weng (Asian pasqueflower root from the foothills of Inner Mongolia and North China), Portulacca Ma Chi Xian (the common Purslane herb) and Fraxinus Chin Pi (Korean ash bark from Northeast Asia). Then there are less well known, yet equally effective remedies such as Pteris Feng Wei Cao (Phoenix-tail fern from the Hong Kong territories and Taiwan).

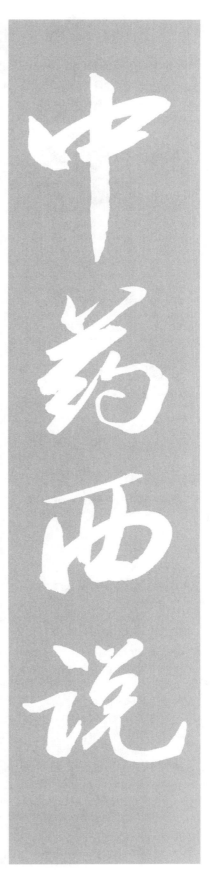

Gastrointestinal Restoratives

REMEDIES TO RESTORE DIGESTION, PROMOTE ABSORPTION AND RELIEVE FATIGUE

➧ BENEFIT THE SPLEEN AND TONIFY THE QI

Sweet digestants, anastative nutritives

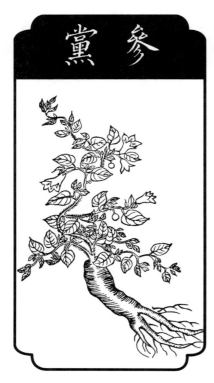

Codonopsis Dang Shen
Downy Bellflower Root *

Botanical source: *Codonopsis pilosula* (Franchet) Nannfeldt or *C. nervosa* (Chipp.) Nannfeldt or *C. tangshen* Oliver (Campanulaceae)
Pharmaceutical name: Radix Codonopsis
Chinese names: Dang Shen, Fang Dang (Shen), Shan Dang Shen, Tai Dang Shen (Mand); Fong Dong Sam (Cant)
Other names: Shan Dang bellflower, "Shan Dang ginseng"; Tojin (Jap)
Habit: Northeast Asian twining perennial vine growing in thickets, in forest perimeters, mountain woods and gullies; in late summer, bell-shaped, pale viridian solitary axillary/terminal flowers with violet streaks appear.
Part used: the root

Therapeutic category: mild remedy with minimal chronic toxicity
Constituents: saponins (incl. codonopsine, codonopsinine), alkaloids (traces), carbohydrates, proteins, mucilage, resin, inulin, saccharides and polysaccharides, tenshenoside I, glucose, taraxeryl acetate, furaldehyde, friedelin, taraxerol, stigmasterol, choline, 17 amino acids 3%, trace elements (incl. iron, manganese, zinc), vitamins B1, B2
Effective qualities: sweet, neutral, moist
    restoring, nourishing, thickening, stabilizing
Tropism: digestive, respiratory, cardiovascular, immune systems
    Spleen, Lung channels; Fluid, Air bodies

ACTIONS AND INDICATIONS

gastrointestinal restorative: sweet digestant: digestive deficiency with poor absorption; malnutrition, malabsorption syndrome, metabolic acidos
anastative nutritive, hemogenic: metabolic/nutritive deficiencies; anemia, anorexia, chlorosis, leukemia, debility
liver restorative: low glycogen reserve, infection proneness, toxicosis, asthenia, chronic nephritis, eczema
gastrointestinal demulcent, anti-inflammatory: chronic enteritis
antacid antisecretory: acid dyspepsia from hyperchlorhydria, gastric ulcer
respiratory restorative: shallow breathing, dyspnea, chronic cough, weak voice
mucogenic: dehydration, thirst (incl. in diabetes)
antiprolapse: rectal and uterine prolapse
hypotensive: high blood pressure
immune enhancer/stimulant, leokocytogenic, phagocyte stimulant: immune deficiency conditions with freqent or chronic infections; leukopenia
radiation protective: radiation damage
interferon inducent, antitumoral: cancer (incl. breast)

SYMPTOM PICTURES

stomach and small intestine Qi deficiency (Spleen Qi deficiency): fatigue, weakness, no appetite, underweight

liver Yin and Blood deficiency: fatigue (esp. evenings), thirst, moodiness, weight loss, frequent infections

Blood deficiency: dizziness, palpitations, tiredness, weakness, thirst, pale complexion

PREPARATION

Use: The root Codonopsis Dang Shen is decocted or used in tincture form.

Dosage: Decoction: 6-14 g
Tincture: 1-4 ml

Caution: None.

NOTES

This mainstay of many a tonifying herb formula was originally called Shan Dang Ren Shen, meaning the ginseng from Shan Dang, the ancient name of the town Lujou in Shaanxi. Although not actually a member of the *Panax* family, the Downy bellflower was considered one of the five *shen,* or ginsengs, with a bias for the Spleen (mainly digestive functions).

This prime sweet, moist-natured *digestive restorative* from the bonnet bellflower family addresses both functional and nutritional digestive deficiencies. However, Downy bellflower root is also a *nutritive blood* and *liver builder* in every sense. The saponins have been shown to increase hemoglobin and erythrocyte levels. The root's content in simple and complex sugars and amino acids (like that of Rehmannia and Wolfberry) is also evidence of its efficacy in anabolic deficiencies. These saccharides also play out *anti-ulcer* and *immunostimulant* activities, which operate by increasing reticuloendothelial phagocytosis.

Tradition has it that Downy bellflower root beautifies and freshens the skin; eczema might well benefit from this valuable remedy.

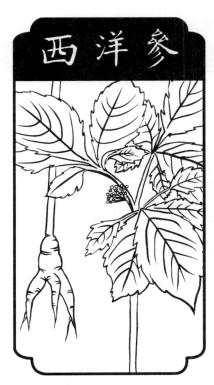

Panax Xi Yang Shen
American Ginseng Root

Botanical source: *Panax quinquefolius* L. (Araliaceae)
Pharmaceutical name: Radix Panacis quinquefolii
Chinese names: Xi Yang Shen, Hua Qi Shen, Xi Shen, Yang Shen (Mand); Sei Yang Sam (Cant)
Other names: Five fingers, Sang, Manroot, Five-leaf ginseng, "Western sea ginseng"; Siyojin (Jap)
Habit: Perennial herb from Northeast North America; likes cool, shady wooded slopes with rich, moist, rocky soil; also cultivated in China; blooms in July with small, pale yellow flowers on a single terminal umbel.
Part used: the root

Therapeutic category: mild remedy with minimal chronic toxicity
Constituents: saponin glycosides ginsenoside and panaxoside c. 5-7%, polysaccharides, essential oil 3% (incl. farnesene, hexadecane, gurjunene), camphoraceous substance, resin, arabinose, mucilage, starch, glucose, saccharides, panaxin, panacic acid, panaquilin, panacene, ginsenin, sapogenin, beta-sitosterol, 18 amino acids, organic acids, traces of trace minerals (incl. copper, zinc, manganese, selenium, iodine)
Effective qualities: a bit sweet and bitter, cool, moist
restoring, raising, relaxing, nourishing
Tropism: digestive, nervous, respiratory, endocrine, immune systems
Stomach, Spleen, Lung, Kidney, Chong, Du channels

ACTIONS AND INDICATIONS

gastrointestinal restorative: sweet digestant: digestive deficiency with poor absorption; malnutrition, metabolic acidosis, malabsorption syndrome, anorexia

anastative nutritive, liver restorative: nutritive and metabolic deficiencies with fatigue, low stamina, frequent infections, weight loss, debility, anemia

central nervous trophorestorative: cerebral deficiency, chronic fatigue, depression, poor concentration and memory, nervous exhaustion, insomnia; convalescence, neurasthenia, cerebral ischemia

pituitary-adrenal restorative: low stamina and endurance, low stress tolerance; menopause, convalescence

pituitary-gonadal restorative, estrogenic: estrogen insufficiency conditions

immune enhancer, adaptogenic: low resistance, debility, low stamina and vitality

demulcent respiratory restorative: shallow breathing, chronic or dry cough, hoarseness, voice loss, hemoptysis; lung TB in initial stage

nervous relaxant/sedative: unrest, tension; insomnia, neurosis, muscular tension, stress

antipyretic: remittent low-grade fevers

SYMPTOM PICTURES

stomach and small intestine Qi deficiency (Spleen Qi deficiency): chronic weakness, fatigue, poor appetite, loose stool, weight loss

liver Yin deficiency: poor stamina, evening tiredness, infection proneness, underweight

nerve and brain deficiency: mental dullness, absent-mindedness, depression, nervous behavior, poor sleep

lung Qi deficiency: shallow or difficult breathing, fatigue, deep cough

lung Yin deficiency: dry cough, voice loss, low-grade fever, coughing up blood

PREPARATION

Use: The root Panax Xi Yang Shen is decocted or used in tincture form.

Dosage: Decoction: 3-10 g
Tincture: 1-4 ml

Caution: Forbidden in indigestion from intestines damp cold, and in high fever.

NOTES

In 1716, this valuable member of the ginseng family was discovered north of Montreal, Canada by the Jesuit missionary, Francois Lafitau. It was introduced to China shortly after that date by Lafitau's confrere, Father Pierre Jartoux. Since then, the Chinese have rightly compared the therapeutic value of this root to that of Asian ginseng, supreme panacea of restorative remedies.

American ginseng is difficult to classify because of the wide spectrum of its effects. It has been valued in both North America and Asia mainly as a *gastrointestinal restorative*. Interestingly, both the original users of this medicinal—which include such Native American tribes as the Seneca, Cherokee, Menominee, Seminole and Penobscots—and Chinese medical herbalists also came to value it as a systemic *restorative*. These discoveries were made quite independently.

American ginseng root is a significant remedy for functional states of metabolic deficiency involving the nervous, endocrine, immune and digestive systems. In terms of channel energetics it can be said to tonify Chong Mai and Du Mai as it brings Blood and Jing to the brain, thereby treating a cluster of endocrine deficiencies that may variously present insomnia, memory loss, physical and mental fatigue, depression, weight loss and a propensity to infection. With its unusual cool and moist qualities, this root is also called for in Yin deficiency conditions, both respiratory and systemic. The remedy is a prime *restorative* to the adrenal cortex, after all.

Far from proving inferior to its Asian cousin, American ginseng root has, in fact, turned out to be more widely applicable for Western conditions than the former. It is more readily acceptable to the Western constitution, especially for the stress-related, adrenal deficient conditions that generate empty heat, so endemic in the West.

Atractylodes Bai Zhu
White Atractylodes Root

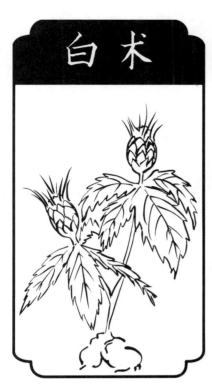

Botanical source: *Atractylodes macrocephala* Koidzumi (Compositae)
Pharmaceutical name: Rhizoma Atractylodis macrocephalae
Chinese names: Bai Zhu, Bai Shu, Yu Zhu, Dong Zhu (Mand); Paak Sat (Cant)
Other names: Large-headed atractylodes, "White Shu"; Byakujutsu (Jap)
Habit: Perennial north Asian herb found in mountain valleys, especially Zhejiang; also cultivated; blooms in autumn with terminal magenta corolla.
Part used: the rhizome

Therapeutic category: mild remedy with minimal chronic toxicity
Constituents: essential oil 1.5% (incl. atractylol, atractylone, humulene, elemol, cucrcumene, palmitic acid, eudesmol, butenolide A), sesquiterpenes (incl. atractylone, hinesol), furfurol, crystals juniper camphor and atractylolide, atractylentriol and methylbutyryl derivatives, vitamin A
Effective qualities: sweet, bitter, a bit pungent and astringent, warm, dry
  restoring, stimulating, decongesting, relaxing
Tropism: digestive, hepatic, urinary, glandular systems
  Spleen, Stomach channels
  Fluid, Air bodies

ACTIONS AND INDICATIONS

gastrointestinal restorative: sweet digestant, anastative: digestive deficiency with poor absorption; malnutrition, malabsorption syndrome, anorexia, metabolic acidosis
digestive stimulant, choleretic, carminative: gastrointestinal and biliary dyspepsia; gastroenteritis
liver restorative: low stamina, weakness, weight loss; hypoglycemia
hypoglycemiant
draining diuretic: edema (incl. during pregnancy)
diuretic detoxicant: dysuria, polyuria; metabolic toxicosis with eczema, rheumatism
antitumoral resolvent: tumors of cervix, uterus, breast, stomach
immunostimulant, phagocyte/lymphocyte stimulant: infections in general
bronchial stimulant: bronchitis, cough
astringent, anhydrotic: chronic diarrhea, copious sweating
fetal relaxant: fetal unrest

SYMPTOM PICTURES

stomach and small intestine Qi deficiency (Spleen Qi deficiency): appetite loss, fatigue, weakness, indigestion

intestines mucous damp (Spleen damp): abdominal distension and gurgling, heaviness of body, head pressure

liver Yin and Yang deficiency: fatigue, low stamina, poor appetite, feeling of general congestion, weight loss

liver fluid congestion: generalized water retention, fatigue, headache, scanty urination, rough skin

PREPARATION

Use: The root Atractylodes Bai Zhu is decocted or used in tincture form.
Dosage: Decoction: 3-10 g
  Tincture: 1-4 ml
Caution: Forbidden in Yin deficiency conditions with deficiency heat signs.

NOTES

In classical Chinese medicine, both White and Black atractylodes types are used as *digestive* and *urinary stimulant* remedies, and in that sense are fairly interchangeable. White atractylodes root, however, is said to be additionally a *Spleen Qi tonic*, i.e., an all-round *metabolic restorative* that increases nutrition, generates flesh, enhances energy production and regulates fluid transformation. The remedy's very well-balanced taste qualities—sweet and bitter, with slight spiciness and astringency—are signs of its *restorative, normalizing* effects on both gastrointestinal and liver functions. In one gesture White atractylodes root increases intestinal absorption, hepatic assimilation, toxin neutralization and nutrient dispatch.

If required, the equally aromatic **Elecampane root,** *Inula helenium* (another composite), could be used as a good general therapeutic equivalent to White atractylodes root for the majority of its functions.

Dioscorea Shan Yao
Mountain Yam Root

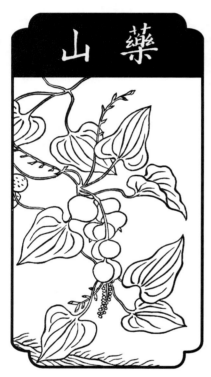

Botanical source: *Dioscorea opposita* Thunberg or *D. batatas* Decaisne (Dioscoreaceae)
Pharmaceutical name: Radix Dioscoreae oppositae
Chinese names: Shan Yao, Shu Yu, Wai San, Huai Shan (Yao) (Mand); Wai San (Cant)
Other names: Cinnamon vine, "Mountain medicine"; Sanyaku (Jap)
Habit: Perennial herbaceous vine from East China, growing on sunny mountain valley hillsides; also cultivated; lavender-colored flower spike blooms in summer.
Part used: the root

Therapeutic category: mild remedy with minimal chronic toxicity
Constituents: saponins, choline, abscisin, bitamin, mannan, phytic acid, allantoin, amino acids arginine, leucine, tyrosine 4%; glutamic and aspartic acids, diosginin, phenols (incl. batatasin), chlorogenic acid, mucilage, vitamin C, trace elements (incl. iron, zinc, chromium, copper), calcium, amylase, glutamine, starch
Effective qualities: sweet, bland, neutral
  restoring, astringing, solidifying, nourishing
Tropism: digestive, hepatic, respiratory, urogenital systems
  Spleen, Lung, Kidney channels
  Fluid body

ACTIONS AND INDICATIONS

gastrointestinal restorative: sweet digestant: digestive deficiency with poor absorption, debility; malabsorption syndrome
anastative nutritive: nutritive and metabolic deficiencies; anemia, malnutrition, convalescence
antidiarrheal: chronic diarrhea; chronic enteritis
respiratory restorative: chronic cough, thirst, shallow breathing, wheezing
urogenital astringent, mucostatic: incontinence with pollakiuria, chronic leucorrhea, spermatorrhea
astringent (topically): boils, incipient abscesses, carbuncles
hypoglycemiant: diabetes mellitus
interferon inducent

Symptom Pictures

stomach and small intestine Qi deficiency (Spleen Qi deficiency): appetite loss, fatigue, exhaustion, weight loss, loose stool

lung Qi deficiency: fatigue, chronic dry cough with thin watery sputum, shallow breathing

genitourinary damp cold: frequent urination, seminal discharges, white vaginal discharges

Preparation

Use: The root Dioscorea Shan Yao is decocted or used in tincture form.

Dosage: Decoction: 10-30 g
Tincture: 2-4 ml

Caution: Contraindicated in full heat conditions and intestinal mucous damp.

Notes

Traditionally classified as a *Qi tonic* because of its tonifying action on both digestive and respiratory functions, this "mountain medicine" is somewhat different from other yam varieties used in herbal medicine (including the Mexican wild yam root). Mountain yam root is essentially *restorative* and *regulative* of processes in the digestive tract. High in amino acids that enhance nutrition and saponins that increase intestinal nutrient assimilation, the sweet root addresses deficiency conditions that display the keynote symptoms of chronic loose stool, weight loss and fatigue. Mountain yam is clearly as contemporary a remedy today in the West as it was in pre-industrial China.

This botanical's *astringent restorative* effect on the urogenital system is similar to that of Dioscorea Bi Xie (Long yam root). Damp cold (mucous damp) conditions such as chronic clear vaginal discharges and frequent urination are treated as Mountain yam tones the mucosa through its *anticatarrhal (mucostatic)* action. However, unlike Long yam which is a *metabolic detoxicant,* Mountain yam is purely a *metabolic restorative:* It should be considered in formulas addressing the long-term types of deficiencies outlined above.

Pseudostellaria Tai Zi Shen
Prince Ginseng Root *

Botanical source: *Pseudostellaria heterophylla* (Miq.) Pax ex Pax et Hoffmann (Caryophyllaceae)
Chinese names: Tai Zi Shen, Hai Er Shen (Mand); Yi Sam (Cant)
Habit: Perennial herb from shady, cool, damp forested mountain slopes and hillsides with loose, sandy fertile soil; small white lanceolate flowers open in late spring.
Category: mild remedy with minimal chronic toxicity
Constituents: saponins, fructose, starch
Effective qualities: sweet, neutral, moist; restoring
Tropism: digestive, respiratory, glandular systems; Spleen, Lung, Heart channels

Actions: *Sweet digestant, anastative, demulcent, mucolytic, expectorant, secretory*

Indications: Digestive deficiency with fatigue; stomach and small intestine Qi deficiency (Spleen Qi deficiency) syndrome; poor absorption, malnutrition; weak lungs, fatigue, dry cough, difficult expectoration with scanty sputum; dehydration, thirst (esp. during or after fevers).

Dosage: Decoction: 10-30 g
Tincture: 2-5 ml

Caution: None.

Notes: Like all others in this section, Prince ginseng root is a sweet and moist-natured remedy traditionally classed as a *Qi tonic*. As it builds up the small intestines' assimilatory processes, appetite, energy and weight improve. The root's good *secretory* action relieve thirst of any type, including that caused by dryness in the lungs.

Campanumoea Tu Dang Shen
Java Bellflower Root

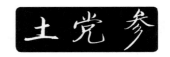

Botanical source: *Campanumoea javanica* Blume (Campanulaceae)

Chinese names: Tu Dang Shen, Man Jie Geng (Mand)

NOTE: This remedy has identical nature, functions and uses to Codonopsis Dang Shen, Downy bellflower root (p. 258). Java bellflower root is additionally employed for insufficient breast milk in nursing mothers.

Dosage: Decoction: 15-30 g
Tincture: 2-5 ml

Codonopsis Yang Ju
Goat's-Tit Bellflower Root

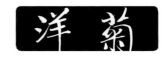

Botanical source: *Codonopsis lanceolata* Bentham and Hooker (Campanulaceae)

Chinese names: Yang Ju, Shan Hai Luo (Mand); Yang Guk (Cant)

NOTES: This remedy has similar effective qualities, tropism, functions and uses as Codonopsis Dang Shen (p. 258). Goat's-tit bellflower root is in addition *detoxicant, detumescent, emmenagogue* and *galactagogue,* being used for acute abscesses (incl. lung abscess and mastitis), acute boils, lymph gland swelling, amenorrhea and insufficient breast milk.

Oryza Jing Mi
Rice Grain

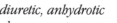

Botanical source: *Oryza sativa* L. (Gramineae)
Chinese names: Jing Mi (Mand); Ging Muk (Cant)
Category: mild remedy with minimal chronic toxicity
Constituents: starch, lipids

Effective qualities: sweet, neutral; restoring, nourishing, decongesting
Tropism: digestive, urinary systems; Spleen, Heart channels

ACTIONS: *Nutritive, sweet digestant, antidiarrheal, draining diuretic, anhydrotic*
INDICATIONS: Appetite loss, diarrhea, dyspepsia; oliguria, edema; spontaneous sweating and thirst from Yin deficiency; hepatoma with ascites.
Dosage: Decoction: 10-30 g
Tincture: 2-5 ml
Caution: None.

Hordeum Yi Tang
Barley Malt Sugar

Botanical source: *Hordeum vulgare* L. (Gramineae)
Chinese names: Yi Tang, Jiao Yi (Mand); Yi Tang (Cant)
Category: mild remedy with minimal chronic toxicity
Constituents: saccharides (maltose), trace minerals, albumin
Effective qualities: sweet, somewhat warm; restoring, nourishing, calming
Tropism: digestive, respiratory systems; Stomach, Spleen, Lung channels

ACTIONS: *Sweet digestant, nutritive, analgesic, demulcent, antitussive*
INDICATIONS: Dyspepsia and poor absorption from deficiency cold; chronic abdominal pain (esp. with excesss saliva), constipation; dry cough; thirst, sore throat; malaise.
Dosage: Decoction: 30-40 g
Tincture: 2-4 ml
Caution: Forbidden in internal damp heat and vomiting.
NOTES: Maltose is another name for this remedy.

Changium Ming Dang Shen
Bright Changium Root

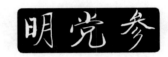

Botanical source: *Changium smyrnioides* Wolff, syn. *Conopodium smyrnoides* (Umbelliferae)
Chinese names: Ming Dang Shen (Mand); Ming Dong Sam (Cant)

NOTES: This remedy is identical in nature, functions and uses to Codonopsis Dang Shen, Downy bellflower root (p.   ). It has additional *antitussive, mucolytic expectorant, antiemetic* and *detoxicant* actions used for coughing with hard sputum, vomiting and boils.

REMEDIES TO MOISTEN THE INTESTINES AND RELIEVE DRYNESS AND CONSTIPATION
➢ MOISTEN THE INTESTINES AND UNBLOCK THE BOWELS
Gastric and intestinal demulcents, demulcent laxatives

Dendrobium Shi Hu
Stonebushel Stem *

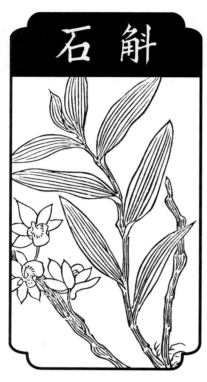

Botanical source: *Dendrobium nobile* Lindley or *D. linawianum* Reichenbach f. or *D. officinale* K. Kimura et Migo and spp. (Orchidaceae)
Pharmaceutical name: Herba Dendrobii
Chinese names: Shi Hu, Huang Tsao, Diao Lan Hua, Xiang Huan Chai, Chuan Shi Hu, Jin Shi Hu (Mand); Sek Hap (Cant)
Other names: Noble orchid; Sekkoku (Jap)
Habit: Perennial evergreen epiphytic alpine herb from the Himalayas, Burma, Taiwan and mid and southwest China; grows in woods on tree trunks and rocky cliffs; racemes of small cream, magenta and lilac flowers bloom in summer.
Part used: the herb or stem

Therapeutic category: mild remedy with minimal chronic toxicity
Constituents: alkaloids (dendrobine, dendranime, nobilonine, dendroxine, dendrin, hydroxydendroxine), polysaccharides, mucilage, starch
Effective qualities: sweet, bland, a bit salty, cool, moist
  restoring, thickening, calming
Tropism: digestive, respiratory systems
  Stomach, Lung, Kidney channels
  Fluid, Warmth bodies

ACTIONS AND INDICATIONS
gastric restorative: gastric demulcent, mucogenic: gastric mucosal deficiency with dry dyspepsia, dry heaving; chronic gastritis, gastric/duodenal ulcer ulcer
antipyretic, secretory: dehydration, hot spells, low-grade fever, sunstroke; convalescence, diabetes; dry cough
analgesic: arthralgia
interferon inducent
Miscellaneous: insects in the ear canal

SYMPTOM PICTURES
stomach dryness: stomachache improved by eating, feeling of abdominal lumps, dry heaving, dry tongue and mouth
Yin and fluids deficiency: hot spells, dry mouth and throat, thirst, dry cough

PREPARATION
Use: The stem Dendrobium Shi Hu is decocted or used in tincture form.
Dosage: Decoction: 8-20 g
  Tincture: 2-4 ml
Caution: Contraindicated in high fever, deficiencies without heat signs, and abdominal distension due to mucous damp in the intestines.

NOTES
Stonebushel stem derives from several varieties of orchid naturally occurring in central and southern China. Its sweet, moist, *demulcent, mucus-forming* and *secretory* properties relieve a

variety of dry conditions, especially those affecting the stomach. Prized by early Daoist recluses, Stonebushel stem later became adopted by the imperial elite as a welcome addition to their pantheon of longevity agents. Current research shows *interferon inducing* activity in this plant. In East Asia the herb is widely nicknamed "honeymooners' tea" because it is thought to quickly replace spent *jing* or sexual fluids.

The quality of this botanical can be determined by its sweetness, stickyness on the teeth and lack of residue with chewing. Research has confirmed this appraisal by correlating it directly with the polysaccharide content of the stem.

Note that the South China substitute for *Dendrobium* spp. is *Ephemerantha fimbriata*, which through importation is commonly the North American source for the remedy Shi Hu.

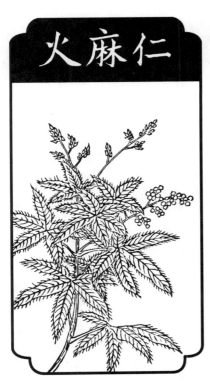

Cannabis Huo Ma Ren
Cannabis Seed

Botanical source: *Cannabis sativa* L. (Moraceae)
Pharmaceutical name: Semen Cannabis
Chinese names: Huo Ma Ren, Da Ma Ren, Huang Ma Ren, Ma Ren (Mand); Fa Ma Yan (Cant)
Other names: Marijuana, Hemp, "Fire hemp"; Kamanin (Jap)
Habit: Annual panglobal subtropical herb; blooms in summer with axillary or terminal viridian flowers.
Part used: the seed

Therapeutic category: medium-strength remedy with some chronic toxicity
Constituents: lipids 30% (incl. saturated fats, cannabinol, phytin, oleic/linoleic/linolenic acids), choline, essential oil cannabidiol, vitamin B
Effective qualities: sweet, mild, moist
　　　　　　　　　　restoring, moistening
Tropism: digestive system
　　　　　Spleen, Stomach, Large Intestine channels
　　　　　Fluid body

ACTIONS AND INDICATIONS
intestinal restorative: demulcent laxative: intestinal dryness with constipation
anti-inflammatory: skin and mouth sores, ulcerations with redness and pain
hypotensive, diuretic: high blood pressure
detoxicant: aconite and mineral poisoning
Miscellaneous: topically for hair loss, wounds, ulcers

SYMPTOM PICTURES
intestines dryness: constipation, small, hard dry stools, dry mouth and throat
Yin and fluids deficiency: fatigue, unrest, afternoon hot spells, dry hard stools, mild dehydration

PREPARATION
Use: The seed Cannabis Huo Ma Ren is decocted or used in tincture form. Crush the seeds before use.
Dosage: Decoction: 10-25 g
　　　　　Tincture: 2-4 ml
Caution: Prolonged use may lead to vaginal discharges or seminal incontinence. Dosages must be respected as overdosing or prolonged use can lead to nausea, vomiting, numb extremities, etc.

Notes

Although in Chinese medicine every single part of the marijuana plant is used medicinally, it is the white seeds that find most frequent use. They are mainly used for their highly reliable *demulcent laxative* effect. Today the remedy deserves research for a potential *heavy metal detoxicant* action.

Cannabis **seeds** are also prepared as congees or gruels. The extracted cannabis **seed oil** is applied topically for hair loss.

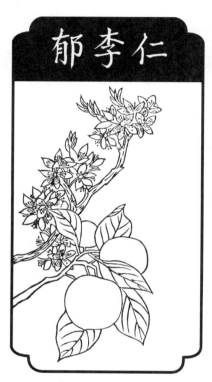

Prunus Yu Li Ren
Bush Cherry Kernel

Botanical source: *Prunus japonica* Thunberg or *P. humulis* Bunge (Rosaceae)
Pharmaceutical name: Semen Pruni japonicae
Chinese names: Yu Li Ren, Tang Di, Zhe Xia Li (Mand); Wat Lei Yan (Cant)
Other names: Dwarf flowering cherry, Japanese bush cherry/plum, "Elegant plum"; Ikurinin (Jap)
Habit: Small mountain shrub from Northeast China, Inner Mongolia, Korea and Japan; much cultivated; blooms in spring with abundant pink flowers.
Part used: the seed

Therapeutic category: mild remedy with minimal chronic toxicity
Constituents: lipids 60-75%, amygdalin, organic acid, protein, cellulose, starch, oleic acid, saponin, vitamins B1, C
Effective qualities: pungent, bitter, sweet, neutral, moist
  restoring, softening, decongesting
Tropism: digestive, urinary systems
  Spleen, Large Intestine, Small Intestine channels
  Fluid body

Actions and Indications

intestinal restorative: demulcent laxative: dry intestinal conditions with constipation
draining diuretic: edema, dysuria
analgesic, antipyretic: heart and rheumatic pain, fever
hypotensive: high blood pressure

Symptom Pictures

intestines dryness and Qi stagnation: small, hard dry stools, constipation, abdominal hardness

general fluid congestion: water retention, difficult urination, constipation

Preparation

Use: The seed Prunus Yu Li Ren is either decocted or used in tincture form.
Dosage: Decoction: 3-12 g
  Tincture: 2-4 ml
Caution: Use with care during pregnancy and in Yin and fluids deficiency conditions.

Notes

The gentle *demulcent laxative* seed of this cherry-like fruit from the mountain valleys of Jiangsu is mainly used in formulas treating the two symptom pictures above.

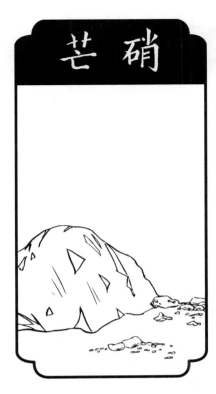

Mirabilitum Mang Xiao
Glauber's Salt

Geological name: Mirabilitum
Pharmaceutical name: Mirabilitum
Chinese names: Mang Xiao, Pu Xiao, Fen Xiao; Xuan Ming Fen (Mand); Mong Siu (Cant)
Other names: Mirabilite, Sodium sulfate, "Spiky niter"; Bosho (Jap)
Source: The raw sulphate mineral mirabilite is obtained in Hebei, Shandong and Henan provinces in eastern China, where it is prepared into Glauber's salt by distillation.
Part used: the mineral salt

Therapeutic category: mild remedy with minimal chronic toxicity
Constituents: sodium tetrasulfate, calcium/magnesium/potassium tetrasulfate, sodium chloride (traces)
Effective qualities: salty, bitter, a bit pungent, very cold, moist
　　　　　　　　　restoring, dissolving
Tropism: digestive, urinary systems
　　　　　Stomach, Large Intestine, Triple Heater channels

ACTIONS AND INDICATIONS
intestinal demulcent restorative, laxative, diuretic: constipation from dryness
anti-inflammatory, detumescent: acute dermatitis, stomatitis, mastitis, conjunctivitis with redness, swelling and pain; swollen mouth and throat ulcers
Topically: mastitis, breast abscess

SYMPTOM PICTURE
intestines heat dryness: hard dry stool, constipation, dehydration, thirst

PREPARATION
Use: Because it dissolves easily, the mineral salt Mirabilitum Mang Xiao is usually added to a decoction or infusion at the end of cooking or steeping time. It may also be infused on its own. Topical applications (e.g., swab, compress) can be made for breast infections.
Dosage: Infusion: 4-14 g
Caution: This *saline laxative* is only to be used in full heat conditions. Contraindicated in digestive deficiency (especially with diarrhea present), during menstruation, pregnancy and postpartum, and for the elderly. Fluid intake should be increased when using this remedy as it causes more water to pass out through the stool.

NOTES
Glauber's salt is one of several mineral remedies still employed in Chinese medicine today. Two general forms of this mineral are distinguished. First, the crude native mirabilite, variously known as **Mang Xiao, Pu Xiao, Pi Xiao, Yen Xiao** or **Fen Xiao,** depending on the degree of purity and the specific form it possesses. All forms of crude mirabilite, whether powder (*fen*) or crystal (*mang*), are mainly sodium sulphate with varying small amounts of sodium chloride, calcium and iron. Second, the purified mirabilite, which is known as **Xuan Ming Fen** after the Tang era alchemist Liu Xuan-qin. Xuan Ming Fen, or purified sodium sulphate, is identical to Glauber's salt in the West (named after the German nineteenth century chemist Glauber). Confusingly, it is this purified form that is generally used in prescriptions whenever the name Mang Xiao appears. The more accurate term Xuan Ming Fen is more often used in the herbal trade itself.

REMEDIES TO PROMOTE ASTRICTION AND STOP DIARRHEA

➥ RESTRAIN LEAKAGE FROM THE INTESTINES
Astringent antidiarrheals

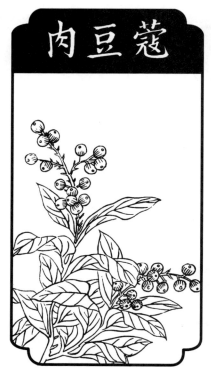

Myristica Rou Dou Kou
Nutmeg Seed

Botanical source: *Myristica fragrans* Houttuyn (Myristicaceae)
Pharmaceutical name: Semen Myristicae
Chinese names: Rou Dou Kou, Rou Guo, Rou Kou (Mand); Yok Dau Chau (Cant)
Other names: "Fleshy cardamom"; Nikuzuku (Jap)
Habit: Perennial (sub)tropical southeast Asian tree; small pale yellow blossoms appear in spring
Part used: the seed

Therapeutic category: medium-strength remedy with some chronic toxicity
Constituents: essential oil (incl. camphene, pinene), myristicin, lipids, tannins
Effective qualities: pungent, astringent, a bit bitter, warm, dry
  restoring, astringing, relaxing, stimulating, raising
Tropism: digestive, central nervous systems
  Stomach, Spleen, Large Intestine channels
  Fluid, Air, Warmth bodies

ACTIONS AND INDICATIONS

gastrointestinal restorative/relaxant: astringent antidiarrheal, anti-infective (antibacterial, antiparasitic): chronic digestive deficiency with loose stool or diarrhea; chronic gastroenteritis and colitis, amoebic dysentery, intestinal dysbiosis, microbial toxicosis
analgesic, spasmolytic: abdominal pain, intestinal colic, IBS, spasmodic dysmenorrhea
nervous stimulant: cerebral deficiency with mental dullness, memory loss, hypochondria, agoraphobia

SYMPTOM PICTURES

intestines cold (Spleen Yang deficiency): chronic diarrhea, fatigue, chilliness, indigestion, abdominal pain
stomach cold: nausea, vomiting, belching, painful distended epigastrium or abdomen

PREPARATION

Use: The seed Myristica Rou Dou Kou is decocted or used in tincture form.
Dosage: Decoction: 3-10 g
  Tincture: 1-3 ml
Caution: Forbidden in acute diarrhea or dysentery, and during pregnancy because of a *uterine stimulant* action. Do not use continuously because of some cumulative toxicity.

NOTES

A native of the Moluccan islands, Nutmeg seed is an essential oil-based remedy, primarily addressing chronic diarrhea and colic with cold or damp cold. Its pungent, warm, *astringent* and *spasmolytic* effects exert a comprehensive action on atonic and dysbiotic digestive states. Formulas treating children and the elderly are the ones most frequently containing Nutmeg seed.

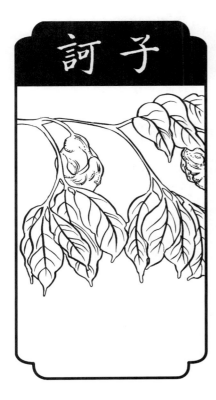

Terminalia He Zi
Myrobalan Fruit

Botanical source: *Terminalia chebula* Retzius or *T. cheb.* var. *gangetica* Roxburgh (Combretaceae)
Pharmaceutical name: Fructus Terminaliae
Chinese names: He Zi, He Zi Rou, Ke Zi Rou, Cang Qing Guo, Xi Cang, He Li Le (Mand); Ngau Ji (Cant)
Other names: Chebulic/Black myrobalans, Inknut tree; Kashi (Jap); Haritaki (Sans)
Habit: Large tropical Asian shade tree, mainly cultivated; fragrant pale yellow flowers bloom in summer.
Part used: the unripe fruit

Therapeutic category: mild remedy with minimal chronic toxicity
Constituents: alkaloids, tannins, organic acids (incl. chebulinic/chebulagic/ellagic acids, terchebin, glucose, glucogallin, saccharose, sennoside A, chebulin, tannin, polyphenol oxidase
Effective qualities: sour, astringent, a bit sweet and bitter, neutral, dry
astringing, solidifying, stabilizing, restoring
Tropism: digestive, respiratory, urogenital, nervous systems
Stomach, Spleen, Large Intestine, Lung, Kidney channels

ACTIONS AND INDICATIONS

intestinal restorative: astringent antidiarrheal, antibacterial, anthelmintic: chronic digestive deficiency with diarrhea, rectal prolapse, blood in stool (melena); bacillary dysentery
analgesic, spasmolytic: abdominal pain, intestinal colic, IBS, heartburn
antiemetic: hiccough, vomiting
genital astringent, mucostatic: incontinence with spermatorrhea, leucorrhea; hemorrhoids, menorrhagia
anhydrotic: excessive sweating, night sweats
respiratory restorative, antitussive: wheezing, voice loss, chronic cough, hoarseness
nervous restorative: fatigue

SYMPTOM PICTURES

intestines damp cold (Spleen Qi deficiency): chronic loose stool, abdominal pains, indigestion, weakness

genitourinary damp cold: clear vaginal discharges, premature ejaculation, sperm loss

lung Qi deficiency: chronic coughing, fatigue, wheezing, voice loss, copious sweating

PREPARATION

Use: The fruit Terminalia He Zi is decocted or used in tincture form. The fresh fruit alone should be used for chronic cough and hoarseness.
Dosage: Decoction: 3-10 g
Tincture: 2-4 ml
Caution: Forbidden in acute diarrhea, the initial stage of dysenterial conditions, dehydration, severe exhaustion or emaciation, and in cough due to infection.

NOTES

A valued remedy in Chinese, Greek and Ayurvedic medicine, Myrobalan fruit originated in the Middle East and was imported into China via the southern sea lanes by early Persian traders. As the most important of the Indian compound, Triphala (the "three fruits"), Myrobalan was attributed in Ayurvedic and Tibetan medicine with truly marvelous properties.

Since the Ming, however, Myrobalan's medicinal effects have been described in more sober and secular terms. The sour, puckery fruit is considered a versatile *intestinal* and *genital astringent* and *mucostatic*, with a secondary *antispasmodic* action on the gut, checking both discharges and secretions. As the syndromes above suggest, for best results it should be used only with chronic cold and deficient conditions.

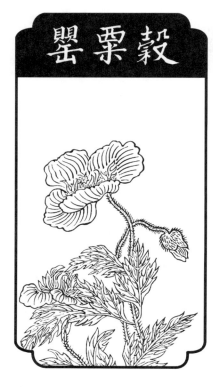

Papaver Ying Su Ke
Opium Poppy Husk

Botanical source: *Papaver somniferum* L. (Papaveraceae)
Pharmaceutical name: Pericarpium Papaveris
Chinese names: Ying Su Ke, Ying Su Qiao, Yu Mi Ke (Mand); Ying So Hok (C)
Other names: Ozokukoku (Jap)
Habit: Annual or biennial subtropical Eurasian herb; flowers in summer with solitary terminal white, pink, red or scarlet flowers.
Part used: the flower husk (capsule) with the opium latex removed

Therapeutic category: medium-strength remedy with some chronic toxicity
Constituents: alkaloids (incl. morphine, codeine, thebaine, papaverine, narcotine, narcotoline), narcein, sedoheptulose, mannoheptulose, mycinositol, erythritol, sanguinarine, choline, protopine
Effective qualities: sour, astringent, neutral, dry
astringing, solidifying, stabilizing, relaxing, calming
Tropism: digestive, respiratory, central nervous systems
Spleen, Large Intestine, Kidney, Lung channels
Fluid, Air bodies

Actions and Indications
intestinal restorative/relaxant: astringent antidiarrheal: chronic digestive weakness with diarrhea; chronic dysentery and enteritis, rectal prolapse
urogenital mucostatic, astringent: incontinence with enuresis, spermatorrhea, leucorrhea
analgesic: pain in general (esp. of abdomen, epigastrium, rectum, chest, sinews, bones, head, teeth)
bronchodilator, antitussive: chronic cough, wheezing; asthma
vasodilator, parasympathetic stimulant

Symptom Pictures
intestines damp cold (Spleen Qi deficiency): loose stool, chronic diarrhea, abdominal pain
genitourinary damp cold: frequent or dribbling urination, clear vaginal discharges, seminal incontinence

Preparation
Use: The husk Papaver Ying Su Ke is decocted or used in tincture form. For chronic coughs it should first be toasted. Traditionally the husk or capsule is prepared by washing, removing the outer skin, drying in the shade, slicing and macerating in rice vinegar or honey (Porter Smith 1871).
Dosage: Decoction: 2-9 g
Tincture: 0.5-3 ml
Caution: Forbidden with acute dysentery-like conditions or acute coughs. Being a medium-strength remedy, Opium poppy husk should be discontinued every two weeks or so if used on its own.

NOTES

An early import from India, the opium poppy was originally cultivated during the Song period purely for its lovely vermilion flowers. The sour, astringent fruit husk, or capsule, displays excellent *astringent, relaxant* and *analgesic* effects on digestive and urogenital functions. Being an alkaloidal plant, its strong *antitussive* action with chronic coughs should not be misused through continuous use.

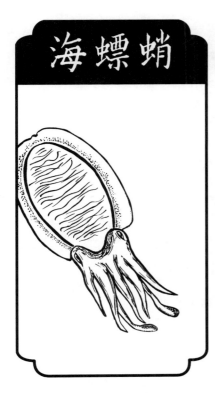

Sepia Hai Piao Xiao
Cuttlefish Bone

Zoological source: *Sepia esculenta* Hoyle and *Sepiella maindroni* de Rochebrune (Sepiidae)
Pharmaceutical name: Os Sepiae
Chinese names: Hai Piao Xiao, Wu Zei Gu, Dan Yu Gu, (Mo) Yu Gu (Mand); Hoi Piu Siu (Cant)
Other names: Uzokukotsu (Jap)
Source: China's coastal provinces.
Part used: the internal shell

Therapeutic category: mild remedy with minimal chronic toxicity
Constituents: calcium carbonate and phosphate c. 87-91%, sodium and magnesium chloride, chitin, gelatin, 17 amino acids 1.5-3%
Effective qualities: salty, astringent, warm, dry
     astringing, solidifying, stabilizing
Tropism: digestive, urogenital, nervous systems
     Stomach, Spleen, Liver, Kidney channels
     Fluid, Air bodies

ACTIONS AND INDICATIONS

intestinal restorative: astringent antidiarrheal: chronic digestive deficiency with diarrhea, umbilical pain; dysentery
antacid antisecretory: acid dyspepsia from hyperchlorhydria, peptic ulcer, bleeding ulcer
genital mucostatic, astringent: incontinence with spermatorrhea (incl. wet dreams), pollakiuria, leucorrhea
hemostatic: passive bleeding (esp. uterine), bloody stools
detoxicant, detumescent: suppurative infections, abscesses, goiter
vulnerary, styptic: chronic ulcers, sores, tissue trauma (with bleeding), eczema, burns
antimalarial

SYMPTOM PICTURES

intestines damp cold (Spleen Qi deficiency): chronic diarrhea, navel pain

genitourinary damp cold: seminal emissions, frequent urination, clear vaginal discharges

PREPARATION

Use: Sepia Hai Piao Xiao is decocted. In powdered form, the remedy is an excellent *vulnerary* and *styptic* for topical use in injuries, eczema, ulcers, nosebleed, tooth extraction and other surgeries.
Dosage: Decoction: 6-12 g
     Powder: 2-6 g
Caution: Avoid longterm use which may lead to constipation. Forbidden in deficiency heat and constipation.

NOTES

Although traditionally also used to nourish the Blood, Cuttlefish bone now is a commonly used ingredient in formulas treating intestinal and genital discharges. The remedy's strong astringency has also proven highly effective for gastric ulcers arising from hyperacidity, as well as in passive hemorrhage. Modern experiments in malaria treatment have also achieved a high success rate.

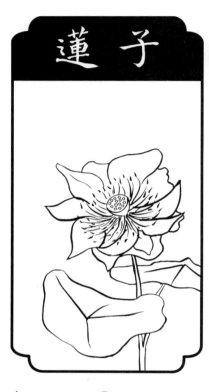

Nelumbo Lian Zi
Lotus Seed

Botanical source: *Nelumbo nucifera* Gaertner (Nymphaeaceae)
Pharmaceutical name: Semen Nelumbinis
Chinese names: Lian Zi, Shi Lian Zi, Lian Shi, Tian Shi Lian, Jian Lian Ru (Mand); Ling Ji (Cant)
Other names: Renshi (Jap)
Habit: Perennial South Asian water plant mainly cultivated in ponds; produced in China's central and mid-coastal provinces; opens in summer with fragrant, large pink or white terminal capitate flowers.
Part used: the seed

Therapeutic category: mild remedy with minimal chronic toxicity
Constituents: raffinose, oxoushinsonine, norarmepavine, protein, starch, asparagin, calcium, phosphorus, iron
Effective qualities: sweet, astringent, neutral, dry
    restoring, astringing, solidifying, stabilizing, calming
Tropism: digestive, urinary, reproductive, cardiovascular systems
    Spleen, Kidney, Heart, Dai channels; Fluid, Air bodies

ACTIONS AND INDICATIONS

gastrointestinal restorative: astringent antidiarrheal: chronic digestive deficiency with diarrhea; enteritis, malabsorption
genital mucostatic, astringent: incontinence with spermatorrhea, leucorrhea, menorrhagia
neurocardiac sedative: unrest, irritability, insomnia, nightmares, anxiety states

SYMPTOM PICTURES

intestines damp cold (Spleen Qi deficiency): chronic diarrhea, fatigue

genitourinary damp cold: wet dreams, clear vaginal discharges

heart and Kidney Yin deficiency/heart Qi constraint with **nerve excess:** irritability, unrest, sleep loss, dry mouth, dark urine, wet dreams

PREPARATION

Use: The seed Nelumbo Lian Zi is decocted or used in tincture form.
Dosage: Decoction: 9-18 g
    Tincture: 2-4 ml
Caution: Forbidden in constipation or abdominal distension.

NOTES

Considered exotic by the Chinese ever since its first ancient importation from India, few plants have been discussed, painted and written about as frequently as the lotus. In keeping with its superlative nature, neither has any plant yielded as many medicinal products: A total of nine distinct parts of the lotus plant are employed in Oriental medicine: root node, stem, leaf, flower, plumule, stamen, receptacle, seed and seed heart. Lotus seed is an auxilliary remedy useful for its essentially *astringing, stabilizing* and *calming* actions on urogenital, intestinal and nervous functions.

Taken alone, the green center of the lotus seed, **Lotus seed heart, Lian Zi Xin** (Mand.) or **Ling Ji Sam** (Cant.), treats fever with thirst, palpitations, sleep loss and high blood pressure. Dose: 1.5-3 g by decoction.

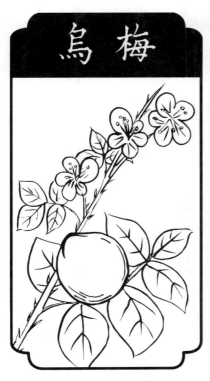

Prunus Wu Mei
Black Plum Fruit

Botanical source: *Prunus mume* Siebold et Zuccarini (Rosaceae)
Pharmaceutical name: Fructus Pruni mume
Chinese names: Wu Mei, Wu Mei Rou, Mei Shi (Mand); Ng Mak (Cant)
Other names: Chinese/Japanese apricot; Ubai (Jap)
Habit: Common large deciduous bush or tree found throughout China; likes warm, humid, sunlit conditions and fertile sandy soil; fragrant, light pink or white, small urceolate sessile flowers bloom in early spring.
Part used: the unripe green fruit

Therapeutic category: mild remedy with minimal chronic toxicity
Constituents: citric/malic/succinic/tartaric/oleanolic acid, sitosterol, carbohydrates
Effective qualities: sour, sweet, salty, warm, dry
astringing, stabilizing, solidifying
Tropism: digestive, respiratory, reproductive systems
Spleen, Large Intestine, Liver, Lung channels
Fluid body

ACTIONS AND INDICATIONS
intestinal restorative: astringent antidiarrheal, antibacterial, antifungal: digestive deficiency with diarrhea; enteritis, bacillary/amoebic dysentery
genital hemostatic: uterine bleeding, menorrhagia
anthelmintic: ascariasis (roundworm), hookworm (esp. with vomiting and abdominal pain)
antitussive respiratory restorative: chronic cough
hydrogenic: dehydration with dry mouth, thirst (incl. in diabetes), achlorhydria
choleretic, cholagogue
antiallergic
anthelmintic: tinea, ascariasis
Topically: callous, corn, psoriasis

SYMPTOM PICTURES
intestines damp cold (Spleen Qi deficiency): chronic diarrhea, fatigue
lung Qi deficiency: chronic coughing, fatigue, dry mouth, thirst

PREPARATION
Use: The fruit Prunus Wu Mei is decocted or used in tincture form. For gynecological bleeding, the hemostatic action is enhanced when the herb is first toasted or partially charred. A plaster of the ground fruit (usually mixed with salt and vinegar) is used to treat calluses, corns, warts, etc. The unripe plums are also pickled as a condiment.
Dosage: Decoction: 3-10 g
  Tincture: 2-4 ml
Caution: Contraindicated in excess conditions.

NOTES
The domesticated black plum tree is one of the "three winter friends" alongside the bamboo and the pine. Its exquisite, fragrant flowers are frequently depicted in Chinese and Japanese art. In medicine, the fruit is an *astringent anti-infective* for the keynote symptoms chronic diarrhea, chronic cough and thirst. Intestinal parasites (roundworm, hookworm) are also treated with it.

Elsholtzia Xiang Ru
Aromatic Madder Herb

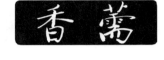

Botanical source: *Elsholtzia splendens* or *E. stauntonii* (Labiatae)
Chinese names: Xiang Ru (Cao), Mu Xiang Ru (Mand); Heung Yu (Chou) (Cant)
Category: mild remedy with minimal chronic toxicity
Constituents: essential oil (incl. ketones, elshotzianic acid, furane, cineol, pinene, terpene, camphorquinone, transcaryophyllene)
Effective qualities: pungent, warm; stimulating, decongesting
Tropism: digestive, urinary systems; Lung, Stomach channels

ACTIONS: *Astringent antidiarrheal, antipyretic, draining diuretic, anti-infective*
INDICATIONS: Diarrhea and fever from food poisoning (summer heat syndrome); nausea, vomiting, water retention, onset of infections (including typhoid).
Dosage: Decoction: 3-10 g
  Tincture: 1-3 ml
Caution: None.

Dolichos Bai Bian Dou
Hyacinth Bean

Botanical source: *Dolichos lablab* L. (Leguminosae)
Chinese names: Bai Bian Dou, Bian Dou, Yen Li Dou (Mand); Baak Bin Dou, Bin Dou (Cant)
Category: mild remedy with minimal chronic toxicity
Constituents: phytin, calcium, phosphorus, iron, zinc, pantothenic acid, hemaglutinin A and B, protein, lipids)
Effective qualities: sweet, neutral, dry; restoring, astringing, stabilizing
Tropism: digestive, reproductive systems; Spleen, Stomach channels

ACTIONS: *Astringent antidiarrheal, detoxicant, antiemetic, genital mucostatic astringent, antipyretic*
INDICATIONS: Chronic diarrhea from intestines damp cold (Spleen Qi deficiency); colic, food poisoning with vomiting (esp. from fish), infantile malabsorption and malnutrition, alcohol intoxication; leucorrhea, gonorrhea; fever, sunstroke.
Dosage: Decoction: 8-18 g
  Tincture: 2-4 ml
  For strengthening digestive functions, this remedy is first toasted.
Caution: Forbidden in all cold conditions, and intermittent fevers and chills.
NOTES: The main use of Hyacinth bean is for summer fevers/heat with diarrhea caused by food poisoning.

Punica Shi Liu Pi
Pomegranate Husk

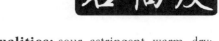

Botanical source: *Punica granatum* L. (Punicaceae)
Chinese names: Shi Liu Pi (Mand); Sek Lao Pei (Cant)
Category: medium-strength remedy with some chronic toxicity

Effective qualities: sour, astringent, warm, dry; astringing, relaxing, solidifying
Tropism: digestive, reproductive systems; Large Intestine channel

ACTIONS: *Astringent antidiarrheal, anthelminthic, antibacterial, antifungal, antiviral*
INDICATIONS: Chronic diarrheal and painful conditions, including dysentery (incl. amoebic), intestinal colic and colitis from intestines damp cold and Intestines Qi constraint syndromes; leucorrhea, menorrhagia, rectal prolapse with bleeding,, intestinal parasites (incl. roundworms, tapeworms).
Dosage: Decoction: 3-10 g
Tincture: 2-4 ml
Caution: Never to be taken with oils or fats as these cause toxins to be absorbed. **Pomegranate root bark, Punica Shi Liu Gen Pi,** may also be used for the above indications, but is cumulatively more toxic than the husk.

Nelumbo He Ye
Lotus Leaf

Botanical source: *Nelumbo nucifera* Gaertner (Nymphaeaceae)
Chinese names: He Ye (Mand); Ho Yip (Cant)
Category: mild remedy with minimal chronic toxicity

Effective qualities: bitter, somewhat sweet, neutral, astringing
Tropism: digestive, respiratory, vascular systems; Spleen, Heart, Liver channels

ACTIONS: *Astringent antidiarrheal, disinfectant, hemostatic, digestive stimulant*
INDICATIONS: Diarrhea from food poisoning, dyspepsia, hemoptysis, congestive urinary and rectal bleeding.
Dosage: Decoction: 3-10 g
Tincture: 1-3 ml
Caution: None.
NOTES: Lotus stem, Lian Geng, is used in a similar way to Lotus leaf. In addition, it relieves stifling sensations in the chest by circulating lung Qi.

Halloysitum Chi Shi Zhi
Red Kaolin

Geological source: *Halloysitum rubrum*
Chinese names: Chi Shi Zhi (Mand); Chek Sek Ji (C.)
Other names: Red halloysite, Red bole
Category: mild remedy with minimal chronic toxicity
Constituents: hydrated aluminium silicate, ferric/manganese/magnesium/calcium oxides, alumina, silica
Effective qualities: sweet, astringent, warm, dry; stabilizing, astringing, solidifying
Tropism: digestive, vascular systems; Spleen, Somach, Large Intestine channels

ACTIONS: *Astringent antidiarrheal, hemostatic, antiprolapse, vulnerary*
INDICATIONS: Chronic dysentery, diarrhea, rectal prolapse with bleeding; chronic, cold and deficient conditions with blood in the stool, uterine bleeding, menorrhagia; mercury and phosphorus poisoning, heavy metal toxicosis
Topically for chronic ulcers.
Dosage: Decoction: 8-26 g

Caution: Forbidden in damp heat in the intestines, i.e. acute dysentery, and during pregnancy.

NOTES: There are two types of Kaolin, or Halloysite, red and white. **White kaolin** is called **Bai Shi Zhi** or **Gao Ling Tu,** and is similarly used as **Red kaolin, Chi Shi Zhi.** Both types belong to the five siliceous clays, Wu Si Shi Zhi, which also include **Jing Shi Zhi,** or **Turquoise siliceous clay, Huang Shi Zhi,** or **Fuller's earth** (literally "Yellow siliceous clay"), and **Hei Shi Zhi,** or **Graphite.**

Kaolin has shown to chelate toxins, including those from intestinal dysbiosis and fermentation, and to possess a *protective* effect on the digestive mucous membrane.

Limonitum Yu Liang Shi
Clay Ironstone

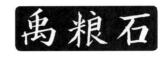

Geological source: *Limonitum*
Chinese names: Yu Liang Shi, Yu Yu Liang, Wu Ming Yi (Mand); Yu Ling Sek (Cant)
Source: China's southeastern provinces
Category: mild remedy with minimal chronic toxicity
Constituents: hydrated ferric oxide, hemotite, goethinite, quartz, clay minerals
Effective qualities: sweet, astringent, neutral; stabilizing, astringing, solidifying
Tropism: digestive, reproductive systems; Large Intestine, Stomach channels

ACTIONS: *Astringent antidiarrheal, hemostatic, mucostatic*
INDICATIONS: Obstinate chronic diarrhea, enteritis, blood in stool, rectal prolapse with bleeding, uterine bleeding, leucorrhea.
Dosage: Decoction: 10-18 g
Caution: Use cautiously during pregnancy.

Gastrointestinal Stimulants

REMEDIES TO PROMOTE DIGESTION, STIMULATE SECRETIONS AND RELIEVE FATIGUE

Bitter digestants

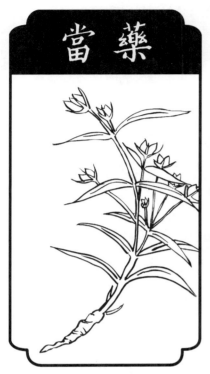

Swertia Dang Yao
Asian Green Gentian Root

Botanical source: *Swertia pseudochinensis* Hara and spp. (Gentianaceae)
Pharmaceutical name: Radix Swertiae pseudochinensis
Chinese names: Dang Yao (Mand); Dong Yok (Cant)
Other names: Senburi (Jap)
Part used: the root

Therapeutic category: mild remedy with minimal chronic toxicity
Constituents: bitter substances, secoiridoid glycosides (incl. sweroside, swertiamarin, gentiopicroside, amarogentin, amaroswering), xanthones (swertianol, swertianolin), flavonoids (swertisin, swertiajaponin), oleanolic acid
Effective qualities: bitter, cold, dry
　　　　　　　　　　stimulating
Tropism: digestive system
　　　　　Liver, Gallbladder channels
　　　　　Warmth body

ACTIONS AND INDICATIONS

gastric stimulant: bitter digestant: gastric deficiency with appetite loss, dyspepsia; anorexia
choleretic, cholagogue: biliary dyspepsia, jaundice, constipation, chronic hepatitis
hepatic sedative/decongestant, liver protective: liver congestion; acute infectious, (viral) hepatitis
antibacterial: acute and chronic bacterial dysentery
dermal and cuticular stimulant: hair loss (alopecia)

SYMPTOM PICTURES

gallbladder and stomach Qi stagnation: appetite loss, slow painful digestion, epigastric bloating, constipation
liver and galbladder damp heat: painful sides, nausea, bitter taste in mouth, jaundice, constipation

PREPARATION

Use: The root Swertia Dang Yao is either decocted or used in tincture form.
Dosage: Decoction: 3-12 g
　　　　　Tincture: 2-4 ml
Caution: Forbidden with diarrhea from digestive weakness.

NOTES

Like other members of the Gentian family, this valuable remedy is used both as a bitter *digestive stimulant* in small doses and a damp-heat-clearing remedy in larger ones. Chinese green gentian root in particular excells with its *liver protective* action, a synergism of its chemical constituents (Chang and But 1987).

REMEDIES TO PROMOTE DIGESTION, RELIEVE COLIC AND RELIEVE ABDOMINAL PAIN

➥ WARM THE MIDDLE AND DISPEL COLD

Pungent analgesic digestants

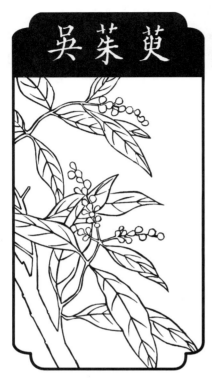

Evodia Wu Zhu Yu
Evodia Berry

Botanical source: *Evodia rutaecarpa* (Juss.) Bentham (Rutaceae)
Pharmaceutical name: Fructus Evodiae
Chinese names: Wu Zhu Yu, Wu Zhu (Mand); Min Jiu Yi (Cant)
Other names: Goshuyu (Jap)
Habit: Small deciduous tree from central and southwestern China, growing on upland slopes and forest outskirts; also cultivated; corymbs of small yellowish white terminal flowers bloom in summer.
Part used: the unripe fruit

Therapeutic category: medium-strength remedy with some chronic toxicity
Constituents: essential oil 0.4% (incl. evodin, ocimene, evodin), alkaloids (incl. rutaevine, evodiamine, rutaecarpine, wuchyine), methoxytriptamine, synephrine, goshyunic acid
Effective qualities: pungent, bitter, astringent, warm, dry
   stimulating, calming, relaxing, sinking
Tropism: digestive, nervous, reproductive systems
   Stomach, Spleen, Liver, Kidney, channels ; Warmth, Air bodies

ACTIONS AND INDICATIONS

gastrointestinal stimulant: pungent digestant, carminative, astringent: spasmodic digestive deficiency with dyspepsia, diarrhea; intestinal colic, IBS, dysbiosis/fermentation, gastroenteritis, hernia
uterine stimulant, emmenagogue: delayed menstruation, amenorrhea
analgesic: abdominal pain, dysmenorrhea, postpartum pain, myalgia, headache from hypertension
antiemetic: vomiting, nausea, sour belching
hypotensive: high blood pressure
anti-infective: antiviral, antibacterial, antifungal, antiparasitic, interferon inducent: viral, bacterial, fungal and parasitic infections (incl. microbial toxicosis, dermatitis, eczema, cholera); pinworms (ascariasis), liver flukes; aphthous stomatitis

SYMPTOM PICTURES

stomach cold: epigastric pain and distension, nausea, sour belching and regurgitation, vomiting

intestines cold (Spleen and Kidney Yang deficiency): early morning diarrhea, fatigue, chilliness

liver cold: headache at vertex, fatigue, right flank pain, indigestion, delayed menses

uterus cold: menstrual cramps, difficult flow, delayed onset

PREPARATION

Use: The berry Evodia Wu Zhu Yu is briefly decocted or used in tincture form.
Dosage: Decoction: 3-10 g
   Tincture: 2-4 ml
Caution: Forbidden in Yin deficiency with empty heat and during pregnancy. It is not to be combined with Licorice root if used for high blood pressure, as Licorice cancels its *hypotensive* effect. Evodia berry should not be taken on its own at full doses over long periods due to some cumulative chronic toxicity.

NOTES
The small, five-sided, sea-green Evodia berry has a unique fresh, leafy and mossy scent, and a pungent, bitter taste. These qualities signals an essential oil responsible for warming, stimulant effects that treat internal cold conditions. Specifically, Evodia addresses digestive and reproductive deficiencies characterized by stagnation, toxin accumulation and pain. Its *carminative*, *analgesic* and *emmenagogue* results are clear in the above four types of cold symptom pictures.

Because of Evodia's additional *broad-spectrum anti-infective* action, the remedy should find increasing usage for disorders involving intestinal dysbiosis. and microbial toxicosis, as well as for actual infections.

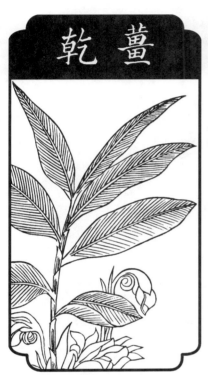

Zingiber Gan Jiang
Dried Ginger Root

Botanical source: *Zingiber officinalis* (Willd.) Roscoe (Zingiberaceae)
Pharmaceutical name: Rhizoma Zingiberis
Chinese names: Gan Jiang, Bai Jiang, Dan Gan Jiang (Mand); Gaan Geung (Cant)
Other names: Shokyo (Jap)
Habit: Perennial tropical East Asian herb cultivated in China's southwest coastal provinces; terminal spikes of viridian flowers bloom in summer.
Part used: the rhizome

Therapeutic category: mild remedy with minimal chronic toxicity
Constituents: essential oil (incl. zingiberine, sesquiterpene alcohols shogaol and gingerol, phellandrene, camphene, zingiberone, borneol, citral), oleoresin, acetic acid, sulphur
Efective qualities: very pungent, a bit sweet and bitter, hot, dry
　　　　stimulating, relaxing, restoring, dispersing
Tropism: digestive, respiratory, reproductive systems
　　　　Stomach, Spleen, Lung, Kidney channels; Warmth, Air bodies

ACTIONS AND INDICATIONS
gastrointestinal stimulant/relaxant: pungent digestant, carminative: spasmodic digestive deficiency with gastrointestinal dyspepsia, nausea; intestinal colic, IBS, chronic gastritis, anorexia
antiemetic: nausea, vomiting, morning sickness, travel sickness
arterial stimulant: cold extremities and limbs
spasmolytic: spasmodic and painful conditions in general
uterine stimulant/relaxant, emmenagogue: spasmodic dysmenorrhea, scanty flow, lochial retention
stimulant expectorant: chronic bronchitis, catarrh
immune regulator: immune stress with immune complex disorder (incl. bronchial asthma, rheumatoid arthritis)
antiviral, antibacterial, interferon inducent: respiratory, intestinal and other infections
detoxicant: food or herb poisoniong
hemostatic: chronic uterine bleeding, menorrhagia

SYMPTOM PICTURES
stomach cold: dull epigastric pain and distension, belching, flatulence, vomiting clear sour liquid, cold extremities
uterus cold: delayed or absent menses, menstrual cramps, chills
lung phlegm cold: coughing with watery, foamy white sputum, cold hands and feet

PREPARATION
Use: The root Zingiber Gan Jiang is decocted or used in tincture or essential oil form. For uterus cold conditions with passive menstrual or intermenstrual bleeding, it should be dry roasted (quick-fried) or baked first to increase the *hemostatic* action. The quick-fried root is called **Pao Jiang** (Mandarin) or **Bou Geung** (Cantonese).

Dosage: Short decoction: 3-10 g
Tincture: 1-2 ml

Caution: Only to be used for passive bleeding with cold conditions. Avoid in heat in the stomach or lungs and during early pregnancy (morning sickness excepted).

NOTES
Originally only cultivated by Inner Mongolian tribes in North China, Ginger root has long since become a classic pungent, warming, relaxing remedy. The spicy essential oil's *stimulant* action on the arterial circulation is the basis for use in the three cold-type symptom pictures above. Dried ginger is a minor component of more prescriptions than it is a major component. In these it lends warmth, movement and increased tropism of the whole formula.

Ginger root skin, Jiang Pi (Mandarin) or **Geung Pei** (Cantonese), is considered pungent, cool in nature. It treats edema and abdominal fullness. Dose: 3-10 g in short decoction.

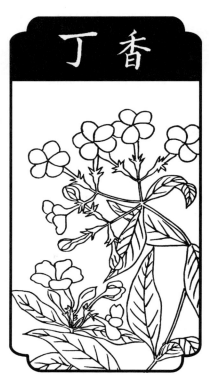

Eugenia Ding Xiang
Clove Bud

Botanical source: *Eugenia caryophyllata* Thunberg (Myrtaceae)
Pharmaceutical name: Gemma Eugeniae
Chinese names: Ding Xiang, Ding Zi Xiang, Gong Ding Xiang (Mand); Ding Heung (Cant)
Other names: Carnation clove, "Nail aromatic"; Choko (Jap)
Habit: Evergreen tropical Southeast Asian tree with white tubular flowers in
Part used: the flower bud

Therapeutic category: mild remedy with minimal chronic toxicity
Constituents: essential oil (incl. 70-85% eugenol, furfurol, pinene, vanillene, caryophyllene, methyl salicylate), tannins, gum, lipids, wax
Effective qualities: pungent, a bit bitter, hot, dry
stimulating, relaxing
Tropism: digestive, urogenital systems
Stomach, Spleen, Kidney, Ren, Dai channels
Warmth, Air bodies

ACTIONS AND INDICATIONS
gastrointestinal stimulant/relaxant: pungent digestant, carminative, analgesic, spasmolytic: spasmodic digestive deficiency with dyspepsia; intestinal colic, IBS, dysbiosis, halitosis, toothache, headache
antiemetic: nausea, belching, hiccups, vomiting
anti-infective: antibacterial, antifungal: preventive in epidemics; microbial toxicosis, fungal infections
reproductive stimulant/restorative, emmenagogue, parturient: sluggish menses or labor; frigidity, sterility, impotence
genital mucostatic: leucorrhea
anthelmintic (vermifuge): intestinal parasites (esp. roundworm)
leukocytogenic: leukopenia
anesthetic (local)

Symptom Pictures
stomach cold: loss of appetite, nausea, abdominal pain, flatulence, hiccups, vomiting

genitourinary damp cold (Kidney Yang deficiency with damp cold): loss of sexual interest, clear vaginal discharges, scanty delayed menses

Preparation
Use: The bud Eugenia Ding Xiang is briefly decocted or used in tincture or essential oil form. The latter brings out its *antiseptic, anti-infective, antiparasitic, analgesic* and *anesthetic* properties the most.

Dosage: Decoction: 1.5-4 g
Tincture: 0.25-2 ml
Essential oil: 1-2 drops in a gel cap topped with olive oil

Caution: Forbidden in fevers, Yin deficiency conditions and pregnancy.

Notes
Originating in the Moluccan islands of northeast Indonesia, the exotic "nail aromatic" *(ding xiang)* has long been an ingredient in Chinese perfumes, incenses and herbal formulas.

Clove bud, and its extracted essential oil, is both a good symptomatic remedy (parasites, pain, fungal infections, vomiting) and a systemic one for two types of cold deficiency symptom patterns. These syndromes are most likely to involve microbial toxicosis. Here clove's pungent, warm, *stimulant/relaxant* effective qualities and its *antifungal* and *antibacterial* actions are outstanding.

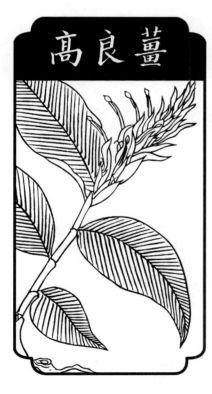

Alpinia Gao Liang Jiang
Galangal Root

Botanical source: *Alpinia officinarum* Hance (Zingiberaceae)
Pharmaceutical name: Rhizoma Alpiniae officinari
Chinese names: Gao Liang Jiang, Man Jiang, Liang Jiang (Mand); Gou Leung Geung (Cant)
Other names: Lesser galangal, "Gao liang ginger"; Koryokyo (Jap)
Habit: Perennial herb with leafy stems growing in subtropical East Asian grassland, thickets and woods; also cultivated; blooms in summer with panicles of ivory and scarlet flowers.
Part used: the rhizome

Therapeutic category: mild remedy with minimal chronic toxicity
Constituents: essential oil (incl. carineole, methyl cinnamate, eugenol, pinene, cineol, cadimene), galangin, kaempferide, quercetin, pungent resin galangol
Effective qualities: pungent, hot, dry
stimulating, relaxing
Tropism: digestive, reproductive systems
Stomach, Spleen channels; Warmth, Air bodies

Actions and Indications
gastrointestinal stimulant: pungent digestant, carminative: spasmodic digestive deficiency with dyspepsia, epigastric or abdominal pain; intestinal colic, IBS, acute and chronic gastroenteritis, cholera
antiemetic: nausea, vomiting, travel sickness, hiccups
uterine spasmolytic: spasmodic dysmenorrhea
antipyretic: remittent fevers

immune regulator: immune stress with immune complex disorders (incl. chronic hepatitis)
anti-infective, interferon inducent: food poisoning
Miscellaneous: hepatomegaly, fainting

SYMPTOM PICTURE
stomach and intestines cold (Spleen Yang deficiency): epigastric or abdominal pain, thirst, nausea, belching, vomiting, diarrhea

PREPARATION
Use: The root Alpinia Gao Liang Jiang is decocted or used in tincture form.
Dosage: Decoction: 2-10 g
Tincture: 1-4 ml
Caution: Contraindicated in Yin deficiency patterns with empty heat.

NOTES
Once used only by southwestern Chinese aboriginal tribes, the essential oil-laden Galangal root has "from ancient times been held in much esteem by Chinese physicians" (Porter Smith 1871). This esteem is now more understandable in light of its new-found regulating action on immune functions. The remedy's current Western image as a poor relation to ginger is regrettable. Galangal's unique aroma—a combination of peppery and gingery—is the key to its classic *digestive stimulant/relaxant* nature, addressing painful, cold dysfunctions of the digestive and reproductive systems.

The root of *Alpinia galanga* (L.) Swartz, **Da Liang Jiang** (Mand.) or **Daai Leung Geung** (Cant.), is used interchangeably with this remedy, although it is less strong. It is less aromatic and spicy, and because of that is extensively used in Malayan cooking (Burkill 1935).

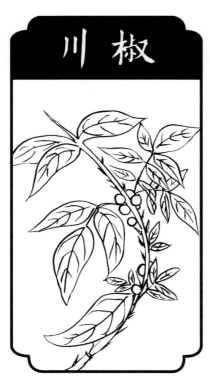

Zanthoxylum Chuan Jiao
Sichuan Peppercorn *

Botanical source: *Zanthoxylum bungeanum* Maximovicz and spp. (Rutaceae)
Pharmaceutical name: Fructus Zanthoxyli bungeani
Chinese names: Chuan Jiao, Shu Jiao, Ba Jiao, Hua Jiao, Jiao Mu (Mand); Chuen Jiu, Chan Jiu (Cant)
Other names: Sichuan prickly ash berry; Sensho (Jap)
Habit: Large spiny shrub or small tree from the mountain valleys of Sichuan, Gansu and Hubei; corymbs of viridian flowers bloom in summer.
Part used: the fruit

Therapeutic category: mild remedy with minimal chronic toxicity
Constituents: essential oil 0.7-9% (incl. geraniol, limonene, cumic alcohol, phellandrene), organic acids
Effective qualities: pungent, hot, dry
stimulating, relaxing
Tropism: digestive, nervous systems
Stomach, Spleen, Kidney channels
Warmth, Air bodies

ACTIONS AND INDICATIONS
gastrointestinal stimulant: pungent digestant, carminative: spasmodic digestive deficiency with dyspepsia; intestinal colic, IBS
relaxant, analgesic: diarrhea or loose stool, abdominal pain (incl. from parasites); chronic enteritis, dysentery, dysmenorrhea
urogenital astringent diuretic: pollakiuria, spermatorrhea
agalactic: weaning, excessive breastmilk
dermatropic: moist skin sores
anthelmintic, parasiticide: roundworm, tapeworm, skin parasites
antibacterial, antifungal

SYMPTOM PICTURE
stomach and intestines cold (Spleen Yang deficiency): epigastric and abdominal pain and distension, nausea, flatulence, fatigue, loose stool, cold extremities

PREPARATION
Use: The berry Zanthoxylum Chuan Jiao is decocted or used in tincture form.
Dosage: Decoction: 2-7 g
Tincture: 0.5-2 ml
Caution: Contraindicated in Yin deficiency conditions with empty heat. Use cautiously during pregnancy.

NOTES
A variety of native *jiao,* or prickly ash berry, Sichuan peppercorn is used throughout Asia in cookery and medicine in the same way as the black peppercorn of Burma and Assam. At once *stimulant* and *relaxant,* this remedy from the Western kingdom of Shu (Sichuan) is ideal for those intestinal conditions with colic and diarrhea that present an overall cold condition.

The berry of the American prickly ash may be used in a similar way to the Sichuan variety. Both contain more volatile oil than the bark, hence are more *warming, stimulating* and *pain relieving,* and less *astringent* than the bark.

Alpinia Cao Dou Kou
Katsumada's Galangal Seed *

Botanical source: *Alpinia katsumadai* Hayata (Zingiberaceae)
Chinese names: Cao Dou Kou, Dou Kou (Mand); Chou Dau Kau (Cant)
Category: mild remedy with minimal chronic toxicity

Constituents: essential oil (incl. camphor), alpinetin, cardamonin
Effective qualities: pungent, warm, dry; stimulating, relaxing
Tropism: digestive system; Spleen, Stomach channels

ACTIONS: *Pungent digestant, carminative, antiemetic, antimalarial, antivenomous, immune regulator*
INDICATIONS: Dyspepsia, colic with epigastric or abdominal pain, flatulence with intestines mucous damp (Spleen damp) and stomach and intestines cold (Spleen Yang deficiency) syndromes; vomiting, acid regurgitation; malaria; poisoning in general; immune complex disorders (incl. bronchial asthma, rheumatoid arthritis).
Dosage: Decoction: 2-7 g.
Tincture: 1-3 ml
The crushed seeds should be decocted covered for 5 minutes. When decocting with other herbs, add the whole seeds 10 minutes before cooking time ends.
Caution: Contraindicated in Yin deficiency conditions; only to be used with damp cold present.
NOTES: A deeply warming herb from the ginger family, Katsumada's galangal seed treats Yang deficiency of the digestive tract manifesting as cold. The volatile oil's spicy, aromatic, dry quality also transforms mucous damp.

Ferula A Wei
Asafoetida Resin

Botanical source: *Ferula foetida* L. (Umbelliferae)
Chinese names: A Wei (Mand); A Ngai (Cant)
Category: mild remedy with minimal chronic toxicity
Constituents: essential oil, resins, gums, calcium sulphate/carbonate, iron oxide, glycosides (incl. kaempferol, quercetin, apigenin)
Effective qualities: pungent, warm, dry; stimulating, relaxing, calming
Tropism: digestive, respiratory, reproductive systems; Spleen, Stomach, Lung channels

ACTIONS: *Pungent digestant, carminative, spasmolytic, antibacterial, anthelmintic, antipyretic, mucolytic expectorant, bronchodilator, antitussive, emmenagogue, anticoagulant*
INDICATIONS: Dyspepsia, intestinal colic with epigastric/abdominal pain, swelling and and flatus in stomach; stomach and intestines Qi stagnation with cold; abdominal lumps, food stagnation (esp. from meat), roundworm, enteritis, fever; chronic bronchitis, croup, whooping cough from lung phlegm cold; amenorrhea, spasmodic dysmenorrhea.
Dosage: Decoction: 0.5-1.5 g in powder form as medicine or cooking spice.
Tincture: 0.25-1 ml
Caution: Contraindicated during pregnancy.

Litsea Bi Cheng Qie
Cubeb Fruit

Botanical source: *Litsea cubeba* (Lour.) Persoon
Chinese names: Bi Cheng Qie (Mand); Dou Sai Geun (Cant)
Category: mild remedy with minimal chronic toxicity
Constituents: fatty oil (incl. lauric/capric/oleic acids), essential oil (incl. citral, cineole, citronellal, furfurol, formaldehyde, acetaldehyde, acetone, methylpepetenone, limonene), cubebin, resins
Effective qualities: pungent, warm, dry; stimulating, calming
Tropism: digestive, respiratory, urinary systems; Stomach, Spleen, Kidney, Bladder channels

ACTIONS: *Pungent digestant, carminative, analgesic, antiemetic, diuretic*
INDICATIONS: Stomch cold syndrome with epigastric and umbilical abdominal pain, appetite loss; nausea, vomiting, hernia, turbid urine in children.
Dosage: Decoction: 1-3 g by short decoction
Tincture: 0.5-1 ml
Caution: None.

Piper Bi Ba
Long Pepper Fruit Spike

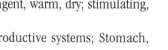

Botanical source: *Piper longum* L. (Piperaceae)
Chinese names: Bi Ba, Bi Bo (Mand)
Category: mild remedy with minimal chronic toxicity
Constituents: essential oil, alkaloids (pipernonaline, piperundecalidine, piperine, chavicine), palmitic acid, sesamin, tetrahydropiperic acid
Effective qualities: pungent, warm, dry; stimulating, calming, relaxing
Tropism: digestive, reproductive systems; Stomach, Large Intestine channels

ACTIONS: *Purgent digestant, analgesic, antiemetic, antibacterial*
INDICATIONS: Abdominal pain from colic or parasites; flatulence, heartburn; stomach and intestines (damp) cold syndrome with nausea or vomiting; gastroenteritis, cholera; menstrual pain, toothache, headache, berberi, infertility.
Dosage: Decoction: 1-3 g
Tincture: 0.5-1 ml
Caution: None.

Foeniculum Xiao Hui Xiang
Fennel Seed

Botanical source: *Foeniculum vulgare* Miller (Umbelliferae)
Chinese names: Xiao Hui Xiang, Shi Lo (Mand); Siu Wui Heung (Cant)
Category: mild remedy with minimal chronic toxicity
Constituents: essential oil 1.75-4.62% (incl. anethone, fenchone, estragol, terpenes, anesic aldehyde, cineol), fixed oil, silica
Effective qualities: pungent, sweet, warm, moist; stimulating, relaxing
Tropism: digestive, urinary, respiratory systems; Stomach, Spleen, Kidney, Liver, Lung, Chong, Ren chan.

ACTIONS: *Pungent digestant, carminative, spasmolytic, antiemetic, uterine stimulant, emmenagogue, estrogenic, galactagogue, stimulant expectorant, interferon inducent*

INDICATIONS: Stomach or intestines cold syndrome with dyspepsia, flatulence, sour regurgitation; intestinal colic, hernia, nausea, vomiting; dysmenorrhea, amenorrhea from uterus cold; insufficient lactation, bronchial asthma; wheezing, voice loss.

Dosage: Decoction/Infusion: 4-12 g. Crush and decoct the seeds for 3 minutes and then infuse for 10 minutes.
Tincture: 2-4 ml
Essential oil: 2-4 drops in a little warm water

Caution: Use cautiously in Yin deficient conditions with empty heat, and during pregnancy.

NOTES: Fennel seed was one of the many botanical gifts of Persian Tebb-e-Yunani medicine to Asian medicine during the Tang period. High in essential oils, the seed is commonly used for digestive and menstrual problems arising from cold.

Trigonella Hu Lu Ba
Fenugreek Seed

Botanical source: *Trigonella foenum-graecum* L. (Leguminosae)
Chinese names: Hu Lu Ba (Mand); Wu Lou Ba (Cant)
Category: mild remedy with minimal chronic toxicity
Constituents: mucilage, choline, alkaloid trigonelline, glycosides (incl. diosgenin, yamogenin, gitogenin, vitexin, orientin, quercetin, luteolin, gentianin, carpaine), phytosterols, vitamin B1
Effective qualities: bitter, pungent, warm, moist; stimulating, decongesting
Tropism: digestive, urinary, endocrine systems; Kidney, Liver channels

ACTIONS: *Pungent digestant, carminative, demulcent laxative, draining diuretic, urinary demulcent, galactagogue, hypoglycemiant, antinematodal*

INDICATIONS: Deficiency cold digestive conditions with abdominal pain and distension; flank pain, hernial pain, water retention in legs, arthritis, urinary irritation, insufficient lactation, high blood sugar, weight loss.

Dosage: Decoction: 3-10 g
Tincture: 1-3 ml

Caution: Forbidden in Yin deficiency conditions with deficiency heat, and during pregnancy.

NOTES: The compound trigonelline has shown *antitumoral* activity, especially in cervical and liver cancer.

Diospyros Shi Di
Persimmon Calyx

Botanical source: *Diospyros kaki* L. f. (Ebenaceae)
Chinese names: Shi Di (Mand); Chi Tai (Cant)
Category: mild remedy with minimal chronic toxicity
Constituents: hydroxytriterpenic acid, oleanic/betulinic/ursolic acid, tannin, glucose, fructose
Effective qualities: bitter, astringent, neutral; calming, sinking
Tropism: digestive systems; Stomach, Lung channels

ACTIONS: *Antiemetic*
INDICATIONS: Hiccups and belching in any condition, including stomach cold.
Dosage: Decoction: 4-10 g
   Tincture: 2-3 ml
Caution: None.
NOTES: Ripe persimmon fruit is eaten for thirst, cough and spitting of blood.

REMEDIES TO PROMOTE DIGESTION, RESOLVE MUCUS AND RELIEVE ABDOMINAL FULLNESS

➥ TRANSFORM SPLEEN DAMP WITH AROMATIC REMEDIES

Pungent, dry digestants

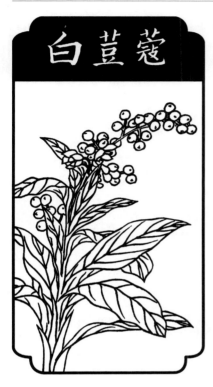

Amomum Bai Dou Kou
Cluster Cardamom Pod

Botanical source: *Amomum cardamomum* L., syn. *A. krervanh* Pierre ex Gagnepain (Zingiberaceae)
Pharmaceutical name: Fructus Amomi cardamomi
Chinese names: Bai Dou Kou, Dou Kou, Bai Kou Ren (Mand); Bak Dou Kou (Cant)
Other names: Round/Ribbed/Siam cardamom, "White cardamom"; Byakuzuku (Jap)
Habit: Perennial leafy-stemmed herb from humid tropical East Asia; dense white/red-white flower spikes spring directly from the rootstock in summer.
Part used: the fruit

Therapeutic category: mild remedy with minimal chronic toxicity
Constituents: essential oil (incl. borneol, camphor, humulene, pinene, caryophillene, carvone, cineol, terpineol, sabinine), trace minerals
Effective qualities: pungent, warm, dry
    stimulating, relaxing, restoring
Tropism: digestive, respiratory, nervous systems
    Spleen, Stomach, Lung channels
    Air, Warmth bodies

ACTIONS AND INDICATIONS
gastrointestinal stimulant: pungent digestant, carminative: mucogenic digestive deficiency with gastrointestinal dyspepsia; gastroenteritis, heartburn
antiemetic: nausea, vomiting
nervous restorative: fatigue, mental dullness, depression
stimulant expectorant: bronchitis
mucolytic: nasal and sinus congestion
antipyretic: remittent fever
immune regulator, antiallergic: immune stress with immediate allegies and immune complex disorders (incl. rhinitis, bronchial asthma, rheumatoid arthritis, nephritis)

SYMPTOM PICTURES
intestines mucous damp (Spleen damp): lethargy, head pressure, appetite loss, indigestion, depression, allergies
stomach cold: vomiting clear, sour fluid, epigastric distension and pain, gurgling abdomen
stomach Qi stagnation: epigastric pain and distension, appetite loss, sour belching, regurgitation

PREPARATION
Use: The pod Amomum Bai Dou Kou should be briefly decocted (5-10 minutes) or added at the end of decoction time if part of a formula.
Dosage: Short decoction: 2-6 g
    Tincture: 1-3 ml

Caution: Contraindicated in Blood (metabolic) and Yin deficiency conditions.

NOTES

So-called because the ripe white seeds cluster like grapes inside the ribbed capsule, the Javanese cluster cardamom is one of three cardamom types routinely included in Chinese prescriptions. This spice enjoys the distinction of having been written about in elegiac terms by the Song poet Si Dong-po from his Hainan island hideout.

Pungent, dry and warm, its *digestive stimulant/relaxant* actions relieve pain and clear sub-infectious mucous damp and cold of the digestive tract. Cluster cardamom is also frequently added to formulas for bronchial conditions of the lung phlegm cold variety. Note that nervous deficiency with mental and physical fatigue also benefits from its use.

Areca Da Fu Pi
Betel Husk

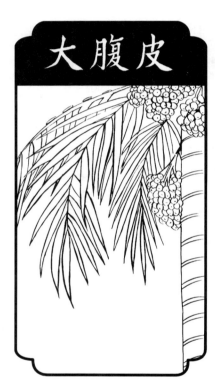

Botanical source: *Areca catechu* L. or *A. dicksonii* Roxburgh (Arecaceae)
Pharmaceutical name: Pericarpium Arecae
Chinese names: Da Fu Pi (Mand); Daai Fuk Pei (Cant)
Other names: Areca nut, "Large abdomen peel"; Daifukuhi (Jap)
Habit: Solitary tall palm tree commonly cultivated throughout the Asian tropics.
Part used: the husk

Therapeutic category: mild remedy with minimal chronic toxicity
Constituents: arecoline, arecolidine, tannin
Effective qualities: pungent, a bit warm, dry
　　　　　　　　　　stimulating, decongesting, sinking
Tropism: digestive, urinary systems
　　　　　Spleen, Stomach, Small Intestine, Large Intestine channels
　　　　　Air, Fluid bodies

ACTIONS AND INDICATIONS

gastrointestinal stimulant: pungent digestant, carminative: mucogenic digestive deficiency with chronic gastrointestinal dyspepsia; acute and chronic gastroenteritis, beriberi
antiemetic: nausea, vomiting
draining diuretic: edema, dysuria, oliguria; chronic hepatitis
hypotensive
anthelmintic: tapeworm, pinworm
Miscellaneous: glaucoma

SYMPTOM PICTURES

intestines mucous damp (Spleen damp): abdominal distension, flatulence and gurgling, head pressure

food stagnation with **stomach and intestines Qi stagnation:** swollen distended epigastrium and abdomen, sour belching, constipation or diarrhea

liver fluid congestion: abdominal or general water retention, indigestion, scanty urination

PREPARATION
Use: The husk Areca Da Fu Pi is decocted or used in tincture form.
Dosage: Decoction: 4-10 g
Tincture: 1-3 ml
Caution: Use cautiously in Qi deficiency conditions.

NOTES
Areca Da Fu Pi is the husk of the betel nut which is mainly used as an *antiparasitic* remedy. The husk is a very versatile *drying digestive stimulant* that will reduce all forms of indigestion due to mucous damp or food stagnation. It is usually reserved for more severe and acute manifestations of long-term digestive disorders involving intestinal dysbiosis or parasitosis, tharby treating the acute manifestation of these condition more than their root.

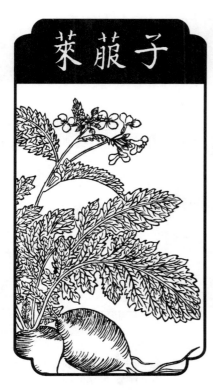

Raphanus Lai Fu Zi
Radish Seed

Botanical source: *Raphanus sativus* L. (Cruciferae)
Pharmaceutical name: Semen Raphani
Chinese names: Lai Fu Zi (Mand); Laai Fuk Ji (Cant)
Other names: Raifukushi (Jap)
Habit: Annual or perennial temperate Eurasian herb, growing wild and cultivated; flowers in spring with racemes of yellow, violet or pink blossoms.
Part used: the seed

Therapeutic category: mild remedy with minimal chronic toxicity
Constituents: fatty oil 35% (incl. erucic/linoleic/oleic acid, glycerol sinapate, raphanin, sinapine), essential oil (incl. methylmercaptan, hexanal, phenols), alkaloids, flavonoids
Effective qualities: pungent, a bit sweet, a bit warm
stimulating, decongesting, relaxing
Tropism: digestive, respiratory, cardiovascular systems
Stomach, Spleen, Lung, Yin Wei channels
Air, Fluid bodies

ACTIONS AND INDICATIONS
gastrointestinal stimulant: pungent digestant, carminative: digestive deficiency with chronic gastrointestinal dyspepsia; intestinal dysbiosis, intestinal fermentation with acid regurgitation
anti-infective: antiviral, antibacterial, antifungal: enteritis, dysentery, microbial toxicosis
intestinal relaxant: diarrhea, enteritis, dysentery with abdominal pain, rectal tenesmus
stimulant expectorant: chronic bronchitis
bronchodilator: asthma with tight chest
thyroid inhibitor: mild hyperthyroid conditions
hypotensive: high blood pressure
diuretic

SYMPTOM PICTURES
food stagnation with **stomach and intestines Qi stagnation:** indigestion, abdominal bloating and pain, sour belching, diarrhea or constipation

lung phlegm damp: chronic cough with white sputum, wheezing, tight chest

Preparation

Use: The seed Raphanus Lai Fu Zi is decocted or used in tincture form. It is usually toasted first when used for productive coughing. Fresh radish juice is strongly *antifungal* and *antibacterial* and has been used to treat trichomonas vaginalis, bronchial conditions such as silicosis, and lung TB with hemoptysis. Used in enemas, it will treat allergic colitis, diarrhea and chronic ulcerative colitis.

Dosage: Decoction: 6-12 g
Tincture: 2-3 ml

Caution: Use with caution in Qi deficiency conditions.

Notes

Radish seed is another remedy common in the West, the many uses of which have been virtually forgotten. Containing both fatty and essential oils, the seed is at once a *digestive stimulant* removing stagnant food, dysbiosis and toxicosis in the gut, and a *relaxant* relieving both diarrhea (infectious and simple) and constipation. Horseradish root is therapeutically similar to Radish seed, but somewhat milder.

In the Orient, dried **radish leaf, Luo Bo Ye,** is used for diarrhea and dysentery. A decoction of the **fresh root, Luo Bo,** is given for digestive distress, hoarseness, thirst, dysentery, migraine, nosebleed and blood in the sputum. A decoction of the **dried, shrunk root, Di Gu Luo,** is a soothing *diuretic* used for urinary irritation and water retention.

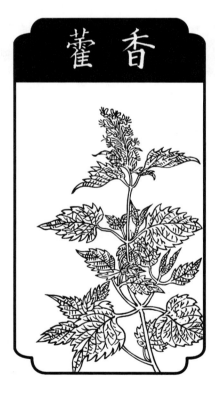

Agastache Huo Xiang
Rugose Giant Hyssop Herb *

Botanical source: *Agastache rugosa* (Fisch. et Mey.) O. Kuntze and *Pogostemon cablin* (Blanco) Bentham (Labiatae)
Pharmaceutical name: Herba Agastachis seu Pogostemis
Chinese names: Huo Xiang, Xiang Ren Hua (Mand); Fuk Heung (Cant)
Other names: *A. rug.:* Kakko (Jap) *P. cab.:* Guang Huo Xiang; Patchouli herb
Habit: *A. rug.:* Fragrant common annual temperate and subtropical East Asian herb growing wild on streamsides and hillsides; also cultivated; small violet blossoms flower in summer and autumn in spike-like raceme clusters.
P. cab.: Annual subtropical herb from the Philippines, Malaysia, India and South China.
Part used: the herb

Therapeutic category: mild remedy with minimal chronic toxicity
Constituents: *A. rug.:* essential oil (incl. methylchavicol, limonene, pinene, humulene, ylangene, anethole, anisaldehyde)
P. cab.: essential oil (incl. cinnamic aldehyde, pogostol, benzaldehyde, eugenol, caryophyllene, patchoulipyridine, epiguaipyridine, elemene, patchoulene)
Effective qualities: pungent, a bit sweet and bitter, warm, dry
stimulating, relaxing, dispersing
Tropism: digestive, nervous systems
Spleen, Stomach, Lung channels
Air, Warmth bodies

ACTIONS AND INDICATIONS

gastrointestinal stimulant: pungent digestant, carminative, astringent: mucogenic digestive deficiency with chronic gastrointestinal dyspepsia; intestinal dysbiosis, gastroenteritis, food poisoning
anti-infective: antibacterial, antifungal, antispirochetal
stimulant diaphoretic: common cold (esp. onset), fever
spasmolytic: abdominal pain, intestinal colic, chest distension
nervous sedative, analgesic: unrest, anxiety, headache, angina pectoris pains
antiemetic: vomiting (incl. from morning sickness)

SYMPTOM PICTURES

intestines mucous damp (Spleen damp): abdominal distension and discomfort, nausea, appetite loss, fatigue, head pressure, loose stool

external wind cold with **intestines damp:** sneezing, headache, chills, feverishness, nausea, indigestion, abdominal distension

PREPARATION

Use: The short 5 to 10 minute decoction is best for the herb Agastache Huo Xiang, unless the tincture is used. The volatile oil—known as Patchouli essential oil—is distilled from *Pogostemon cablin* in Canton, Hainan, India, Sumatra and Malaysia.

Dosage: Decoction: 4-10 g
 Tincture: 2-4 ml

Caution: Forbidden in Yin deficiency with empty heat, and stomach fire.

NOTES

Literally called "bean-leaf aromatic" by the Chinese, Rugose giant hyssop in the lip-flower family was named by botanists *agastache,* meaning "many-spiked" in Greek, refering to the plant's numerous flower spikes. The fragrant, essential oil-laden remedy addresses symptom patterns of mucous damp in the intestines. The specific symptoms that indicate the use of this herb are restlessness, fatigue and nausea—regardless of whether due to indigestion, intestinal dysbiosis, food poisoning or gastroenteritis. The remedy's mild *nervous sedative* and *analgesic* actions are perfect in simple and infectious acute digestive complaints made worse from stress. Traditional formulas also make use of Rugose giant hyssop's *anti-infective* and *diaphoretic* effects for treating the onset of common colds.

Patchouli herb, from *Pogostemon cablin,* although considered a replacement for the remedy Huo Xiang and used identically, is properly called **Guang Huo Xiang** (Mand.) or **Gwong Fuk Heung** (Cant.). Cultivated in warm, moist regions of the Far East and India, patchouli leaves have long been used to scent clothing and protect it from insects. They are now also distilled into essential oil of patchouli for perfumery, food flavoring and aromatherapy industries.

Atractylodes Cang Zhu
Black Atractylodes Root *

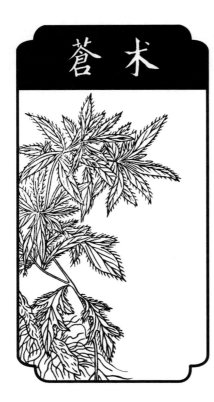

Botanical source: *Atractylodes lancea* (Thunb.) De Candolle or *A. chinensis* (De Cand.) Koidz. and spp. (Compositae)
Pharmaceutical name: Rhizoma Atractylodis lanceae
Chinese names: Cang Zhu, Cang Shu, Zi Shu, Shan Ji, Mao Zhu (Mand); Chong Sat, Chang Sat (Cant)
Other names: Grey/Red atractylodes; Sojutsu (Jap)
Habit: Perennial herb from northeast and coastal China, and Inner Mongolia, growing in dry mountain areas; blooms in autumn with terminal white and purple-tinged flower corollas.
Part used: the rhizome

Therapeutic category: mild remedy with minimal chronic toxicity
Constituents: essential oil 5-9% (incl. eudesmol, hinesol, atractylodin, atractylol, atractylone, atractylin), carotenoids, vitamin A, B1, C
Effective qualities: bitter, pungent, astringent, warm, very dry
  stimulating, dispersing, relaxing, decongesting
Tropism: digestive, hepatic, urinary systems
  Spleen, Stomach channels
  Fluid, Air bodies

ACTIONS AND INDICATIONS

gastrointestinal stimulant: pungent digestant, carminative: mucogenic digestive deficiency with gastrointestinal dyspepsia; acute/chronic gastroenteritis, intestinal dysbiosis
anti-infective, interferon inducent: viral, bacterial and fungal infections (incl. gastroenteritis, influenza, microbial toxicosis, candidiasis); skin infections, operations; prophylaxis for varicella, mumps, scarlet fever, cold, bronchitis, etc.
diaphoretic: onset of cold, flu and respiratory infections
antiemetic: nausea, vomiting
mucostatic astringent: leucorrhea
draining/detoxicant diuretic, analgesic: edema, metabolic toxicosis with rheumatism, arthritis, headache
hypoglycemiant: diabetes
immune regulator: immune stress with immune complex disorders (incl. food allergies, glomerulonephritis, rheumatoid arthritis)
anti-night blindness

SYMPTOM PICTURES

intestines mucous damp (Spleen damp): appetite loss, loose stool, epigastric pain or distension, nausea, pressure in the head

external wind/cold/damp: sneezing, headache, aches and pains, no sweating

metabolic toxicosis (wind damp obstruction): soreness, stiffness and swelling in joints of the extremities

liver fluid congestion: general water retention, headache, tiredness

PREPARATION

Use: The root Atractylodes Cang Zhu is decocted or used in tincture form.
Dosage: Decoction: 4-10 g
  Tincture: 2-4 ml

Caution: Forbidden in Qi deficiency, in profuse sweating and in Yin deficiency with internal heat. Also use with care with loose or watery stool.

NOTES

Black atractylodes is a thistle-like plant in the sunflower family from Northeast China. Its root provides a classic remedy that has always been considered an essential one in the category of damp resolving remedies. Today, the therapeutic profile of Black atractylodes moreover suggests a medicinal that may be even more relevant now than it was in the past.

The field of therapeutic action of Black atractylodes root is fairly typical for a composite, addressing as it does mainly metabolic and digestive disorders, especially on the fluid level. Its extremely high volatile oil content gives the root aromatic, pungent and bitter effective qualities. These in combination exert excellent *stimulant, anti-infective* and *detoxicant* actions, especially on all digestive and respiratory functions.

Black atractylodes root tackles a wide spectrum of gastrointestinal problems. Accumulated mucus or damp with key symptoms of appetite loss and chronic forms of indigestion are highlight indications from the energetic perspective. In physiological terms, Black atractylodes addresses the results of chronic digestive dysbiosis, such as microbial toxicosis and candidiasis. It is very likely that *antiviral, antibacterial* and *antifungal* actions would be demonstrated of this remedy's essential oil once tested, as it promotes regressive development of microbes along their cyclogeny. In view of its general *immune-regulating* and *antiallergic* effect, Black atractylodes is likely also to prove beneficial in the managment of food allergies.

The liver/kidney axis is typically also stimulated by this composite plant, resulting additionally in an extremely reliable *diuretic* effect. This manifests first as a *draining diuretic* action relieving fluid congestion with edema, and second as a deeper *detoxicant diuretic* action addressing metabolic forms of toxicosis, such as rheumatic disorders (traditionally defined by the syndrome wind damp painful obstruction). As a result, not only digestive but also arthritic and even influenza pains may be relieved through its use.

Black atractylodes root is often used in smudging or fumigation sticks together with **Asian mugwort herb, Artemisia Ai Ye,** for topical infections. It is also given together with pig's or sheep's liver for night blindness. Although both remedies are high in vitamin A, in view of the above it is clearly unlikely that this factor alone would be operative as far as Black atractylodes is concerned.

REMEDIES TO PROMOTE DIGESTION, STIMULATE SECRETIONS AND RELIEVE ABDOMINAL FULLNESS

➥ REDUCE FOOD STAGNATION AND TRANSFORM ACCUMULATION

Enzymatic digestants

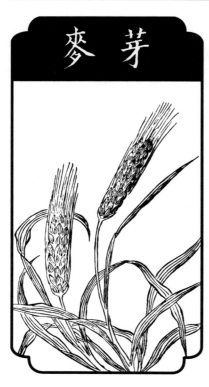

Hordeum Mai Ya
Barley Sprout

Botanical source: *Hordeum vulgare* L. (Gramineae)
Pharmaceutical name: Fructus Hordei germinati
Chinese names: Mai Ya (Mand); San Man Nga (Cant)
Other names: Bakuga (Jap)
Habit: Temperate cultivated cereal herb
Part used: the sprouted grain

Therapeutic category: mild remedy with minimal chronic toxicity
Constituents: enzymes (incl. amylase, invertase, diastase, peptidase, protease, lipase), dextrin, betain, choline, hordenine, vitamin A, B, C, D, phospholipid, maltose up to 45%, glucose
Effective qualities: sweet, warm, moist
  stimulating, restoring, nourishing
Tropism: digestive system
  Spleen, Stomach channels
  Fluid body

ACTIONS AND INDICATIONS

gastrointestinal stimulant: enzymatic digestant: digestive enzyme deficiency with dyspepsia, (esp. of carbohydrates); intestinal fermentation, infantile nutritional disorders
nutritive: debility (esp. in convalescence)
analgesic: epigastric pain worse with stress
antigalactagogue: excessive breast milk with engorged breasts; discontinuation of nursing

SYMPTOM PICTURE

food stagnation and accumulation with **stomach Qi stagnation:** epigastric fullness and distension, nausea, belching, sour regurgitation

PREPARATION

Use: The sprouted grain Hordeum Mai Ya is best taken directly in powder form, but may also be gently decocted.
Dosage: Powder: 6-14 g
  Decoction: 10-30 g
  Up to 120 g may be used for malnutrition and to stop lactation.
Caution: Forbidden in nursing mothers.

NOTES

Sprouted barley is a much-used *enzymatic digestant* remedy that works mainly on starch digestion.

Gallus Ji Nei Jin
Chicken Gizzard Lining

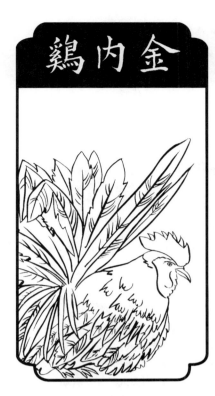

Zoological source: *Gallus domesticus* Brisson (Phasianidae)
Pharmaceutical name: Endothelium corneum gigeriae Galli
Chinese names: Ji Nei Jin, Nei Jin, Ji Zhun Pi (Mand); Gei Loi Gam (Cant)
Other names: Keinaikin (Jap)
Part used: the gizzard mucosa

Therapeutic category: mild remedy with minimal chronic toxicity
Constituents: ventriculin, keratin, bilatriene, vitamin B1 and B2, 17 amino acids, ammonium chloride
Effective qualities: sweet, astringent, mild
restoring, astringing, stabilizing, dissolving
Tropism: digestive, urinary, reproductive systems
Spleen, Stomach, Small Intestine, Bladder channels
Fluid body

ACTIONS AND INDICATIONS
gastrointestinal stimulant: secretory, enzymatic digestant: gastric hypoacidity and enzyme deficiency with dyspepsia; hypochlorhydria, intestinal fermentation, halitosis, infantile nutritional disorders
anti-inflammatory: acute gastroenteritis, laryngitis, acute tonsilitis, ulcerative gingivitis, apthous stomatitis
intestinal astringent: diarrhea, undigested food in stool, dysentery
urogenital astringent: incontinence with enuresis (incl. nocturnal), spermatorrhea (incl. with wet dreams)
antiemetic: nausea, vomiting, regurgitation
antilithic: urinary stones, gallstones

SYMPTOM PICTURE
food stagnation and accumulation with **stomach Qi stagnation:** epigastric fullness and distension, nausea, hiccups, sour regurgitation, pasty unformed stool

PREPARATION
Use: Gallus Ji Nei Jin is most effective when taken in powder or tincture form, since heat tends to destroy the active components.
Dosage: Powder: 3-10 g
Tincture: 1-3 ml
Caution: None.

NOTES
In treating deficiency gastric disorders, Chicken gizzard lining has the advantage of increasing both gastric acidity and enzyme release. The remedy works slowly but effectively to relieve acute and chronic indigestion in the above conditions, where its *anti-inflammatory* and *astringent* actions also contribute.

Chicken gizzard lining is often combined with other *enzymatic digestants* such as Hawthorn berry, Barley sprout, Black atractylodes root and Ripe tangerine rind for conditions of digestive accumulation and food stagnation.

Massa Fermentata Shen Qu
Medicated Leaven

Chinese names: Shen Qu, Liu (Shen) Qu (Mand); Sam Chau (Cant)
Category: mild remedy with minimal chronic toxicity
Constituents: enzymes, lipids, ergosterol, albumin, B complex vitamins
Effective qualities: sweet, pungent, warm; restoring, nourishing
Tropism: digestive system; Spleen, Stomach channels

This remedy is a fermented mixture of wheat flour and six herbs, hence the name *liu shen qu*. The herbs are Artemisia Qing Hao (Celery wormwood herb), Xanthium Cang Er Zi (Cocklebur), Prunus Xing Ren (Bitter apricot kernel), Polygonum La Liao Cao (Knotweed herb), Phaseolus Chi Xiao Dou (Aduki bean) and wheat bran.

ACTIONS: *Enzymatic digestant*
INDICATIONS: Chronic dyspeptic complaints from enzymatic deficiency, especially in accumulation and food stagnation conditions; abdominal distension and discomfort, belching, irregular stool; gastritis.
Dosage: Decoction: 6-16 g
    Tincture: 1-3 ml
Caution: Caution during pregnancy and forbidden in stomach fire.
NOTES: Medicated leaven is often found in formulas to aid the absorption of mineral remedies. A common variation on Shen Qu is the remedy **Shen Qu Cha** ("fermented leaven tea"), which is also available in patent remedy form. It consists of thirteen or more herbs, including Artemisia Qing Hao, Scutellaria Huang Qin, Coptis Huang Lian, Magnolia Hou Po, Poria Fu Ling, Dioscorea Shan Yao, Platycodon Jie Geng, Angelica Du Huo, Amomum Bai Dou Kou, Citrus Chen Pi and several other ingredients. In addition to resolving food stasis and accumulation, Shen Qu Cha is also generally *relaxant* (*spasmolytic, anti-inflammatory,* etc.), and *stimulant* (*mucostatic, carminative,* etc.) to digestive functions, and is better suited for indigestion arising from stress and dysbiosis as well as enzymatic insufficiency. In traditional terms this remedy circulates Qi and clears damp heat in the Middle Warmer. The classic remedy Shen Qu and the expanded version Shen Qu Cha should clearly be differentiated.

Oryza Gu Ya
Sprouted Rice Grain

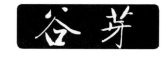

Botanical source: *Oryza sativa* L. (Gramineae)
Chinese names: Gu Ya (Mand); Gu Nga (Cant)
Category: mild remedy with minimal chronic toxicity
Constituents: saccharides, proteins, lipids, protease, peptidase, vitamin B
Effective qualities: sweet, neutral; restoring, nourishing
Tropism: digestive systems; Spleen, Stomach channels

ACTIONS: *Enzymatic digestant, nutritive*
INDICATIONS: Dyspepsia from enzymatic deficiency; food stagnation with poor appetite, abdominal discomfort.
Dosage: Decoction: 10-20 g
    Tincture: 2-4 ml
Caution: None.
NOTES: This enzymatic remedy is somewhat weaker than Hordeum Mai Ya, Sprouted barley grain; the two are usually prescribed together.

REMEDIES TO PROMOTE BOWEL MOVEMENT AND RELIEVE CONSTIPATION

➥ DRAIN DOWNWARD

Stimulant laxatives, purgatives

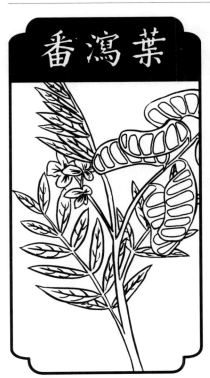

Senna Fan Xie Ye
Senna Leaf

Botanical source: *Senna acutifolia* Delavay or *S. angustifolia* Vahl (Legimunosae)
Pharmaceutical name: Folium Sennae
Chinese names: Fan Xie Ye, Xie ye (Mand); Faan Sie Yip (Cant)
Other names: "Barbarian purge leaf"; Banshayo (Jap)
Habit: Small herb or shrub from tropical East Africa and India; racemes of yellow flowers bloom in spring.
Part used: the leaf

Therapeutic category: mild remedy with minimal chronic toxicity
Constituents: anthraquinone glycosides 4% (sennosides A, B, C, D, rhein, aloe-emodin), chrysophanic acid, mannitol, mucilage, resin, acetic acid salts
Effective qualities: bitter, a bit sweet, warm with cooling potential
  stimulating, relaxing, thickening
Tropism: digestive, reproductive systems
  Large Intestine meridian
  Air, Fluid bodies

ACTIONS AND INDICATIONS

intestinal stimulant: laxative: constipation, acute intestinal obstruction with abdominal distension
uterine stimulant, emmenagogue: delayed or absent menses
spasmolytic, muscle relaxant: acute pancreatitis, cholecystitis
hemostatic: bleeding (esp. gastrointestinal)
antibacterial: bacterial dysentery

PREPARATION

Use: For the least intestinal discomfort, the leaf Senna Fan Xie Ye should be prepared with a 10-hour cold water infusion (maceration). The short 10-15 minute decoction and the tincture are also acceptable, however.
Dosage: Short decoction: 3-8 g
  Tincture: 10-40 drops or 0.5-2 ml
Caution: Being a warm *stimulant,* Senna leaf is forbidden during menstruation, pregnancy, breast-feeding and with congestive, inflammatory and catarrhal conditions such as intestines damp heat/cold and uterus blood congestion. Dosages should not be exceeded and long-term use should be avoided. A *carminative* such as Ginger or Fennel is usually added to Senna leaf to reduce intestinal griping (discomfort).

NOTES

A variety of other remedies in this and other families also go by the name of Senna. The leaf of **American senna**, *Cassia marylandica*, is reputed to be as good as this remedy, while **Bladder senna**, *Colutea arborescens*, and **Wild senna**, *Globularia alypum*, are both milder in effect.

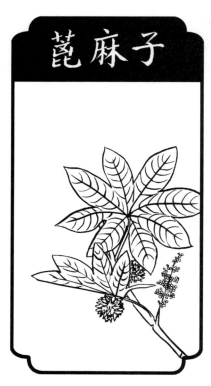

Ricinus Bi Ma Zi
Castor Bean

Botanical source: *Ricinus communis* L. (Euphorbiaceae)
Pharmaceutical name: Semen Ricini
Chinese names: Bi Ma Zi, Hung Bi (Mand); Bei Ma Ji (Cant)
Other names: "Tick hemp bean"; Togoma, Hima (Jap)
Habit: Wild and cultivated annual shrub-like (sub)tropical herb; in summer and autumn, racemes of light yellow terminal flowers appear.
Part used: the seed and the extracted oil

Therapeutic category: medium-strength remedy with some chronic toxicity
Constituents: ricinic oil 40-50% (incl. glycerides of ricinoleic acid, oleic/stearic/linoleic acid), phosphorus, beta-sitosterol, ricin, ricinine
Effective qualities: sweet, pungent, neutral
    stimulating, decongesting, stabilizing, calming
Tropism: digestive, respiratory, lymphatic systems
    Spleen, Liver channels
    Fluid body

ACTIONS AND INDICATIONS

intestinal stimulant: laxative: constipation with hard abdominal distension
uterine stimulant, parturient: labor induction, stalled labor (uterine dystocia), miscarriage, retained placenta
resolvent detoxicant, anti-inflammatory, detumescent: sores, boils, carbuncles, abscesses, acute dermatitis, laryngitis, edema, cysts, benign tumors
lymphatic decongestant: lymphadenitis, lymph gland TB
analgesic: headache, earache, arthralgia
antiprolapse: rectal, uterine prolapse
cytophylactic: scar tissue, adhesions
Miscellaneous: scabies, tinea, scrofula, deafness, facial palsy, pyoderma, tuberculous adenitis, strabismus

PREPARATION

Use: The bean Ricinus Bi Ma Zi is mainly used externally in swabs, compresses, etc., for all the above conditions. The extracted oil, castor oil, may be used in the same way as the seed (use hexane-free cold-pressed oil if possible). External applications have derivative as well as topical effects. Thus, the crushed seeds or the oil are applied to the crown of the head for organ prolapse (acupoint GV 20), to the center of the foot soles for uterine stimulation (acupoint Ki 1), to the opposite side of the face for facial palsy, and so on.

For internal use, the seeds should be boiled for 2 hours to remove their toxicity and then decocted in fresh water. One-time internal use is fine with conditions such as stalled labor, with placental retention and acute constipation, even if the raw castor seed is used.

Bi Ma Zi literally means "tick hemp seed" from its resemblance to cattle ticks.

Dosage: Preboiled seeds: 4-10 g
    Oil: 4-16 ml

Caution: For internal use it is best to use only pre-boiled Castor seeds, and to limit their use to acute conditions needing treatment over two or three days only. The raw seeds are designed to be taken internally only once or twice because of their fairly rapid cumulative toxicity. Do not use the seeds or the oil either internally or topically during pregnancy, except in the obstetrical conditions mentioned above.

Gastrointestinal Relaxants

REMEDIES TO RELAX DIGESTION, REDUCE COLIC AND RELIEVE ABDOMINAL PAIN

➥ CIRCULATE THE QI IN THE MIDDLE AND RELEASE CONSTRAINT

Intestinal spasmolytics, analgesics

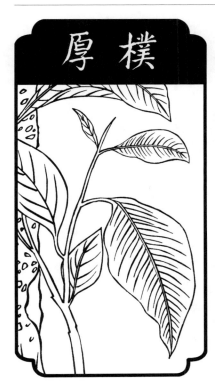

Magnolia Hou Po
Magnolia Bark

Botanical source: *Magnolia officinalis* Rehder et Wilson or *M. biloba* R. et W. or *M. obovata* R. et W. (Magnoliaceae)
Pharmaceutical name: Cortex Magnoliae officinalis
Chinese names: Hou Po, Chuan Po, Hou Bu, Hou Pi (Mand); Hau Pok, Chyun Pok (Cant)
Other names: Koboku (Jap)
Habit: Large deciduous tree growing in the foothills and mountains of Central China; also cultivated; large, cream white, fragrant solitary terminal flowers bloom in spring.
Part used: the bark; also the flower

Therapeutic category: mild remedy with minimal chronic toxicity
Constituents: essential oil 1% (incl. beta-eudesmol, machilol, magnolol, honokiol, pinenes, phenols magnolol, isomagnolol), alkaloids magnocurarine, magnoflorine, salicifoline, tannin
Effective qualities: pungent, bitter, a bit astringent, warm, dry
    relaxing, stimulating
Tropism: digestive, respiratory, reproductive systems
    Spleen, Stomach, Lung, Large Intestine channels
    Air body

ACTIONS AND INDICATIONS
intestinal relaxant: analgesic, spasmolytic, carminative: spasmodic and mucogenic digestive disorders with intestinal dyspepsia; acute intestinal colic, IBS, enteritis, diarrhea
broad-spectrum anti-infective: antibacterial, antiviral, antiprotozoal: gastroenteritis, bacterial and amoebic dysentery, malaria, hepatitis, pneumonia, streptococcal infections, microbial toxicosis
aperitive, stimulant laxative: anorexia, constipation
diuretic: dysuria
stimulant emmenagogue: amenorrhea
antiemetic: nausea, vomiting
bronchodilator, expectorant: cough, asthma, bronchitis
hypotensive, muscle relaxant
immune regulator: immune stress with cell-mediated allergies (incl. chronic hepatitis, peptic ulcer, food allergies)

SYMPTOM PICTURES
intestines Qi constraint: abdominal pain, poor appetite, feeling stressed, constipation and/or diarrhea
intestines mucous damp (Spleen damp) / microbial toxicosis: abdominal distension, indigestion, appetite loss, head pressure, vomiting, diarrhea, food allergies
lung Qi constraint with **phlegm damp:** wheezing, chest tightness, coughing up thick white sputum

PREPARATION

Use: The bark Magnolia Hou Po is decocted or used in tincture form. When decocted with other herbs, it is added half way through decocting time.

Dosage: Decoction: 3-10 g
Tincture: 1-4 ml

Caution: Use with caution during pregnancy.

NOTES

Cultivated for its valuable bark in the provinces of the upper Chang Jiang river valley, the magnolia tree yields an important systemic *relaxant* remedy. Magnolia bark is called for when the predominant symptoms are abdominal pain, distension and nausea. The bitter-pungent bark's secondary *laxative* and *astringent* actions are useful when constipation or diarrhea either predominate or alternate—a common occurrence with stress-induced constrained digestive Qi.

Arising from essential oils and alkaloids, the *anti-infective* and *antiallergic* effects of Magnolia bark further extend its range of applications, which includes microbial toxicosis, viral infections and cell-mediated allergies.

Magnolia flower, called **Hou Po Hua** (Mandarin) and **Chyun Pok Fa** (Cantonese), is collected from the same tree. Containing essential oils, it is pungent, bitter, warm and dry in quality, and enters the Spleen and Stomach channels. Magnolia Hou Po Hua is a *gastrointestinal stimulant* and *carminative* that resolves mucous damp in the intestines (Spleen), thereby relieving indigestion, abdominal fullness and pain, and flatulence. Its *emmenagogue* action also treats amenorrhea. It is forbidden in Yin and fluids deficiency conditions. Dose: 3-6 g by infusion.

Magnolia flower should not be confused with **Yulan magnolia bud, Xin Yi Hua,** in the Nose, Throat and Eyes section, which is obtained from entirely different species of *Magnolia*.

Amomum Sha Ren

Wild Cardamom Pod

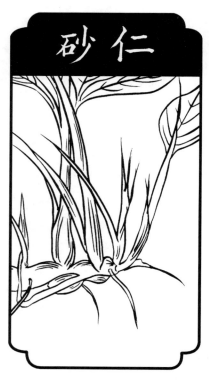

Botanical source: *Amomum villosum* Loureiro or *A. xanthioides* Wallace (Zingiberaceae)
Pharmaceutical name: Fructus seu semen Amomi villosi
Chinese names: Sha Ren, Chun Sha Ren, Yang Chun Sha (Mand); Chan Jai Yan (Cant)
Other names: Tavoy/Bastard cardamom, Grain of paradise, "Sand seed"; Sanin, Shukusha (Jap)
Habit: Perennial subtropical East Asian herb growing in wooded mountain valleys; also cultivated in Guangdong and Hainan; prefers shady, damp conditions; in spring, round flowers grow in a spike pattern diagonally above the rhizome.
Part used: the fruit or seed

Therapeutic category: mild remedy with minimal chronic toxicity
Constituents: essential oil 3.66% (incl. camphor, limonene, linalool, nerodiol, borneol, terpene, bornylacetate)
Effective qualities: pungent, warm, dry
relaxing, stimulating, astringing
Tropism: digestive, reproductive systems
Spleen, Stomach, Kidney channels; Air body

ACTIONS AND INDICATIONS
intestinal relaxant: analgesic spasmolytic, carminative: spasmodic and mucogenic digestive disorders with abdominal and epigastric pain and dyspepsia; intestinal colic, IBS, gastroenteritis, chronic diarrhea, dysentery
antiemetic: nausea, vomiting, morning sickness
fetal relaxant: fetal unrest, imminent miscarriage
interferon inducent

SYMPTOM PICTURES
stomach and intestines Qi constraint: appetite loss, epigastric or abdominal pain and distension, loose stool
intestines mucous damp (Spleen damp): flatulence, abdominal pain, head pressure, belching, diarrhea
intestines cold (Spleen Yang deficiency): chronic loose stool with mucus, fatigue, chilliness

PREPARATION
Use: A short decoction or long infusion is best for the fruit pod Amomum Sha Ren; the tincture is a good alternative.
Dosage: Short decoction (2-5 minutes) or long infusion (20 minutes): 2-7 g
　　　Tincture: 1-3 ml
Caution: Contraindicated in Yin deficiency with empty heat.

NOTES
Like other cardamom types used in Chinese medicine, this commonly used variety has a very high aromatic oil content. Wild cardamom's *spasmolytic, analgesic* actions address abdominal and epigastric pain—keynote symptoms to guide us in its formula applications.

The fruit Sha Ren consists of seeds and pod. When the **seeds** alone are used, the remedy is called **Guang Sha Ren.** It is somewhat stronger than the whole fruit. Dose: 2-5 g

The **shell** alone is called **Sha Ren Ke;** it is somewhat weaker than the fruit. Dose: 3-7 g.

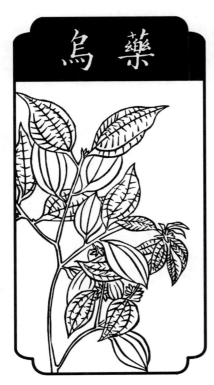

Lindera Wu Yao
Lindera Root

Botanical source: *Lindera strychnifolia* (Sieb. et Zucc.) Villars (Lauraceae)
Pharmaceutical name: Radix Linderae
Chinese names: Wu Yao, Tai Wu, Mei Zi (Mand); Toi Wu (Cant)
Other names: Tien-tai spicebush, "Black medicine"; Uyaku (Jap)
Habit: Evergreen shrub or small tree from Central and South China and Taiwan, growing in thickets along exposed mountain slopes; umbels of small, aromatic, pale viridian flowers bloom in summer.
Part used: the root

Therapeutic category: mild remedy with minimal chronic toxicity
Constituents: essential oil, incl. furanosesquiterpenes (incl. linderol, linderane, lindenenol, lindenene, lindestrene, linderalactone, linderoxide, lindestrenolide, lendrene, lindenenone, linderene acetate), lindereic acid, linderazulene, laurolitsine
Effective qualities: pungent, astringent, warm, dry
　　　relaxing, stimulating, astringing
Tropism: digestive, reproductive, urinary systems
　　　Spleen, Stomach, Lung, Kidney channels
　　　Air body

ACTIONS AND INDICATIONS
digestive relaxant: spasmolytic, analgesic, anti-inflammatory: spasmodic digestive disorders with abdominal, epigastric and chest pain; intestinal colic, IBS, hernia, gastritis, colitis, backache, rheumatic bone and joint pains
digestive stimulant, carminative: gastrointestinal dyspepsia
antiemetic: vomiting, nausea
diaphoretic
uterine stimulant/relaxant: amenorrhea, delayed menses, spasmodic dysmenorrhea
sympathetic nervous stimulant, hypertensive
urogenital restorative, astringent: urinary incontinence with enuresis, pollakiuria; leucorrhea, gonorrhea
hemostatic: hemorrhage
metabolic stimulant: weight loss
antibacterial, antiviral, interferon inducent: herpes simplex, cold sores

SYMPTOM PICTURES
stomach and intestines Qi constraint: epigastric or abdominal pain and distension, flatulence, cold in the lower abdomen

uterus cold: delayed, scanty or absent menses, menstrual cramps

PREPARATION NOTES
Use: The root Lindera Wu Yao is decocted or used in tincture form.
Dosage: Decoction: 3-10 g
Tincture: 2-4 ml
Caution: Being a *uterine stimulant,* this remedy is forbidden during pregnancy. Because of its *hypertensive* action, it is contraindicated also in high blood pressure, and in conditions presenting internal heat and Qi deficiency.

NOTES
Lindera root from the southern province Guangxi is both *relaxing* and *stimulating* to digestive, urinary and reproductive functions. Constrained Qi conditions with cold are the root's main energetic indication in clinical practice, as the two symptom pictures above make clear. In physiologic symptom terms, Lindera treats pain arising from spasm and inflammation caused by chronic metabolic and sympathetic nervous insufficiency. A long string of sesquiterpenes can be seen among its volatile oil components, which are clearly *spasmolytic, analgesic* and *inflammatory* by nature.

Lindera root's *analgesic* property is not limited to relieving pain from digestive disorders, however. Musculoskeletal and menstrual pain also thereby find relief, and are often treated with other pain-relieving remedies from those respective categories. Because of its additional *uterine stimulant* action, Lindera is particularly often used for spasmodic dysmenorrhea as well as amenorrhea.

Lindera root shares many therapeutic similarities with the Western remedies Wild ginger root, Hazelwort root and Juniper berry.

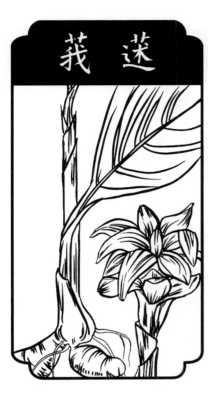

Curcuma E Zhu
Zedoary Root

Botanical source: *Curcuma zedoaria* (Berg) Roscoe or *C. kwangsiensis* S. Lee et C.F. Liang (Zingiberaceae)
Pharmaceutical name: Rhizoma Curcumae zedoariae
Chinese names: E Zhu, Peng Er Zhu, Yu Jin Xiang (Mand); Ou Sat (Cant)
Other names: Gajutsu (Jap)
Habit: Aromatic perennial herb found throughout southern Asia; grows in damp soil; also cultivated.
Part used: the rhizome

Therapeutic category: mild remedy with minimal chronic toxicity
Constituents: essential oil 1-2.5% (incl. sesquiterpenes curcumenol, cucurmol, cucurmadiol, procurcumenol, zedorene, zedoarone, curzerene, furanodienone, curzerenone, curdione, pinenes), starch
Effective qualities: pungent, bitter, warm, dry
relaxing, stimulating, dissolving, diluting
Tropism: digestive, reproductive, nervous, immune systems
Liver, Spleen channels; Air, Fluid bodies

ACTIONS AND INDICATIONS

digestive relaxant: analgesic, spasmolytic: spasmodic digestive disorders with epigastric and abdominal pain; intestinal colic, IBS, colitis

digestive stimulant: gastrointestinal dyspepsia, liver and spleen enlargement

uterine relaxant/stimulant: spasmodic dysmenorrhea, amenorrhea

anticontusion, vulnerary, anticoagulant, anti-inflammatory, antibacterial: injuries, wounds, sprains, strains with pain and swelling; thrombosis

antitumoral, interferon inducent: tumors, incl. cancer (esp. cervical, vulval, uterine, lymphatic [lymphosarcoma], dermal)

leukocyte stimulant: leukopenia

immune regulator: immune stress with immune complex disorders

SYMPTOM PICTURES

stomach and intestines Qi constraint with **food stagnation:** epigastric or abdominal distension, pain and fullness, nausea, abdominal lumps

uterus Qi constraint and Blood congealed: painful, difficult menses, absent menses with cramping pains, clotted flow

PREPARATION

Use: The root Curcuma E Zhu is either decocted or used in tincture form. The essential oil may also be extracted (see below).
Dosage: Decoction: 3-10 g
Tincture: 1-4 ml
Caution: Being a strong *uterine stimulant*, this remedy is forbidden during pregnancy. Zedoary should also be used with circumspection in heavy menses, and in Blood and Qi deficiency conditions.

NOTES

The main Western medical use of the highly aromatic Zedoary root in the Far East is in the treatment of cervical, skin and lymph cancer. The root contains three *antitumoral* compounds, curzeronone and the essential oil fractions curcumol and curdione, and additionally produces interferon. The essential oil extract, used by preference, is thought to be most effective in the early stages when it can prevent surgical or radiotherapeutic intervention (Chang and But 1987).

In terms of vitalistic medicine, the *relaxant* and *stimulant* Zedoary root covers both Qi constraint and Blood congealed symptom patterns, especially those affecting menstrual and digestive functions presenting pain.

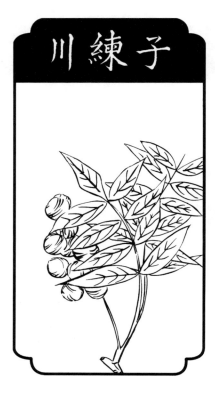

Melia Chuan Lian Zi
Sichuan Beadtree Berry

Botanical source: *Melia toosendan* Siebold et Zuccarini (Meliaceae)
Pharmaceutical name: Fructus Meliae toosendanis
Chinese names: Chuan Lian Zi, Jin Ling Zi, Ku Lian Zi (Mand); Chyun Ling Ji (Cant)
Other names: Sichuan chinaberry; Senrenshi (Jap)
Habit: Deciduous tree from Sichuan, growing wild by roadsides and waste places; also cultivated; blooms in summer with panicles of terminal/axillary purple flowers.
Part used: the fruit

Therapeutic category: medium-strength remedy with some chronic toxicity
Constituents: toosendanin, resin, tannin, fatty oil (incl. stearic/palmitic/lauric/valerianic acids)
Effective qualities: bitter, astringent, cold, dry
relaxing, calming, sinking
Tropism: digestive system
Liver, Stomach, Small Intestine channels
Air body

ACTIONS AND INDICATIONS
digestive relaxant: analgesic spasmolytic: spasmodic digestive disorders with abdominal, epigastric and right subcostal pain; intestinal colic, IBS, hepatitis, hernia, intestinal parasites
anthelmintic (vermifuge): intestinal parasites (esp. roundworm and tapeworm [ascariasis, enterobiasis])
parasiticide: tinea of scalp, earthworm, leech
antifungal: candidiasis; *Crytococci, Blatomyces*
antibacterial

SYMPTOM PICTURE
intestines Qi constraint with **damp heat:** epigastric or abdominal pain, general heaviness, thirst

PREPARATION
Use: The fruit Melia Chuan Lian Zi is decocted or used in tincture form.
Dosage: Decoction: 4-10 g
Tincture: 1-3 ml
Caution: Forbidden in stomach cold conditions. Do not take on its own continuously because of some cumulative toxicity.

NOTES
The dark, shrunken fruits of the beadtree from Sichuan are a supplementary remedy for pain in the main trunk, whatever the cause. The berry is especially indicated for pain generated by Qi constraining the intestines, or from parasites. Its *vermifuge* action, good as it is, is not as reliable as the bark of the related Melia Ku Lian Pi, Beadtree root bark.

Santalum Tan Xiang
Sandalwood

Botanical source: *Santalum album* L. (Santalaceae)
Chinese names: Tan Xiang, Bai Tan Xiang (Mand); Tang Heung (Cant)
Category: mild remedy with minimal chronic toxicity
Constituents: essential oil (incl. santalol, santene, santalene, santenone, santalic acid, santaldehyde)
Effective qualities: pungent, warm, dry; calming, astringing, restoring, relaxing
Tropism: digestive, respiratory, reproductive systems; Spleen, Stomach, Lung, Heart channels

ACTIONS: *Spasmolytic, analgesic, astringent, mucostatic, anti-inflammatory, demulcent, anti-infective, detoxicant, antidepressant, reproductive restorative*
INDICATIONS: Qi constraint syndromes with abdominal pain; intestinal colic, IBS, gastroenteritis, cholera, chest pain, angina pectoris; acute and chronic infections (e.g. urinary tract and venereal infections, incl. gonorrhea); bronchitis, catarrhal discharges, lung TB, dry cough; impotence, frigidity, infertility.
Dosage: Decoction: 1-3 g
Tincture: 0.25-2 ml
Essential oil: 8-12 drops in some water
Caution: Forbidden in hot conditions due to Yin deficiency.

Aquilaria Chen Xiang
Aloeswood

Botanical source: *Aquilaria agallocha* Roxburgh or *A. sinensis* (Lour.) Gilg (Aquilariaceae)
Chinese names: Chen Xiang, Luo Shui Chen (Mand); Chan Heung (Cant)
Other names: Lign aloes, Calambac, Eaglewood; "Sinking aromatic"; Jinko (Jap)
Habit: Large evergreen pan-Asian tree growing in forests; small greenish flowers bloom in early summer on slim pilose pedicels.
Category: mild remedy with minimal chronic toxicity
Constituents: oleoresin with agarospirol, agarol, agarofuran, selinane, sesquiterpenes (bauimuxinol and dehydrobaimuxinol) benzylactone, hydrocinnamic acid
Effective qualities: bitter, a bit pungent and sweet, warm, dry; relaxing, stimulating, calming
Tropism: digestive, respiratory systems; Spleen, Stomach, Lung, Kidney channels

ACTIONS: *Spasmolytic, analgesic, laxative, antiemetic, bronchodilator, diuretic, antimicrobial*
INDICATIONS: Spasmodic digestive disorders with epigastric and abdominal pain and lumps (stomach and intestines Qi constraint, and stomach cold syndromes); intestinal colic, chronic enteritis, colitis, IBS, constipation; nausea, vomiting, morning sickness, hiccups, belching; wheezing, tight chest, asthma, emphysema.
Dosage: Decoction: 1-4 g
Tincture: 1-2 ml
Caution: Use with care in prolapsed conditions due to Qi deficiency, and in Yin deficiency with signs of empty heat.
NOTES: The Aloeswood tree, now possibly an endangered species, is found in a region stretching from Iran to the southern Chinese province Guangdong. The heartwood—the finest coming from the island of Hainan—went into the most select Daoist incense blends, and aloeswood fragrance reached its apotheosis during the Tang era. In Chinese medicine, Aloeswood is used as a *relaxant/stimulant* remedy for the same Qi constraint conditions of the digestive tract as it was in Greek/Galenic medicine. The highly effective *antibacterial* property perfectly complement its *analgesic* action for chronic intestinal infections, clinical and preclinical.

Citrus Fo Shou Gan
Finger Lemon Fruit

Botanical source: *Citrus medica* var. *sarcodactylis* Swingle (Rutaceae)
Chinese names: Fo Shou Gan, Fo Shou, Chen Fo Shou (Mand); Fut Sau Gam, Fut Sau (Cant)
Habit: Small thorny evergreen tree from China and Indochina; cultivated in gardens; flowers in summer.
Category: mild remedy with minimal chronic toxicity
Constituents: essential oil (incl. limettin, citropten, limonene, steroline), nomilin, flavonoids (incl. traces diosmin and hesperidin), coumarin, sitosterol, daucosterol, cinnamic/palmitic/succinic acids
Effective qualities: pungent, bitter, sour, warm; relaxing, stimulating
Tropism: digestive, respiratory, biliary systems; Liver, Stomach, Lung channels

ACTIONS: *Spasmolytic, cholagogue, carminative, analgesic, antiemetic, bronchodilator, expectorant*
INDICATIONS: Spasmodic digestive disorders with dyspepsia, abdominal and costal pain and distension (stomach Qi constraint syndrome); intestinal and biliary colic, IBS, cholecystitis; nausea, vomiting; wheezing, chest distension (lung Qi constraint syndrome); chronic bronchitis, emphysema.
Dosage: Decoction: 3-10 g
Tincture: 1-2 ml
Caution: Use cautiously when Qi constraint is absent and in Yin deficiency conditions with heat.
NOTES: Finger lemon fruit, whose fragrant odor has graced Chinese interiors for many a millenium, is essentially a *relaxant* remedy. Given for spasmodic Qi constraint conditions affecting gastric, thoracic and biliary functions, the fruit especially relieves distension and pain.
  Finger lemon flower, Fo Shou Hua (Fut Sau Fa in Cantonese), is similarly used and reputedly more effective than the fruit for emphysema.

Aristolochia Qing Mu Xiang
Green Birthwort Root

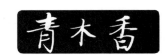

Botanical source: *Aristolochia debilis* Siebold et Zuccarini or *A. contorta* Bunge (Aristolichochiaceae)
Chinese names: Qing Mu Xiang, Tian Xian Teng, Ma Dou Ling Gen, She Shen (Mand); Ching Mok Heung (Cant)
Habit: Perennial vine from temperate China, found on field edges and roadsides; purple-green, trumpet-like single axillary flowers open in summer.
Therapeutic category: medium-strength remedy with some cumulative toxicity
Constituents: magnoflorine, aristolochine, cyclanoline, aristolochic acid, debilic acid, aristolactam, allantoin
Effective qualities: bitter, pungent, cool, dry; relaxing, calming, stimulating
Tropism: digestive, nervous, vascular, respiratory, immune systems; Stomach, Large Intestine, Lung channels

ACTIONS: *Spasmolytic, carminative, antiemetic, analgesic, anti-inflammatory, hypotensive, antitussive, bronchodilator, expectorant, anti-infective (immunostimulant and antiseptic), detoxicant, antivenomous, leukocyte stimulant*
INDICATIONS: Dyspepsia with flatulence, abdominal pain of all types; intestinal colic, rheumatic pain, toothache; hypertension with dizziness; acute bronchitis, wheezing, coughing; boils, chronic abscess, laryngitis, stomatitis, poisonous snake and insect bites; tumors, cancer; chemotherapy and radiotherapy, leukopenia; bruises, bone injury.
Dosage: Decoction: 4-10 g
Tincture: 1-3 ml
Caution: Do not use continuously on its own because of medium-strength status. Normal doses may occasionally produce nausea, vomiting, mouth dryness and constipation. These signs would intensify with high-dosage and/or continuous use.

Allium Xie Bai
Chinese Chive Bulb

Botanical source: *Allium macrostemon* L. (Liliaceae)
Chinese names: Xie Bai, Jiu Bai, Hai Bai (Mand)
Category: mild remedy with minimal chronic toxicity
Constituents: scorodose, trace elements, ascorbic acid

Effective qualities: pungent, bitter, warm, dry; relaxing, stimulating
Tropism: digestive, respiratory systems; Stomach, Large Intestine, Lung channels

ACTIONS: *Spasmolytic, analgesic, expectorant*
INDICATIONS: Dysentery with diarrhea and tenesmus; abdominal pain/colic from intestines Qi constraint or parasites; chest pain, bronchitis, asthma with lung phlegm cold/damp with Qi constraint.
Dosage: Decoction: 4-10 g (30-60 g of the fresh bulb)
  Tincture: 1-4 ml
Caution: None.

Amomum Cao Guo
Cochin Cardamom Fruit

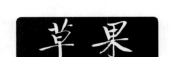

Botanical source: *Amomum Tsao-ko* Crevost et Lemaire (Zingiberaceae)
Chinese names: Cao Guo (Ren) (M.); Chou Gwat (C.)
Category: mild remedy with minimal chronic toxicity

Constituents: essential oil (incl. benzines)
Effective qualities: pungent, warm, dry; relaxing, stimulating
Tropism: digestive systems; Spleen, Stomach channels

ACTIONS: *Spasmolytic, analgesic, antiemetic, antipyretic*
INDICATIONS: Epigastric and abdominal pain/colic with dyspepsia and nausea from stomach and intestines Qi constraint or stomach cold; food stagnation caused by excessive protein intake, dysbiosis or food poisoning; intermittent/remittent fevers (incl. malaria).
Dosage: Decoction: 3-10 g
  Tincture: 1-4 ml
Caution: Forbidden in Blood and Qi deficiency. Do not use without cold and damp present.

Litchi Li Zhi He
Lychee Seed

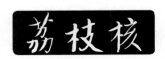

Botanical source: *Litchi chinensis* Sonnerat (Sapindaceae)
Chinese names: Li Zhi He (Mand); Lai Jik Ho (Cant)
Category: mild remedy with minimal chronic toxicity
Constituents: tannins, saponins, glycin

Effective qualities: astringent, warm; calming, astringing
Tropism: digestive, reproductive, nervous systems; Liver, Stomach channels

ACTIONS: *Analgesic, astringent*
INDICATIONS: Painful conditions of various kinds (incl. epigastric, abdominal, hernial, menstrual, orchitic, testicular).
Dosage: Decoction: 0.2-0.4 gm
Caution: Not to be used unless damp and cold are present.
NOTES: The **Lychee fruit** has similar properties and is taken in 4-10 g dosage in decoction or powder form.

Arca Wa Leng Zi
Cockle Shell

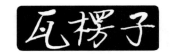

Zoological source: *Arca inflata/subcrenala/granosa* and spp. (Arcidae)
Chinese names: Wa Leng Zi, Kui Ge, Ling Pei (Mand); Ng Leng Ji (Cant)
Category: mild remedy with minimal chronic toxicity
Constituents: calcium carbonate, trace minerals, magnesium, sodium phosphate, iron
Effective qualities: sweet, salty, neutral; calming, dissolving, sinking
Tropism: digestive, reproductive systems; Liver, Spleen, Stomach, Lung channels

ACTIONS: *Analgesic, antacid antisecretory, spasmolytic, detumescent*
INDICATIONS: Epigastric pain with acid regurgitation, acid dyspepsia, peptic ulcer, abdominal lumps (mobile and immobile, incl. phantom tumors); benign tumors (incl. gynecological); goitre; spleen and liver enlargement.
Dosage: Long decoction: 10-30 g
Powder and pill: 3-10 g
The cockle shells should be broken up or powdered before use and decocted alone before any other ingredients are added. The toasted or calcined shell is said to have a greater *antacid* effect in gastric and duodenal ulcers.
Caution: None.

Gastrointestinal Sedatives

REMEDIES TO REDUCE INTESTINAL INFECTION AND STOP DIARRHEA

➥ CLEAR DAMP HEAT FROM THE LARGE INTESTINE

Anti-inflammatory antiseptic astringents

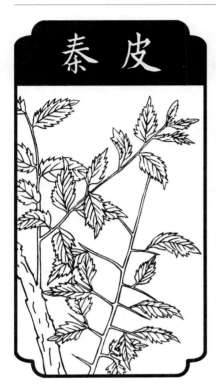

Fraxinus Qin Pi
Korean Ash Bark

Botanical source: *Fraxinus rhynchophyllae* Hance or *F. bungeana* De Candolle or *F. chinensis* Roxburgh or *F. paxiana* Lingelsheim (Oleaceae)
Pharmaceutical name: Cortex Fraxini
Chinese names: Qin Pi, Hua Qu Liu, Jin Pi, Xin Mu (Mand); Ching Pei, Chan Pei (Cant)
Other names: Northern ash; Shinpi (Jap)
Habit: Deciduous tree from Northeast China and Korea, found in forests and on sunny hillsides together with broad-leaved trees; flowers in early summer.
Part used: the branch bark

Therapeutic category: mild remedy with minimal chronic toxicity
Constituents: coumarins (incl. fraxetin, fraxin, aesculin, aesculetin), tannin, alkaloids
Effective qualities: bitter and astringent, cold, dry
    astringing, calming
Tropism: digestive, nervous, muscular, urinary systems
    Large Intestine, Liver, Lung channels
    Warmth, Air bodies

ACTIONS AND INDICATIONS

gastrointestinal sedative: anti-infective, astringent, anti-inflammatory: digestive, respiratory and urogenital infections (incl. acute enteritis, dysentery, conjunctivitis)
urogenital mucostatic: leucorrhea
bronchial relaxant, antitussive, expectorant: asthma, cough, chronic bronchitis
diuretic resolvent detoxicant, analgesic: rheumatism, arthritis, uric acid diathesis
vision restorative, optitropic: poor eyesight, corneal opacity, cataract
anticoagulant: blood hyperviscosity, thrombosis
ultraviolet and infrared protectant

SYMPTOM PICTURES

intestines damp heat: burning, urgent passing of stool, diarrhea, thirst
lung Qi constraint: chronic wheezing, coughing
metabolic toxicosis / wind damp obstruction: muscular or joint pain, swollen red joints

PREPARATION

Use: The bark Fraxinus Qin Pi is decocted or used in tincture form.
Dosage: Decoction: 4-16 g
    Tincture: 1-3 ml
Caution: Contraindicated in diarrhea from deficiency cold.

Notes

The use of Korean ash bark is similar to that of the European ash, *Fraxinus excelsior*, as far as painful uric acid, gouty and rheumatic conditions are concerned (wind damp obstruction syndrome). Unlike the latter, however, Korean ash bark with its astringent, cold, dry qualities is also used to treat acute bacterial intestinal infections with damp heat, and asthmatic conditions.

The coumarins in this remedy (most of which are also present in the Western remedy Horse chestnut) have a *blood-thinning* and *anticoagulant* effect and, therefore, are useful in conditions of hyperviscous blood and a tendency to thromboses.

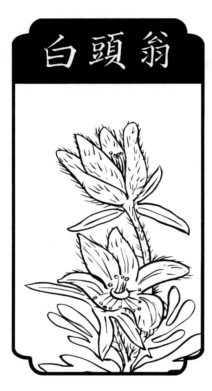

Pulsatilla Bai Tou Weng
Asian Pasqueflower Root

Botanical source: *Pulsatilla chinensis* (Bunge) Regel and spp. (Ranunculaceae)
Pharmaceutical name: Radix Pulsatillae
Chinese names: Bai Tou Weng, Bei Zi Cao (Mand); Baak Toi Yang (Cant)
Other names: Nodding anemone, "White headed grandfather"; Hakutoo (Jap)
Habit: Perennial herb from Inner Magolia and North China, found in foothills on grassy slopes and in thickets; large, purple solitary flowers bloom in summer.
Part used: the root

Therapeutic category: medium-strength remedy with some chronic toxicity
Constituents: glycoside proanemonin, triterpenoid saponins up to 9% (incl. okinalin, okinalein, anemonin), anemoside B4 and A3, stigmasterol, sitosterol, hederagenin, oleanolic acid, anemone camphor
Effective qualities: bitter, astringent, cold, dry
astringing, calming, restoring
Tropism: digestive, cardiovascular, lymphatic systems
Large Intestine, Liver, Stomach channels; Warmth, Fluid bodies

Actions and Indications

intestinal sedative: anti-inflammatory, anti-infective (antibacterial, antiprotozoal, antifungal): acute infections (incl. febrile), incl. enteritis with diarrhea, dysentery (bacterial and amoebic); microbial toxicosis, candidiasis, trichomonas vaginalis
detoxicant, antipyretic: mumps, furunculosis
analgesic, spasmolytic: pain in general (incl. abdominal pain), abdominal lumps, phantom tumors; bone pain, toothache, myalgia
hemostatic: epistaxis, bleeding hemorrhoids
cardiotonic
Miscellaneous: lymph gland TB, goiter

Symptom Picture

intestines damp heat: abdominal pain, painful urgent bowel movement, loose stool, blood in stool

Preparation

Use: The root Pulsatilla Bai Tou Weng is decocted or used in tincture form. Douches and vaginal sponges may be used for vaginal yeast infections.
Dosage: Decoction: 8-18 g
Tincture: 2-5 ml
Caution: Forbidden in diarrhea from intestinal deficiency and cold.

NOTES

Unlike the Western pasqueflower (*Pulsatilla vulgaris*), the Chinese species is valued mainly for its comprehensive action on both acute dysenterial infections (bacterial, amoebic) and chronic dysbiotic subinfections of the terrain, such as microbial toxicosis (bacterial) and "candidiasis" (fungal). Note, in this connection, that only the species *Pulsatilla chinensis* is active against trichomonas vaginalis (Chang and But 1987). Nevertheless, there is a fair degree of therapeutic overlap between Chinese, European and American varieties of *Pulsatilla,* differing health concerns and cultural contexts notwithstanding.

Galla Wu Bei Zi
Chinese Sumac Gallnut

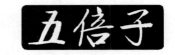

Botanical source: *Rhus sinensis* Miller and *R. potanii* Maximowicz and *R. punjabensis* Stew. var. *sinica* (Diels) Rehder et Wilson (Anacardiaceae)

Chinese names: Wu Bei Zi, Bai Zhong Cang (Mand); Ng Pan Ji (Cant)

Part used: the insect excretion found on the leaves of various Asian sumac trees

Category: mild remedy with minimal chronic toxicity

Constituents: tannic acid 50-70%, resin, starch, wax, lipids

Effective qualities: sour, astringent, salty, cold; astringing, solidifying, stabilizing

Tropism: digestive, respiratory, vascular systems; Large Intestine, Stomach, Lung, Kidney, Liver channels

ACTIONS: *Anti-infective (antibacterial, antiviral), astringent, hemostatic, anhydrotic, vulnerary, detoxicant, antitussive, expectorant*

INDICATIONS: Acute and chronic enteritic conditions with damp heat or damp cold; bacillary dysentery (gram-positive cocci [*Staphylococcus, Streptococcus*], gram-negative bacilli [*Salmonella, Shigella, Pseudomonas*]); chronic diarrhea, blood in stool, rectal prolapse with blood, bleeding hemorrhoids; night sweats, chronic cough, bronchitis, spermatorrhea, leucorrhea, swollen throat.

Topically for boils, sores, hemorrhoids, ringworm, skin and mouth ulcers, oozing sores, scar tissue, burns, bleeding injuries.

Dosage: Decoction: 2-7 g powdered or decocted.
Tincture: 0.5-3 ml

Caution: Forbidden with cough from wind cold/heat invasion (onset of respiratory infection), and with lung heat, or acute bronchial conditions.

Hemsleya Xue Dan
Hemsleya Tuber

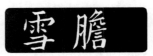

Botanical source: *Hemsleya amabilis* Diels or *H. Macrosperma* C.Y. Wu or *H. chinensis* Cogniaux and spp. (Cucurbitaceae)

Chinese names: Xue Dan, Luo Guo Di, Qu Lian, Jin Gui Lian (Mand); Hat Daam (Cant)

Category: medium-strength remedy with some chronic toxicity

Constituents: tetracyclotriterpenoid bitters (hemsleyadin), dihydrocucurbitacin acetate, dihydrocucurbitacin F, saponins (qingsidai) with aglycone oleanolic acid.

Effective qualities: bitter, dry, cold; calming

Tropism: digestive, cardiovascular, reproductive systems; Large Intestine, Liver, Heart channels

ACTIONS: *Broad-spectrum anti-infective, antibacterial, anti-inflammatory, antipyretic, analgesic, hypotensive, antilipemic, antitumoral*

INDICATIONS: Febrile infections, incl. acute bacillary dysentery, enteritis with diarrhea, abdominal pain, tenesmus; acute cervicitis, tonsilitis, bronchitis, lung TB; epigastric/abdominal pain; coronary deficiency, high blood pressure.

Dosage: Decoction: 6-18 g
Tincture: 2-4 ml
Caution: Not to be used at maximum dosage on its own for any length of time.
NOTES: Hemsleya tuber has shown a very high success rate in treating cervicitis. The simple or compound pill is inserted directly in the vagina as a pessary during the course of seven days.

Portulacca Ma Chi Xian
Purslane Herb

Botanical source: *Portulacca oleracea* L. (Caryophyllaceae)
Chinese names: Ma Chi Xian (Mand); Ma Ji Yin (Cant)
Category: mild remedy with minimal chronic toxicity
Constituents: mucilage, coumarins, flavones, trace minerals, alkoloids, glycosides (cardiac, anthraquinone) omega-3 fatty acids, organic acids, vitamins, minerals
Effective qualities: sour, sweet, salty, cold, moist; calming
Tropism: digestive, reproductive systems; Large Intestine, Spleen, Heart, Liver channels

ACTIONS: *Anti-infective (antibacterial, antifungal, antiparasitic), detoxicant, anti-inflammatory, demulcent, antivenomous, hemostatic*
INDICATIONS: Damp heat and fire toxin conditions (esp. dysentery with blood and pus in stool); intestinal parasites, boils, carbuncles, simple sores, sloughing ulcers, appendicitis, dermatitis, erysipelas, pruritus, urogenital infections with discharge, herpes, postpartum bleeding, snake and wasp bites; eye, mouth, gum and throat inflammation; urinary tract infection.

The fresh herb is highly effective for *Shigella, Salmonella, Staphylococcus*, various fungal infections and hookworm infestation.

Dosage: Decoction: 6-14 g
Tincture: 2-5 ml

Douches, mouthwashes and various external applications are also prepared.

Caution: Forbidden during pregnancy as it is a *uterine stimulant*, and in stomach and intestines cold.

Pteris Feng Wei Cao
Phoenix-Tail Fern

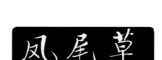

Botanical source: *Pteris multifida* Poiret, *P. ensiformis* Burm. or *P. cretica* L. (Polypodiaceae/Pteridaceae)
Chinese names: Feng Wei Cao (M.); Fun Mai Chou (C.)
Habit: small East Asian tropical fern
Category: mild remedy with minimal chronic toxicity
Constituents: flavonoid, amino acid, phenol
Effective qualities: sweet, bitter, cold; calming, relaxing, astringing, solidifying
Tropism: digestive, respiratory, reproductive systems; Large Intestine, Lung, Liver, Gallbladder channels

ACTIONS: *Anti-infective, anti-inflammatory, analgesic, hemostatic, anthelmintic*
INDICATIONS: Damp heat conditions (incl. enteritis, dysentery, jaundice, hepatitis); tonsillitis, painful laryngitis, mumps, common cold, cough; blood in stool or urine, uterine bleeding; spermatorrhea; cancer (incl. cervical, gastrointestinal); intestinal parasites.

Topically for eczema, nettle rash, boils, injuries, sprains, strains.

Dosage: Decoction: 10-16 g
Tincture: 2-4 ml

External applications are made for traumatic and skin conditions.

Caution: None.

Ailanthus Chun Pi
Tree of Heaven Bark

Botanical source: *Ailanthus altissima* (Miller) Swingle (Simaroubaceae)
Chinese names: Chun Pi, Chu Bai Pi, Chuan Jin Pi (Mand); Chan Pei (Cant)
Habit: Large deciduous tree; blooms in summer in panicles of small greenish-white blossoms.
Part used: the stem bark or root bark
Category: mild remedy with minimal chronic toxicity

Constituents: mersoside, amarolide, quassin, neoquassin, ailantholide, chaparrinone, ailanthine, tannin, oleoresin, resin, mucilage, ceryl alcohol, calcium oxalate crystals, isoquercetin, phlobaphene, ceryl palmitate
Effective qualities: bitter, astringent, dry, cold; astringing, calming, solidifying
Tropism: digestive, reproductive systems; Large Intestine, Liver channels

ACTIONS: *Antibacterial, detoxicant, anti-inflammatory, astringent, hemostatic, mucostatic*
INDICATIONS: Acute and chronic gastroenteritis, dysentery with blood in stool (intestines damp heat syndrome); hemorrhoids; leucorrhea, menorrhagia, congestive dysmenorrhea, premature ejaculation, spermatorrhea.
   Tree of heaven root bark only is also *anthelmintic* and used for tapeworms.
Dosage: Decoction: 3-10 g
   Tincture: 1-3 ml
Caution: Contraindicated in deficiency cold conditions of the stomach and intestines.

Gossampinus Mu Mian Hua
Silk Cotton Tree Flower

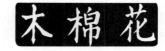

Botanical source: *Gossampinus malabarica* (De Candolle) Merrill (Bombacaceae)
Chinese names: Mu Mian Hua (Mand); Muk Mein Fa (Cant)
Habit: Deciduous tree growing wild along roadsides and on slopes; also cultivated; blooms in spring with single crimson or white flowers.
Part used: the flower
Category: mild remedy with minimal chronic toxicity
Constituents: histamine, proteins, starch
Effective qualities: sweet, cool, dry; astringing, calming
Tropism: digestive system; Large Intestine channel

ACTIONS: *Antibacterial, detoxicant, anti-inflammatory, diuretic, hemostatic, refrigerant*
INDICATIONS: Acute and chronic gastroenteritis, dysentery with blood in stool (intestines damp heat syndrome); functional bleeding, suppuration.
Dosage: Infusion: 6-10 g
   Tincture: 2-4 ml
Caution: None.
NOTES: Silk cotton tree bark, Mu Mian Pi (Mand.) or **Muk Mein Pei** (Cant.) is employed for its *anti-inflammatory* and *analgesic* actions in rheumatic and rheumatoid arthritic conditions (wind damp obstruction syndrome), and for painful sprains and strains. Dose: 15-30 g by decoction, 3-5 ml by tincture.
   The tree root, **Mu Mian Gen** (Mand.) or **Muk Mein Gan** (Cant.) is used to treat epigastric pain and tuberculous lymphadenitis. Dose: 30-60 g by decoction, 4-6 ml by tincture.

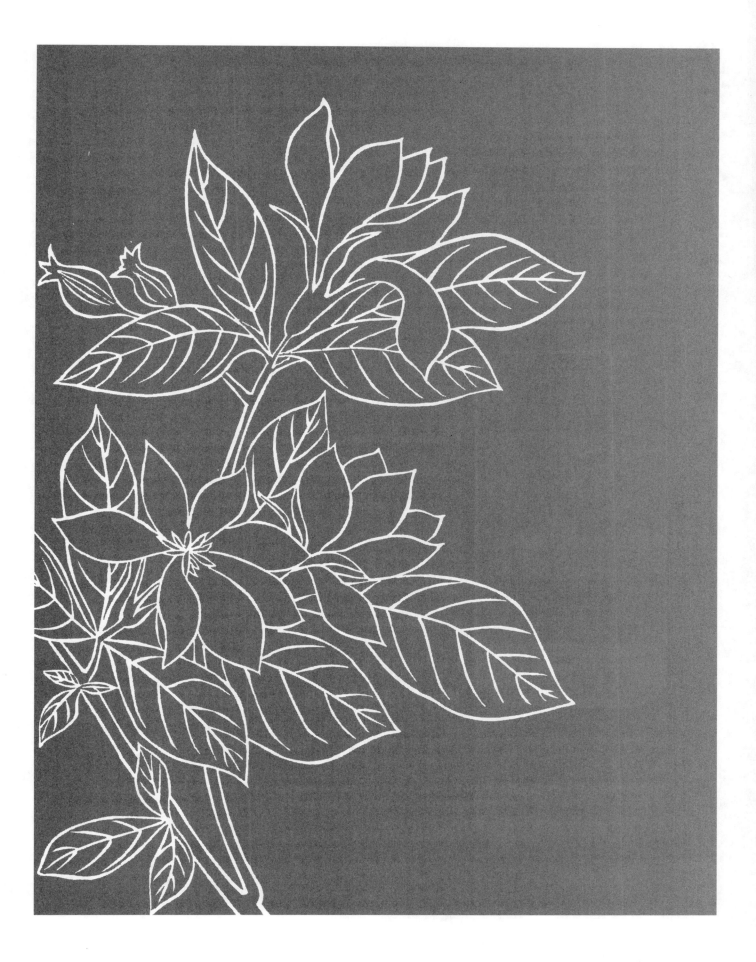

肝胆系统用药

Remedies for the Hepatobiliary System

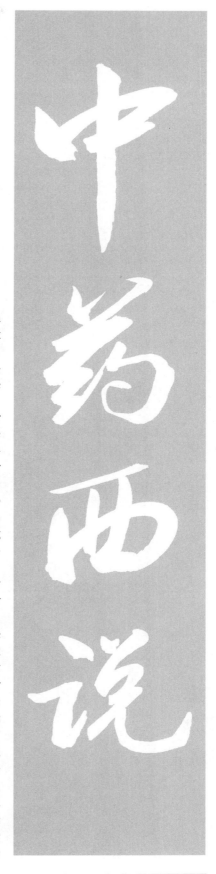

At first glance, the Oriental pharmacy does not seem to contain the same plethora of remedies for the liver and gallbladder that we possess in the West. This impression, however, is misleading. The fact is that the majority of hepatic herbs are found in traditional categories where we would least expect them. There are three reasons for this.

First, Chinese medical terminology does not define the liver exactly as we know it in the West. Many functions of the Chinese organ/channel network "Liver" are in Western physiology neurological and urogenital in nature; hence, looking for hepatic actions in Chinese Liver remedies is often fruitless. Uncaria Gou Teng (Gambir vine twig), for example, is said to "pacify the Liver," but relates to no hepatic pathology as such. It is used for conditions when the "Liver Yang rises," causing dizziness, spasms, convulsions, etc.—clearly neurological disorders.

Second, the traditional Oriental materia medica conversely has many therapeutic categories that include hepatobiliary dysfunctions in different contexts or under different names. Herbs that "clear heat and dry damp," for example, include Scutellaria Huang Qin (Baikal skullcap root), Gentiana Long Dan Cao (Scabrous gentian root) and Sophora Ku Shen (Yellow pagoda tree root), three remedies with a major *choleretic*, or *bile-stimulant*, action. Their *choleretic* effect is simply one action, among others, that contributes to the systemic energetic function of clearing heat and drying damp.

Third, in keeping with Western culture, the Western concept of liver pathology itself leans heavily to the more active Yang aspects of its functions—biliary functions, on one hand, and the active provisioning of nutrients to the bloodstream, on the other. Relatively little thought is given to the more structive Yin aspect of liver functioning which, in contrast, is where Chinese practitioners place most emphasis. We as Westerners are

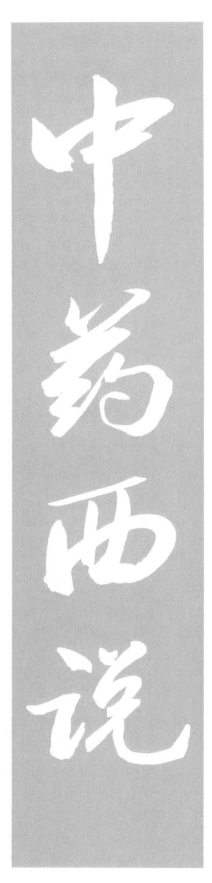

not on the lookout for liver pathology that involves an inability to properly store nutrients. The interesting paradox is that this is precisely where we need to look today for remedies for some of the most serious of contemporary disorders.

With these considerations in mind, we are now in a good position to identify those Chinese botanicals that do, in fact, have Western hepatic and biliary actions. A body of remedies emerges that more than adequately covers the ground of liver and gallbladder pathology. These herbs bring with them a special offering: To the benefit of Western vitalistic medicine, many also do complete justice to the treatment of liver Yin disharmonies.

To this already complex equation we should factor in the following: Herbal medicine with its vitalistic basis and subclinical diagnostic methods is able to detect energetic, preclinical liver and biliary conditions—especially simple Yin and Yang deficiencies of the liver—long before organic tissue pathology results. This accounts for the paucity of Western medical liver conditions in contrast to the six major liver syndromes enumerated by vitalistic medicine.

The liver and gallbladder remedies selected in this text are divided into *restoratives, stimulants* and *relaxants/sedatives*—the four essential herb types of Western energetic herbal medicine.

- ***Hepatobiliary restoratives*** address liver deficiency with blood and nutrient deficiency, presenting weakness, loss of stamina and weight loss.
- ***Hepatobiliary stimulants*** treat deficiencies involving liver congestion and biliary and gastric insufficiency, manifesting epigastric fullness and constipation.
- ***Hepatobiliary relaxants*** and ***sedatives*** address excess conditions such as infection and inflammation of the liver and gallbladder.

The Hepatobiliary Remedies

Restoratives

Because of its roots in ancient, partly prehistoric Daoist culture, Oriental medicine places more value on the Yin than the Yang for health maintenance. In physiological terms, more emphasis is placed on maintaining the Yin than on tonifying the Yang. Nowhere is this emphasis made clearer than in the rich selection of herbs for the liver's anabolic Yin functions of assimilating and storing nutrients. To support these functions, the *hepatobiliary restoratives* actually serve as *hepatic anastative nutritives*. In Oriental texts they are very accurately described as "enriching liver Yin, nourishing the Blood and generating strength."

Liver Yin deficiency is a complex of symptoms typically consisting of low endurance, lack of energy (especially worsening as the day progresses), loss of motivation, excessive introversion, increased appetite, frequent infections and weight loss. If these symptoms are not subclinical, they may be major components of conditions such as malnutrition, anemia, viral infections, chronic hepatitis, endogenous depression, as well as such metabolic disorders as glycogen storage disorders and hypoglycemia. These conditions are precisely where *liver restoratives* would be called for.

The taste of *hepatic anastative nutritives* is invariably quite sweet with mild warmth. Their actions include assisting the liver to filter bacteria, and process and house glycogen, blood and protein. *Hepatic restorative* remedies include Rehmannia Shu Di Huang (Prepared rehmannia root, a type of figwort from the China coast) and four types of fruits rich in minerals, trace elements and vitamins, among them Lycium Gou Qi Zi (Wolfberry, the scarlet berry of a subtropical scrambler) and Zizyphus Da Zao (Jujube berry, from the common South Asian shrub or tree).

Stimulants

Two types of **liver/gallbladder Yang deficiency** conditions are treatable by *hepatobiliary stimulants*. The first, a simple **liver Yang deficiency,** arises from the liver's inability to mobilize glycogen reserves, amino acids, fats and blood—a major aspect of its Yang functions. (This syndrome sometimes becomes **liver cold** because of the signs of coldness it can generate: feeling deeply chilled, cold extremities, etc.) The symptom picture here is one of lethargy and low energy in the morning, afternoon fatigue, drowsiness after meals, feeling congested and heavy, loss of enthusiasm, joint pains worse in the morning and improved with exercise, dizziness and blurred vision made worse from not eating or stress, sugar cravings, weight problems and general improvement with exercise. As the subclinical condition progresses it lays the ground for further organic pathology, beginning, for example, with jaundice, portal congestion and portal hypertension.

Hepatic decongestants, generating energy, lightness and warmth as they decongest, are the herbs of choice for this condition. They include Artemisia Yin Chen Hao (Downy wormwood herb, a relative to the common Wormwood, *Artemisia absinthium*), Curcuma Yu Jin (Turmeric tuber from tropical Asia and Polynesia) and Eupatorium Pei Lan (Orchid-grass herb, a composite from central and coastal China). The *decongestants* are predominantly bitter, as the bitter taste goads the liver into renewed activity.

When digestive functions are impaired due to insufficient or unavailable flow of bile and gastric secretions, the resultant syndrome is **gallbladder and stomach Yang deficiency** (also known as **gallbladder and stomach Qi stagnation).** Keynote symptoms include acute indigestion with epigastric discomfort and distension after eating, heartburn, nausea, belching, hiccups, sour regurgitation, fullness beneath the right ribs, constipation,

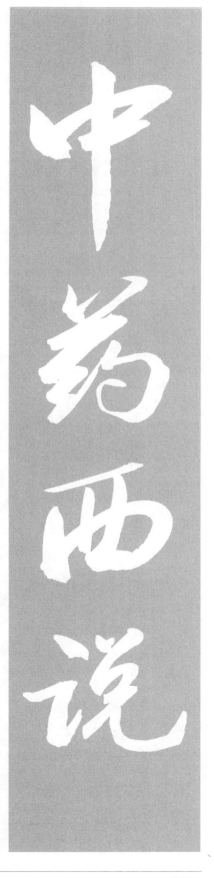

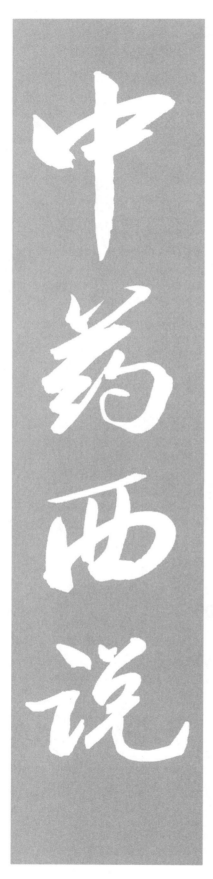

appetite loss, insecurity about health and difficulty making decisions. These symptoms are often found in the context of cirrhosis, and in acute gastritis/gastroenteritis with poor fat digestion.

The type of *hepatobiliary stimulant* preferred for this syndrome is *choleretic* and *cholagogue laxatives;* that is, those that increase bile production or flow, relieve fullness in the epigastrium and promote bowel movement. They include the much used Citrus Chen Pi (Ripe tangerine rind) and the very versatile Saussurea Mu Xiang (Wood aromatic root from the Himalayas), also used in Ayurvedic medicine. Their bitter, pungent, and warm qualities, due to their essential oil content, stimulate the Yang functions of the gallbladder and stomach, relieving fullness and promoting bowel movement.

Note that in strictly traditional Oriental medicine, both the above hepatobiliary syndromes are merged into a single pathology known as **Liver Qi stagnation** or **Liver and Spleen disharmony.** Remedies addressing these symptom pictures are most commonly described as "spreading Liver Qi and transforming accumulation" and "harmonizing the Liver and Spleen." For this and reasons of practical overlap, the botanicals for both syndromes are grouped in a single section.

Relaxants and Sedatives

Because relaxing and sedating the liver are so closely connected, and because the botanical remedies employed are invariably the same, *relaxants* and *sedatives* for the hepatobiliary system are presented as a single group. Specifically, they are *draining hepatic decongestants* that also act on the liver as *anti-inflammatory* and *antiseptic*. Hence they are said in Chinese medical terms to "clear damp heat from the liver and gallbladder channels."

Hepatobiliary relaxants and *sedatives* treat tense and hot conditions of the liver/gallbladder, such as hepatic congestion with heat and damp in vitalistic terms, or infectious and inflammatory conditions in modern medical terms. Two major symptom pictures call for the use of these herbs: **liver and gallbladder damp heat,** and **gallbladder heat.**

The syndrome **liver and gallbladder damp heat** is identified by jaundiced skin and eyes, right subcostal or flank pain, tender sides, unrest, irritability, nausea, vomiting, dark urine, headache and fever. This picture is often found with acute jaundice, hepatitis (all types), fatty liver, liver abscess and lymphoma.

The symptom picture of **gallbladder heat,** on the other hand, includes sharp pain on the right subcostal region (often radiating to below the right shoulder blade), dizziness, nausea, vomiting, bitter taste in the mouth, sour belching, jaundiced eyes and skin, fever with chill shivers, unrest, irritability and fatigue. This pattern usually entails acute gallbladder conditions such as cholangitis, cholecystitis, cholesterolosis and acute gallbladder attack (cholelithiasis) due to gallstone.

Because the overall character of the *hepatobiliary relaxants* and *sedatives* is very much *relaxant,* many remedies in this section are *also relaxant* to the cardiovascular and nervous systems. Variously containing bitters, alkaloids, tannins and glycosides, these herbs include such important broad-acting selections as Gardenia Zhi Zi (the South Chinese Gardenia pod) and Gentiana Long Dan Cao (Scabrous gentian root from Central China). Also in this category are lesser known, more pointedly liver-tropic remedies, such as Canna Mei Ren Jiao (Canna lily root and flower from South Asian grasslands) and Dichondra Ma Di Jin (a bindweed type from Taiwan and South China). Their bitter and astringent taste, and drying and cooling effects are the key qualities that enable these remedies to clear damp heat conditions.

Three remedies stand out for their *biliary sedative* actions, and are frequently used with the syndrome **gallbladder heat.** These are Lysimachia Jin Qian Cao (Chinese moneywort herb, related to the European loosestrife and important for treating urinary as well as biliary stones); the very versatile Rheum Da Huang (Rhubarb root from West and North China); and the very cooling Gardenia Zhi Zi (Gardenia pod from Southeast China and Taiwan).

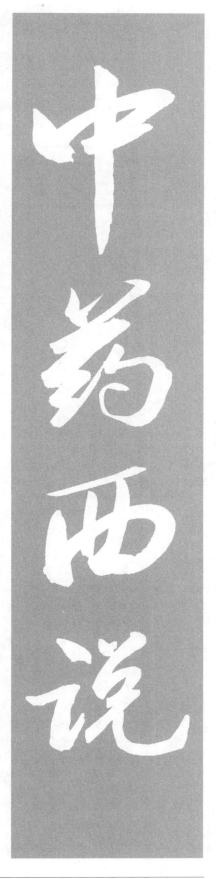

HEPATOBILIARY SYSTEM

Hepatobiliary Restoratives

REMEDIES TO RESTORE THE LIVER, PROMOTE ANABOLISM AND RELIEVE FATIGUE

➥ ENRICH LIVER YIN AND NOURISH THE BLOOD

Hepatic anastative nutritives, metabolic restoratives, hemogenics

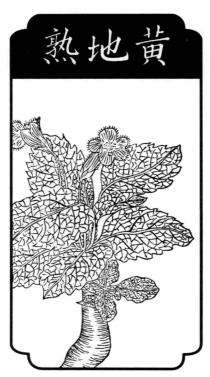

Rehmannia Shu Di Huang
Prepared Rehmannia Root

Botanical source: *Rehmannia glutinosa* (Gaertner) Liboschitz *f. hueichingensis* (Chao et Schih) Hsiao (Scrophulariaceae)
Pharmaceutical name: Radix Rehmanniae preparatae
Chinese names: Shu Di (Huang), Di Sui (Mand); Suk Dei (Wong) (Cant)
Other names: Glutinous rehmannia, Asian foxglove, "Earth yellow"; Jukujio (Jap)
Habit: Hairy perennial herb from coastal and north China; grows in loamy, humid soil on sunny hillsides, roadside wasteground and in marshes; also widely cultivated; terminal maroon-purple or cream flowers emerge in spring.
Part used: the prepared or cured root

Therapeutic category: mild remedy with minimal chronic toxicity
Constituents: alcohols (incl. mannitol, sitosterol, stigmasterol, campesterol), saccharides (glucose, fructose, raffinose), over 20 amino acids (incl. arginine, lysine), aminobutyric acid, iridoid catalpol, 23 glycosides, rehmannin, tannin, resins, stachyose, inorganic ions, iron, phosphorus, selenium, vitamin A
Effective qualities: sweet, oily, warm, moist
    restoring, nourishing, thickening, dissolving
Tropism: digestive, cardiovascular, endocrine, reproductive systems
    Liver, Heart, Kidney channels
    Fluid, Warmth bodies

ACTIONS AND INDICATIONS

liver restorative/protective: liver deficiency with low glycogen reserve and infection proneness; infectious hepatitis, metabolic toxicosis
anastative nutritive: fatigue or debility from poor assimilation, malnutrition, convalescence, anemia
detoxicant, diuretic: metabolic toxicosis, chronic rheumatoid and arthritic conditions, dermatitis, eczema, dysuria
menstrual regulator, hemostatic: amenorrhea, menorrhagia, metrorrhagia, postpartum bleeding
pituitary-adrenocortical restorative: fatigue, poor stamina, dizziness; menopause, convalescence
mucogenic secretory: dehydration, heat exhaustion
hypoglycemiant: diabetes, hyperglycemia, hypoglycemia
cardiotonic: cardiac deficiency
hypotensive, antilipemic: hypertension, hyperlipidemia
anti-inflammatory: hepatitis
radiation-protective: radiation damage
interferon inducent

Symptom Pictures

liver Yin and Blood deficiency: fatigue, loss of stamina, palpitations, dizziness, frequent infections, underweight

metabolic toxicosis: fatigue, malaise, headaches, muscle aches, chronic skin rashes

uterus Blood deficiency: scanty or absent menses, heavy menses, fatigue

Kidney Yin deficiency: thirst, dizziness, ringing in ears, night sweats, nocturnal emissions

Preparation

Use: The root Rehmannia Shu Di Huang is the fresh root prepared by steaming and drying, or by washing or cooking in wine and then drying. The prepared root is decocted, or used in tincture form.

Dosage: Decoction: 10-30 g
Tincture: 2-4 ml

Caution: Overuse may cause loose stool and abdominal bloating (possibly due to inhibited absorption in the colon). This remedy should be used with care in digestive deficiency, Qi stagnation and catarrhal conditions with mucus or phlegm caused by its oily, moist qualities.

Notes

Chinese clinicians long ago discovered that the best *restorative* effects for this plant were obtained when Rehmannia root was washed in millet wine, steamed on a willow frame in a porcelain vessel, then dried and resteamed and redried nine times—in short, until it became as black as ink and as shiny as lacquer. Alternatively, the root could be cooked in wine.

One of the finest remedy for the liver Yin and liver Blood in both an Oriental and a Western sense, Prepared rehmannia root is used overall to restore and regulate, rather than to drain. This is in contrast to the fresh or sun-dried unprepared root, primarily employed for its *heat-clearing* properties. Stamina, endurance and freedom from infections are created through the tonifying actions of the sweet Prepared rehmannia on the blood, liver, pancreas head, adrenal cortex and heart. Blood sugar imbalances both hyper and hypo can be stabilized through its use, for example. It is not surprising to find this important *anastative* and *nutritive* botanical consistently used in traditional and modern herb prescriptions whenever the body's Yin functions as a whole need support. Specifically, Prepared rehmannia is a remedy of choice in any chronic disease process involving adrenal and hepatic insufficiency—chronic infections of all types and generally all conditions involving chronic unproductive stress. Because it provides this Yin endocrine support, formulas that promote longevity have always routinely counted Prepared rehmannia among its ingredients. On a more down-home note, the well-known Mu tea relies for its rich, full-bodied sweetness on this ingredient as much as on Licorice root and Cinnamon bark. These herbs are excellent *adrenal restoratives* that can help see us through the rigors of the winter season.

In a Western sense, Prepared rehmannia root additionally is an *metabolic detoxicant*, working on the liver, interstitial fluids and electrolyte balance to realign metabolic toxicosis conditions such as chronic eczema, rheumatism and arthritis. Noteworthy also are the remedy's widely used applications in menstrual conditions as different as amenorrhea and menorrhagia. Prepared rehmannia is one of the "four substances," the most important formulation for regulating menstruation. Although the pharmacology of these effects is unclear, in a more general sense one could say that this again is the result of the remedy's systemic regulating action on the blood, mediated by the liver.

Lycium Gou Qi Zi
Wolfberry

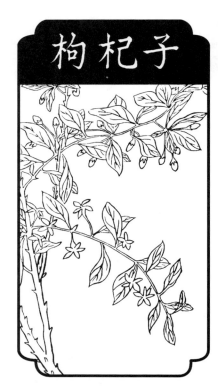

Botanical source: *Lycium chinense* Miller or *L. barbarum* L. (Solanaceae)
Pharmaceutical name: Fuctus Lycii
Chinese names: Gou Qi Zi, Zhou Qi, Gan Qi Zi, Gou Ji Zi, Qi Zi, Xian Ren Zhang (Mand); Gei Ji (Cant)
Other names: Matrimony vine, Boxthorn, Thorn-stalk berry; Kukoshi (Jap)
Habit: Small spinous trailing hardy deciduous shrub from East Asia, growing along roadsides and on hillsides; also cultivated; naturalized in Europe and the U.S.; light purple flowers appear from leaf axils in May through July.
Part used: the fruit

Therapeutic category: mild remedy with minimal chronic toxicity
Constituents: betaine, carotene, thiamin, riboflavin, niacin, organic acids (incl. ascorbic acid, nicotinic acid, linoleic acid), sitosterol, zeaxanthin, physalein, polysaccharide LBP, monosaccharide, crystal scopoletin, amino acids, polyterpene, calcium, trace minerals (incl. iron, potassium, calcium, phosphorus, zinc), vitamins A, B1, B2, C
Effective qualities: sweet, a bit sour, neutral, moist
restoring, nourishing, thickening
Tropism: digestive, respiratory, urogenital, nervous, immune systems
Liver, Kidney, Lung, Chong channels
Fluid body

ACTIONS AND INDICATIONS

liver restorative, metabolic restorative, growth stimulant, cholinergic, liver protective: all chronic functional and organic liver deficiency conditions (incl. deficient storage functions); weight loss, poor stamina, low resistance, hepatitis, liver cirrhosis, toxicosis, rough skin
anastative nututive: fatigue from malassimilation, malnutrition, corvalescence, anemia
cerebral restorative: cerebral deficiency with fatigue, dizziness, tinnitus
vision restorative: poor eyesight, blurred vision
antioxidant (free radical inhibitor): toxicosis, premature aging, vision loss
immune stimulant/enhancer, lymphocyte stimulant: immune deficiency with frequent or chronic infections; epidemics
leukocytogenic: low WBC count (leukopenia)
musculoskeletal and genital restorative: weak knees and legs, backache, seminal incontinence
bronchial demulcent: dry cough, thirst with dry throat, lung TB
hypoglycemiant: diabetes
antilipemic: hyperlipemia, atherosclerosis
interferon inducent

SYMPTOM PICTURES

liver Yin and Blood deficiency: frequent infections, underweight, increased appetite, low energy, introversion, loss of motivation

genitourinary deficiency (Liver and Kidney Yin deficiency): sore or weak back and legs, low-grade abdominal pain, impotence, seminal incontinence

nerve and brain deficiency (Liver and Kidney Essence deficiency): dizziness, impaired or blurred vision, fatigue

Preparation

Use: The berry Lycium Gou Qi Zi is decocted or used in tincture form.
Dosage: Decoction: 6-16 g
Tincture: 2-4 ml
Caution: Not to be used in the onset of infections with wind heat, or in intestines mucous damp. Use cautiously in internal full heat, including high fever.

Notes

The bright scarlet Wolfberry has enjoyed a reputation for enhancing vitality, beauty and long years since prehistory. These effects have been documented and lauded by herbalists, poets and common people alike, including the fastidious Li Shi-zhen himself. Today these claims seem further justified in light of the *antioxidant* and *immune enhancing* activities recently found in this sweet-sour tasting berry. But the whole picture is neccessary if we are to understand the full extent of its *restorative* nature.

The traditional symptom patterns conforming to the use of Wolfberry are Yin and Essence deficiency of the Chinese Liver and Kidney functions. An analysis of these syndromes indicates metabolic deficiencies involving primarily the liver, pancreas, spleen, brain and musculoskeletal system. These deficiencies imply anabolic liver disturbances (for which its polysaccharide has been shown active), toxin catabolism inefficiency, and blood sugar and immunological dysfunctions. This suggests using Wolfberry for liver Yin and spleen Yin deficiencies, as well as for urogenital and musculoskeletal weakness. The *growth stimulant* action, probably due to betaine, is just part of the overall metabolic dynamics of this *anastative* and *nutritive* blood and Yin tonic.

More than other *liver restoratives* in this section, Wolfberry is also renowned for improving skin quality. The beauty it promotes, however, is clearly more than skin deep.

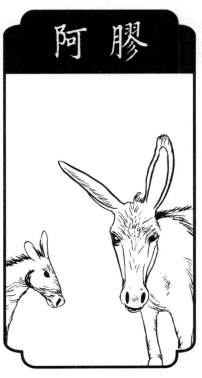

Equus E Jiao
Ass Hide Glue

Zoological source: *Equus asinus* L. or *E. caballus* x *E. asinus* (Equidae)
Pharmaceutical name: Gelatinum (colla) corii Equii asini
Chinese names: E Jiao, A Jiao, Fu Zhi Jiao (Mand); O Gau (Cant)
Other names: Ass hide gel, donkey hide gelatin; Akyo (Jap)
Source: Produced mainly in the mid-coastal provinces of Zhejiang, Jiangsu and Shandong.
Part used: the glue or gel derived from ass hide collagen

Therapeutic category: mild remedy with minimal chronic toxicity
Constituents: 15 amino acids (incl. glycine, arginine, cystine, lysine, histadine), calcium, sulfur, trace minerals, collagen, gelatins, glutins, chondrins
Effective qualities: sweet, mild, moist
restoring, nourishing, thickening
Tropism: digestive, vascular, respiratory, immune systems
Liver, Lung, Kidney channels
Fluid, Air bodies

Actions and Indications

liver/metabolic restorative, calcium metabolism stimulant: liver and metabolic deficiencies with fatigue, weakness; calcium imbalance with deficient calcium uptake, utilization and retention; irritability, insomnia

anastative nutritive: fatigue from malassimilation, malnutrition, convalescence, pregnancy
hemogenic: anemia, amenorrhea, postpartum weakness
immunostimulant, leukocytogenic: low WBC count, frequent infections
muscular restorative: muscular dystrophy and atrophy, hypercalcemia
hemostatic, coagulant: hemorrhage (incl. blood in sputum, stool, urine); intermenstrual bleeding, menorrhagia
bronchial demulcent: chronic dry cough, lung TB, asthma
fetal relaxant: fetal unrest, threatened abortion
Miscellaneous: paralysis, summer dysentery, amenorrhea, dysmenorrhea, purpura

SYMPTOM PICTURES
liver Yin and Blood deficiency: dizziness, fatigue, weak muscles, sallow complexion, frequent infections

lung dryness / lung Yin deficiency: chronic dry cough, blood-tinged sputum, sleep loss, irritability

PREPARATION
Use: Equus E Jiao is the solid glue obtained from the collagen of ass, donkey, horse or ox hide. The hides are first macerated in bitter saline water for four or five days and then washed and scrubbed clean. They are then boiled for a long time in water until the skins come apart. This water is strained, reduced to a glue by boiling and poured into moulds the shape of rectangular ink sticks. The glue stick is usually added directly to a strained decoction in which it readily dissolves. It may also be dissolved on its own in hot water or wine.

Dosage: Dissolved in water or alcohol: 4-16 g
Tincture: 2-4 ml

Caution: Contraindicated in external conditions. Use cautiously in gastric deficiencies and hypercholesterolemia.

NOTES
Ass hide glue is a sweet, moist *nutritive* and *restorative* remedy for metabolic and hepatic deficiencies. An unusual but common ingredient in formulas for Blood deficiencies, it is also much used for respiratory and gynecological conditions, especially with bleeding or weakness present.

Ass hide glue's effect of enhancing calcium metabolism, as well as the resultant *hemostatic* action caused by increased blood clotting, is also noteworthy.

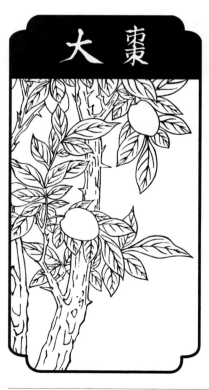

Zizyphus Da Zao
Jujube Berry

Botanical source: *Zizyphus jujuba* Miller var. *inermis* (Bunge) Rehder (Rhamnaceae)
Pharmaceutical name: Fructus Zizyphi jujubae
Chinese names: Da Zao, Mei/Wu Zao (Mand); Daai Jou (Cant)
Other names: Chinese date; Taiso (Jap)
Habit: Spiny, tall deciduous shrub from Southern Asia, cultivated throughout China; axillary cymes of greenish-yellow flowers emerge in spring.
Part used: the fruit

Therapeutic category: mild remedy with minimal chronic toxicity
Constituents: sapogenin, triterpenoid saponins (incl. jujuboside, rutin), organic acids, fatty acids, iron, calcium, phosphorus, vitamins A, B2, C
Effective qualities: sweet, neutral, moist
  restoring, nourishing, calming
Tropism: digestive, nervous systems
  Spleen, Stomach, Heart channels
  Fluid body

ACTIONS AND INDICATIONS

liver restorative/protective: liver deficiency with fatigue, low stamina, weight loss, allergies

anastative nutritive: fatigue from poor nutrient assimilation, malnutrition, anemia

intestinal restorative: digestive deficiency with fatigue, poor nutrient absorption

gastrointestinal demulcent: abdominal pain, dry dyspepsia, gastric ulcer

nervous sedative, analgesic: stress, unrest, abdominal and other pain, insomnia, irritability, neurasthenia, emotional burnout

immune regulator, antiallergic: immune stress with immediate allergies (incl. urticaria, rhinitis, bronchial asthma); cell-mediated allergies (incl. dermatitis, chronic hepatitis, autoimmune disorders [incl. peptic ulcer])

SYMPTOM PICTURES

liver Yin and small intestine Qi deficiency: fatigue, low endurance, loose stool, weight loss

liver and Heart Blood deficiency: unrest, irritability, fatigue, palpitations

stomach dryness: indigestion, epigastric or abdominal pain, feeling stressed

PREPARATION

Use: The fruit Zizyphus Da Zao is best decocted, but may be used in tincture form if account is then taken of its more warming nature. The honey-preserved jujube is used as a medicinal food.

Dosage: Decoction: 10-30 g, or three to ten berries
Tincture: 2-4 ml

Caution: Contraindicated in intestinal mucous damp displaying epigastric distension, in intestinal parasites and dental caries.

NOTES

The sweet, *demulcent* saponin-filled Jujube berry is a *nutritive* botanical frequently added to formulas as a supplementary ingredient for its harmonizing effect on digestion and enhacement of nutrient assimilation as a whole. Traditionally described as Spleen functions, in Western terms these anastate actions clearly involve the small intestine and liver. Jujube berry's tropism for the liver has been experimentally confirmed: The remedy has proven time and again to increase endurance, assist the liver in recoverering from toxic exposure, and reduce serum transaminase levels in a variety of liver disorders. The triterpenoid glycosides likely play an important part in these *restorative* actions.

With its *regulating* and *desensitizing* action on immune functions, Jujube berry strikes a very contemporary note. Japanese research has uncovered successful applications to both type I (immediate) and type IV (cell-mediated) hypersensitivity reaction disorders. Many types of allergies will clearly benefit from inclusion of this remedy in herb combinations.

Jujube berry's general *calming* and *pain-relieving* effect is not as strong as in the related Sour, or Wild, jujube seed. This *nervous sedative* action is good enough, however, to reinforce the berry's tradition-honored profile as an excellent complementary item in formulas for numerous conditions.

There are two varieties of jujubes available, the black and the red fruit (the black fruit is actually an intense dark red on close inspection). Both come from the same botanical species. The name **Da Zao** (Mandarin) or **Daai Jou** (Cantonese) actually refers to the black type of jujube. The red type is called **Hong Zao** (Mandarin) or **Hung Jou** (Cantonese). Although they possess the same functions, the black type is often preferred by many practitioners. In addition, some practitioners use the black jujube in formulas that tonify the Qi, while using the red jujube in formulas that nourish the Blood. In all other cases they simply keep in mind this therapeutic differentiation when selecting this remedy.

Hepatobiliary Stimulants

REMEDIES TO PROMOTE UPPER DIGESTION, REDUCE LIVER CONGESTION AND RELIEVE EPIGASTRIC FULLNESS

➥ SPREAD LIVER QI, HARMONIZE THE LIVER AND SPLEEN, AND TRANSFORM ACCUMULATION

Liver decongestants, cholagogue laxatives

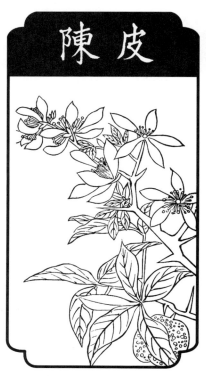

Citrus Chen Pi
Ripe Tangerine Rind

Botanical source: *Citrus reticulata* Blanco or *C. tangerina* Hortorum et Tanaka or *C. erythrosa* Tanaka (Rutaceae)
Pharmaceutical name: Pericarpium Citri
Chinese names: Chen Pi, Ju Pi, Guang Chen Pi, Jie Pi, Guang Gan Pi, Hong Pi (Mand); Chan Pei, Gwat Pei (Cant)
Other names: Satsuma, Mandarin orange, "Aged peel"; Chinpi (Jap)
Habit: Evergreen South Asian tree, also cultivated in Sichuan, Fujian and Guangdong; white flowers in small axillary cymes appear in spring.
Part used: the mature fruit rind

Therapeutic category: mild remedy with minimal chronic toxicity
Constituents: essential oil 1.5-2% (incl. limonene, pinene, myrcene, terpinene, linalol, terpineol, citral, elemene, copanene, humulene, sesquiphellandrene, humulenol acetate), hesperidin, carotene, cryptosanthin, vitamins B1, C
Effective qualities: pungent, bitter, warm, dry
 stimulating, relaxing
Tropism: digestive, respiratory, cardiovascular systems
 Spleen, Stomach, Lung channels; Air body

ACTIONS AND INDICATIONS
hepatobiliary stimulant: choleretic, cholagogue: biliary deficiency with dyspepsia
gastric stimulant, carminative: digestive deficiency with dyspepsia; gastritis
antiemetic: nausea, vomiting, hiccups
stimulant expectorant: bronchitis with cough
cardiac restorative, hypertensive
anti-inflammatory: acute nonpurulent mastitis

SYMPTOM PICTURES
gallbladder and stomach Qi stagnation (Liver Qi stagnation, Liver/Spleen disharmony): epigastric distension and fullness, appetite loss, flatulence, nausea, sour belching
lung phlegm damp: tight chest and diaphragm, wheezing, coughing with production of copious viscous sputum

PREPARATION
Use: The rind Citrus Chen Pi is decocted or used in tincture form. The extracted essential oil is also used internally.
Dosage: Decoction: 3-10 g
 Tincture: 1-4 ml
 Essential oil: 2-3 drops in gelatin cap topped with olive oil

Caution: Do not use in dry coughs due to Yin or Qi deficiency. Also use cautiously for coughing from acute bronchitis (phlegm heat) or dry heat in the lungs, and in cases of spitting up of blood.

NOTES

The citrus family, a genus whose original home was the southern and eastern Himalayan foothills, has since prehistory provided Oriental medicine with numerous remedies. The dried rind of the ripe tangerine is one of the most frequently used Chinese medicinals for indigestion from both biliary and gastric deficiency. It is found in countless formulas of many types, if only as a secondary ingredient in most of them. The characteristic bitter, spicy taste and odor is due to an essential oil, able to remove upper digestive stagnation fundamentally caused by liver, gallbladder or stomach Yang deficiency.

The **rind** of the **ripe red tangerine, Ju Hong** (Mand.) or **Gwat Heung** (Cant.), is derived from the species *Citrus grandis* Osbeck and *C. erythrosa* Tanaka. Although similar to the regular unripe tangerine rind, it is considered somewhat stronger. Because of its superior bitter, dry, warm qualities, Red tangerine rind is especially used for its *stimulant expectorant* action in lung phlegm damp conditions with coughing.

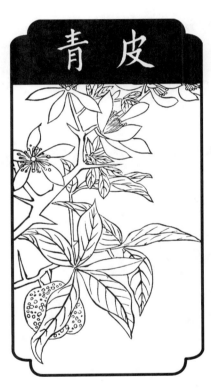

Citrus Qing Pi
Unripe Tangerine Rind

Botanical source: *Citrus reticulata* Blanco or *C. tangerina* Hortorum et Tanaka or *C. erythrosa* Tanaka (Rutaceae)
Pharmaceutical name: Pericarpium Citri reticulatae viride
Chinese names: Qing Pi, Qing Ju Pi (Mand); Ching Pei Cant)
Other names: Satsuma, Mandarin orange, "Green peel"; Jyohi (Jap)
Habit: Cultivated evergreen tree from South Asia; white flowers in small axillary cymes appear in spring.
Part used: the immature green fruit rind

Therapeutic category: mild remedy with minimal chronic toxicity
Constituents: essential oil 1.5-2% (incl. limonene, citral, elemene, copanene, humulene, sesquiphellandrene, humulenol acetate), flavonoids (incl. hesperidin, cryptoxanthin, synephrin, carotene), vitamins B1, C
Effective qualities: pungent, bitter, warm, dry
  stimulating, relaxing, dissolving
Tropism: digestive, respiratory, reproductive systems
  Liver, Gallbladder, Lung, Large Intestine channels
  Air body

ACTIONS AND INDICATIONS

hepatobiliary stimulant: liver decongestant, choleretic, cholagogue: liver congestion with right subcostal pain and hepatobiliary dyspepsia; gastritis, chronic hepatitis
anti-inflammatory: cholecystitis, cholangitis; hepatic and splenic enlargement, liver cirrhosis
intestinal stimulant/relaxant: carminative, spasmolytic: intestinal colic, flatulence, abdominal lumps
uterine relaxant: menstrual cramps; spasmodic dysmenorrhea, uterine fibrosis
stimulant expectorant, antiasthmatic: asthma, bronchitis with cough
immune regulator: immune stress with antibody-mediated cytotoxicity (incl. autoimmune disorders)
Miscellaneous: breast abscess

Symptom Pictures
gallbladder and stomach Qi stagnation (Liver Qi stagnation): slow painful digestion, nausea, flatulence, epigastric bloating and pain, subcostal or chest pain

intestines Qi constraint (Liver/Spleen disharmony): indigestion, flatus, abdominal pain, lumps or distension

Preparation
Use: The rind Citrus Qing Pi is decocted or used in tincture form.
Dosage: Decoction: 3-10 g
Tincture: 1-4 ml
Caution: Use with caution in Qi deficiency conditions with profuse sweating.

Notes
Although primarily a *biliary stimulant*, Unripe tangerine rind overall has a relatively more *relaxant* profile than the ripe peel. It relieves both upper and lower digestive pain, distension and lumps with its *spasmolytic, analgesic* effects. Symptom pictures involving constrained Qi in the intestines, stomach, thorax, bronchi and, even uterus, are thereby addressed.

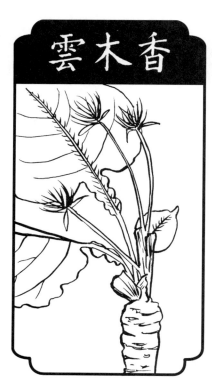

Saussurea Yun Mu Xiang
Wood Aromatic Root *

Botanical source: *Saussurea lappa* Clarke, syn. *Auklandia lappa* Decaisne, and *Vladimiria souliei* (Franchet) Lingelsheim or *V. denticulata* Lingelsheim (Compositae)
Pharmaceutical name: Radix Saussureae
Chinese names: Yun Mu Xiang, Guang Mu Xiang, Mu Xiang (Mand); Muk Heung (Cant)
Other names: Mokko (Jap)
Habit: Large perennial Himalayan mountain herb; also cultivated in Yunnan and Sichuan; likes cool, humid, hilly terrain with deep sandy soil; dark purple terminal flowerheads arise during late spring and summer.
Part used: the root

Therapeutic category: mild remedy with minimal chronic toxicity
Constituents: essential oil 0.3-3% (incl. aplotaxene, costus lactone, costol, costene, camphene, ionone, selinene, costic acid), dehydrocostuslactone, phellandrene), alkaloid saussurine, mono/di/triterpenoids, betulin, saussurin, stigmasterol
Effective qualities: pungent, bitter, warm, dry
stimulating, eliminating, relaxing
Tropism: hepatobiliary, intestinal, respiratory systems
Gallbladder, Spleen, Stomach, Lung channels; Air body

Actions and Indications
hepatobiliary and gastrointestinal stimulant: decongestant, cholagogue, carminative, laxative: liver congestion and gastrointestinal deficiency with dyspepsia, constipation
intestinal relaxant, spasmolytic, analgesic: intestinal colic, diarrhea with tenesmus; colitis, IBS; abdominal pain from intestinal parasites, renal colic
antiemetic: nausea, vomiting
bronchial relaxant, expectorant: bronchial asthma with tight cough, wheezing
antibacterial (incl. Staphylococus, Escherichia coli, bacillus typhi, Bacillus subtilis)

Symptom Pictures

gallbladder and stomach Qi stagnation (Liver Qi stagnation): slow painful digestion, appetite loss, epigastric, subcostal or abdominal pain and distension, nausea, constipation, vomiting

intestines Qi constraint (Liver/Spleen disharmony): nausea, abdominal pain, urgent loose stool

lung Qi constraint with **phlegm damp:** tight chest, wheezing, coughing, scanty viscous sputum production

Preparation

Use: The root Saussurea Yun Mu Xiang should be decocted or used in tincture form. To protect its essential oil content, it should be added only 10 minutes before the end of decocting time.

Dosage: Decoction: 2-10 g
Tincture: 1-4 ml

Caution: Not to be used in Yin or fluids deficiency because of the very dry nature of this remedy.

Notes

With its woody, spicy, resinous fragrance, this root is one of the many *xiang,* or aromatics, that reached China through maritime trade routes from Malasia and India. Originally from Kashmir and Ceylon, Mu Xiang, literally "wood aromatic," was used in incense making and perfumery, as well as in medicine. Here its major *stimulant* and *relaxant* actions on biliary and gastric functions are highly valued.

The remedy is ideal for stagnant and constrained Qi digestive conditions involving gallbladder, stomach and intestines, and presenting pain, distension and diarrhea. Wood aromatic root's *bronchodilatant* action has brought much success in asthmatic conditions. In Chinese medical terms, the remedy is significant for circulating the Qi and relieving constraint in the digestive and respiratory tract. Biochemically it contains a unique combination of essential oils, terpenoids and alkaloids (the latter being especially *spasmolytic*), but with a mild *antiseptic* effect.

This plant is not to be confused with the equally fragrant spiral flag—or *Costus*—a member of the ginger family, also from India.

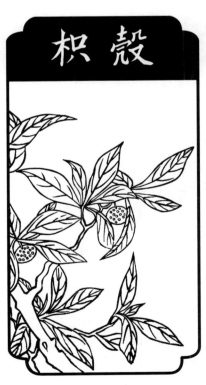

Citrus Zhi Shi
Unripe Bitter Orange Fruit

Botanical source: *Citrus aurantium* L. or *C. wilsonii* Tanaka and *Poncirus trifoliata* Rafinesque (Rutaceae)
Pharmaceutical name: Fructus Citri seu Ponciri immaturi
Chinese names: Zhi Shi, Zhi Qiao (Mand); Jek Sat (Cant)
Other names: Sour orange; Kijitsu (Jap)
Habit: Small evergreen tree from warm, moist, tropical low mountain areas throughout Asia; found along rivers and lakes and in open fields with loose sandy soil; in spring, solitary or clustered white flowers blossom.
Part used: the immature green fruit

Therapeutic category: mild remedy with minimal chronic toxicity
Constituents: essential oil (incl. limonene, linalool, citronellal), flavonoids (incl. poncirin, hesperidin, rhoifolin, naringin, lonicerin), coumarins (incl. umbelliferone, auraptene), synephrin, citric acid, vitamin C
Effective qualities: bitter, a bit pungent and sour, cool, dry
relaxing, stimulating, decongesting, stabilizing
Tropism: digestive, respiratory systems
Spleen, Stomach, Lung channels; Air, Fluid bodies

Hepatobiliary Stimulants

Actions and Indications
hepatobiliary and gastrointestinal stimulant: cholagogue, diuretic, laxative: hepatic and gastrointestinal deficiency with dyspepsia; edema, constipation
carminative, spasmolytic: dyspepsia, flatulence
antiprolapse: uterine, rectal and gastric prolapse
cardiac stimulant, hypertensive: hypotension, (incl. surgical)
analeptic: shock, coma
contraceptive (ovulation inhibitor)

Symptom Pictures
gallbladder, stomach and intestines Qi stagnation (Liver Qi stagnation): indigestion, epigastric, subcostal and abdominal distress and fullness, sour belching, sick headache, flatulence, constipation

intestines Qi constraint (Liver/Spleen disharmony): abdominal pain and distension, constipation

Preparation
Use: The fruit Citrus Zhi Shi is briefly decocted or used in tincture form. The essential oil of the rind is also used.
Dosage: Decoction: 3-10 g (12-30 g is used for organ prolapse).
Tincture: 1-4 ml
Essential oil of bitter orange rind: 2-3 drops
Caution: Use with caution in stomach cold conditions, during pregnancy, and whenever the normal Qi is weak.

Notes
A *cholagogue* and *digestive stimulant* in one (unlike the tangerines), Unripe bitter orange fruit treats two types of upper and lower gastric stagnation: spasmodic and deficient. It is a versatile component of many a traditional prescription, as reflected in the two symptom pictures above.

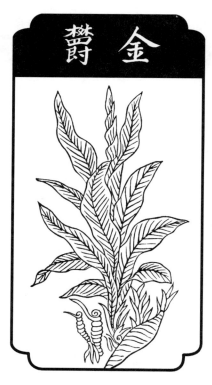

Curcuma Yu Jin
Turmeric Tuber

Botanical source: *Curcuma longa* L. or *C. aromatica* Salisbury (Zingiberaceae)
Pharmaceutical name: Tuber/Radix Curcumae
Chinese names: Yu Jin, Yu Ju, Yu Jin Xiang, Chuan Yu Jin, Guang Yu Jin (Mand); Wat Gan (Cant)
Other names: Wild turmeric, Wild zedoary, "Constrained gold"; Ukon (Jap)
Habit: Aromatic perennial tropical Asian herb found on fertile, loose soil and in mountain grasslands in thickets; also cultivated; blooms in summer with pale green-white or pink tubular flowers.
Part used: the tuberous root

Therapeutic category: mild remedy with minimal chronic toxicity
Constituents: essential oil 5% (incl. camphene, curcumene, phellandrene, camphor, turmerol, turmerone, curcumone, carvone, valeric and caproic acid), dipotassium-magnesium-dioxalate-dihydrate, starch, lipid
Effective qualities: bitter, pungent, neutral with warming and cooling potential
stimulating, decongesting, relaxing, calming, dissolving, astringing
Tropism: hepatobiliary, urogenital, cardiovascular, nervous systems
Liver, Stomach, Heart, Lung, Yin Wei channels
Fluid, Air bodies

ACTIONS AND INDICATIONS

hepatobilary stimulant: liver decongestant, cholagogue, choleretic, laxative: liver congestion with dyspepsia and pain; jaundice, hepatitis, gallstone, cholecystitis
uterine stimulant, emmenagogue, parturient: amenorrhea, miscarriage, prolonged pregnancy
capillary stimulant, coronary restorative: angina pectoris, coronary deficiency/disease, arrhythmia
antilipemic: hyperlipemia, atherosclerosis
nervous sedative, anticonvulsant: agitation, anxiety states, mania, seizures (incl. epileptic)
analgesic: postpartum abdominal pain, dysmenorrhea, pain of trauma
vulnerary, anticontusion, anti-inflammatory, analgesic, detumescent: chronic sores and ulcers, wounds, injuries, contusion; all with pain and swelling; liver enlargment
hemostatic: nosebleed, coughing up blood, blood in urine, postpartum bleeding
anti-infective: antifungal, antibacterial, antiviral: miscellaneous infections (incl. viral hepatits, influenza)
antioxidant (free radical inhibitor), antitumoral

SYMPTOM PICTURES

gallbladder and stomach Qi stagnation (Liver Qi stagnation): epigastric pain and distension, slow painful digestion, constipation

liver and gallbladder damp heat: abdominal/subcostal swellin and pain, nausea, unrest, anxiety, yellow skin

uterus Qi constraint and Blood congealed: painful, difficult or delayed menses, PMS

heart blood and Qi stagnation: feeling stressed, anxiety, chest tightness and pain, labored breathing, cold extremities

phlegm heat heart obstruction: agitation, anxiety, manic speech and behavior, convulsions

PREPARATION

Use: The tuber Curcuma Yu Jin is decocted or used in tincture form.
Dosage: Decoction: 5-15 g
Tincture: 2-5 ml
Caution: Forbidden in conditions not presenting symptoms of Qi or Blood stagnation, and also in Yin deficiency conditions due to blood loss. Use with care during pregnancy as Curcuma Yu Jin is a mild *uterine stimulant*.

NOTES

An aromatic, bitter plant indigenous to Southwest China, Turmeric is employed in the textile industry for its yellow dye and in herbal medicine for its versatile medicinal properties.

Today, treating congestive, swollen, painful conditions of the liver and gallbladder is the focus of this botanical. Turmeric tuber addresses conditions that crystallize around the symptom pictures gallbladder and stomach Qi stagnation, and damp heat of the liver and gallbladder. All forms of jaundice and hepatitis (including viral) can be influenced by this valuable remedy. Because of its *sedative* action on the nervous system and *restorative* effect on the coronary circulation, Turmeric tuber is often used today for anxiety and manic states, especially involving angina. Its *antilipemic* action reinforces the heart's circulation.

Turmeric tuber is a popular remedy for trauma and other local conditions, including those involving pain and swelling. These conditions additionally benefit from its *anti-infective* action, due to the complex essential oil content.

Several *Curcuma* types have, at one time or another, also been used in Greek/Galenic medicine. From India, where it has also been used in Ayurvedic medicine, Turmeric spread west in the Moslem era and was incorporated by Persian doctors practicing Tibb Unani (i.e., Greek) medicine. From the Middle East, it reached central Europe during the late Middle Ages along with Greek medicine itself. Because of its limited availability and high cost, however, Turmeric tuber never achieved Western status as the important liver/gallbladder remedy it is.

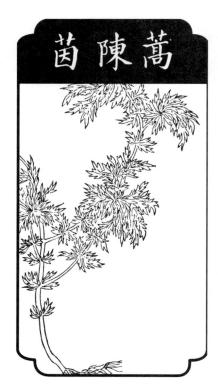

Artemisia Yin Chen Hao
Downy Wormwood Herb *

Botanical source: *Artemisia capillaris* Thunberg or *A. scoparia* Waldstein et Kitag (Compositae)
Pharmaceutical name: Herba Artemisiae capillaris
Chinese names: Yin Chen (Hao), Mian Yin Chen, Xiang Gao (Mand); Yin Chan (Hou), Mai Yin Chan, Min Yin Chan (Cant)
Other names: Evergreen artemisia; Inchinko (Jap)
Habit: Perennial herb from Northeast and Southwest China, Japan and Taiwan, inhabiting grass thickets on roadsides and streamsides; panicles of small, greenish yellow capitulate blossoms open in summer.
Part used: the herb

Therapeutic category: mild remedy with minimal chronic toxicity
Constituents: essential oil 0.3-0.6% (incl. eugenol, capilline, eugenylmethylbutyrate/-propanoate, eugenylvalerate), coumarins (incl. esculetin, scopoletin, dimethoxycoumarin), chromones (incl. capillarisin), flavonoids, scoparone, chlorogenic/caffeic/stearic/palmitic/oleic/linoleic/arachidic/montanic acid
Effective qualities: bitter, pungent, warming/cooling potential, a bit dry
  stimulating, decongesting, relaxing, softening
Tropism: digestive, urinary, vascular systems
  Liver, Gallbladder, Spleen, Stomach channels; Warmth, Fluid bodies

ACTIONS AND INDICATIONS

hepatobiliary stimulant: liver decongestant, cholagogue, choleretic, laxative: liver congestion with dyspepsia and constipation; jaundice, hepatitis, gallstone
liver protective: icteral hepatitis
draining diuretic: edema, dysuria, oliguria
coronary dilator, antilipemic, hypotensive: coronary disease, hyperlipemia, hypertension
antipyretic, anti-inflammatory: fever of all types, cholecystitis
anti-infective: antibacterial, antiviral, interferon inducent: flu, common cold (esp. with alternating chills and fever); viral hepatitis
anthelmintic: ascariasis (roundworm), leptospiriasis (ten types)
antifungal, antipruritic: fungal skin conditions (incl. tinea corporis/pedis, yeast infections); pruritus, vaginitis

SYMPTOM PICTURES

liver and gallbladder damp cold (Liver cold): lethargy, cold extremities, headache, difficult urination, water retention, jaundice, constipation and/or diarrhea

liver fluid congestion: local or general water retention, fatigue, lethargy, thirst

liver and gallbladder damp heat: fatigue, jaundice, fever, difficult or dribbling urination, constipation

external wind heat and **Shao Yang heat:** intermittent feverishness and chills, bitter taste in mouth, poor appetite, nausea, chest tightness, subcostal pain

PREPARATION

Use: The herb Artemisia Yin Chen Hao is either briefly decocted for 5-10 minutes, or infused for 20 minutes. Washes, douches, vaginal sponges, etc., can be prepared for localized infections.
Dosage: Short decoction and infusion: 10-20 g
  Tincture: 2-4 ml
Caution: Forbidden in Qi deficiency jaundice with pale yellow skin, normal urination and a soggy pulse.

NOTES

Like the Western Wormwood and other related species of *Artemisia,* Downy wormwood has a primary tropism for the liver and gallbladder. Having both *stimulant* and *relaxant* characteristics, it will clear congestive, cold conditions of the liver due to Yang deficiency, as well as hot, infectious conditions. The aromatic acetylene capillin (part of its essential oil) is thought to be a key element in Downy wormwood's *cholagogue* action. This *diuretic* remedy also effectively engages the liver and kidneys to mobilize stagnant fluids and promote urination. Like other wormwoods, it also possesses good *antiparasitic* and *antimicrobial* properties.

In general, the common Wormwood would be a good synergistic or substitute remedy for this herb in treating the above three syndromes.

Artemisia Qing Hao
Celery Wormwood Herb

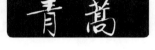

Botanical source: *Artemisia apiacea* Hance (Compositae)
Chinese names: Qing Hao (Mand); Ching Hou (Cant)
Category: mild remedy with minimal chronic toxicity

Constituents: essential oil, abrotanine, vitamin A
Effective qualities: bitter, pungent, cold, dry, stimulating
Tropism: digestive, immune systems; Liver, Gallbladder channels

ACTIONS: *Liver decongestant, cholagogue, antipyretic, anti-infective, phagocyte stimulant, hemostatic, antifungal*
INDICATIONS: Jaundice, dyspepsia from gallbladder and stomach Qi stagnation; food poisoning with summer heat, dysentery; remittent and intermittent fever (including with Yin deficiency and malaria), low-grade fever; nosebleeds, fungal kin conditions.
Dosage: Infusion: 4-10 g
　　　　　　Tincture: 1-4 ml
Caution: Contraindicated in postpartum mothers with Blood (metabolic) deficiency, and in stomach/intestines cold.

Eupatorium Pei Lan
Orchid-Grass Herb *

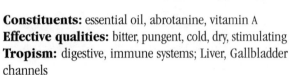

Botanical source: *Eupatorium fortunei* Turczaninow (Compositae)
Chinese names: Pei Lan, Lan Cao, Xiang Cao, Ja Lang (Mand); Poi Laan (Cant)
Other names: "Admiring orchid"; Hairan (Jap)
Habit: Damp-loving perennial East Asian herb found along streams and other wet places; in autumn, cymes of capitate magenta flowers appear.

Category: mild remedy with minimal chronic toxicity
Constituents: essential oil (incl. neryl acetate, cymene, methylthymol ether), coumarin, coumaric acid, thymohydroquinone
Effective qualities: sweet, bitter, pungent, neutral, dry; stimulating, decongesting, dispersing, calming
Tropism: digestive, nervous systems; Stomach, Spleen, Liver channels

ACTIONS: *Hepatobiliary decongestant, cholagogue, digestive stimulant, laxative, diaphoretic, nervous sedative, analgesic, antibacterial, antiviral*
INDICATIONS: Liver congestion with dyspepsia, jaundice, halitosis, constipation; gallbladder and stomach Qi stagnation syndrome; digestive deficiency with loss of appetite, regurgitation; intestines mucous damp (Spleen damp) syndrome with sweet/sticky taste in mouth, head pressure, heaviness of body; early stage of fever with dry skin; unrest, headache, pain in general; food poisoning, hepatitis, influenza; external wind heat with damp syndrome
　　　　Topically for dandruff.
Dosage: Infusion: 4-14 g
　　　　　　Tincture: 2-4 ml

When decocting as part of a formula, add this herb 10 minutes before the end to protect the essential oils.
Caution: Forbidden in Yin deficiency conditions.
Notes: Both upper and lower digestive stagnation are relieved by Orchid-grass' *liver, biliary* and *gastric stimulant* effects. Most typical of its indications is a sweet or sticky taste in the mouth, signaling stagnant digestive dampness.

This species of *Eupatorium* has by nature and usage little in common with either *Eupatorium perfoliatum*, Boneset herb, or *Eupatorium purpureum*, Gravel root. This is a good example of a botanical similarity that bears little relevance to the therapeutic characteristics and practical usage of the plant as a remedy.

Curcuma Jiang Huang
Turmeric Rhizome

Botanical source: *Curcuma longa* L. (Zingiberaceae)
Chinese names: Jiang Huang, Pian Jiang Huang (Mand); Geung Wong (Cant)
Category: mild remedy with minimal chronic toxicity
Constituents: essential oil (incl. zingerene, turmerone, phellandrene, cineole, sabinene, borneol), curcumin, arabinose, lipids
Effective qualities: pungent, bitter, warm, dry; stimulating, calming, dissolving
Tropism: digestive, musculoskeletal systems; Liver, Spleen, Yin Wei channels

Actions: *Biliary and gastrointestinal stimulant, choleretic, laxative, analgesic, coronary decongestant, hemostatic, vulnerary, anti-infective*
Indications: Dyspepsia, jaundice, hepatitis; liver/gallbladder Qi stagnation syndrome; angina pectoris, hyperlipemia, menstrual clots and spasms, rheumatic and arthritic pain with paresthesia and edema (especially of shoulder joint); amenorrhea, traumatic bleeding; bacterial, fungal and viral infections (incl. fungal skin conditions, influenza).
Dosage: Decoction: 3-10 g
　　　　　Tincture: 1-4 ml
Caution: Contraindicated during pregnancy.

Citrus Zhi Ke
Ripe Bitter Orange Fruit

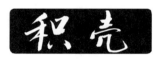

Botanical source: *Citrus aurantium* L. (Rutaceae)
Chinese names: Zhi Ke, Zhi Qiao (Mand); Jek Hok (Cant)
Category: mild remedy with minimal chronic toxicity
Constituents: essential oil, flavonoids (incl. naringin, neohesperidin, rhoifolin, lonicerin), vitamin C
Effective qualities: sour, bitter, pungent, cool, moist; relaxing, stimulating
Tropism: digestive system; Spleen, Stomach channels

Actions: *Liver and gastric stimulant, cholagogue, carminative, antiprolapse*
Indications: Dyspepsia from biliary or gastric deficiency; gallbladder and stomach Qi stagnation syndrome; epigastric and abdominal pain, pressure and distension; constipation; diarrhea from parasites, intestinal and uterine prolapse, constipation due to intestines dryness.
Dosage: Short decoction: 3-10 g
　　　　　Tincture: 1-3 ml
Caution: None.
Notes: The rind and seeds should be removed and the fruit dried before use. This remedy is gentler than Citrus Zhi Shi, Unripe bitter orange fruit.

Cucumis Tian Gua Di
Young Cantaloupe Stalk

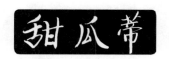

Botanical source: *Cucumis melo* L. (Cucurbitaceae)
Chinese names: Tian Gua Di, Ku Ding Xiang, Gua Di (Mand); Ting Gwa Di (Cant)
Part used: the stalk of the young fruit
Category: medium-strength remedy with some chronic toxicity

Constituents: cucurbitacin B, E and D and pyranoglucosides, isocucurbitacin B
Effective qualities: bitter, cool, dry; stimulating, decongesting
Tropism: digestive, upper respiratory systems; Liver, Lung, Stomach channels

ACTIONS: *Hepatobiliary decongestant, cholagogue, liver protective, draining diuretic, cellular immunostimulant, antitumoral, interferon inducent, nasal decongestant, emetic*

INDICATIONS: Liver congestion, jaundice, acute and chronic hepatitis; liver/gallbladder Qi stagnation syndrome with right subcostal pain and distension, fatigue; hepatomegaly, splenomegaly, severe general edema (anasarca); cancer (incl. hepatoma); acute rhinitis, nasal polyp, anosmia; undigested food accumulation, epilepsy, stroke (whenever emetic therapy is indicated).

Dosage: Infusion and maceration: 2-5 g
Tincture: 0.25-1 ml or 6-25 drops

The maceration is a steeping in cold water for several days. The powdered Cantaloupe stalk is also given as a nasal spray or insufflation. The larger dose will cause vomiting for emetic therapy and is only suited for one-time use for the functions and uses of emetic therapy (see Holmes 1989).

Caution: This remedy is contraindicated in general weakness and heart disease and should not be taken for more than two weeks because of its medium-strength nature. Ten days at the low to medium dose is the average course for liver conditions.

NOTES: Apart from its use as a simple *emetic,* the stalk of the young Cantaloupe melon in the past was a much-vaunted remedy for nasal conditions of all kinds—hence traditional nasal insufflation and the modern nasal spray. Severe liver conditions, such as anasarca and all types of jaundice, have historically also responded well to it. In recent times, Young cantaloupe stalk has found success with most types of hepatitis, presumably because of its *stimulant* action on cellular immunity through increased lymphocyte transformation (Chang and But 1987).

Hepatobiliary Relaxants and Sedatives

REMEDIES TO REDUCE LIVER AND GALLBLADDER INFECTION AND INFLAMMATION
➧ CLEAR DAMP HEAT FROM THE LIVER AND GALLBLADDER
Anti-inflammatory and antiseptic hepatic decongestants

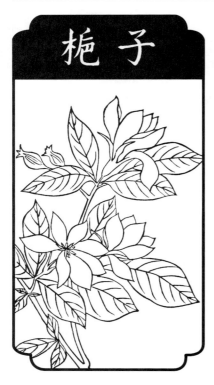

Gardenia Zhi Zi
Gardenia Pod

Botanical source: *Gardenia jasminoides* Ellis (Rubiaceae)
Pharmaceutical name: Fructus Gardeniae
Chinese names: Zhi Zi, Shan Zhi Zi, Huang Zhi Zi (Mand); San Ji Ji (Cant)
Other names: Shishi (Jap)
Habit: Evergreen shrub from southeast China, Taiwan and Japan, growing in damp and warmth on hillsides, streamsides and in thin forests; also cultivated; fragrant, white axillary/terminal flowers appear in early summer.
Part used: the fruit

Therapeutic category: mild remedy with minimal chronic toxicity
Constituents: flavonoids (incl. crocin, crocetin, gardenin), ursolic acid, tannins, mannitol, sitosterol, terpenoid iridoids (incl. gardenoside, geniposide, genipin, shanzhiside), glucosides, nonocosane
Effective qualities: bitter, astringent, cold, dry
  stimulating, decongesting, astringing, calming, sinking
Tropism: hepatobiliary, cardiovascular, nervous systems
  Heart, Lung, Triple Heater, Liver, Gallbladder, Yin Wei channels
  Warmth, Fluid, Air bodies

ACTIONS AND INIDICATIONS

hepatobiliary sedative: liver decongestant, antibacterial: acute liver and gallbladder congestion and/or infections; acute hepatitis and jaundice, liver and other abscesses
cholagogue, choleretic: biliary dyspepsia, jaundice, constipation
antipyretic, anti-inflammatory: high fever, cholangitis, conjunctivitis, mastitis, stomatitis; facial and oral sores and boils; burns, scalds
nervous sedative, hypotensive: insomnia, unrest, toothache; stress, hypertension
parasympathetic nervous stimulant, sympathetic antagonist
astringent, hemostatic: bleeding (incl. blood in saliva, stool, nosebleed); hematemesis, epistaxis, enteritic melena
antifungal: fungal skin conditions
anticontusion: sprains, strains

SYMPTOM PICTURES

liver and gallbladder damp heat: right subcostal pain, unrest, irritability, nausea, vomiting, jaundice
Yang excess and Blood heat: fever, irritability, unrest, nosebleed, blood in urine, stool or vomit

PREPARATION

Use: The pod Gardenia Zhi Zi should be decocted or used in tincture form. The tincture is somewhat less *cooling* and more *sedative* in effect. Gardenia pod is traditionally lightly charred when used for to treat various forms of bleeding. The charred remedy is called **Shan Zhi Zi Tan** (Mand.) or **San Ji Ji Taan** (Cant.).

Dosage: Decoction: 6-12 g
Tincture: 2-4 ml
Caution: Avoid using in loose stool due to digestive deficiency.

NOTES

The scarlet seed pods of the Gardenia plant have always been used for their yield of lustrous yellow dye, while its flowers are valued for their rare fragrance. In medicine this remedy is traditionally classed in the heat-clearing, or *refrigerant,* category, which modern research and experimentation show to consist of significant *choleretic, nervous sedative* and *hypotensive* actions. The *hypotensive* effect is thought to be activated by increased medullary parsaympathetic excitability.

The clinical implications of these main actions are nowhere better described than in the syndrome liver and gallbladder damp heat, where biliary stasis, liver congestion, bacterial (sub)infection, sympathetic nervous hypertonia and pain coalesce. This gives Gardenia pod the profile of a classic *hepatobiliary sedative.*

Gardenia flower, Zhi Zi Hua (Mand.) or **San Ji Ji Fa** (Cant.) and its extracts, such as the triterpenoid gardenolic acid, are used for their *contraceptive* effect.

Bretschneider (1871) a long time ago cleared up the confusion of identity between this Chinese gardenia and the South African cape jasmine.

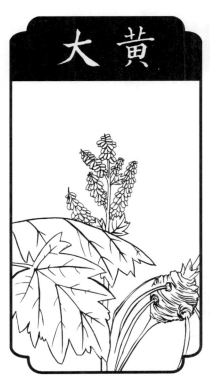

Rheum Da Huang
Rhubarb Root

Botanical source: *Rheum palmatum* L. or *R. tanguticum* Maximoxicz ex Regel or *R. officinale* Baillon (Polygonaceae)
Pharmaceutical name: Rhizoma Rhei
Chinese names: Da Huang, Chuan Jun, Sheng Jun, Huang Liang (Mand); Daai Wong (Cant)
Other names: Chinese rhubarb, "Great yellow"; Daio (Jap)
Habit: Large perennial herb from West and North China; grows in cold, dry, forested mountain regions in somewhat shady, damp locales with moist, deep soil; blooms during summer with small multiple clusters of purple flowers.
Part used: the rhizome

Therapeutic category: mild herb with minimal chronic toxicity
Constituents: anthraquinones and derivatives (incl. emodin, chrysophanic acid, rhein, physcion, sennosides A, B, C, D), tannins, oxalic/cinnamic/gallic acids, iron, magnesium, calcium, vitamins B and C
Effective qualities: bitter, astringent, cold, dry
  calming, stimulating, decongesting, astringing, sinking
Tropism: digestive, vascular system
  Liver, Stomach, Spleen, Large Intestine, Pericardium channels
  Air, Warmth bodies

ACTIONS AND INDICATIONS

biliary sedative: biliary decongestant, anti-infective: acute biliary and pancreatic infections
anti-inflammatory, antipyretic: acute appendicitis, acute enteritis, dysentery; skin inflammations, burns, scalds, stomatitis, mouth ulcers, conjunctivitis
anti-infective: antibacterial, antifungal, antiviral: intestinal infections (acute or chronic), dermatitis, eczema, herpes zoster; gram-positive and gram-negative cocci (esp. *Neisseria gonorrhea* and *Staphylococci;*

Dermatomyces, Nocardia, Epidermophyton); Myxovirus influenzae
antiparasitic: esp. *Trichomonas hominis*
biliary, gastric and pancreatic stimulant, choleretic: liver congestion with acute dyspepsia, jaundice; gastritis, gastroenteritis, anorexia
stimulant laxative, purgative: constipation, hard distended abdomen
astringent, coagulant hemostatic: chronic gastroenteritis, diarrhea; blood in vomit, nosebleed, bleeding hemorrhoids
interferon inducent, antitumoral: female reproductive tumors; acute monocytic leukemia, ascitic cancer, breast cancer, melanoma, lymphosarcoma
antilipemic: hyperlipidemia
anticontusion: injuries, sprains, strains; mentrual clots with delayed menses

Symptom Pictures

gallbladder heat: right subcostal pain, dizziness, sour belching, vomiting, jaundice, fever

gallbladder and stomach Qi stagnation: appetite loss, sour eructations or regurgitation, swollen painful epigastrium

liver Qi stagnation: constipation or pasty unformed stool, nausea, jaundice, right subcostal pain

intestines dry heat: constipation, abdominal distension, high fever, profuse sweating, thirst

intestines damp heat: burning urgent bowel movement with loose stool, abdominal pain, thirst, feverishness

intestines damp cold: indigestion, profuse watery stool, nausea, tender swollen abdomen, unrest, chills

Preparation

Use: The chopped or powdered root Rheum Da Huang is usually decocted or tinctured. Decoction should not exceed 10 minutes, unless the *astringent* or *hemostatic* effect is required. In this case, longer cooking time (e.g. 30-40 minutes) will make the tannins more available.

Dosage: The small dosage has an *astringing* and *calming* effect useful in intestines damp cold/damp heat syndromes. The medium dosage is *stimulant* and *laxative* and should be used for conditions of liver, Gallbladder and stomach Qi stagnation and with acute intestines damp heat. The high dosage is *purgative* and *cooling,* appropriate for full heat or damp heat conditions of the gallbladder, liver and stomach.

Decoction: Small dose: 0.05-0.5 g
Medium dose: 0.5-2 g
High dose: 2-3 g
Tincture: Small dose: 6-12 drops or 0.25-0.5 ml.
Medium dose: 12-50 drops or 0.5-2 ml
High dose: 50-100 drops or 2-4 ml

Caution: Rhubarb root is forbidden during pregnancy and lactation, and in gout, hemorrhoids and oxalic acid stones. It should also not be used for its *choleretic* or *stimulant laxative* action in conditions of Qi or Blood (metabolic) deficiency and stomach/intestines cold, where it usually causes constipation rather than bowel movement. For several reasons Rhubarb should never be used long-term.

Notes

Rhubarb root is one of the few remedies that spans three major systems of medicine, namely Oriental, Ayurvedic and Greek/Western. It is also uncommon in aiding a wide range of digestive dysfunctions associated with the liver, gallbladder, stomach and colon. Rhubarb root's functional versatility arises from its polar constituents: the *dry, astringent,* tannins on one hand, and the *stimulant, decongestant* anthraquinones on the other. This makes Rhubarb's action very dosage dependent, as described under Dosage.

Being equally effective and reliable with all above syndromes, its classification becomes difficult. Cultural-medical preferences have historically determined whether Rhubarb root was seen primarily as an agent for *clearing excess heat* (Chinese medicine), as a *stimulant laxative* (Ayurvedic medicine), or as a *hepatobiliary stimulant* (traditional Greek medicine).

Gentiana Long Dan Cao
Scabrous Gentian Root *

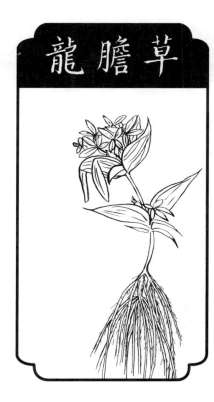

Botanical source: *Gentiana scabra* Bunge or *G. triflora* Pallas or *G. manshurica* Kitagawa (Gentianaceae)
Pharmaceutical name: Radix Gentianae scabrae
Chinese names: Long Dan Cao, Long Dan, Dan Cao (Mand); Lung Daam Chou (Cant)
Other names: Japanese gentian, "Dragon gallbladder weed"; Ryutan (Jap)
Habit: Perennial herb found throughout China; grows on wasted slopes and in grassland thickets; blue single/clustered terminal flowers open in fall/winter.
Part used: the root

Therapeutic category: mild herb with minimal chronic toxicity
Constituents: bitter glycosides (incl. gentiopicrin, gentianose, gentisin, gentiopicroside, swertiamarin, sweroside), alkaloids (incl. gentianine, gentianidine), carbohydrates
Effective qualities: very bitter, a bit astringent, cold, dry
  stimulating, decongesting, astringing, sinking
Tropism: digestive, reproductive systems
  Liver, Gallbladder, Bladder channels; Warmth, Fluid bodies

ACTIONS AND INDICATIONS
hepatobiliary sedative: decongestant: acute hepatobiliary infections with jaundice; liver congestion, hepatitis, cholecystitis, cholangitis
antipyretic, anti-inflammatory: fever, vulvovaginitis, laryngitis, conjunctivitis, tonsilitis; malaria
anti-infective, detoxicant: venereal infections, esp. with discharge, vaginitis, genital pruritus, leucorrhea, metritis; acute intestinal infections; hematuria; eczema, boils, abscesses, sores
cholagogue, laxative: biliary dyspepsia, jaundice, constipation
gastric stimulant: appetite loss, loose stool, fatigue
antiallergic: immune stress with immediate allergies (incl. rhinitis, urticaria, bronchial asthma)
Miscellaneous: sudden deafness, earache

SYMPTOM PICTURES
liver and gallbladder damp heat / gallbladder heat: nausea, vomiting, right subcostal or flank pain, jaundice, constipation

Liver fire: throbbing headache, congested red head, face and eyes, subcostal pain, tremors, fever

genitourinary damp heat: genital itching and swelling, fetid yellow discharge, short, dark painful urination

gallbladder and stomach Qi stagnation: fatigue, appetite loss, epigastric pain and distension, sick headache

PREPARATION
Use: The root Gentiana Long Dan Cao should be decocted or used in tincture form. For moving gallbladder/stomach stagnation, only the smallest dosage is used. The larger the dose, the greater the draining and decongestant effect in damp heat or hot syndromes.
Dosage: Decoction: 3-10 g
    Tincture: 1-3ml
Caution: Forbidden in diarrhea due to digestive weakness.

NOTES
Scabrous gentian root may be used interchangeably with the Western Gentian, *Gentiana lutea*.

The main difference between them lies in their therapeutic use as determined by different cultural contexts and health needs rather than by any intrinsic differences. Both gentians are bitter, cold *refrigerant* and *decongestant cholagogues* with an ultimate *sedative* effect. These actions may be used for treating excess liver and biliary conditions, such as acute hepatitis and cholecystitis, involving damp heat and liver fire.

Like the Western Gentian root, Scabrous gentian root may also be taken in smaller doses for stagnant conditions of the stomach and gallbladder—another application of the bitter taste energy.

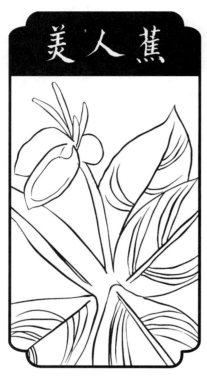

Canna Mei Ren Jiao
Canna Lily Root

Botanical source: *Canna indica* L., syn. *Canna orientalis* Roscoe (Cannaceae)
Pharmaceutical name: Rhizoma Cannae
Chinese names: Mei Ren Jiao (Gen); Feng Wei Hua (M); Muk Yan Jiu (C)
Other names: Indian shot/canna, "Beautiful Jiao"; Dandoku (Jap) Tasbeh (Ar)
Habit: Perennial herb from South Asia, inhabiting damp grasslands; also cultivated; racemes of bright carmine terminal flowers open in summer.
Part used: the rhizome

Therapeutic category: mild remedy with minimal chronic toxicity
Constituents: six phenolic substances, terpenes, coumarins, glucose, alkaloids, gum, calcium, phosphorus
Effective qualities: sweet, bland, cool, dry
    stimulating, decongesting, dispersing, relaxing, astringing
Tropism: digestive, vascular systems
    Liver, Gallbladder, Large Intestine, Lung channels
    Air, Warmth bodies

ACTIONS AND INDICATIONS
hepatic sedative: liver decongestant, liver protective: liver congestion with jaundice; acute hepatitis
antipyretic, diaphoretic, diuretic: fever due to infection, oliguria
cholagogue, choleretic, laxative: biliary dyspepsia, jaundice, constipation
intestinal relaxant, astringent: chronic dysentery, enteritis, IBS with diarrhea
hypotensive: hypertension
astringent, mucostatic, hemostatic: hemoptysis, leucorrhea, menorrhagia
vulnerary: wounds, injuries, boils

SYMPTOM PICTURES
liver and gallbladder damp heat: bitter taste in mouth, constipation, irritability, jaundice, right subcostal pain
external wind heat: feverishness, some chills, sore throat, irritability, dry skin, scanty urination

PREPARATION
Use: The root Canna Mei Ren Jiao is decocted or used in tincture form. The flower may be used in external styptic applications.
Dosage: Decoction: 15-30 g
    Tincture: 2-5 ml
    High doses are mainly used for acute hepatitis.
Caution: None.

NOTES

Canna lily root represents an important remedy today for the treatment of acute hepatitis—the result of *liver protective, cholagogue* and *choleretic* activities in concert.

The overall *sedative/relaxant* character of this important remedy from the tropics, combined with its tropism for the digestive and cardiovascular systems, also ensures relief from other hot and tense conditions. These would include enteritis and high blood pressure, as well as wind heat onset of infections when a *relaxant diaphoretic* is required.

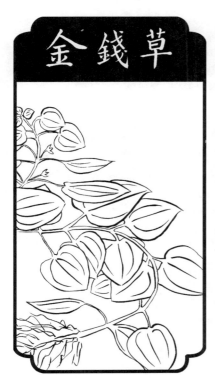

Lysimachia Jin Qian Cao
Asian Moneywort Herb *

Botanical source: *Lysimachia christinae* Hance or *L. hemsleyana* Maximovicz (Primulaceae)
Pharmaceutical name: Herba Lysimachiae
Chinese names: Jin Qian Cao, Da Jin Qian Cao, Guo Lu Huang (Mand); Gam Chin Chou, Gam Chan Chou (Cant)
Other names: "Gold coin weed", Christina's loosestrife; Kinsenso (Jap)
Habit: Perennial herb from south of the Yangtze river, incl. Sichuan; grows in grassy thickets by roadsides; yellow single axillary flowers open in summer.
Part used: the herb

Therapeutic category: mild remedy with minimal chronic toxicity
Constituents: flavonoids (incl. quercetin, rutin, kaempferol), essential oil (incl. phenol, lactones), amino acids, choline, sterols, dymethoxychalcone, potassium and sodium chloride, nitrites, tannins, benzoic acid, uracil, trace elements (incl. zinc, copper, manganese)
Effective qualities: a bit salty, bitter and sour, cool, moist
  calming, stimulating, decongesting, dissolving, sinking
Tropism: digestive, urogenital systems
  Liver, Gallbladder, Bladder, Kidney channels; Warmth, Fluid bodies

ACTIONS AND INDICATIONS

biliary sedative: anti-inflammatory, antiseptic: acute hepatobiliary infections; cholecystitis, cholelithiasis, icteral hepatitis; cystitis, urethritis, mastitis, whooping cough, conjunctivitis, burns, dermatitis
hepatobiliary stimulant: decongestant, cholagogue: hepatobiliary dyspepsia; jaundice, liver congestion
resolvent diuretic, biliary and urinary antilithic: biliary and urinary stones, dysuria, oliguria, anuria
detoxicant, detumescent: boils, abscess, traumatic injury
antivenomous: snake or insect bite, herb and mushroom poisoning

SYMPTOM PICTURES

gallbladder heat: sharp right subcostal pain, sour belching, irritability, bitter taste in mouth, jaundiced skin

liver and gallbladder damp heat: painful subcostal region, nausea, vomiting, jaundice, fever

bladder damp heat: painful burning urination, scanty or obstructed urination, thirst, sharp lower abdominal pains, sand or blood clots in urine

PREPARATION

Use: The herb Lysimachia Jin Qian Cao is infused, briefly decocted or used in tincture form.
Dosage: Infusion and short decoction: 15-30 g
  Tincture: 2-4 ml
Caution: None.

NOTES

Asian moneywort, a species of loosestrife, has proven to be one of the most versatile and outstanding *biliary sedative* remedies in the Chinese pharmacopeia. The herb is much used on its own, or combined with other remedies, drugs or acupuncture. Asian moneywort is specific in programs to expel biliary stones, as well as to offset or treat gallstone attacks and other acute gallbladder conditions. Its *refrigerant, anti-inflammatory, downward moving* qualities are embodied in *cholagogue* and *diuretic* actions, in vitalistic terms addressing hot or damp heat conditions.

Asian moneywort is used in the same way that *Lysimachia nummularia*, **Moneywort**, was in traditional Greek/Galenic medicine. It is interesting to see the same plant (and similar plants) called by virtually the same name in both East and West. Other vicariads of *Lysimachia christinae* are *Desmodium styracifolium*, **Coin-leaf desmodium**, properly known as **Guang Dong Jin Qian Cao** (see below); and species of **Ground ivy** (*Glechoma*) and **Lawn water pennywort** (*Hydrocotyle*): these are considered to a large extent to have the same therapeutic value as Lysimachia Jin Qian Cao.

Desmodium Guang Dong Jin Qian Cao
Coin-Leaf Desmodium Herb *

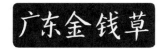

Botanical source: *Desmodium styracifolium* (Osbeck.) Merrill (Leguminosae)
Chinese names: Guang Dong Jin Qian Cao (Mand)
Category: mild remedy with minimal chronic toxicity

Effective qualities: a bit salty and bitter, cool, moist; stimulating, calming, decongesting, softening
Tropism: digestive, urinary systems; Liver, Gallbladder, Bladder channels

ACTIONS: *Hepatobiliary decongestant, anti-inflammatory, antiseptic, choleretic, cholagogue, resolvent diuretic, biliary and urinary antilithic, hypotensive, coronary decongestant, detoxicant*

INDICATIONS: Gallbladder heat syndromes with jaundice, liver congestion, cholecystitis, acute cholelithiasis, acute icteric hepatitis; liver and gallbladder damp heat syndromes, bladder damp heat syndromes with cystitis, urethritis, nephritis, urinary stones, dysuria, oliguria; hypertension, angina pectoris, congestive coronary disease; mastitis; conjunctivitis, burns, dermatitis, boils, abscesses.

Dosage: Short decoction: 15-60 g
Tincture: 2-5 ml

Caution: None.

Acanthus Lao Shu Le
Holly-Leaf Acanthus Root *

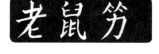

Botanical source: *Acanthus ilicifolius* L. (Acanthaceae)
Chinese names: Lao Shu Le, Lao Shu Pa, Juan Ku Mu Dan, Xie Jua Le (Mand); Lou Syu Laak
Category: mild remedy with minimal chronic toxicity

Constituents: flavonoids vasicine, vasicinol, amino acids
Effective qualities: a bit bitter, cool, dry; stimulating, decongesting, calming, relaxing
Tropism: digestive, reproductive, respiratory systems; Liver, Spleen channels

ACTIONS: *Liver decongestant, anti-inflammatory, antipyretic, analgesic, bronchial relaxant, uterine stimulant, antitumoral*

INDICATIONS: Liver and spleen enlargement, hepatitis with liver damp heat, chronic fever, gastric pain, asthma, therapeutic abortion, lymphadenitis, scrofula, mumps, cancer.

Dosage: Decoction: 30-60 g
Tincture: 2-5 ml

Caution: Forbidden during pregnancy.

Sedum Chui Pen Cao
Stringy Stonecrop Root and Herb

Botanical source: *Sedum sarmentosum* Bunge (Crassulaceae)
Chinese names: Chui Pen Cao, Shi Zhi Jia (Mand); Chai Pan Chou (Cant)
Category: mild remedy with minimal chronic toxicity

Constituents: glycoside sarmentosiin
Effective qualities: sweet, bland, sour, cool; decongesting
Tropism: digestive system; Liver, Gallbladder channels

ACTIONS: *Liver decongestant, liver protective, anti-inflammatory, antipyretic, detoxicant, detumescent*
INDICATIONS: Acute and chronic hepatitis, low-grade Yin deficiency fevers, carbuncles, deep-rooted ulcers.
Dosage: Decoction: 10-20 g
Tincture: 2-5 ml
Caution: None.

Dichondra Ma Di Jin
Dichondra Herb

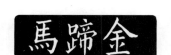

Botanical source: *Dichondra repens* Forst (Convulvulaceae)
Chinese names: Ma Di Jin, Huang Dan Cao, Xiao Jin Qian Cao (Mand); Ma Dei Jing (Cant)

Category: mild remedy with minimal chronic toxicity
Effective qualities: bitter, cool; decongesting, calming
Tropism: digestive system; Liver, Gallbladder, Stomach, Lung channels

ACTIONS: *Liver decongestant, astringent, anti-inflammatory, detoxicant, diuretic, antilithic, hemostatic*
INDICATIONS: Jaundice with damp heat, dysentery, hemoptysis, fever, stomach ulcers, mastitis, scrofula, boils, urinary stones, turbid urine, edema, external and external injuries.
Dosage: Short decoction: 6-16 g
Tincture: 2-4 ml
Caution: None.

Hemerocallis Xuan Cao Gen
Tawny Day Lily Root

Botanical source: *Hemerocallis fulva* L. (Liliaceae)
Chinese names: Xuan Cao, Xuan Cao Gen (Mand); San Chou (Cant)
Category: medium-strength remedy with chronic toxicity

Constituents: asparagin, chrysophanol, alkaloids (incl. colchinin, friedelin, hemerocallin, obtusifolin), rhein, trehalase, beta-sitosterol
Effective qualities: sweet, cool; calming, decongesting

ACTIONS: *Liver decongestant, anti-inflammatory, antiseptic, resolvent and draining diuretic, detoxicant, demulcent laxative, hemostatic, antitumoral*
INDICATIONS: Liver congestion, jaundice, hepatitis; urinary tract infection, urinary stones, dysuria, oliguria; mastitis, parotitis, middle-ear infection, cervical lymphadenitis; dry constipation; nosebleed, coughing up blood, blood in urine or stool; breast tumor.
Dosage: Decoction: 6-10 g
Tincture: 1-2.5 ml
Topical applications are often made with the root for mastitis, breast abscess or tumor.
Caution: Do not take internally on a continuous basis because of some cumulative toxicity. Signs of intoxication include urinary incontinence, dilated pupils, difficult breathing and diarrhea.
NOTES: Day lily flower, Xuan Cao Hua, is considered an effective *analgesic, spasmolytic* and *antipyretic*. The remedy is given especially for pain-relief during labor. It is also high in iron.

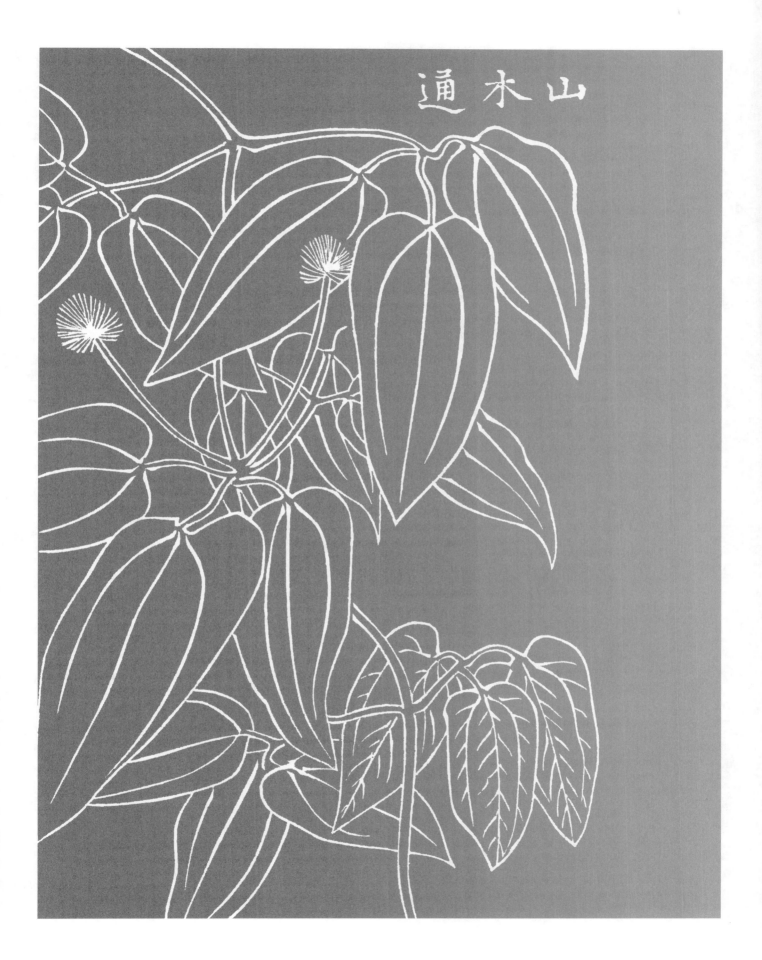

泌尿系统用药

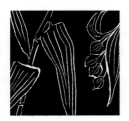

Remedies for the Urinary System

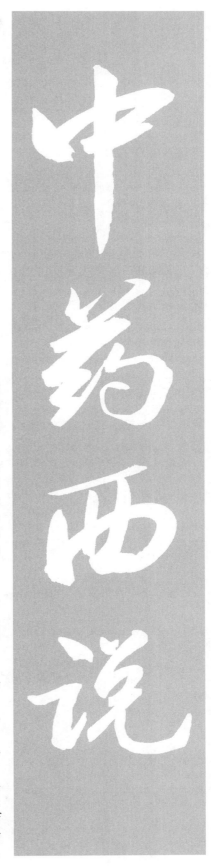

Oriental doctors treat urinary disorders through use of a wide variety of plant parts, including grasses, seeds, berries, herbs, roots and fungi. In traditional Chinese herbals, urinary remedies are found in only two herb classes: those that "strongly astrict" and those that "benefit the fluids and permeate damp" (i.e., drain fluid congestion). Today we can classify these remedies according to *restoration, stimulation, relaxation* and *sedation*—the four essential herb actions in Western energetic phytothe-rapy. This classification allows practitioners not only to more clearly distinguish among the remedies from the Western perspective, but also to make more specific and accurate choices when applying them to various urinary disorders.

- ***Urinary restoratives*** address deficiency conditions involving either:
    - urogenital weakness presenting incontinence and urogenital discharge.
    - kidney and bladder dryness presenting urinary irritation.
- ***Urinary stimulants*** treat deficiency conditions with kidney damp and fluid congestion, presenting edema.
- ***Urinary relaxants*** address tense conditions displaying urinary irritation and pain.
- ***Urinary sedatives*** treat hot conditions involving acute infection, accompanied by pain.

Interestingly, remedies for the urinary tract clearly demonstrate the close link between urinary and reproductive functions. *Urinary astringent restoratives* especially cover a whole range of urinary and genital deficiency conditions at the same time. Many of these are also notable *restoratives* for the reproductive system.

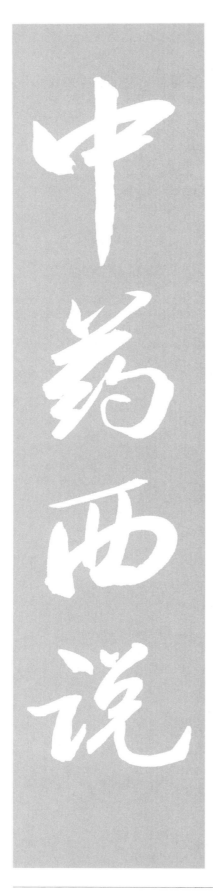

The Urinary Remedies

Restoratives

There are two kinds of *urinary restoratives:*
- *antienuretics* and *antileucorrheals* that restore the bladder and relieve urinary incontinence and genital discharges.
- *moist demulcents* and *hydrogenics* that moisten the kidneys and bladder, and relieve urinary irritation.

Urinary restoratives of the first kind, some of which are *astringents,* relieve urinary incontinence by toning the bladder sphincter muscle. They ameliorate symptoms such as copious, frequent and dribbling urination, bedwetting, and bladder distension without a feeling of fullness. In Western medical terms the symptoms signal polyuria, pollakiuria and enuresis, respectively. Unless strictly preclinical, these keynote symptoms of the syndrome **urinary Qi deficiency** may involve conditions such as renal deficiency, atonic neurogenic bladder and renal tubular acidosis. By toning the mucosa with their astringency they also stop mucus discharges that are considered signs of **urinary damp cold.**

Because of the close connection between functional urinary and genital deficiencies, reproductive system signs such as leucorrhea and seminal incontinence may join these two symptom pictures. *Urinary astringents* may be labelled *mucostatic* and *antileucorrheal* as well as *antienuretic,* as they also arrest white vaginal and seminal discharges in the larger syndrome **genitourinary Qi deficiency** and **genitourinary damp cold.**

It should be noted that in terms of classical Oriental medicine, these remedies are said to operate because of their tonifying action on Kidney Qi and Kidney Yang. A deficiency of these functions—which roughly translates as insufficiencies of kidney/adrenal system functions—then causes the urogenital syndromes described above. Hence, *urinary restoratives* are defined as "promoting astriction, stabilizing the Kidney and retaining urine and essence."

Urinary astringents are for the most part either sweet and mildly astringent in taste, such as Euryale Qian Shi (the common aquatic Foxnut), or sour and astringent, such as Rosa Jin Ying Zi (Cherokee rose hip, another common shrub) and Cornus Shan Zhu Yu (the berry of the montane Japanese dogwood). All contain a variety of chemical constituents presumed accountable for their therapeutic action, including saponins, glycosides, essential oils, organic acids and tannins.

The second type of *urinary restorative* is *demulcent* in nature, and is known as a *hydrogenic* and *urinary demulcent.* It helps the kidneys to retain fluid in the system, provides moisture to the kidneys and bladder, and soothes urinary irritation. Consequently, *hydrogenic demulcents* are given not only for bladder irritation causing urinary discomfort, but also for metabolic acidosis presenting thirst, dehydration, dry itchy skin, and scanty, light urination. This symptom pattern can be defined as **kidney dryness,** because here the kidneys fail to retain sufficient water, sodium, chlorine and bicarbonates, while poorly excreting potassium and hydrogen ions.

Interestingly, *urinary demulcents* include two seeds and two plant piths: the important and common Asian plantain seed (Plantago Che Qian Zi) and Muskmallow seed (Malva Dong Kui zi), as well as the piths of the subtropical Rice paper plant and the aquatic Bulrush (Tetrapanax Tong Cao, Juncus Deng Xin Cao). These *demulcents* have sweet, bland, cool and moist effective qualities because of their high mucilage content: They soothe, cool and moisten the urinary passages.

Stimulants

When the kidneys and/or liver fail to control the transformation of fluids due to functional deficiency, the fluids congest causing tissue swelling (edema) at the peripheries, such as puffy eyes or face on waking in the morning, swollen ankles or legs and, in the case of liver involvement, generalized water retention. The syndrome is called **kidney/liver fluid congestion** and, after the subclinical stage, may involve metabolic alkalosis, acute or chronic nephritis, acute glomerulonephritis, nephrotic syndrome, cirrhosis or ascites.

In the case of metabolic alkalosis the symptom picture may also include frequent urination, calf cramps, stiff muscles and joints, neuromuscular tension, dark circles under the eyes, acute weekly salt cravings, irritability, fearfulness and insecurity. This syndrome can be defined as **kidney damp** since here the kidneys retain excess water, sodium and bicarbonates, while being unable to retain potassium and hydrogen ions.

Urinary stimulants encourage the kidneys and liver to regulate intracellular water balance, promote lymphatic drainage and increase the volume of urine produced, with the net result of draining the tissues of superfluous fluid. In Chinese medicine they are usually referred to as "benefiting the fluids and permeating/draining damp." Fittingly, they are called *draining diuretics* and have mainly sweet, bland and neutral to cool effective qualities. The commonly used Poria Fu Ling (Hoelen fungus, found around coastal pine trees) and Imperata Bai Mao Gen (the subtropical Woolly grass root) are good examples. The *urinary stimulants* contain various constituents thought to be instrumental in their action, notably potassium, polysaccharides and glycosides.

Draining diuretics also play an important part in the treatment of scanty and blocked urination (oliguria, anuria), whether caused by eruptive fever, hydronephrosis, acute or chronic renal failure, renal vein thrombosis, acute glomerulonephritis (the syndrome **kidney fire),** acute tubular necrosis, prostate hyperplasia, etc. This is especially true of the last seven herbs in this section: *purgative draining diuretics,* that have bitter, pungent

URINARY SYSTEM

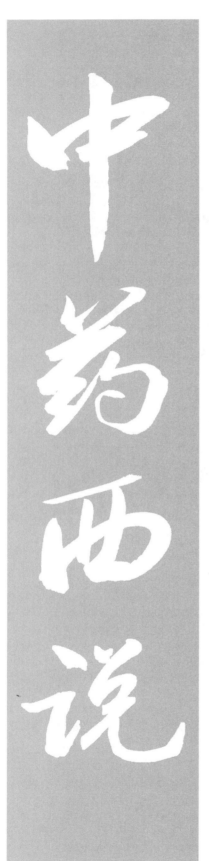

and stimulant qualities. These botanicals quickly eliminate excessive fluid through both the bladder and colon—they "expel fluids downward." Acute nephritis, ascites, pulmonary edema, hydrothorax and acute anuria are conditions most benefited by these strong remedies. They are usually given only once or twice because of both the acute conditions they treat and their strong (toxic) or medium-strength therapeutic status.

Relaxants

Urinary relaxants relieve symptoms such as suppressed, frequent, scanty, dribbling urination without a feeling of fullness, and bedwetting. These symptoms belong to the symptom picture **bladder Qi constraint,** often caused by nervous tension and emotional distress. They may involve, for example, neurogenic bladder, acute renal colic, acute pyelonephritis and Reiter's syndrome.

Urinary relaxants are both *spasmolytic* and *analgesic,* while reducing the incidence of the above symptoms. A good example is the sweet, cool, moist-natured Coix Yi Yi Ren (Job's tears seed from China's lowlands), which also has considerable *demulcent* qualities.

Sedatives

Like *sedatives* for other body systems, *urinary sedatives* treat infectious, inflammatory and painful urinary conditions such as acute pyelonephritis and acute urinary tract infections (cystitis, urethritis). The traditional symptom picture **bladder damp heat** involves painful, burning, urgent and frequent urination, cloudy urine, thirst, fever, backache and nausea.

Urinary sedatives comprise *anti-inflammatory, antiseptic* and *spasmolytic* actions, and are described in Oriental medicine as "clearing damp heat from the bladder." Their primary qualities are bitter, astringent and very cooling, qualities found, for instance, in Aristolochia Bai Mu Tong (Manchurian birthwort stem, from the climbing northeast Chinese vine) and Dianthus Qu Mai (the herb of the common proud pink). These remedies variously contain glycosides, essential oils and tannins, which helps explain not only their strong *antiseptic* action but also their ability to reduce the resultant inflammation and urinary irritation.

An unusual yet important *urinary sedative* is Talcum Hua Shi, the mineral talc mined in the northern provinces. Consisting mainly of hydrous magnesium silicate, this remedy has proven perennially reliable in managing acute urinary tract infections with difficult, painful urination.

Urinary Restoratives

REMEDIES TO RESTORE THE KIDNEYS AND BLADDER, RELIEVE UROGENITAL INCONTINENCE AND STOP DISCHARGE

➥ STABILIZE THE KIDNEY AND RETAIN URINE AND ESSENCE

Antieneuretics, antileucorrheals

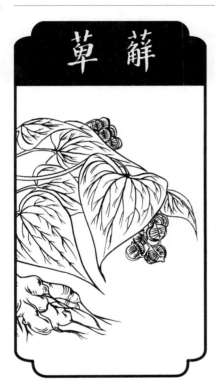

Dioscorea Bi Xie
Long Yam Root

Botanical source: *Dioscorea hypoglauca* Palibin or *D. colletti* Hooker f. or *D. tokoro* Makino or *D. gracillima* Miquel (Dioscoreaceae)
Pharmaceutical name: Rhizoma Dioscoreae hypoglaucae
Chinese names: Bi Xie, Bei Xie, Qi Jie, Chuan Bi Xie (Mand); Bei Gaai, Chyun Bei Gaai (Cant)
Other names: Fish poison yam, Seven-lobed yam; Hikai (Jap)
Habit: Perennial vine-like climbing herb from the mountains of Central and East China; blooms in summer with purplish and viridian flower spikes.
Part used: the rhizome

Therapeutic category: mild remedy with minimal chronic toxicity
Constituents: steroidal saponins (incl. diosgenin, dioscin, gracillin, dioscoreasapotoxin, yononin, tokoronin, tokorogenin), tannins
Effective qualities: a bit bitter and bland, neutral, dry
    restoring, astringing, stabilizing, solidifying
Tropism: urogenital, muscular, dermal systems
    Liver, Stomach, Bladder, Dai channels; Fluid, Air bodies

ACTIONS AND INDICATIONS

urinary restorative: antienuretic: urinary deficiency with incontinence and enuresis, pollakiuria, dysuria, cloudy or mucousy urine; albuminuria, chyluria
stimulant diuretic: anuria
genital mucostatic, astringent: leucorrhea, gonorrhea
anti-inflammatory, analgesic: prostatitis; numbness, stiffness or pain of lower extremities, arthralgia, myalgia, lumbar pain, knee pain, penis pain
detoxicant, dermatropic antifungal: arthritis, eczema, dermatitis, fungal skin conditions, boils, pustular sores, toxic ulcers; hyperlipemia
antiparasitic: intestinal parasites

SYMPTOM PICTURES

genitourinary damp cold: frequent, difficult, painful, cloudy urine, clear vaginal discharges, backache
metabolic toxicosis (wind damp/damp heat obstruction): muscle, joint and lower back pain, numb or stiff lower extremities

PREPARATION

Use: The root Dioscorea Bi Xie is decocted or used in tincture form.
Dosage: Decoction: 10-18 g

Caution: Forbidden in Kidney Yin deficiency.

NOTES

Long yam root is an important *urinary restorative* that directly affects difficult, dribbling or frequent urination, whatever the etiology. It is also one of the few Oriental specific remedies for albuminuria and chyluria. Damp and cold afflicting the Lower Warmer with Dai Mai deficiency is the primary energetic condition that indicates the use of this versatile remedy.

Being a systemic *resolvent detoxicant* that contains the steroidal saponins found in other varieties of medicinal yam, Long yam root also addresses various chronic and acute skin and musculoskeletal conditions, especially with numbness and stiffness of the legs and feet. Arthritic and myalgic conditions benefit from its *anti-inflammatory* and *analgesic* actions.

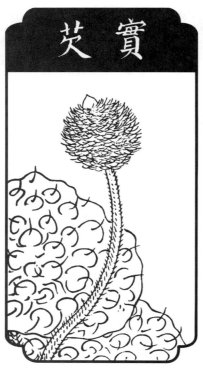

Euryale Qian Shi
Foxnut

Botanical source: *Euryale ferox* Salisbury (Nymphaeaceae)
Pharmaceutical name: Semen Euryalis
Chinese names: Qian Shi, Ji Tou, Yen Hui (Mand); Sui Sat (Cant)
Other names: Prickly water lily, Gorgon, Chickenhead; Kenjitsu (Jap)
Habit: Annual aquatic temperate Asian herb, common in ponds and marshes; blooms in summer and autumn with magenta flowers that open at noon and fade by dusk.
Part used: the seed

Therapeutic category: mild remedy with minimal chronic toxicity
Constituents: thiamine, nicotinic acid, protein 10%, starch, carotene, iron, calcium, potassium, phosphorus, vitamin C
Effective qualities: sweet, astringent, neutral, dry
  restoring, astringing, stabilizing, solidifying
Tropism: urinary, genital, digestive systems
  Kidney, Spleen, Stomach channels
  Fluid body

ACTIONS AND INDICATIONS

urinary restorative: astringent antienuretic: urinary deficiency with incontinence, mucus in urine; enuresis
genital mucostatic, astringent: leucorrhea, premature ejaculation, spermatorrhea, gonorrhea
intestinal astringent: chronic diarrhea (esp. infantile)
analgesic: arthralgia, neuralgia

SYMPTOM PICTURES

genitourinary damp cold: frequent, dribbling, mucousy urination; clear vaginal discharges, nocturnal emissions, premature ejaculation

intestines damp cold (Spleen Qi deficiency): chronic diarrhea, fatigue

PREPARATION

Use: The seed Euryales Qian Shi is decocted or used in tincture form.
Dosage: Decoction: 8-16 g
  Tincture: 2-4 ml
Caution: None.

NOTES
The prickly water lily is cultivated for its starch, and almost the entire plant, including the seed, is used for making flour. The seed, called foxnut, is a versatile *restorative* to the urogenital organs, treating both simple and infectious types of incontinence with discharge. Foxnut is also considered one of the best *astringents* for chronic diarrhea, especially in children.

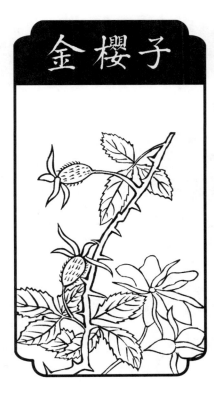

Rosa Jin Ying Zi
Cherokee Rosehip

Botanical source: *Rosa laevigata* Michaux (Rosaceae)
Pharmaceutical name: Fructus Rosae laevigatae
Chinese names: Jin Ying Zi (Mand); Jing Ying Ji (Cant)
Other names: "Gold cherry berry"; Kinoshi (Jap)
Habit: Evergreen Chinese climbing shrub growing on sunny slopes, roadside shrub thickets, in crevices and cliffs; in spring, large, fragrant, white single terminal flowers appear.
Part used: the fruit

Therapeutic category: mild remedy with minimal chronic toxicity
Constituents: citric and malic acids, saponins, tannin, fructose, sucrose, resin, vitamin C
Effective qualities: sour, sweet, a bit astringent, neutral, dry
    astringing, restoring, solidifying, stabilizing
Tropism: urogenital, digestive, respiratory systems
    Kidney, Bladder, Large Intestine channels
    Fluid body

ACTIONS AND INDICATIONS
urinary restorative: astringent antienuretic: urinary deficiency with enuresis, pollakiuria, mucus in urine
genital mucostatic, astringent: leucorrhea, spermatorrhea, menorrhagia, uterine prolapse
intestinal astringent: diarrhea, chronic enteritis, rectal prolapse
anhydrotic: spontaneous sweating, night sweats
antitussive: chronic cough, bronchitis
antilipemic: atherosclerosis
antibacterial, antiviral

SYMPTOM PICTURES
genitourinary damp cold: dribbling, frequent, copious, mucousy urination; clear vaginal discharges, wet dreams

intestines damp cold: chronic loose stool

PREPARATION
Use: The rosehip Rosa Jin Ying Zi is infused or used in tincture form.
Dosage: Decoction: 6-14 g
    Tincture: 1-3 ml
Caution: Forbidden in excess heat syndromes.

NOTES

Because it was introduced to North America at a very early date, this ubiquitous white-flowered rose was for a long time mistakenly assumed to be indigenous and hence called "Cherokee rose." Oriental doctors make use of the sour taste quality of this rosehip to promote astriction in conditions of urinary or genital incontinence. Many types of discharges from below may respond to its generally *mucostatic* and *astringent* effect, including diarrhea.

Cherokee rosehip leaf makes a good *vulnerary*.

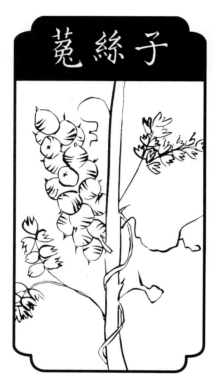

Cuscuta Tu Si Zi
Asian Dodder Seed

Botanical source: *Cuscuta chinensis* Lamarck or *C. japonica* Choisy (Convulvulaceae)
Pharmaceutical name: Semen Cuscutae
Chinese names: Tu Si Zi, Nu Lo, Huang Si Teng, Tu Lu (Mand); To Si Ji (Cant)
Other names: Japanese dodder, "Hare silk seed," Lady's laces; Toshishi (Jap)
Habit: Annual twining parasitic herb from Central China and Japan; grows on shrub branches on slopes, neglected stream banks and old roads; blooms in summer and autumn with short spikes of fragrant (orange-) white flowers.
Part used: the seed

Therapeutic category: mild remedy with minimal chronic toxicity
Constituents: glycoside cuscutin, saccharides, protein, fixed oil, vitamins
Effective qualities: sweet, a bit pungent, a bit warm, neutral
restoring, astringing, solidifying, stabilizing, relaxing
Tropism: reproductive, urinary, cardiovascular systems
Kidney, Liver, Ren, Yin Qiao, Dai channels
Fluid, Air bodies

ACTIONS AND INDICATIONS

urinary restorative: antienuretic: urinary deficiency with chronic urinary incontinence and enuresis
genital mucostatic, reproductive restorative: leucorrhea, spermatorrhea (incl. nocturnal), premature ejaculation; sexual disinterest, impotence, chronic miscarriage
hemostatic: bleeding (esp. uterine)
fetal relaxant, antiabortive: fetal distress, threatened miscarriage
intestinal astringent: chronic diarrhea
hypotensive: hypertension with dizziness, tinnitus
muscular restorative: backache, weak or sore knees, rheumatoid paralysis
vision restorative: blurred vision, poor eyesight and other vision disorders
antioxidant: toxicosis, premature aging
interferon inducent
Miscellaneous: hearing loss

SYMPTOM PICTURES

genitourinary damp cold (Kidney Yang deficiency with damp cold): clear vaginal discharges, nocturnal emissions, sexual disinterest; dribbling, frequent, scanty urination

Liver and Kidney Yin/Essence deficiency: blurred vision, spots in vision, dizziness, ringing in ears

Preparation

Use: The seed Cuscuta Tu Si Zi is decocted or used as a tincture. The tincture brings out its warming potential, especially with musculoskeletal problems.

Dosage: Decoction: 10-18 g
Tincture: 2-5 ml

Caution: None.

Notes

Although Dodder herb, *Cuscuta europea*, was traditionally used as a *urinary* and *hepatic* remedy in Europe, it never acquired the precise specific symptomatology that Dodder seed has in China. This consists mainly of urogenital (Kidney Yang) deficiency conditions with discharges, especially functional weaknesses—including habitual miscarriage and sexual disinterest. The use of Asian dodder seed for the traditional Liver and Kidney Yin deficiency syndrome correlates today with its known *hypotensive* action, yet includes vision and hearing improvement as well.

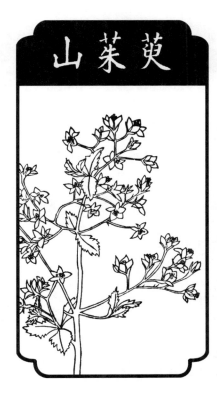

Cornus Shan Zhu Yu
Japanese Dogwood Berry

Botanical source: *Cornus officinalis* Siebold et Zuccarini (Cornaceae)
Pharmaceutical name: Fructus Corni
Chinese names: Shan Zhu Yu, Shan Yu Rou, Rou Zao, Shu Xuan Zao (Mand); San Yi Yak (Cant)
Other names: Japanese cornel, Asian cornelian cherry, "Sour mountain date"; Sanyuniku (Jap)
Habit: Deciduous mountain shrub or small tree from Mid and North China, Korea and Japan; also cultivated; yellow early spring blooms form umbellate clusters; the small drupe matures in November.
Part used: the fruit

Therapeutic category: mild remedy with minimal chronic toxicity
Constituents: verbenalin, cornin, saponins, ursolic/gallic/tannic/malic acids, tannin, iridoid glycosides (morroniside, loganin, sweroside), 17 amino acids, trace minerals, vitamin A
Effective qualities: sour, a bit salty and astringent, a bit warm
restoring, astringing, stabilizing, solidifying, relaxing
Tropism: urinary, reproductive, cardiovascular, nervous systems
Liver, Kidney, Dai channels; Fluid, Air bodies

Actions and Indications

urinary restorative: astringent antienuretic: urinary deficiency with incontinence with enuresis, pollakiuria, polyuria
reproductive restorative: spermatorrhea, impotence
hemostatic: uterine bleeding (metrorrhagia), menorrhagia
anhydrotic: excessive sweating (incl. in shock)
diuretic: hepatitis
hypotensive, parasympathetic nervous stimulant: hypertension; deafness, tinnitus, vertigo
antiallergic (antihistamine)
anti-infective: antibacterial, antifungal, antimalarial: various infections (incl. malaria)
leukocytogenic: leukopenia
Miscellaneous: shock

Symptom Pictures

genitourinary Qi deficiency (Kidney Qi deficiency): dribbling or copious urination, heavy menses, sexual disinterest, premature ejaculation

Liver and Kidney depletion: hard of hearing, ringing in ears; sore, weak lower back and knees, heavy menses

Preparation

Use: The berry Cornus Shan Zhu Yu is made into a short decoction or is used in tincture form.
Dosage: Decoction: 6-12 g; 30-60 g in cases of shock
Tincture: 2-4 ml
Caution: To be used with caution for Kidney Yang deficiency, and contraindicated with painful or difficult urination due to urinary tract infection.

Notes

Various species of dogwood grow all over the world, yet only the Chinese seem to have made extensive use of the berry. Native Americans, for example, used the astringent, bitter bark of *Cornus florida* mainly for intermittent fevers, diarrhea, dysentery and weakness.

No culture but the Chinese has used the sour quality of an herb to restrain urogenital discharges—witness the many *sour astringent* medicinals in this section. Moreover, the small shriveled, deep magenta dogwood berry is considered more than merely a remedy for seminal and urinary incontinence and excessive sweating. Because the fruit does not ripen until winter and, in fact, survives it, this plant is said to possess and impart vital endurance. Energetically, it tonifies the Chinese Kidney and Liver functions, and moreover has a general bracing effect on the Dai extra channel. When these processes are disordered, urogenital, neurological and musculoskeletal symptomatology appear, as seen in the two syndromes above. Note in particular Japanese dogwood's contemporary use as a *parasympathetic nerve stimulant* in cases of chronic sympatheticotonia with hypertension.

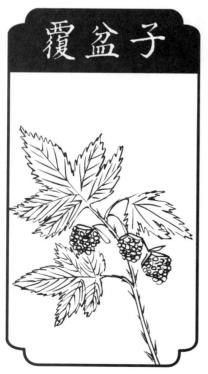

Rubus Fu Pen Zi
Chinese Raspberry Fruit

Botanical source: *Rubus chingii* Hu (Rosaceae)
Pharmaceutical name: Fructus Rubi chingii
Chinese names: Fu Pen Zi (Mand); Fuk Pan Ji (Cant)
Other names: "Overturned bowl berry"; Fukubonshi (Jap)
Habit: Deciduous shrub from temperate East Asia, growing on waste ground; in April, single five-petaled terminal flowers appear.
Part used: the unripe fruit

Therapeutic category: mild remedy with minimal chronic toxicity
Constituents: organic acids, vitamins C and A, glucose, trace minerals
Effective qualities: sour, sweet, astringent, neutral, dry
restoring, astringing, stabilizing, solidifying
Tropism: urogenital, hormonal systems
Liver, Kidney channels
Fluid body

ACTIONS AND INDICATIONS
urinary restorative: antienuretic: urinary deficiency with incontinence with enuresis, polyuria
genital astringent: premature ejaculation, seminal incontinence, spermatorrhea, impotence
vision enhancer: poor vision
estrogenic

SYMPTOM PICTURE
genitourinary Qi deficiency (Kidney Qi deficiency): dribbling or copious urination, bedwetting, premature ejaculation, wet dreams

PREPARATION
Use: The fruit Rubus Fu Pen Zi is briefly decocted or used in tincture form.
Dosage: Decoction: 2-10 g
Tincture: 1-3 ml
Caution: Contraindicated in difficult urination and to be used cautiously in Yin deficiency with empty heat.

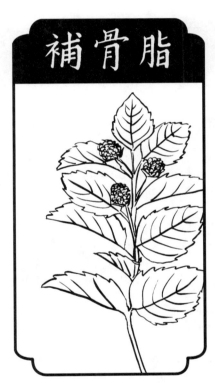

Psoralea Bu Gu Zhi
Scurf Pea Berry

Botanical source: *Psoralea corylifolia* L. (Leguminosae)
Chinese names: Bu Gu Zhi, Po Gu Zhi (Mand); Po Ku Ji (Cant)
Pharmaceutical name: Fructus Psoraleae
Other names: Scuffy pea, Malay tea, "Restore bone resin"; Babchi (Ind); Hokotsushi (Jap)
Habit: Erect annual herb of the (sub)tropical Asian plains, growing in tussocks along streams; also cultivated; peduncled heads of small lilac or yellow flowers appear in spring.
Part used: the fruit

Therapeutic category: mild remedy with minimal chronic toxicity
Constituents: flavonoids (incl. coryfolin, coryfolinin, bavachromene), essential oil (incl. monoterpene, phenol bakuchiol, angelicin, furanocoumarins [psoralidin, psoralen, isopsoralen]), fatty oil, phytosterols, resin
Effective qualities: pungent, bitter, astringent, warm, dry
restoring, astringing, stabilizing, solidifying, relaxing
Tropism: reproductive, urinary, cardiovascular, respiratory, dermal systems
Kidney, Spleen, Pericardium, Yin Qiao channels; Fluid, Air bodies

ACTIONS AND INDICATIONS
urinary restorative: astringent antienuretic: urinary deficiency with enuresis, pollakiauria, nocturia
reproductive restorative, androgenic, estrogenic: spermatorrhea, impotence
uterine and fetal relaxant, antiabortive: threatened miscarriage, fetal unrest
hemostatic, astringent: bleeding (esp. uterine); menorrhagia; diarrhea
coronary dilator, cardiotonic: angina pectoris, coronary deficiency
bronchodilator: acute asthma, cough
antioxidant (free radical inhibitor), antiallergic
anti-infective, leukocytogenic: infections in general; low WBC count (leukopenia)
vulnerary: fractures
photosensitizer: skin pigment loss (leucoderma), vitiligo, psoriasis

dermal, antitumoral (topically): psoriasis, vitiligo, callosities, alopecia, leprosy, skin cancer, solar urticaria, polymorphous light eruption

SYMPTOM PICTURES
genitourinary cold (Kidney Yang deficiency): premature ejaculation, sexual disinterest; frequent, dribbling urination

intestines cold (Spleen Yang deficiency): chronic diarrhea, abdominal pain, rumbling abdomen, fatigue

PREPARATION
Use: The berry Psoralea Bu Gu Zhi is decocted or used in tincture form. In skin conditions such as psoriasis, and in fractures, internal use should be supplemented by topical applications.
Dosage: Decoction: 3-10 g
Tincture: 2-4 ml
Caution: Contraindicated in Yin deficiency conditions with heat, and during pregnancy and breastfeeding. Very large doses of this herb experimentally have shown to possess *teratogenic*, i.e., fetus-injuring, effects.

NOTES
Although Scurf pea berry is "prescribed in all forms of sexual incompetency" (Porter Smith 1871), it is clear from the symptom pictures above that this remedy excels as a *tonifying urogenital astringent* for cold, deficient syndromes. Like Asian dodder seed, Scurf pea's tropism for the reproductive organs, female as well as male, is evinced in its competence in preventing miscarriage and treating metrorrhagia, for example. The presence of phytosterols and purported gonadotropic hormonal activity also reinforce the concept of a first class *reproductive restorative*.

Scurf pea berry is biochemically a loaded plant (including flavonoids and volatile oils), which helps explain the wide range of its traditional and modern applications, even though there are still huge holes in its current pharmacology. The *coronary* and *bronchial relaxant effect,* the *antioxidant* action and the application in various skin disorders are all uses worth watching for..

Scurf pea's *hemostatic* action, while being slow of onset, is still very effective, while the *fracture-healing* action is similar to Comfrey's in every way.

Alpinia Yi Zhi Ren
Sharp-Leaf Galangal Berry *

Botanical source: *Alpinia oxyphylla* Miquel (Zingiberaceae)
Chinese names: Yi Zhi Ren (Mand); Yik Ji Yan, Jek Ji Yan (Cant)
Habit: Perennial herb from subtropical South China and Southeast Asia.
Category: mild remedy with minimal chronic toxicity

Constituents: essential oil (incl. pinene, cineol, notkatone, camphor, zingiberene, zingiberol); phytosterol, trace minerals
Effective qualities: pungent, a bit bitter and astringent, warm, dry; restoring, astringing, stabilizing, stimulating
Tropism: urogenital, digestive systems; Kidney, Spleen, Stomach channels

ACTIONS: *Astringent antienuretic, genital astringent, spasmolytic, analgesic, cerebral restorative*
INDICATIONS: Urinary incontinence with damp cold; enuresis, polyuria; seminal incontinence, menorrhagia, amniorrhea; diarrhea, abdominal pain/colic, vomiting; dysmenorrhea; mental fatigue or impairment.
Dosage: Decoction: 3-10 g
Tincture: 2-4 ml
Caution: Contraindicated in vomiting, diarrhea and spermatorrhea presenting heat.
NOTES: This "intelligence benefitting" (*yi zhi*) remedy was traditionally used to enhance mental faculties. The more common use of the Sharp-leaf galangal berry is for its *restorative astringent* action on waning urinary and seminal functions, and for its *relaxant* effect on abdominal colic due to deficiency cold.

Allium Jiu Cai Zi
Asian Leek Seed

韭菜子

Botanical source: *Allium tuberosum* Rottler (Liliaceae)
Chinese names: Jiu Cai Zi, Jiu Zi (Mand)
Category: mild remedy with minimal chronic toxicity
Constituents: essential oil, sulphates, glycosides, vit. C

Effective qualities: pungent, sweet, warm, dry; restoring, stimulating, astringing
Tropism: urinary, reproductive, digestive systems; Liver, Kidney channels

ACTIONS: *Astringent antienuretic, mucostatic, antiemetic, aphrodisiac, carminative*
INDICATIONS: Urinary incontinence and frequency from damp cold; leucorrhea, spermatorrhea; weak knees and lower back, impotence; vomiting, nausea, flatus, dyspepsia and loose stool from stomach cold.
Dosage: Decoction: 3-10 g
Tincture: 1-3 ml
Caution: None.

Astragalus Sha Yuan Zi
Flat Milkvetch Seed

沙苑子

Botanical source: *Astragalus complanatus* R. Br. or *A. chinensis* L. (Leguminosae)
Chinese names: Sha Yuan Zi, Tong Ji Li, Sha Yuan Ji Li (Mand); Sa Yan Ji (Cant)
Category: mild remedy with minimal chronic toxicity

Constituents: flavanoids (neocomplanoside, myricomplanoside), sitosterol, fatty acids (incl. heptenoic, pentadecanoid, linolenic, eicosanoic acids), tannins
Effective qualities: sweet, warm; restoring, astringing
Tropism: urogenital, nervous s.; Liver, Kidney channels

ACTIONS: *Astringent antienuretic, mucostatic, nervous restorative*
INDICATIONS: Urinary incontinence and frequency from damp cold; leucorrhea, premature ejaculation, spermatorrhea; ringing in ears, poor or blurred vision, dizziness.
Dosage: Decoction: 8-16 g
Tincture: 2-4 ml
Caution: Contraindicated in Yin deficiency with empty heat and in hyperactive sex drive.

Rubus Dao Sheng Gen
Korean Raspberry Fruit

倒生根

Botanical source: *Rubus coreanus* Miq. (Roseaceae)
Chinese names: Dao Sheng Gen (M); Dou Song Gan (C)
Category: mild remedy with minimal chronic toxicity
Constituents: organic acids, trace elements, vitamins

Effective qualities: sour, sweet, astringent, neutral; restoring, astringing
Tropism: urogenital, nervous systems; Kidney, Liver channels

ACTIONS: *Astringent antienuretic, nervous restorative*
INDICATIONS: Incontinence with polyuria, enuresis, spermatorrhea; impotence, sterility, debility, early hair graying; lung TB, diabetes.
Dosage: Decoction: 3-10 g
Tincture: 1-3 ml
Caution: None.
NOTES: Hairy raspberry fruit, *Rubus hirsutus*, is used similarly, with the emphasis on promoting virility, fertility and hair growth.

Nelumbo Lian Xu
Lotus Stamen

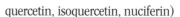

Botanical source: *Nelumbo nucifera* Gaertner (Nymphaeaceae)
Chinese names: Lian Xu (Mand); Ling Sou (Cant)
Category: mild remedy with minimal chronic toxicity
Constituents: alkaloids, glycosides (incl. luteolin, quercetin, isoquercetin, nuciferin)
Effective qualities: sweet, astringent, neutral; astringing, restoring
Tropism: urogenital, vascular systems; Kidney, Heart channels

Actions: *Astringent antienuretic, mucostatic, hemostatic, antiviral*
Indications: Incontinence with enuresis, pollakiuria, leucorrhea, spermatorrhea; coughing up blood, nosebleed, uterine bleeding; influenza.
Dosage: Decoction: 6-10 g
   Tincture: 2-3 ml
Caution: Forbidden in difficult urination.

Paratenodera Sang Piao Xiao
Praying Mantis Egg Case

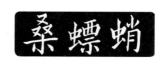

Zoological source: *Paratenodera sinensis* de Saussure or *P. augustipennis* de Saussure and *Hierodula patellifera* Serville and *Mantis religiosa* L. and *Statilia maculata* Thunberg (Mantidae)
Chinese and other names: Sang Piao Xiao (Mand); San Piu Siu, Song Piu Siu (Cant); Sohyosho (Jap)
Part used: the steamed and dried egg case
Category: mild remedy with minimal chronic toxicity
Constituents: glycoprotein, lipoprotein, 18 amino acids (incl. 8 essential), phospholipids, carotin, minerals (incl. iron, calcium)
Effective qualities: sweet, salty, astringent, neutral; astringing, restoring, stabilizing
Tropism: urinary, genital, nervous systems; Liver, Kidney, Dai channels

Actions: *Urinary restorative, astringent antienuretic, mucostatic, anhydrotic*
Indications: Incontinence with enuresis, pollakiuria (esp. in children, elderly); leucorrhea, spermatorrhea (incl. nocturnal, esp. without dreams), genitourinary damp cold syndrome; amenorrhea.
Dosage: Decoction: 3-10 g
   Mantis Sang Piao Xiao is also toasted and used in powder or pill form.
Caution: Contraindicated in Yin deficiency with empty heat, and in bladder damp heat.

Ephedra Ma Huang Gen
Ephedra Root

Botanical source: *Ephedra sinica* Stapf and spp. (Ephedraceae)
Chinese names: Ma Huang Gen (M); Ma Wong Gan (C)
Category: mild remedy with minimal chronic toxicity
Constituents: ephedradines A/B/C/D, feruloylhistamines
Effective qualities: astringent, pungent, sweet, neutral; astringing, restoring
Tropism: cardiovascular systems; Lung, Heart channels

Actions: *Anhydrotic, hypotensive, vasodilator*
Indications: Ecessive sweating of any type in deficiency conditions, including spontaneous sweating (from Qi deficiency), night sweats (from Yin deficiency), postpartum sweating.
Dosage: Decoction: 3-10 g
   Tincture: 1-3 ml
Caution: Not to be used in the onset of infection, i.e., external conditions.

Oryza Nuo Dao Gen
Sweet Rice Root

Botanical source: *Oryza sativa* L. (Gramineae)
Chinese names: Nuo Dao Gen (Xu) (Mand)
No Du Gan (Cant)
Other names: Glutinous rice

Category: mild remedy with minimal chronic toxicity
Effective qualities: astringent, sweet, neutral; astringing, restoring
Tropism: nervous system; Liver, Kidney, Lung channels

ACTIONS: *Anhydrotic, antipyretic, hepatic, anti-infective, antidiabetic*
INDICATIONS: Excessive sweating (e.g. spontanous perspiration, night sweats, low-grade or Yin deficiency fevers, in pneumonia, lung TB); infectious hepatitis, boils, perineal abscesse, filariasis; diabetes; throat obstruction; white or cloudy urine.
Dosage: Decoction: 16-60 g
Tincture: 2-4 ml
Caution: None.

REMEDIES TO MOISTEN THE KIDNEYS AND BLADDER, AND RELIEVE URINARY IRRITATION

Hydrogenics, urinary demulcents

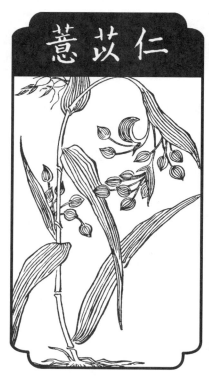

Coix Yi Yi Ren
Job's-Tears Seed

Botanical source: *Coix lachryma-jobi* L. var. *Ma-yuen* (Roman) Stapf (Gramineae)
Pharmaceutical name: Semen Coicis
Chinese names: Yi Yi Ren, Jie Li, Ji Shi, Sheng Yi Ren, Yi Mi, Yi Ren (Mi) (Mand); Yi Yi Yan, San Yi Mai, Sak Yi Mai (Cant)
Other names: False pearl barley, Adlay; Yokuinin (Jap)
Habit: Annual/perennial lowland herb from Mid China and Southeast Asia; grows in fields, along canals and roadsides; much cultivated; blooms in summer with axillary spikelets of blueish white flowers.
Part used: the seed

Therapeutic category: mild remedy with minimal chronic toxicity
Constituents: fatty oil 4.65% (incl. coixol, coixenolide), starch, protein, (incl. amino acids, leucine, tyrosine, lycine, arginine, glutamic acid), polysaccharides, phytosterol, vitamin B1
Effective qualities: sweet, bland, cool, moist
   restoring, relaxing, moistening, decongesting, stimulating
Tropism: urinary, digestive, respiratory, muscular, immune systems
   Kidney, Spleen, Lung, Large Intestine channels
   Fluid, Warmth bodies

ACTIONS AND INDICATIONS

urinary restorative: hydrogenic demulcent: urinary dryness with enuresis, oliguria, dysuria; metabolic acidosis
urogenital relaxant: dysuria, stranguria, neurogenic bladder, cloudy urine, leucorrhea
draining diuretic: edema (incl. of lower limbs); ascites
detoxicant, anti-inflammatory, antipyretic: boils, carbuncles, pulmonary or intestinal abscess (incl. appendicitis), eczema, lung TB, fevers
analgesic, antiarthritic: stiff joints, muscle or joint spasms; arthralgia, myalgia, ostalgia
intestinal demulcent, antidiarrheal: diarrhea, enteritis
lung restorative/relaxant: respiratory deficiency, wheezing; pneumonia, pleurisy
antitumoral, interferon inducent: tumors (incl. cancer, e.g. granuloma, hepatic, gastric, cervical)
immunostimulant, lymphocyte stimulant
antiverrucal: plantar warts, foot tinea

SYMPTOM PICTURES

kidney dryness: scanty urination, thirst, dehydration, dry itchy skin

bladder Qi constraint with **damp:** difficult, irritated urination, cloudy or mucousy urine, vaginal discharges

general fluid congestion: water retention, difficult, scanty urination

intestines damp cold (Spleen Qi Deficiency): mild diarrhea, appetite loss

wind damp obstruction: stiff painful joints, spasms of extremities

PREPARATION

Use: The seed Coix Yi Yi Ren is decocted or used in tincture form. If used for its *antidiarrheal* properties, it may be dry toasted first. The wine is drunk for painful wind damp obstruction syndrome. Job's-tears soup is considered *moistening, nutritious* and *Yin enhancing*.

Dosage: Decoction: 10-30 g
Tincture: 2-4 ml

Caution: Use cautiously during pregnancy.

NOTES

The hard, beadlike Job's-tears seed is a moistening, *hydrogenic kidney restorative* that relieves systemic dryness from an over–alkaline condition. The seed is traditionally held to moisten dry skin and generally beautify any skin. The remedy's *diuretic* action is pivotal in treating water retention and fire toxin signs such as boils and abscesses.

The other aspect of Job's-tears seed, that of a *relaxant* remedy, affects the lungs and sinews as well as the waterworks. The anticomplementary polysaccharides have been found active in its *interferon inducent, antitumoral* and *immunostimulant* activities (Yamada and Kiyohara 1989).

Job's tears root, Yi Yi Gen (Mand.) or **Yi Yi Gan** (Cant.), is given for damp heat urinary tract infections, urinary stones, jaundice, edema and leucorrhea. Dose: 6-18 g.

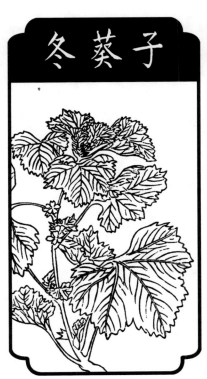

Malva Dong Kui Zi
Musk Mallow Seed

Botanical source: *Malva verticillata* L. (Malvaceae)
Pharmaceutical name: Semen Malvae
Chinese names: Dong Kui Zi, Lu Gui (Mand); Dong Kwai Ji (Cant)
Other names: Cluster mallow, Curly-leaf mallow, "Winter gui"; Tokishi (Jap)
Habit: Common biennial temperate Asian herb growing by roadsides and near villages; also cultivated; pink and magenta flowers bloom in summer.
Part used: the seed

Therapeutic category: mild remedy with minimal chronic toxicity
Constituents: mucilage, protein, fixed oil, saccharose, maltose, glucose, starch
Effective qualities: sweet, cold, moist
restoring, softening, relaxing, decongesting
Tropism: urinary, digestive, hormonal systems
Bladder, Small Intestine, Large Intestine channels
Fluid, Warmth bodies

ACTIONS AND INDICATIONS

urinary restorative/relaxant: hydrogenic demulcent: urinary dryness with irritation or dysuria; metabolic acidosis, urinary stone, urinary tract infection
demulcent laxative: constipation with dryness
anti-inflammatory: urinary tract infection, mastitis; painful swollen breasts, initial stage of breast abscess
draining diuretic: edema (incl. of pregnancy)
galactagogue: insufficient breast milk

Symptom Pictures
kidney dryness: scanty urination, thirst, dehydration, dry itchy skin

bladder damp heat: painful, burning urination, thirst, blood in urine

intestines dryness: dry hard stool, constipation

Preparation
Use: The seed Malva Dong Kui Zi is decocted or used in tincture form.
Dosage: Decoction: 8-14 g
Tincture: 2-4 ml
Caution: Use with caution during pregnancy; forbidden in diarrhea from intestinal deficiency.

Notes
In the past, the young mucilagenous leaves of the musk mallow were commonly eaten as a sweet spring green. Its seed is a cool, *demulcent* remedy that is given in dry, irritated and infective urinary conditions on the one hand and dry constipation on the other. Like the Western mallow varieties, Musk mallow is used to promote breast milk in nursing mothers.

The **seed** of *Abutilon theophrastii*, **Indian mallow, China jute** or **Velvet leaf,** is properly known as **Qing Ma** (Mand.) or **Ching Ma** (Cant.), rather than Dong Kui Zi. It is not *laxative* or *galactagogue* like Dong Kui Zi, but otherwise employed in the same way. Velvet leaf is now a widely distributed weed in the eastern U.S.

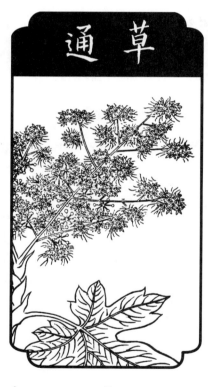

Tetrapanax Tong Cao
Rice Paper Pith

Botanical source: *Tetrapanax papyrifera* (Hooker) K. Koch (Araliaceae)
Pharmaceutical name: Medulla Tetrapanacis
Chinese names: Tong Cao, Tong To Mu (M); Tong Chou, Bai Tong Chou (C)
Other names: Rice paper plant; Tsuso (Jap)
Habit: Small tree or shrub from South China and Taiwan, growing in damp areas near ravines, on hills and slopes; terminal umbels of pale green blossoms bloom in summer.
Part used: the pith

Therapeutic category: mild remedy with minimal chronic toxicity
Constituents: uronuic acid, galacturonic acid, galactose, glucose, xylose, akebin, inositol
Effective qualities: sweet, bland, cold, moist
restoring, softening, relaxing, decongesting, stimulating
Tropism: urinary, respiratory, glandular systems
Bladder, Lung, Stomach channels
Fluid, Warmth bodies

Actions and Indications
urinary restorative/relaxant: hydrogenic demulcent: urinary dryness with dysuria, enuresis; metabolic acidosis, urinary tract infection
draining diuretic: edema, anuria, diabetes
uterine stimulant, parturient: prolonged pregnancy, uterine dystocia
bronchial demulcent: acute bronchitis, cough
antipyretic: fever

galactagogue: scanty or absent breast milk
anthelmintic

Symptom Pictures
kidney dryness: scanty urination, thirst, dehydration, dry itchy skin

bladder damp heat: dark scanty urine; difficult, painful or dribbling urination

Preparation
Use: The pith Tetrapanax Tong Cao is decocted or used in tincture form.
Dosage: Decoction: 3-10 g
Tincture: 1-3 ml
Caution: Use cautiously in all Yin or Qi deficiency conditions; contraindicated during pregnany.

Notes
Tetrapanax, which is found in much of Taiwan, is not only the source of rice paper used in calligraphy, painting and for making paper flowers, but also the remedy Tong Cao. Rice paper pith is a versatile *demulcent restorative/relaxant* remedy for simple or infectious urinary problems signaled by scanty, painful or dribbling urination.

Juncus Deng Xin Cao
Bulrush Pith

Botanical source: *Juncus effusus* L. (Juncaceae)
Chinese names: Deng Xin Cao, Long Xu Cao, Shui Deng Cao (Mand); Ding Sam Chou (Cant)
Habit: Perennial water herb from temperate regions, found along the edges of swamps and other damp terrain.
Part used: the herb; sometimes the root and herb
Category: mild remedy with minimal chronic toxicity

Constituents: cellulose, arabinose, saccharides, xylan, fatty oil, protein
Effective qualities: sweet, bland, cold, moist; restoring, relaxing, calming
Tropism: urinary, nervous systems; Bladder, Lung, Heart, Small Intestine channels

Actions: *Hydrogenic urinary demulcent, anti-inflammatory, draining diuretic, neurocardiac sedative, antipyretic, antitussive, liver decongestant*
Indications: Urinary dryness with irritated, painful or dribbling urination; edema, metabolic acidosis, urinary tract infection, blood in urine; fever; irritability, unrest, sleep loss, anxiety; weeping, crying fits and seizures in babies and infants (esp. nocturnal); dry cough, sore throat; liver congestion, jaundice.
Topically for fistulous sores.
Dosage: Decoction: 2-3 g
Tincture: 1-2 ml
Caution: Forbidden with signs of digestive deficiency and cold.
Note: Bulrush flower, Deng Xin Hua (Ding Sam Fa in Cantonese) is often used for treating dysuria arising from damp heat in the Lower Warmer.

Urinary Stimulants

REMEDIES TO DRY THE KIDNEYS, PROMOTE URINATION, DRAIN FLUID CONGESTION AND RELIEVE EDEMA

➧ BENEFIT THE FLUIDS AND DRAIN DAMP

Draining diuretics

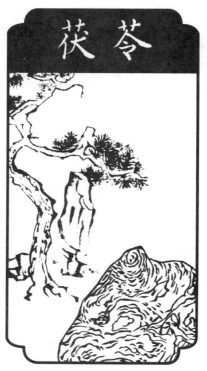

Poria Fu Ling
Hoelen Fungus

Botanical source: *Poria cocos* (Schw.) Wolf (Basidiomycetes)
Pharmaceutical name: Sclerotium Poriae
Chinese names: Fu Ling, Bai Fu Ling, Yun (Fu) Ling (Mand); Fuk Ling, Wong Fuk Ling, Waan Ling (Cant)
Other names: Tuckahoe, Indian bread; Bukuryo (Jap)
Habit: Perennial white or pale pink fungus of various shape and size, growing on the lower trunk of coniferous trees and as much as 30 cm underground; found on sunny, warm, dry hillsides in central and south coastal China, preferring fertile sandy soil; also occurs in Japan and temperate North America.
Part used: the fungus

Therapeutic category: mild remedy with minimal chronic toxicity
Constituents: pachymic and tumulosic acid, polysaccharides (pachyman), ergosterol, choline, histidine, adenine, chitin, hyperin, eburicoic and tumulosic acids, sterols, protein, fats, glucose, lipase, protease, potassium
Effective qualities: sweet, bland, neutral, dry; decongesting, calming
Tropism: urinary, digestive systems
   Bladder, Spleen, Stomach, Heart, Lung channels; Fluid body

ACTIONS AND INDICATIONS

draining diuretic: edema or ascites with thirst, dysuria, oliguria
antidiarrheal: diarrhea, indigestion
antacid antisecretory: acid dyspepsia from hyperchlorhydria
nervous sedative (mild): palpitations, insomnia (esp. infantile)
immune regulator: immune stress with cell-mediated allergies (incl. glomerulonephritis, peptic ulcer)
immunostimulant, phagocyte stimulant: infections in general
interferon inducent, antitumoral

SYMPTOM PICTURES

general fluid congestion: difficult scanty urination, water retention, heaviness of body, nausea, thirst
intestines damp cold (Spleen Qi deficiency): diarrhea, abdominal distension, poor appetite

PREPARATION

Use: The fungus Poria Fu Ling is usually decocted, but may be used in tincture form.
Dosage: Decoction: 10-18 g
   Tincture: 2-4 ml
   Up to 60 g may be used for acute facial edema.
Caution: Forbidden in copious, frequent urination resulting from cold deficiency, and in prolapse.

NOTES

The fungal growth around fir tree roots called Hoelen is ubiquitous in traditional formulas to remove fluid congestion and damp—for removing any type of fluid or mucus accumulation below the diaphragm. Hoelen is a bland *draining diuretic*, rather than a *renal stimulant diuretic*, gentle and safe to use in any damp condition requiring drying out.

The smaller, lighter, looser, younger type of Hoelen is called **Fu Shen** (**Po Fuk Sam** in Cantonese), **"Hoelen spirit."** It is considered a better *nervous sedative* than the regular Hoelen.

Hoelen skin, Fu Ling Pi (Mand.) or **Fuk Ling Pei (Wong Ling Pei)** (Cant.), is the thin brown exterior of the fungus; it is used for edema and scanty urination only. Dose: 9-15 g.

Red hoelen, Chi Fu Ling (Mand.) or **Chek Fuk Ling** (Cant.), is the pink exterior part of the fungus. It is used to treat scanty or cloudy urination, and discharges such as gonorrhea and diarrhea (including dysenterial). Dose: 6-12 g. Forbidden in sperm loss, frequent urination and urogenital prolapse.

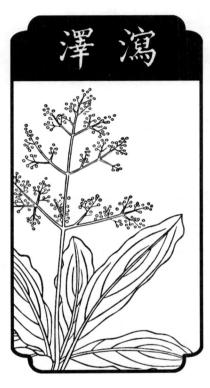

Alisma Ze Xie
Water Plantain Root

Botanical source: *Alisma orientalis* (Sam.) Juzepczuk (Alismataceae)
Pharmaceutical name: Rhizoma Alismae
Chinese names: Ze Xie, Niu Qun, Shui Xie, Yu Sun (Mand); Jaak Se, Jaak Sei (Cant)
Other names: Oriental water plantain, "Marsh drain"; Takusha (Jap)
Habit: Perennial marsh herb from mid China and Fujian, growing in lowland swamps and boggy ground; flowers in summer with small white blossoms in large verticillate divisions.
Part used: the rhizome

Therapeutic category: mild remedy with minimal chronic toxicity
Constituents: triterpenoids (alisol, alisol acetates, epialisol), asparagine, essential oil (incl. furfuraldehyde), alkaloids, biotin, amino acids (lecithin, cholin, valin, acetylvalin), stigmasterol, organic acids, fatty acid, pungent resin, starch, potassium, vitamin B 12
Effective qualities: sweet, bland, a bit bitter, cool
    stimulating, decongesting, sinking, calming, restoring
Tropism: urinary, reproductive, digestive systems
    Kidney, Bladder, Spleen, Ren channels; Fluid, Warmth bodies

ACTIONS AND INDICATIONS

urinary/renal stimulant: draining diuretic: renal deficiency with edema, leg edema, oliguria; nephritis
urinary sedative: urinary tract infections with dysuria, oliguria, hematuria; acute cystitis, nephritis, chyluria
reproductive restorative: infertility, difficult labor (uterine dystocia), irregular menses
astringent: acute diarrhea; enteritis
antilipemic: hyperlipidemia (dizziness, head and chest distension), fatty liver congestion
hypoglycemiant: diabetes
hypotensive: hypertension
immune regulator, antiallergic: immune stress with immediate allergies (incl. rhinitis, urticaria, asthma)
galactagogue
interferon inducent, antitumoral

Symptom Pictures

general fluid congestion: water retention, difficult scanty urination, lethargy

bladder damp heat: painful burning or scanty urination, thirst, fever

intestines damp cold (Spleen Qi deficiency): diarrhea, scanty or difficult urination

Kidney fire: dizziness, ringing ears, thirst, hot spells

Preparation

Use: The root Alisma Ze Xie is decocted or used in tincture form.
Dosage: Decoction: 6-16 g
            Tincture: 2-4 ml
Caution: Contraindicated in damp cold and Kidney Yang deficiency conditions, especially with leucorrhea or spermatorrhea.

Notes

The water-loving Water plantain has proven its strong *diuretic* action through thousands of years of usage in both acute and chronic, simple and infectious urinary dysfunctions. Painful, scanty, difficult urination are the key symptoms for its use.

Both root and seed of *Alisma* are traditionally held to regenerate the womb, promote fertility and ease labor—clearly a contender for use in the last part of pregnancy. Today, Water plantain root is also a frequent ingredient in formulas addressing hypertension and immediate allergies.

Imperata Bai Mao Gen
Woolly Grass Root

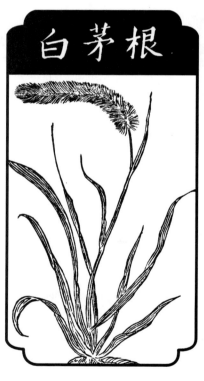

Botanical source: *Imperata cylindrica* Beauvais var. *major* (Nees) C.E. Hubb (Gramineae)
Pharmaceutical name: Rhizoma Imperatae
Chinese names: Bai Mao Gen, (Si) Mao Gen (Mand); Baak Miau Gan (Cant)
Other names: Floss/Cogon/Thatch/White grass, Alang-alang, Lalang; Hakubokon (Jap)
Habit: Perennial (sub)tropical Asian herb; grows in dry, sunny areas, on slopes, grassland, and waste ground; in summer, flower styles form a panicle densely covered by silken, woolly white hairs.
Part used: the rhizome

Therapeutic category: mild remedy with minimal chronic toxicity
Constituents: triterpenoids (cylindrin, arundoin, anemonin, fernenol, isoarborinol, simiarenol, coixol), calcium, potassium, hydroxytryptamine, oxalic acid, sucrose, glucose, fructose, organic acids
Effective qualities: sweet, cold, dry
                    stimulating, decongesting, astringing, thickening, relaxing, sinking
Tropism: urinary, digestive, vascular, respiratory systems
           Bladder, Lung, Stomach, Small Intestine channels; Fluid body

Actions and Indications

urinary/renal stimulant: draining diuretic: renal deficiency with acute nephritic edema; jaundice with edema, anuria, dysuria, urinary tract infections, acute and chronic nephritis

coagulant hemostatic: hemorrhage, nosebleed, coughing or vomiting blood, blood in urine; menorrhagia, epistaxis, hematemesis, hematuria

bronchodilatant: asthma
antipyretic: fever
antiemetic: nausea, vomiting in fever
antiviral: acute viral hepatitis

SYMPTOM PICTURES
general fluid congestion with **heat:** water retention, thirst, fever, nausea
kidney fire: scanty or obstructed urination, thirst, fever, puffy eyes
bladder damp heat: painful, scanty urination, thirst, fever

PREPARATION
Use: The root Imperata Bai Mao Gen is decocted or used in tincture form.
Dosage: Decoction: 10-30 g
 Tincture: 2-5 ml
Up to 60 g may be used when taken alone or if the fresh plant is used.
Caution: Contraindicated in intestines deficiency cold.

NOTES
The root of the Woolly grass, a common reed from China's central plains, is an effective *heat-clearing, stimulant diuretic*. This sweet–cold botanical is best used in kidney edema and acute or chronic nephritis, as well as for general *hemostatic* purposes.
 Woolly grass flower, Bai Mao Hua (Baak Miao Fa), is used for nosebleed, vomiting blood.

Polyporus Zhu Ling
Umbel Polypore Mushroom

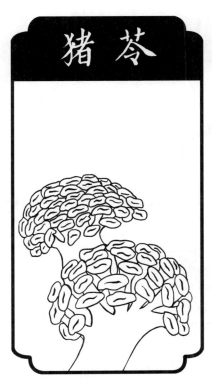

Botanical source: *Polyporus umbellatus* (Pers.) Franchet, syn. *Grifola umbellata* (Pers.) Pilat (Polyporaceae)
Pharmaceutical name: Sclerotium Polypori
Chinese name: Zhu Ling, Ye Zhu Fen, Jia Zhu Shi (Mand); Ju Ling (Cant)
Other names: "Pig fungus"; Chorei (Jap)
Habit: Pantemperate basidiomycetic fungus with multiple grey-brown caps, parasitic on oak, beech, mahogany and maple tree roots and fallen trunks; grows during late summer and autumn.
Part used: the fruiting body

Therapeutic category: mild remedy with minimal chronic toxicity
Constituents: ergosterol, biotin, polysaccharide, crude protein, hydroxytetracosanoic acid, vitamin H
Efective qualities: bland, sweet, neutral, dry
 decongesting, calming, astringing
Tropism: urinary, immune systems
 Kidney, Bladder channels
 Fluid body

ACTIONS AND INDICATIONS
 draining diuretic: edema (alltypes), ascites with liver cirrhosis
 urinary sedative: dysuria, oliguria, anuria; urinary tract infections
 astringent: diarrhea, leucorrhea, gonorrhea

immunostimulant, phagocyte stimulant, antibacterial: infections in general (esp. urinary tract infections)
antitumoral, interferon inducent: cancer (esp. of lung and esophagus)
radiation-protective: radiation damage

SYMPTOM PICTURE
general fluid congestion: severe or chronic water retention, difficult dribbling urination

PREPARATION
Use: The mushroom Polyporus Zhu Ling is decocted or used in tincture form.
Dosage: Decoction: 6-18 g
Tincture: 2-4 ml
Caution: Contraindicated in conditions without damp. Do not use on its own continuously, as it may injure the body's Yin by causing dryness.

NOTES
With a dry, draining nature, Umbel polypore mushroom is a strong *fluid decongesting* remedy. This polypore is mainly used in formulas for severe edema, dysuria and discharges. Modern practice also makes use of this remedy's efficacy in various types of cancer, an action attributable to both its *immune-stimulating* action (mediated by polysaccharides) and its *interferon inducing* effect.

The Umbel polypore is one of the few entirely edible polypores, alongside the **Maitake mushroom** (*Grifola frondosa*) from northeastern Japan, which is now also used for its *immunostimulant, antitumoral* and other related actions.

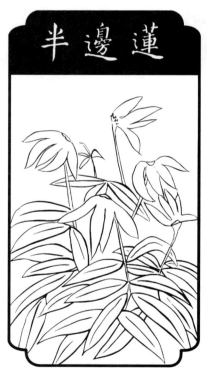

Lobelia Ban Bian Lian
Rooting Lobelia Herb and Root *

Botanical source: *Lobelia chinensis* Loureiro, syn. *L. radicans* Thunberg (Campanulaceae)
Pharmaceutical name: Herba et radix Lobeliae chinensis
Chinese names: Ban Bian Lian, Qi Jie Suo, Xi Mi Cao (Mand);
Bau Bin Ling, Bin Ling (Cant)
Other names: Chinese lobelia, "Half edge lily"; Hanpenren (Jap)
Habit: Perennial vine-like herb from mid-coastal China; grows in damp areas along paddy fields, ditch edges and stream banks; red or violet single axillary flowers appear in summer.
Part used: the herb and root, i.e. the entire plant

Therapeutic category: mild herb with minimal chronic toxicity
Constituents: alkaloids (incl. lobeline, lobelanine, lobelanidine, isolobelanine, lobelinin), polyfructosan, saponins, flavonoids, essential oil (incl. phenols), inulin, succinic/fumaric/hydroxybenzoic acid
Effective qualities: pungent, a bit sweet and bitter, neutral
stimulating, decongesting, relaxing, dissolving
Tropism: urinary, respiratory, cardiovascular, digestive systems
Lung, Small Intestine, Heart channels; Fluid, Air bodies

ACTIONS AND INDICATIONS
urinary/renal stimulant: draining diuretic: renal deficiency with nephritic edema; ascites, acute nephritis
resolvent detoxicant, diuretic: metabolic toxicosis with rheumatism, syphilis, eczema, cirrhosis

cholagogue laxative: biliary dyspepsia, jaundice, constipation
respiratory stimulant/relaxant: asphyxia, asthma
anti-inflammatory, detoxicant, antivenomous: deep boils, tonsilitis, enteritis; snake bites, wasp stings
hypotensive, parasympathetic nervous stimulant: hypertension
antipyretic: fever, malaria
parasiticidal: blood-flukes (schistosomiasis, not early stage), hookworm (ancylostomiasis)
antifungal: fungal skin conditions
Miscellaneous: bruises

Symptom Pictures
general fluid congestion: severe swelling due to water retention, labored breathing

gallbladder and stomach Qi stagnation: epigastric and right flank swelling and discomfort, belching, constipation

metabolic toxicosis with **skin damp heat:** red, weeping skin eruptions, headaches, malaise

Preparation
Use: The herb and root Lobelia Ban Bian Lian are decocted or used in tincture form. External preparations are used in cases of fungal skin conditions, bruising, boils, insect and animal bites, etc.
Dosage: Decoction: 10-30 g
Tincture: 2-4 ml
Caution: Contraindicated in deficiency conditions generally.

Notes
A variety of conditions and symptoms are treatable with this versatile remedy, including some first aid situations. The overall *stimulating* effective quality of Rooting lobelia is mainly applied to water retention and biliary deficiency with congestive upper and lower digestive problems.

Although containing many alkaloids identical to those of the North American Lobelia herb (*Lobelia inflata*), Rooting lobelia's only therapeutic resemblance with the latter lies in the *detoxicant, antivenomous* and *anti-inflammatory* actions. Here is another case where more clinical experience is required to determine whether greater overlap exists.

Euphorbia Jing Da Ji
Peking Spurge Root

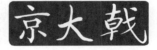

Botanical source: *Euphorbia pekinensis* Ruprecht
Chinese names: Jing Da Ji, Da Ji (Mand); Ging Daai Ji (Cant)
Category: medium-strength remedy with chronic toxicity
Constituents: resin, alkaloids, euphorbon, calcium oxalate/malate, butyric acid
Effective qualities: bitter, cold, dry; decongesting, stimulating
Tropism: urinary, respiratory systems; Lung, Spleen, Kidney channels

Actions: *Renal stimulant, draining diuretic, stimulant expectorant, emmenagogue, antibacterial, antiparasitic, detoxicant*
Indications: Nephritic edema with fluid congestion, ascites, hydrothorax, lung edema, nephritis; chest congestion with sticky sputum, chronic bronchitis; amenorrhea; enteritis, dysentery; schistosomiasis; boils, carbuncles.
Dosage: Decoction: 1-3 g
Tincture: 0.1-1.25 ml
Caution: Forbidden during pregnancy and in edema from deficiency cold. Do not combine with Glycirrhiza Gan cao (Licorice root) nor use longer than three days at a time.

Knoxia Hong Da Ji
Knoxia Root

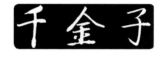

Botanical source: *Knoxia valerianoides* Thorel (Rubiaceae)
Chinese names: Hong Da Ji, Da Ji (Mand); Hong Daai Ji (Cant)
Category: medium-strength remedy with some cumulative toxicity
Effective qualities: bitter, cold; decongesting, stimulating

Actions: *Renal stimulant, draining diuretic, stimulant expectorant*
Indications: Nephritic edema with fluid congestion, ascites, hydrothorax, lung edema, nephritis; chest congestion with sticky sputum; anorexia; epilepsy, boils, carbuncles.
Dosage: Decoction: 1-3 g
Tincture: 0.1-1.25 ml
Caution: Forbidden during pregnancy and in edema from deficiency cold. Do not combine with Glycirrhiza Gan cao (Licorice root) nor use longer than three days because of its medium-strength status.

Euphorbia Qian Jin Zi
Caper Spurge Seed

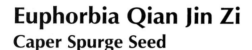

Botanical source: *Euphorbia lathyris* L. (Euphorbiaceae)
Chinese names: Qian Jin Zi, Xu Sui Zi (Mand); Chan Gam Ji (Cant)
Category: medium-strength remedy with chronic toxicity
Constituents: saponins (incl. aesculin, betulin, daphnetin, euphorbetin, kaempferol, quercetin, taraxerol), DOPA
Effective qualities: pungent, warm; stimulating, dissolving
Tropism: urinary, reproductive, epidermal systems; Liver, Kidney channels

Actions: *Renal stimulant, draining diuretic, laxative, emmenagogue, antifungal, antitumoral*
Indications: Edema with fluid congestion, severe abdominal distension, constipation, dysuria, amenorrhea, gynecological tumors, cancer. Topically for scabies, fungal infections, warts, sores, snakebites and cancer (melanoma).
Dosage: Decoction: 1-2 g
Tincture: 0.1-1 ml
Caution: Being a medium-strength remedy, use only short-term. Forbidden during pregnancy.

Phaseolum Chi Xiao Dou
Aduki Bean

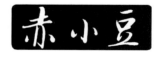

Botanical source: *Phaseolum calcaratus* Roxburgh (Leguminosae)
Chinese names: Chi Xiao Dou (Mand); Sai Siu Dau (C)
Category: mild remedy with minimal chronic toxicity
Constituents: starch, fat, protein, nicotinic acid, vitamins B1, B2, calcium, iron, phosphorus
Effective qualities: sweet, sour, neutral, dry; decongesting, calming
Tropism: urinary, digestive systems; Heart, Small Intestine, Spleen channels

Actions: *Draining diuretic, detoxicant*
Indications: Edema of most kinds from fluid congestion (especially hepatic); suppurative skin infections (incl. boils, carbuncles, toxic swellings, simple sores); diarrhea, food poisoning, oliguria, bladder irritation, beriberi.
Dosage: Decoction: 10-16 g. Aduki beans are also commonly cooked and eaten as food.
Caution: During pregnancy; excessive or prolonged use can cause dryness.

REMEDIES TO PROMOTE URINATION AND BOWEL MOVEMENT, DRAIN FLUID CONGESTION AND RELIEVE EDEMA

➥ EXPEL FLUIDS DOWNWARD
Purgative draining diuretics

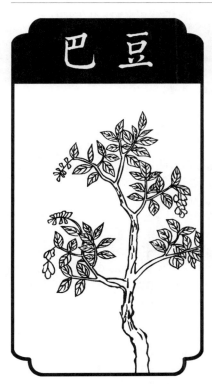

Croton Ba Dou
Croton Seed

Botanical source: *Croton tiglium* L. (Euphorbiaceae)
Pharmaceutical name: Semen Crotonis
Chinese names: Ba Dou, Ba Shu (Mand); Ba Dau (Cant)
Other names: Hazu (Jap)
Habit: Small evergreen tree from Sichuan, Guangdong, Taiwan and other parts of Southeast Asia; grows on stream banks and hillsides; blooms in summer with terminal racemes of small white blossoms.
Part used: the seed

Therapeutic category: strong remedy with acute toxicity
Constituents: croton oil 34-57% (incl. glyceryl crotonate, croton resin, croton cocarcinogens A and B, phorbol formate/butyrate/crotonate), crotin, crotonoside, ricinine-like alkaloid, crotonic and tiglic acid
Effective qualities: pungent, hot, dry
  stimulating, decongesting, relaxing
Tropism: urinary, digestive, respiratory systems
  Large Intestine, Stomach, Lung channels

ACTIONS AND INDICATION:
urinary/renal stimulant, draining diuretic: renal deficiency with edema (incl. lung edema); hydrothorax, ascites
purgative diuretic: acute constipation, edema
uterine stimulant, emmenagogue: obstinate amenorrhea
bronchodilator, expectorant: wheezing, tachypnea, coughing with sputum
biliary and intestinal relaxant, analgesic: biliary colic, biliary ascariasis, intestinal colic, IBS, chronic diarrhea
antiseptic, detoxicant: acute laryngitis, malaria, diphtheria, ulcers, warts, moles; acute mastitis
antifungal: scabies, fungal skin conditions
antitumoral
Miscellaneous: paralysis, stroke, toothache

SYMPTOM PICTURES
lung fluid congestion: acute water retention in the torso or chest with labored breathing, coughing up phlegm
intestines cold: abdominal pain and distension, acute constipation or chronic diarrhea

PREPARATION
Use: The seed Croton Ba Dou is decocted or made into a tincture. The defatted kernel is also made into capsules of 150-300 mg each. Topical applications of seed preparations, including the extracted oil, are used for skin conditions, such as warts, moles and fungal infections.
Dosage: Decoction: 0.1-0.3 g
  Tincture: 0.05-0.1 ml (1-2.5 drops)
  Defatted capsule of 150-300 mg: 1 or 2 capsules, repeated every 4 hours if necessary (Chang & But 1987).

Caution: Only to be used under professional supervision. Croton seed is very toxic and only suitable for one-time use in an acute condition. Dosages must be respected! The remedy is contraindicated during pregnancy and breast-feeding, with weak patients and in all conditions except for the above. Only the defatted kernel may be used in capsules internally with the above dosages.

NOTES

Croton root, Ba Dou Gen, is a remedy in the medium-strength category. It is given for rheumatoid arthritis, hematoma and snakebite. Dosage: 3-10 g in decoction.

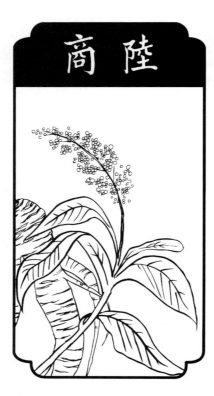

Phytolacca Shang Lu
Asian Poke Root

Botanical source: *Phytolacca acinosa* Roxburgh or *P. esculenta* Van Houtte (Phytolaccaceae)
Pharmaceutical name: Radix Phytolaccae acinosae
Chinese names: Shang Lu, Ye Luo Bo, Ye Hu, Zhang Liu Gen (Mand); Cheun Lok (Cant)
Other names: "Commerce continent"; Shoriku (Jap)
Habit: Perennial herb cultivated in North China; also found wild in fields and uplands; small white or pink terminal/axillary flower racemes open in summer.
Part used: the root

Therapeutic category: strong remedy with acute toxicity
Constituents: oxyristic/jaligonic acid, acidic steroidal saponins, phytolaccine, phytolaccatoxin 4%, potassium nitrate, polysacharides, resin, glucoside
Effective qualities: bitter, a bit sour and pungent, cold
      stimulating, decongesting, astringing, sinking
Tropism: urinary, digestive, respiratory, glandular systems
      Bladder, Lung, Spleen channels; Fluid, Air bodies

ACTIONS AND INDICATIONS

urinary/renal stimulant: draining diuretic: renal deficiency with edema, oliguria or anuria; acute and chronic nephritis, cardiac edema, ascites, lung edema, hydrothorax
purgative diuretic: severe edema with constipation or obstructed urination
stimulant expectorant: acute and chronic bronchitis
detoxicant, dermatropic, diuretic: metabolic toxicosis with chronic psoriasis, eczema, dermatitis
detoxicant, anti-inflammatory: boils, carbuncles, ulcers, pyogenic skin infections, pleuritis; laryngitis with throat numbness, pain and obstruction
antitumoral, immunostimulant: tumors
hemostatic, mucostatic: hemorrhage, purpura, hemoptysis, leucorrhea, cervical erosion
vulnerary: tissue trauma
radiation-protective: radiation damage
antibacterial, antifungal

SYMPTOM PICTURES

general fluid congestion: water retention with swelling, scanty or absent urination, rough skin
lung fluid congestion: wheezing, difficult breathing, water retention
lung phlegm damp: coughing, difficult expectoration, bringing up sticky white sputum

Preparation

Use: The root Phytolacca Shang Lu is decocted or used in tincture form. External preparations can also be made for skin conditions.

Dosage: Decoction: 3-8 g
Tincture: 0.1-1.5 ml

Caution: Only to be used under professional supervision. This remedy should only be used for a short time because of its fairly acute toxicity. Dosages must be respected! Signs of overdosing include rapid heartbeat, nausea, vomiting, colic and diarrhea. Contraindicated during pregnancy.

Notes

As witness to its efficacy in fluid congestion conditions, Asian poke root carries jaligonic acid, a strong *stimulant diuretic* compound. The bitter–pungent remedy is also an effective *stimulant expectorant* when given in phlegm damp respiratory syndromes.

Comparing the Asian and North American species of *Phytolacca* from both biochemical and therapeutic perspectives shows that they have strong similarities as well as significant differences. Both species of contain phytolaccatoxin, for instance. Indications that both types of Poke root have in common—those that justify exchanging one remedy for the other—include a variety of chronic skin conditions, inflammatory and/or pyogenic boils, ulcers and wounds.

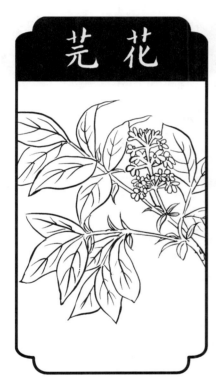

Daphne Yuan Hua
Lilac Daphne Flower *

Botanical source: *Daphne genkwa* Siebold et Zuccarini (Thymelaceae)
Pharmaceutical name: Flos Daphnis genkwae
Chinese names: Yuan Hua, Du Yuan, Du Yu, Dou Teng Hua (Mand); Yan Fa (Cant)
Other names: Bottleneck, "Yuan flower," "Fish poison"; Genka, Fujimodoki (Jap)
Habit: Deciduous shrub from central and mideastern China, growing in river valleys along field edges; spring sees axillary lilac flowers appear.
Part used: the flower

Therapeutic category: strong remedy with acute toxicity
Constituents: flavonoids (incl. aglycone genkwanin, hydroxygenkwanin, apigenin), beta-sitosterol, benzoic acid, pungent oil, diterpenoid orthoesters (yuanhuatine, yuanhuapine, genkwadaphnin), diterpenoid yuanhuacine (in root), chlorogenic acid analogs
Effective qualities: bitter, a bit pungent, warm, dry
stimulating, decongesting, sinking
Tropism: urinary, digestive, respiratory, reproductive systems
Kidney, Lung, Spleen channels; Air, Fluid bodies

Actions and Indications

urinary/renal stimulant: draining diuretic: renal deficiency with edema; ascites, hydrothorax, lung edema; chronic renal failure
purgative diuretic: severe acute edema with constipation or blocked urination
uterine stimulant, oxytocic parturient, abortive: prolonged pregnancy, hypotonic uterine dystocia, miscarriage, retained placenta
stimulant expectorant: bronchitis

dermatropic detoxicant, anti-inflammatory, detumescent: toxicosis, eczema, boils, furuncles, traumatic injuries, acute mastitis; acute and chronic hepatitis; chronic malaria
antiparasitic: tinea, scabies
topical stimulant: frostbite, hair loss
antitumoral
antibacterial, antifungal

Symptom Pictures

general fluid congestion: water retention with swelling in chest and flanks, labored breathing

lung fluid congestion: water retention, wheezing, coughing

lung phlegm damp: coughing, difficult expectoration, bringing up sticky white sputum

Preparation

Use: The flower Daphne Yuan Hua is decocted or used in tincture form. Topical applications, such as washes, can be made for frostbite, inflamed boils, sores, parasites, ets.

Dosage: Decoction: 1.5-3 g
Tincture: 0.1-1 ml

Caution: Only to be used under professional supervision and only for a short time for acute situations. Dosages must be respected! Contraindicated during pregnancy and with weak persons. Daphne Yuan Hua should never be combined with Licorice root: it not only counteracts the *purgative* and *diuretic* effect, but also increases its toxicity.

Notes

With its strong twin *water-chasing* and *purgative* effect, Lilac daphne flower (like other remedies in this section) is said to possess a *sinking* movement. Both the flower and the root also exert an *oxytocic* action on the uterus. In China they are considered safe *parturients* and *abortifacients* in injections of the above preparation forms or, better still, in the form of the extracted yuanhuatine or yuanhuacine—as long as correct dosages are maintained.

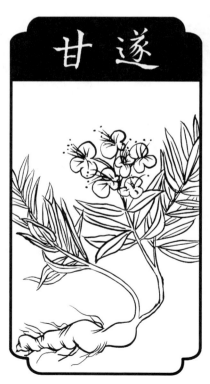

Euphorbia Gan Sui
Sweet Spurge Root *

Botanical source: *Euphorbia kansui* Liou (Euphorbiaceae)
Pharmaceutical name: Radix Euphorbiae kansui
Chinese names: Gan Sui, Jing Da Ji, Gan Gao (Mand); Gam Sai, Gam Jam (Cant)
Other names: "Sweet process"; Kansui (Jap)
Habit: Perennial herb of mid and north China's mild, cool dry climes; racemes of viridian terminal blossoms bloom throughout summer.
Part used: the root

Therapeutic category: strong remedy with acute toxicity
Constituents: diterpene esters, triterpenoids (incl. euphorbon, euphadienol, euphol, tirucallol, euphorbol, euphorbadienol), tannins, resin, palmitic acid, glucose, saccharide, starch, vitamin B1
Effective qualities: bitter, sweet, cold
stimulating, decongesting, sinking
Tropism: urinary, digestive, respiratory systems
Kidney, Lung, Spleen, channels; Fluid body

ACTIONS AND INDICATIONS
urinary/renal stimulant: draining diuretic: renal deficiency with generalized or facial edema, dysuria, anuria; ascites, hydrothorax with dyspnea, lung edema, hydrocele
purgative diuretic: severe acute edema with constipation or blocked urination
stimulant expectorant: bronchitis
uterine stimulant, abortive: miscarriage, retained placenta
antiepileptic: epilepsy
anti-inflammatory, detumescent: swollen painful boils, sores
interferon inducent
Miscellaneous: deafness

SYMPTOM PICTURES
general fluid congestion: water retention with swelling in chest and flanks, labored breathing, difficult urination
lung fluid congestion: water retention, wheezing, coughing
lung phlegm damp: coughing, difficult expectoration, bringing up sticky white sputum

PREPARATION
Use: The root Euphorbia Gan Sui is decocted or used in powder or tincture form. For internal use, the root is best toasted or stir-fried first to reduce its toxic nature. Topical preparations are used for boils.
Dosage: Decoction: 1-3 g
Powder: 0.3-1 g
Tincture: 0.25-0.1 ml (6-25 drops)
Caution: Only to be used under professional supervision, and only once for an acute condition. Contraindicated during pregnancy and in weak people. For best results avoid combining it with Licorice root.

NOTES
Like the other strong *purgative diuretics* in this section, the highly stimulating Sweet spurge root is used in various situations where water needs to be quickly evacuated. These conditions include ascites, hydrothorax and both chronic and acute lung edema.

Lepidium Ting Li Zi
Wood Whitlow Grass Seed

Botanical source: *Lepidium apetalum* Willdenov or *L. virginicum* L. or *Descurainia sophia* (L) Schur (Cruciferae)
Chinese names: Ting Li Zi (Mand); Tang Nek Ji (Cant)
Habit: Perennial herb from North China
Category: mild remedy with minimal chronic toxicity
Constituents: essential oil (incl. benzyl and allyl isothiocyanate, allyl disulfide), linoleic/linolenic/erucic/palmitic/stearic acid, sitosterol, helveticoside
Effective qualities: pungent, bitter, very cold; stimulating, decongesting, relaxing
Tropism: urinary, cardiovascular, respiratory, digestive systems; Lung, Bladder, Large Intestine channels

ACTIONS: *Renal stimulant, draining diuretic, purgative diuretic, cardiotonic, bronchodilator, antitussive*
INDICATIONS: Acute nephritic edema of the head and face, cirrhosis with ascites, hydrothorax, pulmonary edema (Kidney and Lung fluid congestion syndrome), chronic cor pulmonale with cardiac failure; anuria, scanty urination, constipation; acute asthma, pleurisy, cough with phlegm.
Dosage: Decoction: 3-10 g
Tincture: 1-3 ml
Caution: Forbidden in cough due to deficiency and edema from hepatic deficiency.

Pharbitis Qian Niu Zi
Japanese Morning Glory Seed

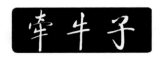

Botanical source: *Pharbitis nil* (L.) Choisy or *P. purpurea* (L.) Voigt (Convulvulaceae)
Chinese names: Qian Niu Zi (Mand); Chan Ngau Ji (Cant)
Habit: Annual (sub)tropical herb from East Asia; pale pink or blue axillary flowers bloom in summer.
Category: medium-strength remedy with chronic toxicity

Constituents: pharbitin, angelic/gallic/nillic acid, chanoclavine, penniclavine, iso- and elimoclavine, cyanoside, pelargoniside, pharbitoside, rhamnose
Effective qualities: bitter, pungent, cold; stimulating, decongesting
Tropism: urinary, respiratory, digestive systems; Lung, Large Intestine, Kidney channels

ACTIONS: *Renal stimulant, draining diuretic, purgative diuretic, anthelmintic, emmenagogue*
INDICATIONS: Acute nephritic edema, cirrhosis with ascites, hydrothorax, lung edema; severe constipation and anuria; roundworm, tapeworm (esp. with edema); amenorrhea.
Dosage: Decoction: 3-8 g
　　　　　Tincture: 0.5-2 ml
Caution: Contraindicated during pregnancy and with weak digestion (Spleen Qi). Never combine with Croton Ba Dou. Do not take for more than ten days because of some cumulative toxicity. Signs of intoxication include blood in the urine and stool, dizziness, abdominal pain and vomiting.

Urinary Sedatives

REMEDIES TO REDUCE URINARY INFECTION AND RELIEVE IRRITATION

➥ DRAIN DAMP HEAT FROM THE BLADDER

Anti-inflammatory urinary antiseptics and spasmolytics

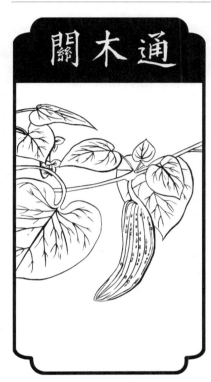

Aristolochia Guan Mu Tong
Manchurian Birthwort Stem

Botanical source: *Aristolochia manshuriensis* Komarov and *A. moupinensis* (Aristolochiaceae)
Pharmaceutical name: Caulis Aristolochiae manshuriensis
Chinese names: Guan Mu Tong, Mu Tong, Tong Cao, Quan Mu Tong (Mand); Gwan Muk Tong, Muk Tong (Cant)
Other names: Mokkutsu (Jap)
Habit: Perennial climbing vine from Northeast China (Manchuria); purple or white flowers appear in spring.
Part used: the stem

Therapeutic category: mild remedy with minimal chronic toxicity
Constituents: aristolochic acids A and D, debilic acid, tannin, aristolocide, magnoflorine hederagenin, calcium
Effective qualities: bitter, astringent, cold, dry
　　　　　　　　　　calming, relaxing, stimulating, sinking
Tropism: urinary, reproductive, glandular systems
　　　　　Bladder, Heart, Small Intestine channels; Warmth, Fluid bodies

ACTIONS AND INDICATIONS
urinary sedative: astringent, anti-inflammatory, antiseptic, antifungal: acute urinary tract infections with oliguria, dysuria, enuresis; cystitis, nephritis, urethritis, leucorrhea, mouth and tongue sores or ulcers, sore throat (esp. with gram-positive bacilli)
antipyretic: fevers
analgesic: urinary pain, arthralgia, pain in general
antitumoral, immunostimulant
uterine stimulant: amenorrhea, dysmenorrhea
galactagogue: insufficient breast milk
antifungal

SYMPTOM PICTURES
bladder damp heat: scanty, painful or dribbling urination, dark yellow or red urine, thirst
bladder Qi constraint: suppressed, scanty, difficult, painful urination

PREPARATION
Use: The stem Aristolochia Guan Mu Tong is decocted or used in tincture form.
Dosage: Decoction: 3-9 g
　　　　　Tincture: 1-3 ml
Caution: Contraindicated during pregnancy. Because of its drying nature, this remedy should be used cautiously in elderly or weak people, especially with signs of Yin or fluids deficiency present.

NOTES

Chinese medicine often uses different plant species and even genuses to supply a single remedy. Consequently, we can now distinguish three types of the remedy Mu Tong commonly in use: **Guan Mu Tong** (Mand.) or **Gwan Muk Tung** (Cant.), *Aristolochia manshuriensis;* **Bai Mu Tong** (M.) or **Baak Muk Tong** (C.), *Akebia quinata* and *A. trifoliata;* and **Chuan Mu Tong** (M.) or **Chyun Muk Tong** (C.), *Clematis montana* and *C. armandii.* (Bai Mu Tong is presented separately below.) Nevertheless, since 150 years at least, the primary botanical material for the remedy commonly known as Mu Tong is *Aristolochia manshuriensis.* This was not always so, however. The records of past dynastic herbals clearly make *Akebia quinata* the main source of this remedy.

Today, having been thoroughly investigated, the actions of all the various plants called Mu Tong are understood more distinctly. It turns out that Manchurian birthwort stem can be relied upon for superior *anti-inflammatory, antiseptic* and *analgesic* effects in acute urinary infections.

Dianthus Qu Mai
Proud Pink Herb

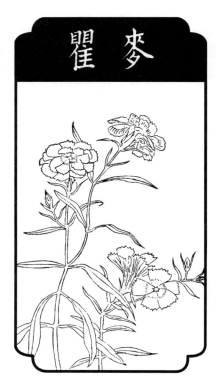

Botanical source: *Dianthus superbus* L., *D. chinensis* L. (Caryophyllaceae)
Pharmaceutical name: Herba Dianthi
Chinese names: Qu Mai, Ye Mai, Gu Gu Mai, Da Lan (Mand); Kui Mok (Cant)
Other names: China/Rainbow/Fringed pink, Carnation; Kubaku (Jap)
Habit: Perennial herb from mid and north China, Siberia and Japan; grows on hillsides and streamsides and in open woods; large, fragrant lilac, pink and white terminal flowers bloom on racemes in late summer.
Part used: the herb

Therapeutic category: mild herb with minimal chronic toxicity
Constituents: saponins, alkaloids, essential oil (incl. eugenol), phenylethyl-alcohol, benzyl benzoate and salicylate, protein, cellulose, vitamin A
Efective qualities: bitter, cold, dry
   calming, relaxing, stimulating, decongesting, sinking
Tropism: urinary, reproductive, digestive systems
   Kidney, Bladder, Heart, Small Intestine, Chong, Ren channels
   Fluid, Warmth bodies

ACTIONS AND INDICATIONS

urinary sedative: anti-inflammatory, antiseptic (antibacterial), analgesic: acute urinary tract infections with dysuria, enuresis; cystitis, urethritis, nephritis, urinary stones or neurogenic bladder with strangury
antipyretic: fever
dermatropic detoxicant, vulnerary: eczema, carbuncles, venereal sores, wounds, purulent running ulcers
stimulant and draining diuretic: urinary retention, edema
uterine stimulant: emmenagogue, parturient, abortive: amenorrhea, dysmenorrhea; prolonged pregnancy, stalled labor, placental retention, miscarriage
intestinal stimulant: dyspepsia
anticoagulant: blood clots
antitumoral: rectal and esophageal cancer
antiparasitic: lumbricoid worms, schistosomiasis (blood flukes)
Miscellaneous: corneal opacity

Symptom Pictures

bladder damp heat: painful or burning, difficult scanty urination, blood in urine, thirst

bladder Qi constraint: suppressed, difficult urination; urinary irritation

uterus Qi stagnation: delayed, difficult or absent menses

metabolic toxicosis with **skin damp heat:** red skin rashes, difficult urination, malaise

Preparation

Use: The herb Dianthus Qu Mai is infused or used in tincture form.
Dosage: Infusion: 4-12 g
Tincture: 2-4 ml
Caution: Contraindicated in pregnancy and in digestive, urinary and reproductive deficiency conditions.

Notes

An excellent *diuretic* and *skin-cleansing* remedy in one, Proud pink herb is similar in this respect to Nettle herb in the West. The bitter, cold dry qualities of Proud pink make it *downward-moving* and *heat-clearing* in acute urinary infections presenting damp heat. Its content in active components such as eugenol (*anti-infective*) and alkaloids corroborates this usage. The saponins could also play a part in relieving dysuria, while almost certainly being involved in resolving eczema from metabolic toxicosis. Among its secondary and special applications, note this remedy's use for promoting contractions in case of prolonged pregnancy or uterine dystocia.

Talcum Hua Shi
Talc

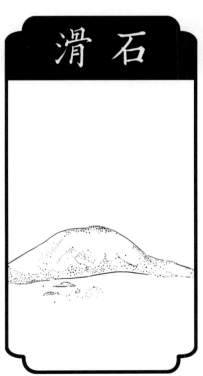

Geological source: Talcum
Pharmaceutical name: Talcum
Chinese names: Hua Shi, Ye Shi, Liao Shi (Mand); Waat Sek (Cant)
Other names: Steatite, Soapstone, "Slippery stone"; Kasseki (Jap)
Source: China's northern provinces Shaanxi, Shanxi, Shandong, Jiangxi and Jiangsu.
Part used: the mineral clay

Therapeutic category: mild remedy with minimal chronic toxicity
Constituents: hydrous magnesium silicate, traces of iron oxide, aluminum
Effective qualities: sweet, bland, cold
calming, astringing, solidifying, stimulating
Tropism: urinary, digestive systems
Bladder, Stomach channels
Warmth, Fluid bodies

Actions and Indications

urinary sedative: antiseptic (antibacterial), analgesic, astringent: urinary tract infections with dysuria, oliguria, enuresis; cystitis, urethritis, nephritis

diuretic urinary/renal stimulant: anuria

astringent, hemostatic: diarrhea, coughing up blood, nosebleed, vomiting; gastritis, food poisoning

vulnerary: traumatic wounds, weeping eczema

Symptom Pictures
bladder damp heat: dark, burning scanty urine, thirst, dribbling urination

summer heat: diarrhea, irritability, thirst, fever, difficult urination

Preparation
Use: Talc is decocted. When decocting, first wrap the mineral separately in a cotton bag before adding to other ingredients. External prepararations are used for traumatic and eczematous conditions.
Dosage: Decoction: 10-18 g
Caution: Contraindicated in digestive deficiency, spermatorrhea, excessive urination, fluid depletion or dehydration due to fever and pregnancy.

Notes
The mineral talc is commonly found in formulas for acute urinary infections—bladder damp heat conditions. With its strong affinity for renal and urinary functions—embodied in its *diuretic* and *astringent* actions—Talc also treats a variety of urination problems.

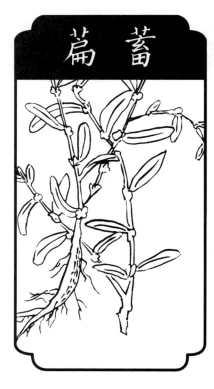

Polygonum Bian Xu
Knotgrass Herb

Botanical source: *Polygonum aviculare* L. (Polygonaceae)
Pharmaceutical name: Herba Polygoni avicularis
Chinese names: Bian Xu, Bai Huo La, Bian Zhu (Mand); Bin Chok (Cant)
Other names: Knotweed; Henchiku (Jap)
Habit: Annual temperate Eurasian herb growing in waste places, fields and on roadsides; blooms in summer with green flower clusters.
Part used: the herb

Therapeutic category: mild remedy with minimal chronic toxicity
Constituents: tannins, avicularin, quercetrin, rutin, gallic/caffeic/oxalic silicic/chlorogenic/coumaric acid, mucilage, catechol, glucose, fructose, sucrose
Effective qualities: bitter, astringent, cold, dry
calming, astringing, solidifying, stimulating
Tropism: urogenital, digestive systems
Bladder channel
Fluid, Warmth bodies

Actions and Indications
urinary astringent sedative/restorative: acute urinary tract infections with dysuria, oliguria, enuresis; cystitis, urethritis, nephritis
astringent: diarrhea, enteritis, bacillary dysentery, leucorrhea, hemorrhoids, diabetes
hemostatic: uterine bleeding, postpartum hemorrhage, blood in sputum
diuretic, resolvent antilithic: urinary and biliary stones, albuminuria, jaundice
dermatropic detoxicant, antipruritic: weeping eczema, dermal and vaginal pruritus
vermifuge, antiparasitic, antifungal: tapeworm, hookworm, pinworm (threadworm), roundworm; tinea, scabies, trichomonas vaginalis
vulnerary: genital/venereal ulcers

Symptom Picture
bladder damp heat: painful, burning, scanty dribbling urination, thirst

Preparation
Use: The herb Polygonum Bian Xu is infused or used as a tincture. Externally, washes, compresses, douches and the like are used for itching, ulcerative and parasitic skin conditions.
Dosage: Infusion: 8-16 g
Tincture: 2-4 ml
Caution: Use carefully in difficult urination arising from abdominal weakness.

Notes
Damp heat urinary conditions with difficult, dribbling urination are the focus of Knotgrass, which has the potential to both *drain* and *tonify*. Itching of whatever kind also falls under its beneficial influence, as do a large spectrum of parasitic and fungal infections.

Knotgrass is also a traditional remedy in Western herbal medicine where, in addition to the above uses, it is also considered a *diuretic detoxicant* for toxicosic and depository conditions, including gout and rheumatism.

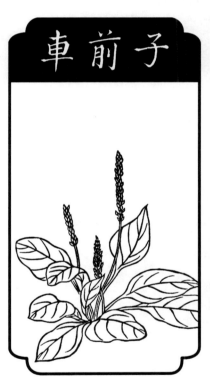

Plantago Che Qian Zi
Asian Plantain Seed

Botanical source: *Plantago asiatica* L. or *P. depressa* Willdenow and spp. (Plantaginaceae)
Pharmaceutical name: Semen Plantaginis asiaticae
Chinese names: Che Qian Zi, Dang Dao, Niu Yi (Mand); Che Ching Ji (Cant)
Other names: Asian plantain, "Cart-track herb"; Shazenshi (Jap)
Habit: Perennial temperate Asian herb growing along roadsides, in fields and waste ground; in summer, tall spikelets of minute greenish white flowers appear.
Part used: the seed

Therapeutic category: mild remedy with minimal chronic toxicity
Constituents: plantagin, aucubin, adenine, ursolic/planterolic/succinic/palmitic/stearic acid, oleic acids, choline, proteins, lipids, mucilage, vits. A, B1
Effective qualities: sweet, bland, cool, moist
calming, relaxing, restoring, softening
Tropism: urinary, digestive, respiratory systems
Bladder, Kidney, Liver, Small Intestine, Lung, Yin Qiao channels
Fluid body

Actions and Indications
urinary sedative/relaxant: demulcent: acute urinary tract and prostate infections with dysuria, enuresis, strangury; cystitis, nephritis, urethritis, prostatitis, metabolic acidosis, neurogenic bladder
anti-inflammatory: urinary and intestinal infections; conjunctivitis with dry, red, swollen eyes
draining diuretic, renal stimulant, antilithic: nephritic edema, kidney stones
antitussive expectorant: coughing with sputum, bronchitis
spasmolytic: abdominal pain from intestinal colic
reproductive restorative: insufficient semen, premature ejaculation, difficult labor
vision restorative, optitropic: photophobia, cataract, poor eyesight, nebula, blood-shot eyes
fetal regulator: fetal malposition
interferon inducent

Symptom Pictures

bladder damp heat: burning, scanty, difficult urination, thirst

kidney dryness: scanty urination, thirst, dehydration, dry itchy skin

bladder Qi constraint: difficult, suppressed, scanty urination with irritation

intestines damp heat: diarrhea, painful bowel movement

lung phlegm heat: coughing with copious sputum production, thirst, dryness

Preparation

Use: The seed Plantago Che Qian Zi is decocted or used in tincture form.
Dosage: Decoction: 4-12 g
Tincture: 2-4 ml
Caution: Contraindicated in urogenital deficiency conditions with leucorrhea and urinary and seminal incontinence, as well as during pregnancy.

Notes

Asian plantain seed commonly occurs in Oriental prescriptions for acute urinary, intestinal and respiratory infections—damp heat syndromes of these organs. The seed is primarily a bland, moist, cool, i.e., *demulcent sedative* remedy for the urinary tract. Moreover, it relieves conditions genreally signaled by dryness and irritation, especially renal dryness with metabolic acidosis. Asian plantain seed's other specialty is in dealing with a variety of eye and vision complaints.

The seeds from the plantains used in the Western tradition, Lance-leaf plantain and Round-leaf plantain, can be used as fair substitutes for the Asian variety.

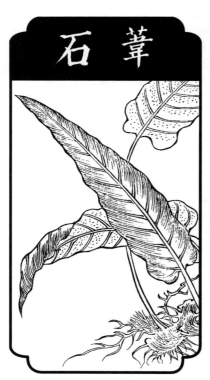

Pyrrosia Shi Wei
Felt Fern Leaf

Botanical source: *Pyrrosia sheareri* (Baker) Ching or *P. lingua* (Thunb.) Farwell or *P. petiolosa* (Christ) Ching (Polypodiaceae)
Pharmaceutical name: Folium Pyrrosiae
Chinese names: Shi Wei, Shi Pi, Jin Xing Cao (Mand); Sek Wai (Cant)
Other names: Tongue fern, "Rock thong," "Golden star-grass"; Sekii (Jap)
Habit: Perennial creeping fern from temperate China; the leathery, willow-shaped leaves grow under dank, dark conditions in rock crevices on hilly slopes and cliff edges, as well as on tree trunks and branches.
Part used: the leaf

Therapeutic category: mild remedy with minimal chronic toxicity
Constituents: flavonoids, saponins, tannins, diploptene, sitosterol, organic acids, caffeeic acid, isomangiferin, saccharose, fructose, glucose
Effective qualities: bitter, a bit sweet, cold, dry
calming, stimulating, astringing
Tropism: urinary, respiratory, vascular systems
Bladder, Lung channels
Fluid, Warmth bodies

Actions and Indications

urinary sedative: antibacterial, anti-inflammatory: acute urinary tract infections with dysuria, enuresis; cystitis, urethritis, nephritis

renal stimulant diuretic, antilithic: urinary stones, gravel; albuminuria, acute and chronic nephritis (all types), nephritic edema
hemostatic: blood in urine (hematuria), uterine bleeding (metrorrhagia), coughing and vomiting blood (hemoptysis, hematemesis)
stimulant expectorant, antitussive: chronic bronchitis, bronchial asthma, cough
antiviral: herpes simplex (genital herpes)
Miscellaneous: leucopenia

SYMPTOM PICTURES
bladder damp heat: painful, difficult, dribbling urination, blood in urine

lung phlegm heat: cough with sputum, wheezing, thirst

PREPARATION
Use: The leaf Pyrrosia Shi Wei is decocted or used in tincture form.
Dosage: Decoction: 8-16 g
 Tincture: 2-4 ml
Caution: None.

NOTES
A variety of felt fern species furnish the remedy Shi Wei, a reliable agent for clearing both acute urinary and lung heat, especially with blood present. Felt fern's affinity for calming down and healing the body's waterworks—signalled by bitter-cold qualities—extends to conditions such as pyelo- and glomerulonephritis and albuminuria.

The compound isomangiferin has shown *antiviral* activity in herpes simplex.

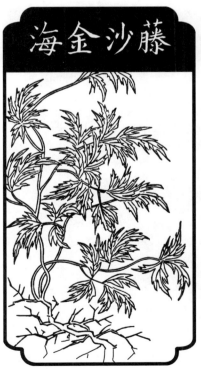

Lygodium Hai Jin Sha Teng
Japanese Climbing Fern Herb

Botanical source: *Lygodium japonicum* (Thunb.) Sweet (Schizaeaceae)
Pharmaceutical name: Herba Lygodii
Chinese names: Hai Jin Sha (Teng), Hai Jin Sha Cao (Mand); Hoi Gam Sa (Cant)
Other names: Climbing fern, "Sea gold sand vine"; Kinshato (Jap)
Habit: Perennial vine-like climbing fern from East Asia, growing on hillsides, in woods and by roadsides in shrub thickets.
Part used: the herb or whole plant

Therapeutic category: mild remedy with minimal chronic toxicity
Constituents: lygodin, lipids
Effective qualities: sweet, bitter, cold
 calming, decongesting, sinking
Tropism: urinary, digestive systems
 Bladder, Small Intestine channels
 Warmth body

URINARY SEDATIVES

ACTIONS AND INDICATIONS
urinary sedative: astringent, anti-inflammatory, antiseptic: acute urinary tract infections with dysuria and hematuria; cystitis, urethritis, nephritis
antilithic: urinary stones or gravel
draining diuretic, renal stimulant: nephritic edema
anti-infective, detoxicant: common cold, flu, epidemic encephalitis, hepatitis, enteritis, dysentery, laryngitis, parotitis, mastitis

SYMPTOM PICTURE
bladder damp heat: painful, burning dark urination, blood or sand in urine, thirst

PREPARATION
Use: The herb Lygodium Hai Jin Sha Teng is briefly decocted or used in tincture form.
Dosage: Decoction: 10-30 g
Tincture: 2-4 ml
Caution: None.

NOTES
Gathered primarily from the hills of the Yangze river provinces, the Japanese climbing fern furnishes an excellent remedy for acute urinary infections and stone formation. The *draining* effect of this botanical—clear from its bitter, cold qualities—also goes beyond this to address a variety of infections characterized by damp heat or fire toxins.

If alone the **spores** of the Japanese climbing fern are used, the remedy is called **Hai Jin Sha** (Mand.) or **Hoi Gam Sa** (Cant.) (literally "sea gold sand"). Its actions and indications are the same as for the herb or whole plant. Dose: 6-10 g.

Akebia Bai Mu Tong
Akebia Stem

Botanical source: *Akebia quinata* (Thunb.) Decaisne (Lardizabalaceae)
Chinese names: Bai Mu Tong, Mu Tong, Ba Yue Sha (Mand); Baak Mok Tong (Cant)
Habit: Deciduous vine growing in thickets in dark, damp or forested places; blooms in spring with racemes of fragrant purple flowers.
Category: mild remedy with minimal chronic toxicity

Constituents: akeboside (akebin), potassium, sapogenins, oleanolic acid, glucose, aristolochine, rhamnoside, oleanolic acid, sapogenins (eugein, hederagenin)
Effective qualities: bitter, astringent, cold, dry; calming, relaxing, stimulating, decongesting, sinking
Tropism: urinary, reproductive, cardiovascular, nervous systems; Bladder, Heart, Small Intestine, Yin Qiao channels

ACTIONS: *Antiseptic, anti-inflammatory, antipyretic, draining diuretic, uterine stimulant, nervous sedative, analgesic, galactagogue, antifungal*
INDICATIONS: Acute urinary tract infections (bladder damp heat) with oliguria, dysuria, enuresis with dark color; leucorrhea, oliguria, dysuria, strangury; esp. gram-positive bacilli; edema, ascites, cardiac edema; mouth or tongue sores/ulcers; fevers, arthralgia, dysmenorrhea, amenorrhea; irritability, palpitations, insomnia; insufficient breast milk.
Dosage: Decoction: 3-10 g
Tincture: 1-4 ml
Caution: Contraindicated during pregnancy. Because of its drying nature, to be used cautiously in elderly or weak people, especially with signs of Yin or fluids deficiency with dryness.
NOTES: Also called Chocolate vine, this botanical today is rarely the source of the remedy Mu tong, as it was over two centuries ago (see also Aristolochia Guan Mu Tong at the start of this section).

Lopatherum Dan Zhu Ye
Bamboo Grass Leaf

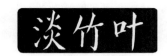

Botanical source: *Lopatherum gracile* Brongnart (Gramineae)
Chinese names: Dan Zhu Ye, Dan Zhu Xie, Shui Zhu Ye, Zhu Ye (Mand); Daam Jok Yip (Cant)
Habit: Perennial herb from Asia and Australia, found on slopes and in damp, shady wooded roadsides.

Category: mild remedy with minimal chronic toxicity
Constituents: taraxerol, friedelin, arundoin, cylindrin, phenol, amino acid, organic acids, saccharides
Effective qualities: sweet, bland, cold, moist; calming
Tropism: urinary, respiratory, digestive systems; Bladder, Heart, Stomach, Small Intestine channels

ACTIONS: *Anti-inflammatory, antipyretic, nervous sedative*
INDICATIONS: Acute urinary tract infection from damp heat; scanty, difficult or irritated urination, blood in urine; fever with unrest, anxiety and thirst; heatstroke, measles, flu; pharyngitis; stomatitis, mouth and tongue sores, swollen gums from stomach fire syndrome.
Dosage: Decoction: 10-16 g
　　　　　Tincture: 2-4 ml
Caution: Use carefully during pregnancy.
NOTES: Bamboo grass root, Dan Zhu Gen (Mand.) or **Daam Jok Gan** (Cant.), is a *uterine stimulant* employed for stalled labor (uterine dystocia) and miscarriage.

野梔子

生殖系统用药

Remedies for the Reproductive System

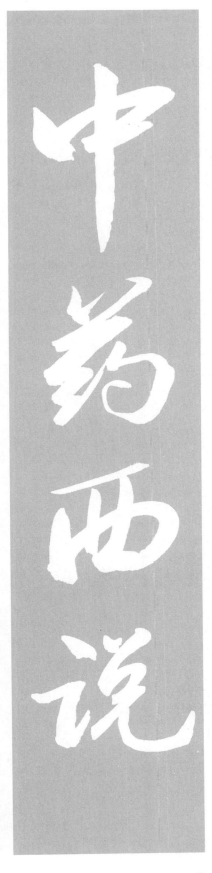

The Chinese mainland offers an abundance of plant remedies for managing female and male reproductive problems. Conditions affecting the uterus, ovaries, prostate and external female and male genitalia are readily treatable with traditional remedies, whether the disorders are functional or organic, and tissue-based or hormonal. In the People's Republic of China, botanicals are also commonly used in obstetrics and gynecology, and combined with Western medicine when necessary.

In traditional Oriental herbals, remedies for reproductive conditions are divided into female and male classifications. The female herb classes "nourish the Blood" and "vitalize the Blood." The male category includes remedies that "fortify the Yang." While these classes confirm the greater diversity of female reproductive problems as compared to the male, they also point to the perennial link of woman with the Blood, and man with the Yang principle. The use of the term Blood, *xue,* in this context refers to the actual red fluid. Woman loses blood monthly; therefore her periodic discomforts are considered disharmonies of the Blood.

Traditional Chinese herb categories tend by nature to be polyvalent. The class of remedies for "fortifying the Yang," for example, consists of remedies that treat all-male problems such as impotence, premature ejaculation, urinary incontinence, lower back pain and weak knees. Here, our first task is to sift out those *Yang tonics* that truly address reproductive conditions from those that mainly treat urinary, musculoskeletal and other dysfunctions. Likewise, in the class of remedies that "vitalize the Blood"—*relaxant* and *spasmolytic* herbs for the most part—we need to apportion them to the main system of their tropism.

Next, the fourfold differentiation of remedies—*restoring, relaxing, stimulating, sedating*—gives us a clearer understanding and overview of these remedies from the vitalistic perspective. It also helps clarify appropriate use alongside comparable Western herbs.

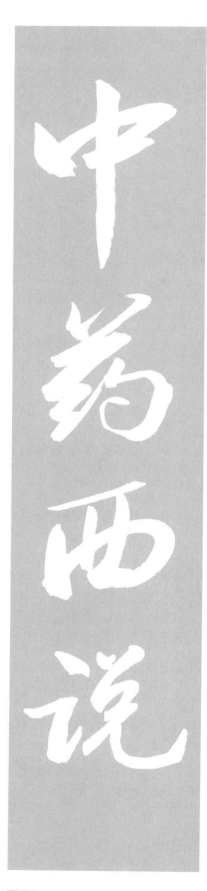

- **Reproductive restoratives** treat two types of functional reproductive deficiencies:
  - deficiency with hormonal insufficiency, presenting infertility, sexual disinterest and impotence.
  - deficiency with pelvic blood congestion, displaying heavy menstrual or intermenstrual bleeding.
- **Reproductive stimulants** address deficiency conditions involving hormonal or uterine insufficiency, presenting delayed, scanty or absent menses.
- **Reproductive relaxants** treat excess conditions with autonomic nervous stress, presenting delayed, scanty or absent menses and tension.
- **Reproductive sedatives** include herbs for treating infectious and inflammatory (i.e., **damp heat**) conditions of the reproductive organs, as well as conditions involving sexual overstimulation. However, because infectious conditions are treated for the most part with *broad-spectrum anti-infectives,* the remedies for these are found in the section on infection and toxicosis. Likewise, remedies reducing sexual overstimulation can be found among the *reproductive restoratives, urinary restoratives* and *neurocardiac sedatives*. Stegodon Long Gu (Dragon bone) and Ostrea Mu Li (Oyster shell), for instance, are frequently used *sexual sedatives* in herbal formulation.

Although *reproductive restoratives* contain remedies for both the female and male systems, *stimulants* and *relaxants* include only gynecological remedies. This is because only women menstruate and are therefore predisposed to its cyclical disrhythmias and disharmonies.

The Reproductive Remedies

Restoratives
Two types of herbs are used to restore the reproductive system and its functions:
- *fertility* and *aphrodisiac restoratives* that address infertility, sexual disinterest and impotence.
- *astringent uterine decongestants* that remove congested blood in the uterus and pelvis, moderating excessive or prolonged menstruation (menorrhagia).

Although all *reproductive restoratives* of the first type increase male sexual potency, the majority also promote fertility and treat functional sterility. This is especially true of Curculigo Xian Mao (Golden eye-grass root from tropical Asia) and Cistanche Rou Cong Rong (the parasitic Fleshy broomrape herb). Containing phyto-androgens and -estrogens, the majority of these *fertility* and *aphrodisiac restoratives* operate through hormonal and other dynamics to enhance sexual desire, promote depth and frequency of orgasm, strengthen male erection, and increase both the quantity and quality of the male sperm and female sexual fluids. In this way they may cause reversal of functional infertility and impotence. Whether actually *aphrodisiac* or not, these *fertility* and *aphrodisiac restoratives* have little in common from either the energetic or the biochemical pharmacological point of view. Notably they include several maritime animal products, such as Sea horse (Hippocampus Hai Ma), and various forms of deer antler (Cervus Lu Rong, Cervus Lu Jiao, Cervus Lu Jiao Jiao).

Traditionally described in Oriental medicine as **Kidney Yang deficiency,** the collection of symptoms just enumerated is better understood as **genitourinary cold** and **genitourinary Qi deficiency,** especially as it may include signs of incontinent urination, premature ejaculation and leucorrhea. The phrase "tonifying the Kidney and fortifying the Yang" that traditionally describes these remedies should now be clearer.

Astringent uterine decongestants, the second type of *reproductive restorative,* primarily address women's problems. Blood has a tendency to stagnate in the capillary bed of the pelvic basin, and in woman this congestion easily leads to congestive dysmenorrhea, expressed in the symptom pattern **uterus blood congestion.** Symptoms include a feeling of heaviness or downward pressure in the lower abdomen before onset of menstruation, PMS, clots in the flow and heavy or prolonged flow. This syndrome may include etiological factors such as venous blood stasis, liver congestion, leiomyomas (fibroids), inadequate tissue oxygenation, adrenal cortex deficiency, excess estrogen in the system and low progesterone. **Venous blood stagnation** counts as a separate, although overlapping syndrome, and includes fatigue, varicose veins and hemorrhoids.

By astricting the capillaries, *uterine decongestants* in this section promote venous return, reduce pelvic and uterine congestion and so reduce menorrhagia. In traditional Oriental medicine these herbs are said to "vitalize the Blood and disperse Blood stasis in the Lower wWrmer." They include an Oriental variety of mugwort, Artemisia Ai Ye (Asian mugwort leaf), much used for passive functional bleeding, and two remedies acting strongly on the venous circulation, Biota Ce Bai Ye (Oriental arborvitae twig, related to the cypress tree whose essential oil is similarly employed) and Sophora Huai Hua (Japanese pagoda tree flower, common throughout China). These *uterine decongestants* are dominated by their bitter and astringent taste which, from the vitalistic viewpoint, accounts for their *decongestant* action.

Stimulants

Gynecological conditions that require stimulation are characterized by stagnation of the Qi and Blood, and may involve cold and deficiency. They are seen in functional amenorrhea and dysmenorrhea, and may involve factors such as thyroid deficiency, and estrogen and progesterone deficiencies or excess. The syndromes **uterus Qi and Blood stagnation**, **uterus Blood**

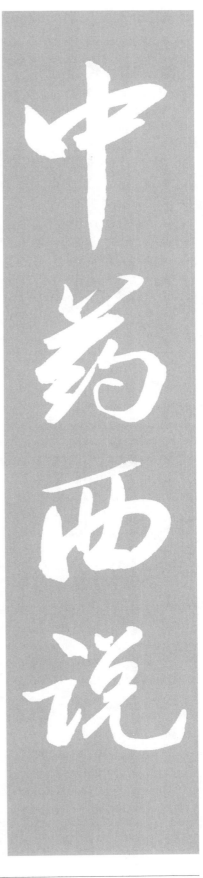

REPRODUCTIVE SYSTEM

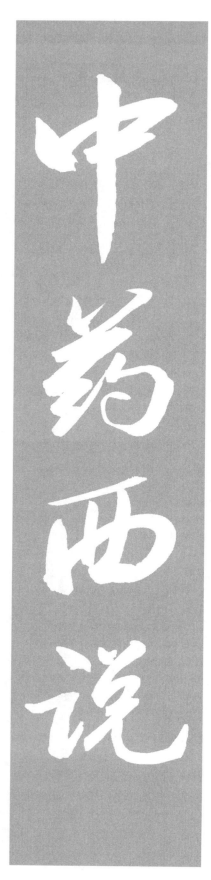

congealed and **uterus cold** summarize these conditions. The first symptom picture is dominated by delayed, absent or slow-starting menses, and the second is characterized by blood clots causing delayed, difficult, painful or absent menses. With **uterus cold** the symptomatology of **uterus Qi stagnation** is augmented by cold signs, including chills and cold extremities.

Uterine stimulants stimulate the uterus and promote menstruation, hence their alternative name, *emmenagogues*. These remedies also are traditionally described as "circulating the Qi and vitalizing the Blood in the Lower Warmer." They tend to be high in essential oils—imparting them their characteristic spicy, warm nature—and are found, for example, in the important remedies Angelica Dang Gui (Dong quai root, an alpine umbellifer from Central China) and Paeonia Mu Dan Pi (tree peony root bark, a much cultivated shrub originally from the East China mountains). In obstetrics, *uterine stimulants* are frequently employed to stimulate uterine contractions in prolonged pregnancy, stalled labor (uterine dystocia) and after miscarriage. They can also help discharge the lochia during the puerperal period. *Uterine stimulants* are normally forbidden during pregnancy as they may cause fetal unrest or abortion.

Because *stimulant* herbs are often also *relaxant* by nature, there is considerable overlap between remedies in this and the next section. A case could be made for placing botanicals such as Cyperus Xiang Fu (Purple nutsedge root) and Impatiens Ji Xing Zi (Garden balsam seed) in either category.

Relaxants

The emphasis of *reproductive relaxants* is on relieving spasmodic dysmenorrhea (i.e., menses with cramps before or during onset). This is often accompanied by irritability, unrest and clots in the flow, forming a symptom pattern that may be called **uterus Qi constraint.** The underlying dynamics may include hormonal imbalances such as estrogen deficiency, estrogen accumulation and progesterone excess, as well as autonomic nervous stress. In the energetic terminology of Chinese medicine, *uterine spasmolytics* relieve menstrual pain by "circulating the Qi" or "releasing constrained Qi in the Lower Warmer," thereby relaxing the uterus and promoting smoother menstruation.

These *relaxants* contain alkaloids, glycosides and essential oils as their main chemical constituents, and are chiefly pungent and bitter by nature. Paeonia Bai Shao (White peony root from Northeast Asia) typically contains essential oil and an assortment of glycosides. By far the most commonly used *uterine relaxant*, White peony root is also ubiquitous in Chinese herb formulating for its systemic *relaxant* effect. The same is true, to a lesser extent, of Cyperus Xiang Fu (Purple nutsedge root from China's coastal marshes) and Leonorus Yi Mu Cao (Asian motherwort herb from Northeast China).

The key constituents contained in two *relaxant* animal remedies often used for spasmodic dysmenorrhea are unique in that they are not found in plants. Trogopterum Wu Ling Zhi (Flying squirrel dropping) and Manis Chuan Shan Jia (Pangolin scale) chemically contain clusters of acids such as dicarbolic and hydroxybenzoic acids. Both remedies are important *spasmolytics* and *analgesics* found in numerous formulas addressing painful and/or spsmodic conditions.

Traditionally, many Chinese remedies are held to relieve menstrual pain by "vitalizing the Blood and dispersing Blood stasis." Today we know that the majority of remedies that relieve spasmodic dysmenorrhea relax the uterine muscle with a *spasmolytic-analgesic* action, rather than a literal *anticoagulant* effect. As a result, included in this section of *uterine relaxant* are many remedies traditionally called "Blood vitalizers."

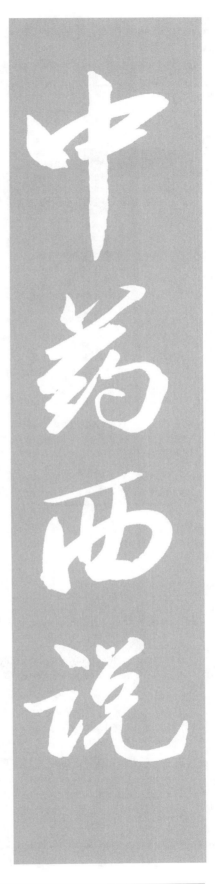

Reproductive Restoratives

REMEDIES TO RESTORE REPRODUCTION AND RELIEVE INFERTILITY AND IMPOTENCE

➺ TONIFY THE KIDNEY AND FORTIFY THE YANG

Fertility and aphrodisiac restoratives

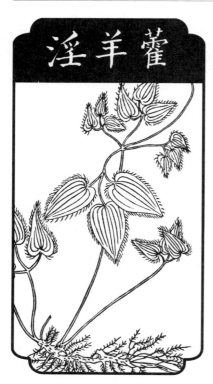

Epimedium Yin Yang Huo
Horny Goat Weed Leaf

Botanical source: *Epimedium saggitatum* (Sieb. et Zucc.) Maximowicz or *E. macranthum* Morris et Decne or *E. brevicornum* Maximowicz and spp. (Berberidaceae)
Pharmaceutical name: Folium Epimedii
Chinese names: Yin Yang Huo, Xian Ling Pi, Yin Ying Cao, Gang Jian (Mand); Gan Yeng Fuk, Seun Ling Pei (Cant)
Other names: Barrenwort; Inyokaku (Jap)
Habit: Perennial woody evergreen herb from temperate and subtropical Asia; grows on slopes, in cliff crevices, under trees and shrubs, and in shady, humid bamboo groves; small, pale yellow terminal flowers open in summer in racemes or panicles.
Part used: the leaf

Therapeutic category: medium-strength remedy with some chronic toxicity
Constituents: flavonoids 4-5% (incl. icariin, methylicariin, anhydrocaritin), polysaccharides, olivil, icariresinol, epimidine, alkaloid magnoflorine, benzene, sterols, tannin, fixed oil, palmitic/linoleic acid, vitamin E
Effective qualities: pungent, sweet, warm, dry
restoring, astringing, solidifying, raising, stimulating, relaxing
Tropism: reproductive, endocrine, urinary, musculoskeletal, nervous, cardiovascular, respiratory systems
Liver, Kidney, Du, Yang Qiao, Yin Qiao channels
Fluid, Air bodies

ACTIONS AND INDICATIONS

reproductive restorative: androgenic aphrodisiac: reproductive deficiency with male sexual disinterest, impotence, sterility, low sperm count, infertility, sexual neurasthenia
pituitary-gonadotropic stimulant, estrogenic: irregular menses, menopausal syndrome; estrogen deficiency
urogenital astringent restorative: enuresis, polyuria, spermatorrhea; chronic prostatitis
neuromuscular stimulant/relaxant, spasmolytic: paresthesia and spasms of limbs and extremities; spasms, seizures, hemiplegia, paraplegia; acute poliomyelitis; chronic tracheitis
analgesic, anti-inflammatory: arthralgia, lumbar pain
nervous restorative: cerebral deficiency with memory loss, depression, fatigue; neurasthenia
coronary restorative/dilator, antilipemic: coronary deficiency with angina pectoris; hyperlipemia, coronary disease, myocardial ischemia
hypotensive, capillary stimulant, vasodilator, diuretic: hypertension, peripheral arterial disorder
stimulant expectorant, antitussive: coughing with phlegm; chronic bronchitis
anti-infective: antiviral, antibacterial, immunostimulant, antigenic, lymphocyte stimulant: infections (incl. enteritis, HIV infection, poliomyelitis)

Miscellaneous: eye ulcerations and corneal conditions after eruptive fever

Symptom Pictures

genitourinary cold (Kidney Yang deficiency): sexual disinterest, impotence, irregular menses, frequent urination

wind/damp/cold obstruction: joint, lower back and knee pain; cramps, spasms or numbness in hands and feet

nerve and brain deficiency: fatigue, absent-mindedness, forgetfulness, numbness of extremities

heart blood and Qi stagnation with **Qi constraint:** fatigue, palpitations, dizziness, chest tightness or pain, shortness of breath

lung phlegm cold: productive coughing, coughing up white sputum, mental dullness

Preparation

Use: The leaf Epimedium Yin Yang Huo is infused or used in tincture form. It may be decocted if part of a formula.

Dosage: Infusion: 3-14 g
Tincture: 2-4 ml

Caution: Epimedium Yin Yang Huo is contraindicated in signs of dryness, and deficiency heat accompanied by excessive sexual drive or wet dreams.

This remedy should not be taken on its own over long periods of time (e.g., several months) because of mild cumulative toxicity. It may also cause idiosyncratic reactions at any time. Such reactions include vomiting, dizziness, dry mouth, nosebleed and injury to the body's Yin in general.

Notes

Derived from various species of *Epimedium* in the barberry family, Horny goat weed leaf is an essential ingredient in many a longevity formula from China's past, such as the Kangbao Pill from the Ming dynasty. Like most other stellar remedies, this botanical also exhibits a variety of images. Deep down, however, Horny goat weed is by nature systemically *tonifying* and *regulating*. Classical medical texts rank it among the *warming Yang tonics* because—as the name literally implies—it promotes comprehensive tonification of reproductive functions. Deficiency of the Kidney Yang—essentially a deficiency cold condition of the urogenital organs—is thereby addressed, with the keynote symptoms impotence and irregular menses. Horny goat weed has recently been proven a *gonadotropic hormonal regulator* with *androgenic* and *estrogenic* actions. Among its other interesting chemical components, the plant's phytosterols have shown activity in this connection. Hence the successful use of this remedy in a large range of male and female reproductive conditions, including infertility, menopausal syndrome and chronic prostatitis.

Another aspect of its *restorative* nature is evident in Horny goat weed leaf's benefits in nervous, and specifically cerebral, deficiencies. Memory loss, chronic tiredness and numbness or tingling of the extremities are prominent symptoms here. The *cerebral restorative* action of this botanical may include a stimulation of the cerebral circulation, similar to Ginkgo leaf. This would be a fruitful area for research, as a *peripheral vasodilatory* action has been confirmed.

In traditional Chinese terms, this remedy's deep, systemic neuroendocrine tonification amounts to an activation of the Du and Yin Qiao extra meridians.

Modern medicine also makes use of the reliable *cardiovascular relaxant* effect of Horny goat weed for conditions such as hypertension and angina; its *bronchial stimulant* action for bronchitis; and its *immune modulating* action for viral and bacterial diseases (note its polysaccharide content). These properties are generally more available when an alcoholic extract rather than a water preparation is used.

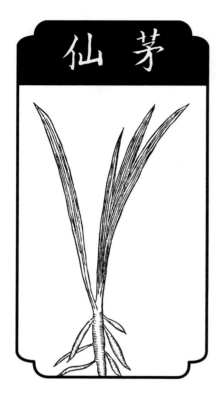

Curculigo Xian Mao
Golden Eye-Grass Root

Botanical source: *Curculigo orchioides* Gaertner (Amaryllidaceae)
Pharmaceutical name: Rhizoma Curculigonis
Chinese names: Xian Mao, Tian Xian Mao, Po Lo Men Shen (Mand); Sin Maau (Cant)
Other names: Black musli, "Immortal grass," "Brahma root"; Senbo (Jap)
Habit: Perennial tropical herb from South China, Malaysia and India, growing on sunny hillsides and in wild spots; yellow terminal flowers open in summer.
Part used: the rhizome

Therapeutic category: medium-strength remedy with some chronic toxicity
Constituents: glycodies (incl. curculigoside, orcinol), tannins 4%, resin, fixed oil, starch
Effective qualities: pungent, sweet, astringent, a bit bitter, warm, very dry
 restoring, astringing, stabilizing, relaxing
Tropism: reproductive, urinary, musculoskeletal, nervous, cardiovascular systems
 Kidney, Liver, Spleen, Dai, Yang Wei channels
 Fluid, Air bodies

ACTIONS AND INDICATIONS
reproductive restorative: aphrodisiac: sexual disinterest, infertility, impotence
urogenital restorative, astringent: incontinence with enuresis, spermatorrhea (incl. nocturnal), premature ejaculation
analgesic: lumbar pain, bone pains, joint pains, generalized pain; myalgia, arthralgia, neuralgia, ostalgia
hypotensive: hypertension
diuretic: chronic nephritis
digestive stimulant: gastrointestinal dyspepsia
Miscellaneous: menopausal syndrome

SYMPTOM PICTURES
genitourinary cold (Kidney Yang deficiency): loss of sexual desire, premature ejaculation, dribbling or frequent urination, infertility, impotence

damp cold obstruction: painful, cold, weak lumbars and legs, chronic muscle and joint pains and spasms

PREPARATION
Use: The root Curculigo Xian Mao is decocted or used in tincture form.
Dosage: Decoction: 3-10 g
 Tincture: 2-4 ml
Caution: This warm and dry-natured botanical is forbidden in all dry conditions and in Yin deficiency with empty heat. It is not be used continuously on its own because of some slight cumulative toxicity.

NOTES
Golden eye-grass was officially introduced to the Middle Kingdom when an Indian missionary monk presented the root to the Tang monarch Xuan Zong. In the late part of the last century Dr. Porter Smith, a keen resesearcher in Oriental materia medica, translated this plant's Buddhist name, Po Lo Men Shen, as "Brahminical ginseng." This venerable name points not only to the Indian Buddhist origins of this medicinal, but also to the esteem in which it was held as a

warming reproductive and *systemic restorative* that "fortifies the Yang." Infertility, impotence and urogenital incontinence are the main conditions for which it is traditionally used.

This is one of several remedies in the Oriental pharmacy whose action on the reproductive system has not, as yet, received much research. However, as with other remedies in this section, one suspects that hormonal mechanisms are involved.

Golden eye-grass root owes its usage for chronic muscle and joint pains to the outstanding *analgesic* effect.

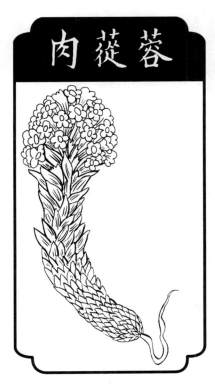

Cistanche Rou Cong Rong
Fleshy Broomrape Herb *

Botanical source: *Cistanche salsa* (C.A. Meyer) G. Beck or *C. deserticola* Y.C. Ma or *S. ambigua* (Bge.) G. Beck (Orobanchaceae)
Pharmaceutical name: Herba Cistanchis
Chinese names: Rou Cong Rong, Dan Cong Rong, Rou Song Yong (Mand); Yak Sung Yan (Cant)
Other names: Beechdrops, Ghost plant; Nikujuyo (Jap)
Habit: Perennial parasitic herb from West China, Tibet and Inner Mongolia, gowing in sandy, dry river beds; terminal spikes of white or violet flowers bloom in early summer.
Part used: the herb

Therapeutic category: mild remedy with minimal chronic toxicity
Constituents: alkaloids, orobanchin, phytosterols, beta-sitosterol, succinic acid, betaine, glucose
Effective qualities: sweet, salty, sour, astringent, warm, moist
  restoring, astringing, solidifying, softening
Tropism: reproductive, urinary, digestive, musculoskeletal, cardiovascular systems
  Kidney, Liver, Large Intestine, Ren, Dai channels; Fluid body

ACTIONS AND INDICATIONS
reproductive restorative: androgenic, estrogenic, aphrodisiac: reproductive deficiency with sexual disinterest, infertility, impotence; menopausal syndrome
astringent urogenital restorative: incontinence with enuresis, spermatorrhea; leucorrhea
analgesic: lower back pain, knee pain
mucogenic, demulcent laxative: insufficient secretions, dehydration, constipation from dryness
hypotensive: hypertension

SYMPTOM PICTURES
uterus cold: infertility, clear vaginal discharges, uterine bleeding, cold extremities

genitourinary cold (Kidney Yang deficiency): sexual disinterest, impotence, urinary dribbling, premature ejaculation

PREPARATION
Use: The herb Cistanche Rou Cong Rong is decocted or used in tincture form.
Dosage: Decoction: 6-18 g
  Tincture: 2-4 ml
Caution: Contraindicated in diarrhea due to stomach Qi deficiency, and in Yin deficiency conditions with empty heat.

NOTES

The scaly, pliant, fleshy stem of the broomrape is traditionally considered to address Kidney Yang deficiency conditions, including deficient reproductive and urinary functioning. In Oriental medicine the remedy is mainly applied to the two symptom patterns above. From the Western biomedical perspective, however, it is Fleshy broomrape stem's *restorative* action on both male and female reproductive systems that is foremost. Interestingly, Fleshy broomrape stem also has its Yin-fostering side, as a *demulcent* and *mucogenic* that promotes and restores mucus.

The root of various broomrape species in the American mountain West may be similarly used.

Morinda Ba Ji Tian
Morinda Root

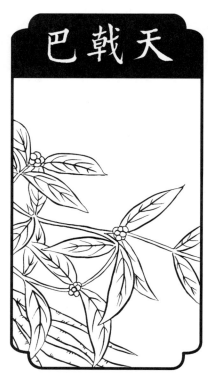

Botanical source: *Morinda officinalis* How (Rubiaceae)
Pharmaceutical name: Radix Morindae
Chinese names: Ba Ji Tian, Ba Ji, San Man Cao, Ji Rou (Mand); Ba Gek Tin (Cant)
Other names: Indian mulberry; Hagekiten (Jap)
Habit: Herbaceous climbing vine found throughout the (sub)tropics; grows along valley streams and under sparse trees in hills; flowers in summer with terminal white umbels.
Part used: the root

Therapeutic category: mild remedy with minimal chronic toxicity
Constituents: anthraquinone morindone, rubichloric acid, morindadiol, soranjidiol, rubiadin, monotropein, asperuloside tetraacetate, sitosterol, asperuloside, phytosterols, tannin, saccharides, resin, vitamin C
Effective qualities: sweet, a bit astringent and pungent, warm, dry
　　　　　　　　　　restoring, astringing, solidifying, raising
Tropism: reproductive, urinary, musculoskeletal, nervous, endocrine systems
　　　　　Liver, Kidney, Ren, Yin Qiao channels
　　　　　Fluid, Air bodies

ACTIONS AND INDICATIONS

reproductive restorative: androgenic, aphrodisiac: reproductive deficiency with sexual disinterest, impotence, infertility
astringent urogenital restorative: enuresis, pollakiuria, spermatorrhea
analgesic: painful knees, legs, lumbars, back; rheumatoid arthritis
adrenocortical restorative: stamina loss, fatigue; metabolic deficiencies, menopause
musculoskeletal restorative: weakness due to weak muscles and bones (incl. lumbar weakness); muscular atrophy
cerebral restorative: cerebral deficiency, impaired thinking
hypotensive, diuretic
interferon inducent
Miscellaneous: beriberi

SYMPTOM PICTURES

genitourinary cold (Kidney Yang Deficiency): sexual disinterest, seminal incontinence; frequent, dribbling urination

wind/damp/cold obstruction: painful or sore muscles and joints, esp. leg and lower back muscles

musculoskeletal deficiency (Liver and Kidney depletion): weak legs and knees, weak muscles, fatigue

PREPARATION

Use: The root Morinda Ba Ji Tian is decocted or used in tincture form.
Dosage: Decoction: 6-16 g
Tincture: 2-4 ml
Caution: Forbidden in Yin deficiency conditions with deficiency heat, and in difficult urination.

NOTES

To the long-lived Manchu emperor Qian Long, this warming tonic was one of the secrets of longevity. A systemic *restorative* effect is evident when considering the tonifying action on reproductive, urinary, musculoskeletal and adrenal functions. In this respect, Morinda root is therapeutically similar to Dipsacus Xu Duan and Cibotium Gou Ji, but carries more emphasis on inadequacies of sexual functions—an area in which a Son of Heaven could not afford to be ailing.

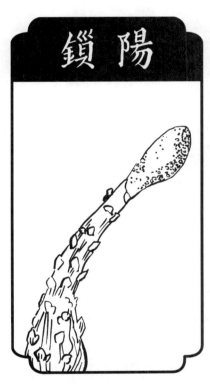

Cynomorium Suo Yang
Lock Yang Stem *

Botanical source: *Cynomorium songaricum* Ruprecht (Cynomoriaceae)
Pharmaceutical name: Herba Cynomorii
Chinese names: Suo Yang (Mand); Soi Yeung (Cant)
Other names: Sayo (Jap)
Habit: Perennial parasitic herb growing in the dry, sandy desert regions of Mongolia and East and North China; dark purple flowers bloom in midsummer.
Part used: the stem

Therapeutic category: mild remedy with minimal chronic toxicity
Constituents: anthocyanic glycosides, triterpenoid saponins, enzyme, tannin, fixed oil, saccharide, essential oil (incl. hexa/octa-decanoic acid)
Effective qualities: sweet, warm, moist
restoring, solidifying, stimulating
Tropism: reproductive, muscoloskeletal, digestive, nervous systems
Liver, Kidney, Large Intestine, Ren, Dai channels
Fluid bodies

ACTIONS AND INDICATIONS

reproductive restorative, aphrodisiac: reproductive deficiency with sexual disinterest, impotence
urogenital astringent restorative: polyuria, enuresis, spermatorrhea
neuromuscular restorative/stimulant: weakness due to weak sinews; lumbar weakness, muscular atrophy, paralysis, motor impairment/ataxia, myasthenia gravis
demulcent laxative: constipation with dry stool

SYMPTOM PICTURES

genitourinary cold (Kidney Yang deficiency): impotence, frequent urination, premature ejaculation
neuromuscular deficiency (Liver and Kidney depletion): weak muscles and tendons, difficulty of movement, paralysis, fatigue

PREPARATION

Use: The stem Cynomorium Suo Yang is decocted or used in tincture form.

Dosage: Decoction: 6-16 g
Tincture: 2-4 ml
Caution: Contraindicated in Kidney Yin deficiency with deficiency heat, and in diarrhea.

NOTES

In the past, Lock yang stem was considered a medicinal for life extension. Although its *restorative* and *aphrodisiac* effects on reproductive functions are acknowledged, today the botanical is possibly applied more for the *restorative* action on muscular innervation—note that motor impairment and paralysis are among its uses. In both functions Lock yang stem closely resembles the Brazilian remedy Marapuama bark and wood.

Like other tonics in this section, the remedy is frequently used during later life, when its *demulcent laxative* property makes a welcome contribution.

Cervus Lu Jiao
Mature Deer Antler

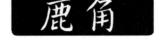

Zoological source: *Cervus nippon* Temminck or *C. elaphus* L. (Cervidae)
Chinese names: Lu Jiao, Lu Rong Lao (Mand); Lok Jiu (Cant)
Category: mild remedy with minimal chronic toxicity
Constituents: amino acids, gelatin, trace minerals, calcium phosphate, calcium carbonate
Effective qualities: salty, warm, dry; restoring, nourishing, astringing
Tropism: reproductive, musculoskeletal, endocrine systems; Kidney, Liver, Chong, Dai channels

ACTIONS: *Reproductive restorative and stimulant, aphrodisac, urogenital astringent, musculoskeletal restorative, metabolic restorative, nutritive, vulnerary, detumescent*
INDICATIONS: Impotence, loss of sexual drive; sperm loss, leucorrhea (Kidney Yang deficiency syndrome); fatigue, debility; weak bones and muscle, weak lumbars and knees, connective tissue deficiency, pain in bones, joints, lumbars; bleeding during pregnancy; whooping cough; breast pain, traumatic wounds, severe boils, carbuncles.
Dosage: Decoction: 3-10 g
Powder: 1-1.5 g
Caution: In people with Yin deficiency with empty heat.
NOTES: Mature deer antler's functions are similar, but lesser, than those of Velvet deer antler.

Cervus Lu Jiao Jiao
Mature Deer Antler Glue

Zoological source: *Cervus nippon* Temminck or *C. elaphus* L. (Cervidae)
Chinese names: Lu Jiao Jiao (Mand); Lok Jiu Jiu (Cant)
Part used: the glue or colloid obtained when the antler is cooked over a long period
Category: mild remedy with minimal chronic toxicity
Constituents: amino acids, gelatin, trace minerals
Effective qualities: salty, oily, warm, moist; restoring, nourishing, astringing
Tropism: reproductive, musculoskeletal, endocrine systems; Kidney, Liver, Chong channels

ACTIONS: *Reproductive restorative and stimulant, aphrodisac, urogenital astringent, musculoskeletal restorative, metabolic restorative, nutritive, vulnerary, hemostatic*
INDICATIONS: Impotence, loss of sexual drive; sperm loss (Kidney Yang deficiency syndrome); fatigue, debility, nutritional and metabolic deficiencies (Blood and Essence deficiency syndrome); weak bones and muscle, weak lumbars and knees, connective tissue deficiency; traumatic wounds/fractures, hemorrhage, coughing up blood, menorrhagia

Dosage: Decoction: 4-12 g
Caution: In people with Yin deficiency with empty heat.
NOTES: Mature deer antler glue is said to possess superior *nutritive* and *anastative* effects to the raw antler itself.

The residue obtained from the cooking process of mature deer antler, once the colloid gel has formed, is called **Lu Jiao Shuang** (Mand.) or **Lok Jiu Shuen** (Cant.). This residue is then prepared into a powder.

Mature deer antler powder, Lu Jiao Shuang, has the same properties as the raw antler itself, but is less tonifying to the Kidney Yang, bones and sinews. It is especially *astringent, mucostatic* and *hemostatic*, however, and is often used for white vaginal discharge, seminal emission and uterine bleeding. Moreover, unlike Mature deer antler gel, the powder has the advantage of not being oily in quality, being easily digested by those intolerant of oily herbs and foods. It is also applied topically to stop bleeding.

Stichopus Hai Shen
Sea Cucumber

Zoological source: *Stichopus japonicus* Selenka
Chinese names: Hai Shen (Mand); Hoi Sam (Cant); "Sea kidney"
Category: mild remedy with minimal chronic toxicity
Effective qualities: salty, warm, moist; restoring, nourishing, thickening
Tropism: reproductive, digestive, respiratory, nervous, urinary systems; Kidney, Heart, Lung channels

ACTIONS: *Reproductive restorative, aphrodisiac, nervous restorative, urinary restorative, antienuretic, nutritive, demulcent*
INDICATIONS: Impotence, loss of sexual drive from Kidney Yang deficiency; pollakiuria; nocturnal spermatorrhea; malnutrition, anemia, exhaustion, postpartum debility, neurasthenia, hemophilia, lung TB, constipation from dryness.
Dosage: Decoction: 10-30 g
Sea cucumber is also cooked in soups.
Caution: Contraindicated in diarrhea from digestive deficiency and copious bronchial sputum.

Hippocampus Hai Ma
Sea Horse

Zoological source: *Hippocampus kelloggi* Jordan et Snyder, *H. histrix* Kaup and spp. (Syngnathidae)
Chinese names: Hai Ma (Mand); Hoi Ma (Cant)
Category: mild remedy with minimal chronic toxicity
Effective qualities: sweet, salty warm; restoring, calming
Tropism: reproductive, urinary, respiratory, endocrine systems; Kidney, Liver channels

ACTIONS: *Reproductive restorative, androgenic, estrogenic, aphrodisac; adrenocortical restorative, antiasthmatic, urinary restorative, antienuretic, hemostatic, dissolvent*
INDICATIONS: Impotence, loss of sexual drive, low estrogen conditions; uterine dystocia; Kidney Yang deficiency syndrome; urinary incontinence with enuresis; wheezing from adrenal deficiency; fatigue (esp. in the elderly), lumbar pain; bleeding, pain, swollen sores and boils, scrofula.
Dosage: Decoction: 2-10 g
Caution: Caution during pregnancy and in Yin deficiency with empty heat.

Callorhinus Hai Gou Shen
Seal Genitals

Zoological source: *Callorhinus ursinus* L. and *Phoca vitulina* L.
Chinese names: Hai Gou Shen (Mand); Hoi Gau Sam (Cant)

Category: mild remedy with minimal chronic toxicity
Effective qualities: salty, hot; restoring, calming
Tropism: reproductive, digestive, musculoskeletal systems; Kidney, Liver channels

ACTIONS: *Reproductive restorative, aphrodisac, analgesic*
INDICATIONS: Impotence; fatigue, weak knees and lumbars (Kidney Yang deficiency); abdominal pain with chills.
Dosage: Decoction and powder: 3-10 g
Caution: Forbidden in Yin deficiency with heat and chronic cough, in dyspepsia from gastrointestinal deficiency and cold, and with sexual overstimulation.

Actinolitum Yang Qi Shi
Actinolite

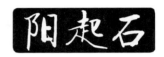

Geological source: *Actinolitum*
Chinese names: Yang Qi Shi (Mand); Yong Chak Sek (Cant); "Yang raising stone"
Other names: Actinolite asbestos, tremolite
Source: Hebei, Henan, Hubei and Shandong provinces

Category: mild remedy with minimal chronic toxicity
Constituents: calcium and magnesium silicate
Effective qualities: salty, warm; restoring, stimulating, astringing
Tropism: reproductive system; Kidney, Chong channel

ACTIONS: *Reproductive restorative and stimulant, aphrodisac, emmenagogue, astringent*
INDICATIONS: Impotence and infertility with Yang deficiency, amenorrhea, dysmenorrhea, uterine bleeding from deficiency, premature ejaculation, spermatorrhea, prostate obstruction (protatism); cold lower limbs.
Dosage: Decoction: 3-8 g
Caution: Do not use in Yin deficiency with empty heat present.

REMEDIES TO REMOVE UTERINE BLOOD CONGESTION AND RELIEVE MENORRHAGIA
➧ VITALIZE THE BLOOD AND DISPERSE BLOOD STASIS IN THE LOWER WARMER
Astringent uterine decongestants

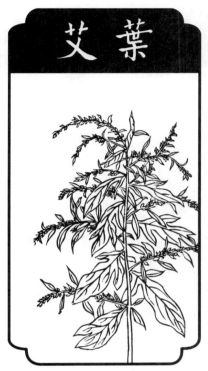

Artemisia Ai Ye
Asian Mugwort Leaf

Botanical source: *Artemisia argyi* Leveillé et Vant. (Compositae)
Pharmaceutical name: Folium Artemisiae argyi
Chinese names: Ai Ye, Wu Yue Ai, Ai Hao, Qi Ai (Mand); Ai Yip, Ai Yang (Cant)
Other names: Gaiyo (Jap)
Habit: Fragrant, hairy perennial herb from temperate Asia; also cultivated in mid China; grows on grassland, waste ground and roadsides; small, pale yellow panicles of capitulate terminal flowers blossom in summer and autumn.
Part used: the leaf

Therapeutic category: mild remedy with minimal chronic toxicity
Constituents: essential oil (incl. cineol 30%, terpineol, carveol, caryophyllene, phellandrene, artemisia alcohol, adenine, camphor, borneol, linalol), tannins, bitter glycosides, 2 acidic polysaccharides, vitamins A, B1, B2, C, D
Effective qualities: bitter, pungent, astringent, warm, dry
    decongesting, astringing, solidifying, stimulating, relaxing
Tropism: urogenital, vascular, digestive, respiratory systems
    Liver, Spleen, Kidney, Lung, Dai, Yang Wei, Ren channels
    Warmth, Fluid bodies

ACTIONS AND INDICATIONS
uterine restorative: astringent decongestant: pelvic congestion with congestive dysmenorrhea, menorrhagia
hemostatic, coagulant: passive uterine bleeding (incl. postpartum); rectal hemorrhage, vomiting blood, nosebleed, leucorrhea
reproductive restorative: infertility, irregular menstruation
spasmolytic, analgesic: dysmenorrhea, postpartum pain, epigastric and abdominal pain, diarrhea, colitis
fetal relaxant, antiabortive: fetal unrest (esp. with vaginal bleeding), threatened miscarriage
bronchial relaxant, antitussive: asthma, chronic bronchitis
immune regulator, antiallergic: immune stress with immediate allergies (incl. bronchial asthma, asthmatic bronchitis, urticaria, rhinitis, otitis, angioedema, drug allergy, atopic dermatitis)
antibacterial, antivenomous, immunostimulant, interferon inducent: infections (incl. bacterial dysentery, malaria), insect and snake bites
antifungal, antiparasitic: tinea, scabies

SYMPTOM PICTURES
uterus blood congestion with **cold:** prolonged menses with scanty clotted flow, intermenstrual uterine bleeding, cramps, sexual disinterest

intestines Qi constraint with **damp cold:** diarrhea, abdominal pain, blood in stool

PREPARATION
Use: The leaf Artemisia Ai Ye is infused or used in tincture form. Its *hemostatic* action is said to be increased after charring, when it is known as **Ai Ye Tan** (Mand.) or **Ai Yip Taan** (Cant.). Cleaned of stems and twigs and rolled into cigar-shaped sticks, the punk or down of Asian mugwort is known as "moxa," and when ignited, is used to

stimulate acupuncture points and warm and relax tissues. This procedure is called "moxibustion."

Like numerous *Artemisias* of the American southwest, this variety also has a powerful cleansing action, both vibrationally and as a *disinfectant;* it is frequently used to fumigate or smudge. It is often mixed with powdered Atractylodes Cang Zhu root, which enhances its action as a *fumigant,* and is used as such to prevent or treat local fungal infections, herpes sores, wounds, etc. This indirect form of moxibustion should be applied topically to conditions such as these, making sure that the smoke wafts directly onto the affected area (blow if neccessary).

The essential oil of Asian mugwort leaf has been found particularly effective for bronchitis and asthma, using the oral spray (nebulizer) method of internal delivery.

Dosage: Decoction: 3-10 g
Tincture: 1-4 ml

Caution: Use with caution during pregnancy and in Blood heat and Yin deficiency conditions.

NOTES

Asian mugwort is not the same botanical species as the Western mugwort, which is *Artemisia vulgaris.* The latter was once confused with the former (Chang and But 1987). Moreover, the two herbs cannot be substituted across the board. With its *astringent, decongestant* and *relaxant* actions, Asian mugwort leaf is used primarily to stop uterine bleeding, relieve pain, disinfect and relieve cold and Qi constraint conditions of the uterus. Western mugwort herb, conversely, mainly stimulates the uterus and generally disinfects.

Like most remedies in this subsection, Asian mugwort leaf can be seen to activate the Dai and Yang Wei extra meridians in its *blood decongestant, astringent* and *hemostatic* action on the pelvic/uterine area. This herb, moreover, has the distinction of also entering the Ren meridian. This is suggested by its historical use for dysmenorrhea, irregular cycles and infertility, as well as in its use for asthmatic and eczematous conditions.

Two strongly anticomplementary polysaccharides have been recently found in Asian mugwort leaf (Yamada and Kiyohara 1989), providing theoretical support for its *immune stimulating* and *interferon producing* activities. The use of this remedy for a range of type I or immediate allergic conditions is today also well documented.

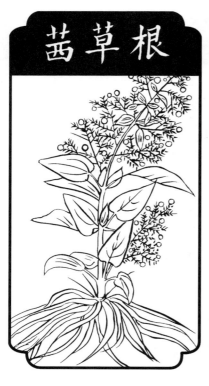

Rubia Qian Cao Gen
Heart-Leaf Madder Root *

Botanical source: *Rubia cordifolia* L. and spp. (Rubiaceae)
Pharmaceutical name: Radix Rubiae
Chinese names: Qian Cao Gen, Xi Cao, Hong Si Xian, Qian Gen, Di Xue (Mand); Chan Chou Gan, Sai Chou Gan (Cant)
Other names: Indian madder, "Earth blood"; Seisokon, Akane (Jap)
Habit: Perennial climbing mountain herb from Central Asia and West China; grows in damp, shady upland forests, woods, ravines and bush; cymes of light yellow terminal/axillary flowers bloom in summer.
Part used: the root

Therapeutic category: mild remedy with minimal chronic toxicity
Constituents: anthraquinones (incl. purpurin, pseudopurpurin, alizarin, munjistin, purpuroxanthin, rubimallin), tannins, sitosterol, daucosterol
Effective qualities: bitter, astringent, cold, dry
decongesting, astringing, thickening, stimulating, dissolving
Tropism: reproductive, respiratory, vascular, nervous systems
Heart, Liver, Lung, Dai, Yang Wei channels; Fluid, Air bodies

Actions and Indications

uterine restorative: astringent decongestant: pelvic congestion with congestive dysmenorrhea, menorrhagia
hemostatic, coagulant: uterine bleeding; passive or active hemorrhaging, blood in stool and urine, nosebleed, coughing or vomiting blood
astringent: early stage of carbuncle or throat abscess, diarrhea, dysentery
analgesic, vulnerary: chest and flank pain, joint pain, abdominal pain, trauma pain; traumatic injuries (incl. fractures)
uterine stimulant, emmenagogue, parturient: amenorrhea, prolonged pregnancy, retained placenta
stimulant expectorant, antitussive: chronic bronchitis, cough
urinary restorative, antilithic, diuretic: urinary incontinence with enuresis, urinary sand and stones, gallstones (also preventively), hyperuricemia, albuminuria; eczema, rickets
liver decongestant, cholagogue, laxative: liver congestion with dyspepsia, jaundice, liver and spleen enlargement, chronic hepatitis
antibacterial, antiviral: miscellaneous infections (incl. influenza, hepatitis)
antitumoral: tumors (incl. cancer)

Symptom Pictures

uterus blood congestion: heavy or prolonged menses, clotted flow, intermenstrual bleeding, lower abdominal pressure

uterus Qi stagnation: absent, delayed or difficult menses, abdominal pain

liver Qi stagnation: indigestion, epigastric discomfort and bloating, constipation, appetite loss

Preparation

Use: The root Rubia Qian Cao Gen is decocted or used in tincture form. Charring the root first is said to increase its astringency.

Dosage: Decoction: 8-16 g
            Tincture: 2-3 ml

Caution: Contraindicated in indigestion due to cold and during pregnancy. Harmless orange discoloration of the urine may be caused by the dye alizarin contained in the root.

Notes

Heart-leaf madder is one of many imports from the Himalayas, and has a long history of use in Chinese medicine for gynecological disorders. The root is an excellent *astringent decongestant* that "vitalizes the Blood," and a good tannin-based *coagulant hemostatic* remedy that is as much part of the Western herbal tradition as the Eastern. Besides shortening bleeding time, it primarily addresses menstrual conditions caused by pelvic blood congestion. Other related uses include tissue trauma presenting pain and bleeding.

Paradoxically, because of its content in glycosides, Heart-leaf madder also acts as an effective *uterine stimulant* for amenorrhea. As a *parturien* it can also play an important role during the third phase of childbirth to help expel the lochia, contract the uterus, stop bleeding and relieve pain.

This plant's celebrated preventive and remedial action on stone formation is also well documented in both Ayurvedic and Greek medical systems. The anthraquinones have shown significant activity in this respect—as they have in Cascara sagrada bark *(Rhamnus purshiana)*, for instance. Other *restorative* benefits on urinary functions include relief of albuminuria and hyperuricemia.

All species of Madder root are therapeutically fairly interchangeable. This species, like its Western counterpart, may also be used for its *decongestant* effect on the liver, which includes *cholagogue* and *laxative* actions. Liver Qi stagnation presenting acute indigestion and constipation, and chronic liver disorders, are addressed here.

Gossypium Mian Hua Gen
Cotton Root Bark

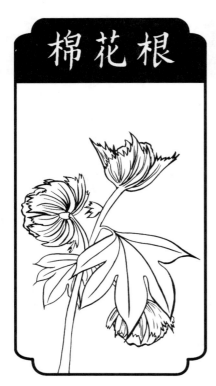

Botanical source: *Gossypium hirsutum* L. or *G. herbaceum* L. (Malvaceae)
Pharmaceutical name: Cortex radicis Gossypii
Chinese names: Mian Hua Gen, Cao Mian (Mand); Mai Fa Gan (Cant)
Habit: Annual temperate and subtropical herb or shrub; widely cultivated in China and North America; five-petaled yellow flowers with pale purple centers flower in late summer.
Part used: the root bark

Therapeutic category: mild remedy with minimal chronic toxicity
Constituents: phenolic glycoside gossypol 0.56-2.05%, asparagine, arginine, tannin, salicylic acid, resin
Effective qualities: sweet, astringent, warm, dry
astringing, stabilizing, decongesting, stimulating, relaxing
Tropism: reproductive, respiratory, digestive systems
Liver, Lung, Spleen, Dai, Yang Wei channels
Fluid, Air bodies

ACTIONS AND INDICATIONS

uterine restorative: astringent decongestant: pelvic congestion with menorrhagia, congestive dysmenorrhea
hemostatic: uterine bleeding (metrorrhagia)
antitumoral: benign and malignant tumors (incl. uterine fibroids, endometriosis, ovarian cancer)
uterine stimulant, emmenagogue, parturient, abortive: delayed menses, amenorrhea; uterine subinvolution, miscarriage, prolonged pregnancy
spermicidal male contraceptive: contraception in men
respiratory stimulant: expectorant, antitussive: chronic bronchitis with cough
gastrointestinal restorative: diarrhea, malabsorption, fatigue
antiviral: influenza
Miscellaneous: epididymis swelling

SYMPTOM PICTURES

uterus blood congestion: early or heavy menses, lower abdominal pressure before onset, uterine bleeding

lung phlegm cold: chronic coughing, expectoration of white phlegm, wheezing, tight chest

PREPARATION

Use: The root Gossypium Mian Hua Gen is decocted or used in powder or tincture form. For temporary male contraception, two months of daily use is required to decrease sperm count to virtually zero.
Dosage: Decoction and powder: 10-20 g
Tincture: 2-5 ml
For contraception, the oral dosage of the active extract, gossypol, is 20 mg per day for two months, then 20-28 mg twice a day. High dosages of the decoction or tincture are equivalent to this amount.
Caution: Forbidden during pregnancy because of its *uterine stimulant* effect.

NOTES

Cotton root bark and its extract gossypol are a *decongestant, hemostatic* and *antitumoral* remedy for the female reproductive organs. The remedy's success rate with various types of congestive female disorders—heavy menses, uterine bleeding, fibroids and endometriosis—has been very high. Conversely, Cotton root bark can also exert a *stimulant* action on female reproductive and respiratory organs.

The remedy's male contraceptive aspect, however, has received the most attention. The *antifertility* effect is due to a general inhibition of sperm production, damage to and eventual atrophy of the spermatids in the seminiferous tubules, and immobilization of their forward motility. No hormonal mechanism has ever been observed, and with discontinuation of the remedy, normal fertility is usually resumed within three months (Leung and Tso 1989). Cotton root bark can, therefore, be said to be a safe producer of temporary and reversible infertility for men.

Cotton seed, Mian Zi (Mand.) or **Mai Ji** (Cant.), may also be used for male contraceptive purposes. Pungent-warm by nature, the seed additionally has *muskuloskeletal restorative, analgesic, hemostatic, galactagogue, demulcent* and *emollient* properties useful for weak back and knees, epigastric and abdominal pain, hemorrhage and insufficient lactation. It is also applied topically for dry, irritated skin conditions, scabies and leprosy. Dose: 8-16 g by short decoction.

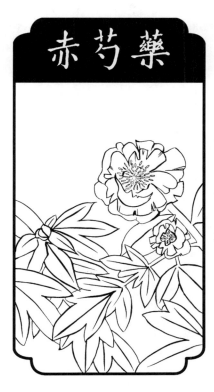

Paeonia Chi Shao Yao
Red Peony Root

Botanical source: *Paeonia lactiflora* Pallas, *P. obovata* Maximowicz or *P. veitchii* Lynch (Compositae)
Pharmaceutical name: Radix Paeoniae rubrae
Chinese names: Chi Shao (Yao), Cao Shao Yao, Chuan Shao Yao (Mand); Chek Cheuk Yeuk, Chek Chat (Lai) (Cant)
Other names: Sekishaku (Jap)
Habit: Perennial wild and cultivated herb from temperate Northeast Asia; also cultivated; blooms in summer with large, solitary magenta or purple flowers.
Part used: the root

Therapeutic category: mild remedy with minimal chronic toxicity
Constituents: monoterpene paeoniflorin, paeonol, tannins, benzoic acid, resin, alliflorine, fatty oil and acids, gallic acid, catechin, protein, glucose, mucilage, starch
Effective qualities: bitter, sour, astringent, cool, dry
  decongesting, astringing, solidifying, stimulating, relaxing, calming
Tropism: reproductive, digestive, vascular systems
  Liver, Spleen, Dai, Yang Wei channels; Air, Warmth bodies

ACTIONS AND INDICATIONS
uterine restorative: astringent decongestant: pelvic congestion with congestive dysmenorrhea, early menstrual onset, menorrhagia
hemostatic: intermenstrual bleeding, coughing up blood, nosebleeds (hematemesis, epistaxis)
uterine stimulant/relaxant, emmenagogue: amenorrhea, spasmodic dysmenorrhea, spasmodic uterine dystocia
nervous sedative/relaxant: analgesic, spasmolytic: PMS, unrest and pain in general (esp. menstrual and intestinal colic)
coronary dilator, anticoagulant: coronary thrombosis, atherosclerosis, menstrual clots
antacid antisecretory: acid dyspepsia with hyperchlorhydria
anticontusion, detumescent: strains, sprains, swelling and pain of traumatic injury
anti-inflammatory: early stage boils and carbuncles; conjunctivitis
anti-infective: antibacterial, antifungal, antiviral: dysentery, typhoid, septicemia; fungal skin infections; flu, herpes

Symptom Pictures

uterus blood congestion: early or heavy menses, feeling of weight and bearing down before onset

uterus blood congealed and Qi constraint: painful or delayed menses, thick purple clots in flow, abdominal or flank pain, unrest, irritability, stress

Blood and Nutritive level heat: skin eruptions, bleeding, fever, unrest, irritability

Preparation

Use: The root Paeonia Chi Shao Yao is decocted or used in tincture form.
Dosage: Decoction: 6-14 g
Tincture: 2-4 ml
Caution: Use cautiously in Blood deficiency and during pregnancy.

Notes

Being the most *astringent* and *decongestant* of the "three peony sisters," Red peony root is also the most effective for relieving uterine and pelvic blood congestion. Although very similar in all respects to White peony root and Tree peony root bark, this botanical nevertheless stands out for its vitalizing effect on the coronary circulation and for its *antithrombotic* action.

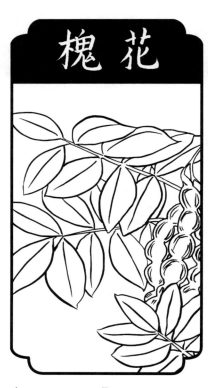

Sophora Huai Hua
Japanese Pagoda Tree Flower

Botanical source: *Sophora japonica* L. (Leguminosae)
Pharmaceutical name: Flos seu gemma Sophorae japonicae
Chinese names: Huai Hua, Huai Hua Mi (Mand); Wai Fa, Wai Fa Mai (Cant)
Other names: Chinese scholar tree; Kaikamai (Jap)
Habit: Deciduous spreading tree found throughout China and Korea in country and towns; terminal panicles of white flowers bloom in summer.
Part used: the flower; also the flower bud (Huai Hua Mi)

Therapeutic category: mild remedy with minimal chronic toxicity
Constituents: flavonoids (incl. rutin, quercetin), triterpenoid saponins (betulin, sophoradiol), glucuronic acid, tannins, vitamin A
Effective qualities: bitter, astringent, cool
  restoring, astringing, solidifying, decongesting, relaxing
Tropism: reproductive, cardiovascular, digestive systems
  Liver, Large Intestine, Dai, Yang Wei channels
  Fluid, Air, Warmth bodies

Actions and Indications

uterine restorative: astringent decongestant: pelvic congestion with congestive dysmenorrhea, menorrhagia
venous decongestant, capillary restorative: venous deficiency with varicose veins, hemorrhoids, phlebitis; blood congestion (any type)
hemostatic: bleeding, hemorrhage; uterine, menstrual and hemorrhoidal bleeding; blood in urine, stool and spittle, nosebleed
astringent, anti-inflammatory: phlebitis, enteritis, dysentery, conjunctivitis, leucorrhea
gastric mucosal restorative: acid dyspepsia from hyperchlorhydria, peptic ulcer
nervous sedative, hypotensive: anxiety, agitation, irritability, dizziness; stress; hypertension
amtibacterial, antifungal

Symptom Pictures

uterus blood congestion: heavy menses with early flow, lower abdominal pressure before onset, intermenstrual bleeding

venous blood stagnation: hemorrhoids, varicose veins, fatigue

intestines damp heat: urgent bowel movement, loose stool with blood and pus

Preparation

Use: The flower Sophora Huai Hua is decocted or used in tincture form.
Dosage: Decoction: 8-16 g
Tincture: 2-4 ml
Caution: Forbidden in bleeding from Qi deficiency, and in deficiency cold of the stomach and intestines.

Notes

The yellow-green flowers of this common Asian ornamental tree furnish an effective *blood decongestant* remedy that benefits both the capillary bed and venous circulation. Through *astringent* capillary shrinkage and *toning*—note its prominent glycosides, saponins and tannin content—Japanese pagoda tree flower effectively removes blood stasis and prevents hemorrhage, especially of the uterus. Its *hemostatic* and *anti-inflammatory* actions combine to treat enteritic conditions presenting bloody stool.

Japanese Pagoda tree bud, Huai Hua Mi (Mand.) or **Wai Fa Mi** (Cant.), possesses the same actions as the flower. The remedy is mainly used for its good *hemostatic* action that can stop most types of bleeding. Dose: 6-16 g by decoction, 1-4 ml in tincture.

Japanese pagoda tree fruit, Huai Jiao (Mand.) or **Wai Jiu** (Cant.), is used mainly as a *hemostatic*. It is additionally *uterine stimulant, parturient, abortifacient, laxative* and *hypotensive*. The *hemostatic* action is considered less strong than that of the flower, but the *anti-inflammatory* effect is greater. It is used especially for uterine bleeding, blood in the urine, inflamed hemorrhoids, venereal sores, milk fever, stalled labor and abortion. Dose: 10-16 g, by decoction.

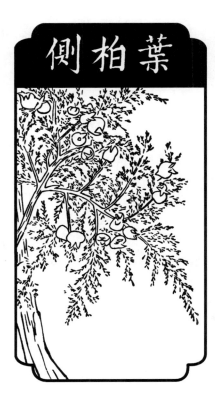

Biota Ce Bai Ye
Oriental Arborvitae Tip

Botanical source: *Biota orientalis* (L.) Endicher, syn. *Thuja orientalis* L. (Cupressaceae)
Pharmaceutical name: Cacumen Biotae orientalis
Chinese names: Ce Bai Ye, Ce Bo Ye, Ce Bai (Mand); Jak Baak Yip (Cant)
Other names: "Flat fir leaf"; Sokuhakuyo (Jap)
Habit: Aromatic evergreen tree or pyramidal shrub from temperate China and Korea, found on dry slopes; also cultivated; catkins flower in spring.
Part used: the leafy end twigs or tips

Therapeutic category: mild remedy with minimal chronic toxicity
Constituents: essential oil (incl. pinene, thujene, thujone, fenchone), flavonoids (aromadendrin, quercetin), isopimaric acid, tannins, lignans, resin, bitter pinipicrin
Effective qualities: bitter, astringent, cold, dry
decongesting, astringing, relaxing, calming
Tropism: reproductive, nervous, vascular, respiratory, digestive, systems
Heart, Liver, Large Intestine, Dai, Yang Wei channels

ACTIONS AND INDICATIONS

uterine restorative: astringent decongestant: pelvic congestion with congestive dysmenorrhea, menorrhagia
venous decongestant: venous deficiency with varicose veins, hemorrhoids (incl. with bleeding), phlebitis
hemostatic: coughing or vomiting blood, nosebleed, blood in stool or urine, uterine bleeding
astringent: acute and chronic bacillary dysentery, gastric/duodenal ulcer
neurocardiac sedative: unrest, irritability, insomnia, palpitations; neurosis, neurocardiac syndrome; arthralgia
bronchial relaxant, expectorant: cough with bloody sputum, wheezing; asthma, acute and chronic bronchitis, lung TB, whooping cough
antipyretic, anti-inflammatory: fevers, burns, dermatitis, pruritus with oily skin, erysipelas, parotitis
antibacterial, antiviral: enteritis, bronchitis; herpes
hair growth stimulant: alopecia (hair loss)

SYMPTOM PICTURES

uterus blood congestion: early or heavy menstrual flow, bearing-down pressure and aching in lower abdomen, irritability

venous blood stagnation: fatigue, varicose veins, spider veins, hemorrhoids

heart Qi constraint with **nerve excess:** stress, palpitations, unrest, worry, sleep loss

lung Qi constraint with **phlegm heat:** wheezing, difficult cough with scanty, fetid blood-streaked sputum, fever

intestines damp heat: blood in stool, painful urgent bowel movement, diarrhea, feverishness

PREPARATION

Use: The twig Biota Ce Bai Ye is used in decoction (raw or charred) or tincture form. Ointments for burns can be prepared with this remedy, and a tincture extract rubbed in topically promotes hair growth.
Dosage: Decoction: 6-15 g
    Tincture: 2-4 ml
Caution: Avoid using during pregnancy and breastfeeding, as it contains the toxic ketone thujone.

NOTES

A widely used remedy for stagnant blood conditions, Oriental arborvitae twig is essentially a *blood decongestant, hemostatic* and *neurocardiac sedative*. This astringent, bitter botanical is invaluable when blood stasis and Qi constraint appear simultaneously.

There is not much in common between the use of this herb and the related *Thuja occidentalis*, **Arborvitae** or **Yellow cedar:** The latter is used mainly for its *stimulant* action on the heart, lungs, uterus, kidneys and muscular system, as well as its *mucous resolvent* and *anti-discharge* effects. Both remedies do, however, have *antiviral* activity in common, particularly as regards the treatment of herpes, as well as an *expectorant* action for infectious bronchial disorders.

Oriental arborvitae twig is therapeutically much closer to another related remedy in the Cypress family, **essential oil of Cypress** (*Cupressus sempervirens*) (see Holmes 1989). Both have *relaxant* actions, particularly on the bronchi, and both vitalize the blood and remove venous stagnation through their *decongestant* action.

Reproductive Stimulants

REMEDIES TO PROMOTE MENSTRUATION AND RELIEVE AMENORRHEA

➜ CIRCULATE THE QI AND VITALIZE THE BLOOD IN THE LOWER WARMER

Uterine stimulants, emmenagogues

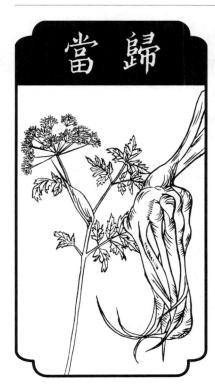

Angelica Dang Gui
Dong Quai Root

Botanical source: *Angelica sinensis* (Oliv.) Diels (Umbelliferae)
Pharmaceutical name: Radix Angelicae sinensis
Chinese names: Dang Gui, Qin Gui, Yun Gui, Quan Dang Gui (Mand); Dong Gwai (Cant)
Other names: "State of return"; Toki (Jap)
Habit: Perennial herb from Gansu and Shanxi provinces with a preference for cold, damp, high, forested mountain terrain and rich, deep sandy soil; also very widely cultivated; flowers in summer with compound white umbels.
Part used: the root

Therapeutic category: mild remedy with minimal chronic toxicity
Constituents: essential oil (45% ligustilide, butylidine phthalide, safrol, carvacrol, valerophenone carboxylic acid; coumarins bergapten, scopoletin, umbelliferone), falcarinol, sitosterol, 6 polysaccharides, nicotinic and folic acid, sodium ferulate, ferulic/palmitic/linolenic acid, sesquiterpenes and their alcohols, cadinene, dodecanol, sucrose, carotene, 24 minerals and trace elements (incl. magnesium, iron, selenium, manganese, silica, vanadium), vits A, B12, E
Effective qualities: a bit sweet, pungent and bitter, warm, moist
  stimulating, restoring, relaxing, calming, diluting, softening
Tropism: reproductive, cardiovascular, digestive, nervous, endocrine systems
  Liver, Spleen, Heart, Chong, Yin Wei, Ren, Yin Qiao channels
  Fluid, Warmth, Air bodies

ACTIONS AND INDICATIONS

uterine stimulant/relaxant: emmenagogue: deficient and spasmodic menstrual conditions with delayed or scanty menses; amenorrhea, spasmodic dysmenorrhea, infretility
estrogenic, progesteronic: estrogen and progesterone deficiency conditions; PMS
fetal relaxant: fetal unrest, threatened miscarriage
metabolic/liver restorative, anastative hemogenic, liver protective: metabolic deficiencies with weakness, fatigue; liver glycogen deficiency, anemia, vitamin E deficiency
nervous sedative, analgesic, anti-inflammatory: unrest, anxiety, menstrual and postpartum pain, epigastric and abdominal pain, headache, backache, myalgia, neuralgia, pain of trauma; neurocardiac syndrome
cardiovascular relaxant, hypotensive vasodilator: palpitations; arrhythmia, peripheral arterial deficiency, hypertension
coronary restorative: coronary deficiency/disease, angina pectoris
antilipemic: hyperlipemia, atherosclerosis
anticoagulant: thrombosis, traumatic contusion, old injuries
immunostimulant, phagocyte/lymphocyte stimulant: infections in general
antitumoral, interferon inducent: women's reproductive myoma, fibroids

antifungal: fungal infections

immune regulator, antiallergic: immune stress with immediate allergies (incl. rhinitis, urticaria, angioedema, bronchial asthma, drug allergies)

radiation-protectant: radiation damage

demulcent laxative: constipation, hard dry stool

Miscellaneous: post-traumatic edema

SYMPTOM PICTURES

uterus Qi stagnation with **Blood deficiency:** delayed, irregular, scanty or absent menses; fatigue, pale complexion, chills

uterus Qi constraint: painful, difficult menses; cramps, clots with flow, irritability, unrest

heart blood and Qi stagnation with **Qi constraint:** stress, anxiety, palpitations, chest tightness or pain, shortness of breath

Blood deficiency: fatigue, palpitations, dizziness, dry skin and hair, pale ashen complexion, cold extremities

PREPARATION

Use: The root Angelica Dang Gui should be decocted in the standard way or used in tincture form.

Dosage: Decoction: 4-12 g
Tincture: 2-4 ml

Caution: Being a *uterine stimulant*, this remedy is contraindicated during pregnancy, as it also is in Yin deficiency syndromes with empty heat. Use cautiously in diarrhea or abdominal distension caused by intestinal mucous damp.

NOTES

The sweet-spicy Dong quai root fully deserves the reputation it enjoys for managing a variety of women's problems. The net regulating effect on menstruation and PMS of this very versatile remedy is due to several actions: *stimulating* and *relaxing* on the uterus, and enhancing both estrogen and progesterone hormonal levels, as required. These actions suggest applications to Blood deficiency, Qi stagnation and Qi constraint conditions of the uterus. No wonder that Dong quai root is a major ingredient in the quintessential Chinese gynecological formula, the Four Substances Decoction. Metabolic deficiencies centered around the liver—Blood deficiency in traditional terms—are also improved through its sweet, *restorative* qualities. In the energetic terms of Oriental medicine, the extra channels Chong and Ren and their coupled channels are engaged.

Like the botanically related Sichuan lovage root, Chinese hospitals also routinely make use of Dong quai root's multifaceted *cardiovascular* and *coronary relaxant* actions for treating conditions such as hypertension, thromboangiitis and neurogenic cardiac disorders. In energetic terms, these conditions would be attributed to blood and Qi stagnation in the chest impairing coronary circulation—again note the Chong and Yin Wei connection.

More recently, interesting anticomplementary activity has been demonstrated by Dong quai's pectic polysaccharides. These modulate *antitumoral, interferon-inducing* and *immune-stimulating* actions (Li Zhong 1988). Ferulic acid is also thought to be instrumental in the last-mentioned effect. In addition, immune regulation has been shown in immediate hypersensitivity disorders such as allergic rhinitis, hives and drug allergies.

Although Dong quai root has no exact equivalent in the West, Lovage root, *Levisticum officinale*, also in the carrot family, shares not only its *uterine stimulant* and *estrogenic* actions, but also major essential oil components such as ligustilide, n-butylthalide and n-butylidene phthalide. Not surprisingly, in China Lovage root is known as "European Dang Gui." From the larger therapeutic perspective, however, the two remedies need to be clearly distinguished. The two actions just mentioned apart, the two remedies are very different and should not substitute for each other in any other way.

Paeonia Mu Dan Pi
Tree Peony Root Bark

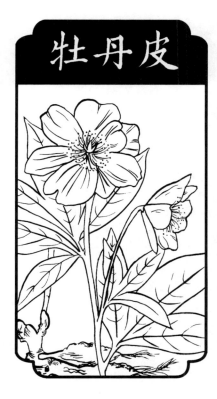

Botanical source: *Paeonia suffruticosa* Andrews (Compositae)
Pharmaceutical name: Cortex radicis Paeoniae suffruticosae
Chinese names: Mu Dan Pi, Dan Pi, Mu Dan, Fen Dan Pi (Mand); Maau Daan Pei, Daan Pei (Cant)
Other names: Moutan, "Male red"; Botanpi (Jap)
Habit: Small perennial deciduous mountain shrub from mid and east China; fond of warm, sunny climes of around 1600 feet and fertile soil; also cultivated; solitary magenta-purple or white flowers appear in late spring.
Part used: the root bark

Therapeutic category: mild remedy with minimal chronic toxicity
Constituents: essential oil (incl. ketone paeonol, monoterpenes paeoniflorin and oxypaenyflorin), glycosides (apiopaenoside, paeonoside, paeonolide), steroids (campesterol, beta-sitosterol), benzoic acid
Effective qualities: pungent, bitter, a bit astringent, cool, dry
stimulating, calming, decongesting, astringing, softening, dissolving
Tropism: reproductive, cardiovascular, respiratory systems
Kidney, Liver, Heart, Chong channels; Air, Warmth, Fluid bodies

ACTIONS AND INDICATIONS

uterine stimulant: emmenagogue: deficient menstrual conditions with amenorrhea, delayed or scanty menses
antipyretic: dry fever, hot spells
anti-inflammatory, detoxicant: macula and papula, appendicitis, scarlet fever, typhus, skin rashes/ulcers/cancer, boils, carbuncles, appendicitis, dermatitis, gynecological tumors
anticontusion, vulnerary: bruises, strains, sprains, fractures, blood clots
hemostatic: hemorrhage (incl. coughing up blood, nosebleeds, bloody stool, subcutaneous bleeding)
nervous sedative, analgesic, anticholinergic: dysmenorrhea, headache, arthralgia, pruritus; PMS, agitation, insomnia, seizures (incl. febrile)
hypotensive: hypertension
immune regulator, antiallergic: immune stress with allergic conditions (incl. rhinitis, eczema); antibody-mediated cytotoxicity (incl. hemolytic anemia, autoimmune disorders, thrombocytopenic purpura)
broad-spectrum antibacterial: dysentery, typhoid, whooping cough, strep throat; fungal infections

SYMPTOM PICTURES

uterus Qi stagnation with **Blood congealed:** absent, delayed, difficult or painful menstruation, painful clotted flow, headache, irritability

Qi constraint with **nerve excess (Liver and Heart fire):** painful irregular menses, headache, irritability, stress, sleep loss

Blood and Nutritive level heat: hot spells or fever, irregular menses, skin rashes, blood in urine, sputum or vomit, subcutaneous bleeding

PREPARATION

Use: The root bark Paeonia Mu Dan Pi is decocted or used in tincture form.
Dosage: Decoction: 6-12 g
Tincture: 2-4 ml
Caution: Avoid use during pregnancy, in menorrhagia, in Yin deficiency conditions with excessive sweating, and in cold conditions.

REPRODUCTIVE STIMULANTS

NOTES

Along with chrysanthemums, magnolias, lotuses and several other plants elevated to the status of a cultural emblem, the "thousand-petaled" tree peony is one of China's most beloved flowers. From its cultivation centers, which included Changan, Fengxien (in the Tibetan foothills), Loyang and Caozhou (in Shandong), the tree peony has through the centuries generated more horticultural and literary extravaganzas than any other ornamental.

In tree peony's root bark coexist two opposing therapeutic tendencies: stimulation and astringency. When applied to its main tropism, the female reproductive organs, the *stimulant emmenagogue* effect wins out. Unlike its sisters Red peony and White peony, Tree peony can only be used with sluggish or absent menses—as in the syndrome uterus Qi stagnation—but not for menstrual flooding.

Recent research has shown that this remedy produces excellent results in bronchial and intestinal infections—apparently due to strong *antiseptic* activity—as well as in various types of allergic/hypersensitivity conditions. The unique spicy and somewhat floral scent of the root bark indicates the presence of an essential oil that is implicated in these actions.

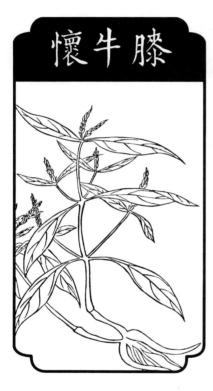

Achyranthes Huai Niu Xi
White Oxknee Root *

Botanical source: *Achyranthes bidentata* Blume or *A. longifolia* Makino or *A. aspera* L. or *Cuccubala Baccifer* L. (Amaranthaceae)
Pharmaceutical name: Radix Achyranthis
Chinese names: Huai Niu Xi, Tan Niu Xi, Bo Bei (Mand); Wai Ngau Sat, (Cant); *A. long*: Tu Niu Xi (Mand); To Ngau Sat (Cant); *A. asp.*: Wei Niu Xi, Ju Niu Xi (M); Wai Ngau Sat (C); *C. bac.*: Bai Niu Xi (M); Baak Ngau Sat (C)
Other names: "Huai river oxknee", Twin-tooth chaff-flower; Goshitsu (Jap)
Habit: Perennial herb common in Mid China, esp. Henan; grows on roadsides, waste ground and in damp, shady areas like streams and forests; also cultivated; tall, slender terminal spikes of small green flowers appear in summer.
Part used: the root

Therapeutic category: mild remedy with minimal chronic toxicity
Constituents: triterpenoid saponins (sapogenin, oleanolic acid), ecdysterone, inokosterone, peptic polysaccharide, mucilage, calcium oxalate, potassium
Effective qualities: a bit sweet, bitter, sour, cool, dry
    stimulating, astringing, restoring, relaxing
Tropism: reproductive, hepatic, musculoskeletal, vascular, urinary systems
    Liver, Kidney, Ren channels; Air, Fluid bodies

ACTIONS AND INDICATIONS

uterine stimulant: emmenagogue: deficient menstrual conditions with amenorrhea, dysmenorrhea
puerperial, parturient, abortive: prolonged pregnancy, puerperal cervical rigidity, hypotonic uterine dystocia, miscarriage, retained placenta
musculoskeletal restorative: weakness/atrophy of ligaments, bones; lumbar and knee atrophy, limb contraction
protein anabolism stimulant: deficient protein synthesis
draining diuretic, antilithic: nephritic edema, urinary stones, gravel
hypotensive: hypertension
immune regulator: immune stress with antibody-mediated cytotoxicity (incl. autoimmune hemolytic anemia, thrombocytopenic purpura)

analgesic, anti-inflammatory: dysmenorrhea, postpartum pain, dysuria, arthralgia, lumbago, sciatica, toothache, gingivitis, laryngitis
vulnerary, anticontusion: traumatic injuries, sprains, strains, fractures
detoxicant: boils, carbuncles, cystitis
hemostatic, astringent: blood in urine/stool, coughing up blood, nosebleed, bleeding gums, urinary incontinence
Miscellaneous: diptheria prevention; beriberi

SYMPTOM PICTURES

uterus Qi stagnation: delayed, absent, difficult or painful menstruation

musculoskeletal deficiency (Liver and Kidney depletion): weak, sore lower back and knees, fatigue

Liver Yang rising: headache, dizziness, blurred vision, nosebleeds

PREPARATION

Use: The root Achyranthes Huai Niu Xi is decocted or used as a tincture. The latter, like the wine-treated root itself, is more pain-relieving and relaxing.
Dosage: Decoction: 6-16 g
Tincture: 2-4 ml
Caution: Forbidden during pregnancy, in diarrhea due to intestinal deficiency, and in menorrhagia and spermatorrhea.

NOTES

This plant in the amaranth family is so called because its large joints resemble the knees of oxen. It originates in central China's river Huai area. Millenia of gynecological and obstetrical experience show White oxknee root to be a reliable *labor-inducing* agent at any stage of gestation, an *expeller of the lochia* and an *emmenagogue*—in short, a very versatile *uterine stimulant*.

With its *astringent* and *analgesic* properties, White oxknee root is also an important trauma medicine, especially when bleeding and pain are involved. In recent years the remedy has also shown to increase protein anabolism in the liver and kidneys.

Vaccaria Wang Bu Liu Xing
Cowcockle Seed

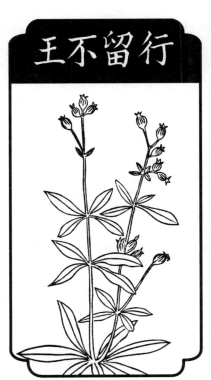

Botanical source: *Vaccaria segetalis* (Neck.) Garcke (Caryophyllaceae) L. (Moraceae)
Pharmaceutical name: Semen Vaccariae
Chinese names: Wang Bu Liu Xing, Jin Gong Hua (M); Wong Bo Lau Chin (C)
Other names: Cowherb, Dairy pink, "Forbidden in the palace"; Ofurugyo (Jap)
Habit: a) Annual/biennial temperate Eurasian herb growing in corn fields and on hillsides; also cultivated; terminal cymes of small pink to crimson flowers appear in late spring.
Part used: the seed

Therapeutic category: mild remedy with minimal chronic toxicity
Constituents: saponins (vacsegoside, gypsogenin, isosaponarin, saponaretin, vitexin), glucuronic acid, glucose, arabinose, xylose, protein, starch, lipids
Effective qualities: bitter, astringent, neutral, dry
stimulating, astringing
Tropism: reproductive, glandular systems
Liver, Stomach channels; Fluid, Air bodies

ACTIONS AND INDICATIONS
uterine stimulant: emmenagogue, parturient: amenorrhea, prolonged pregnancy, stalled labor
galactagogue: insufficient or absent lactation
detumescent: painful swellings, boils, abscesses (esp. of breasts/testicles); mastitis, lymphadenitis, prostate hyperplasia
astringent, vulnerary: ulcers, traumatic wounds
diuretic, antilithic: urinary stones
antiviral: herpes zoster

PREPARATION
Use: The seed Vaccaria Wang Bu Liu Xing is decocted or used in tincture form. In the latter form it strongly promotes menstruation. For herpes the toasted and powdered seeds are mixed with a fatty oil into a paste and applied topically. Simple washes are prepared for external use.
Dosage: Decoction: 5-15 g
   Tincture: 2-4 ml
Caution: This *uterine stimulant* is forbidden during pregnancy.

NOTES
Cowcockle seed is usually seen in formulas addressing the above menstrual and obstetrical conditions. It is also a special remedy for benign prostate congestion.

In South China and often in the U.S., this remedy is represented by the fruit of *Ficus pumila,* **Creeping fig,** properly known as **Bi Li** or **Mu Man Tou.** Although *Vaccaria* and *Ficus* share the first two functions above, Ficus Bi Li also treats urogenital incontinence, diarrhea and arthritic and rheumatic pain

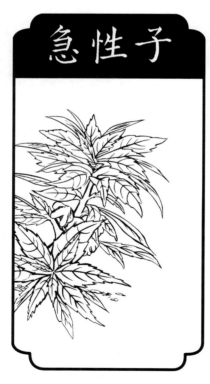

Impatiens Ji Xing Zi
Garden Balsam Seed

Botanical source: *Impatiens balsamina* L. (Balsaminaceae)
Pharmaceutical name: Semen Impatiensis
Chinese names: Ji Xing Zi, Feng Xian Zi (Mand); Jek Chin Ji (Cant)
Other names: Rose balsam, "Quick-temper seed"; Hosenka (Jap)
Habit: Annual herb growing in moist ground along streams and field margins; also cultivated; blooms in summer with white, yellow, magenta or purple axillary flowers.
Part used: the seed

Therapeutic category: medium-strength remedy with some chronic toxicity
Constituents: saponins, fixed oil (incl. balsaminasterol, parinaric acid), essential oil, glycosides (quercetin, kaempferol derivatives), naphthaquinones
Effective qualities: bitter, pungent, warm
   stimulating, relaxing, softening
Tropism: reproductive, digestive systems
   Liver, Chong channels
   Air body

ACTIONS AND INDICATIONS
uterine stimulant/relaxant, emmenagogue: deficient and spasmodic menstrual conditions (amenorrhea, etc.)
parturient, abortive: prolonged pregnancy, stalled labor, miscarriage
ovulation inhibitor, contraceptive: contraception
digestive relaxant: dyspepsia with painful hard abdomen, intestinal colic

throat relaxant: esophageal obstruction, choking due to inadvertent swallowing of bones; dysphagia
antitumoral: esophageal cancer

SYMPTOM PICTURE
uterus Qi stagnation and Qi constraint: scanty, difficult or absent menses, abdominal lumps

PREPARATION
Use: The seed Impatiens Ji Xing Zi is decocted or used in tincture form.
Dosage: Decoction: 3-12 g. For cancer 15-60 g should be used.
Tincture: 2-4 ml
Caution: Being *uterine stimulant* and having some cumulative toxicity, this remedy is contraindicated during pregnancy and breastfeeding. It should not be used continuously on its own.

NOTES
The ornamental garden balsam from the jewelweed family, with its variegated flowers and dramatic popping sound when the seed pods are burst—its quick temper—was incorporated into Chinese medicine from India at an early date. The seed has been consistently used as a general symptom-relief remedy for amenorrhea and dysmenorrhea. Its *contraceptive* effect is said to be due to an inhibitory action on ovulation.

Garden balsam seed contains powerful glycosides and naphthoquinones, known experimentally to possess various actions different from this remedy's traditional usage. The exception to this is the use for esophageal cancer. Garden balsam seed deserves extensive research for potential *anti-inflammatory, antiallergic* and *antioxidant* activities, among others.

Garden balsam flower, Ji Xing Hua (Mand.) or **Jek Chin Fa** (Cant.), is used for amenorrhea, traumatic injury, sprains, arthralgia, furuncles, ringworm and snake bites. Dose: 3-6 g in infusion.

Saussurea Xue Lian
Snow Lotus Root *

Botanical source: *Saussurea laniceps* Handel-Mazzetti, *S. medusa* Maximowicz, *S. involucrata* Karelin et Kirilov ex Maximovicz, *S. tridactyla* Schultz-Bipontinus and *S. eriocephala* Franchet (Compositae)
Chinese names: Xue Lian (Mand); Hat Ling (Cant)
Habit: Perennial alpine herb from East China (Xinjiang and Xizang [Tibet]) found at 4,000 meters (the snow line) in the Tianshan and Kunlun range.
Category: mild remedy with minimal chronic toxicity

Constituents: *S. medusa*: alkaloids, flavonoids, lactones, sterols, essential oil, acidic polysaccharide with calcium chloride
S. involucrata: syringin, butylpyranofructoside
Effective qualities: sweet, a bit bitter, warm; stimulating, astringing, decongesting, relaxing
Tropism: reproductive, circulatory, musculoskeletal, respiratory systems; Kidney, Liver, Lung, Chong, Dai, channels

ACTIONS: *Emmenagogue, parturient, abortive; spasmolytic, analgesic, anti-inflammatory, astringent, hemostatic, mucostatic, reproductive restorative, aphrodisiac, antirheumatic, antitussive*
INDICATIONS: Amenorrhea with uterus Qi stagnation; stalled labor, miscarriage, prolonged pregnancy, retained placenta; spasmodic and congestive dysmenorrhea, menorrhagia, uterine bleeding; uterus blood congestion syndrome; impotence; abdominal cramps; rheumatism; cough with thin sputum.
Dosage: Decoction: 5-16 g
Tincture: 1-3 ml
Caution: Contraindicated during pregnancy unless used for the disorders above.
NOTES: Snow lotus root is an important gynecological remedy from East China. The root contains components that both *stimulate* the uterus and *promote astriction* and *blood decongestion*. The net result is very much a regulating one on uterine functions, especially regarding menstruation and childbirth.

Rosa Yue Ji Hua
Moonseason Rose Bud *

Botanical source: *Rosa chinensis* Jacqet (Roasaceae)
Chinese names: Yue Ji Hua, Yue Yue Hong (Mand)
Other names: Monthly/Bengal/Climbing/Chinese tea rose; Gekkika (Jap)
Habit: Cultivated evergreen shrub blooming all year round; the red or pink flowers are terminally clustered.

Category: mild remedy with minimal chronic toxicity
Constituents: essential oil (incl. terpenes)
Effective qualities: sweet, warm, moist; stimulating, calming, softening
Tropism: reproductive, digestive systems; Liver, Large Intestine channels

ACTIONS: *Emmenagogue, analgesic, demulcent laxative, detumescent, detoxicant, anti-inflammatory*
INDICATIONS: Amenorrhea, delayed menses; uterus Qi stagnation syndrome; dysmenorrhea, abdominal or thorassic pain and distension; constipation with dryness, neck swellings, boils, carbuncles, scrofula.
Dosage: Infusion: 5-10 g
　　　　　Tincture: 2-4 ml
　　External applications for boils and swellings are also prepared with these preparations.
Caution: Can cause diarrhea in intestinal deficiency conditions; forbidden during pregnancy.
NOTES: One of the classical Chinese roses that transformed the dowdy European cultivars, this species was first grown in England as the "blush tea" rose in 1759. As a remedy, Moonseason rose is a simple *uterine stimulant* with similar functions to essential oil of Rose.
　　　Moonseason rose root, Yue Ji Gen, is given for leucorrhea, nocturnal emmission and traumatic injury. Dose: 6-20 g by decoction.

Caesalpinia Su Mu
Sappanwood

Botanical source: *Caesalpinia sappan* L. (Leguminosae)
Chinese name: Su Mu (Mand); So Mok (Cant)
Other names: Soboku (Jap)
Habit: Prickly large shrub or small evergreen tree from (sub)tropical Asia (incl. South China); flowers in early summer with yellow terminal panicles.
Part used: the heartwood

Category: mild remedy with minimal chronic toxicity
Constituents: sappanin, essential oil (incl. phellandrene, ocimene), tannins, brasilin, brasilein, tannic and gallic acid
Effective qualities: sweet, salty, astringent, neutral; stimulating, astringing, calming
Tropism: reproductive, digestive, vascular systems; Heart, Liver, Chong channels

ACTIONS: *Emmenagogue, analgesic, anticontusion, detumescent, hemostatic, antitumoral*
INDICATIONS: Amenorrhea, dysmenorrhea with severe pain; uterus Qi stagnation syndrome; postpartum pain, epigastric and abdominal pain; chronic pain and swelling from sprains, strains, fractures, injuries, abscesses; postpartum bleeding.
Dosage: Decoction: 3-10 g
　　　　　Tincture: 2-4 ml
Caution: Contraindicated during pregnancy because of its *uterine stimulant* property.
NOTES: Named after the Javanese island of its origin, Sumbawa, the sulphur yellow-flowered sappanwood tree has been used for both its yield of bright red dye—the bresil wood of the European Middle Ages—and its medicinal properties. Both Chinese and Greek medicine make use of the reliable pain-relieving and menses-promoting action of the heartwood. Stagnant conditions with painful cramps due to spasms, not blood clots, are its specific indications. Several of Sappanwood's properties come together in relieving postpartum pain and bleeding.

Campsis Ling Xiao Hua
Asian Trumpet Creeper Flower

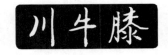

Botanical source: *Campsis grandiflora* (Thunb.) K. Schumann (Bignoniaceae)
Chinese names: Ling Xiao Hua, Yun Xiao Teng (Mand); Ling Siu Fa (Cant)
Habit: Deciduous woody climbing vine from Mid and South China, found on roadsides and hillsides; cymes of red terminal flowers open during summer.

Category: mild remedy with minimal chronic toxicity
Constituents: dextrose, sucrose, cyanidin-rutinoside
Effective qualities: sour, astringent, pungent, dry, cool; stimulating, relaxing, decongesting
Tropism: reproductive, nervous, digestive, urinary systems; Liver, Spleen, Heart channels

ACTIONS: *Emmenagogue, spasmolytic, analgesic, mucostatic, hemostatic, hypoglycemiant, diuretic, antipyretic*
INDICATIONS: Amenorrhea, spasmodic dysmenorrhea with abdominal lumps from uterus Qi stasis; leucorrhea, menorrhagia, uterine and rectal bleeding; diabetes; fevers; infantile appetite loss; pruritic and allergic skin conditions (incl. urticaria, eczema; also topically).
Dosage: Short decoction: 4-10 g
Tincture: 1-3 ml
Caution: Forbidden during pregnancy and in weak people.
NOTES: Aian trumpet creeper root, Ling Xiao Gen (Mand.) or **Ling Siu Gan** (Cant.), is used for rheumatic pain, acute gastroenteritis and traumatic injury. Dose: 10-30 g in decoction.

Cyathula Chuan Niu Xi
Hookweed Root

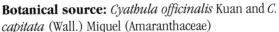

Botanical source: *Cyathula officinalis* Kuan and *C. capitata* (Wall.) Miquel (Amaranthaceae)
Chinese names: Chuan Niu Xi (Mand); Chyun Ngau Sat (Cant)
Category: mild remedy with minimal chronic toxicity
Constituents: ecdysones (nine types: cyasterone, isocyasterone, sengosterone, epicyasterone, amaras-terones A and B, capisterone, precyasterone)
Effective qualities: bitter, sour, neutral; stimulating, relaxing, calming
Tropism: reproductive, musculoskeletal, epidermal systems; Liver, Kidney channels

ACTIONS: *Emmenagogue; contraceptive; hemostatic, diuretic, analgesic*
INDICATIONS: Amenorrhea from uterus Qi stagnation; contraception; hematuria; rheumatism, arthritis, eczema.
Dosage: Decoction: 6-15 g
Tincture: 2-5 ml
Caution: Forbidden in pregnancy and in menorrhagia, spermatorrhea and wet dreams.

Reproductive Relaxants

REMEDIES TO RELAX THE UTERUS AND RELIEVE DYSMENORRHEA

➥ CIRCULATE THE QI IN THE LOWER WARMER AND RELEASE CONSTRAINT

Uterine spasmolytics

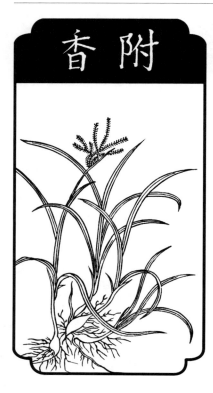

Cyperus Xiang Fu
Purple Nutsedge Root

Botanical source: *Cyperus rotundus* L. (Cyperaceae)
Pharmaceutical name: Rhizoma Cyperi
Chinese names: Xiang Fu, Xian Fu Zi, Suo Cao (Mand); Heung Fu (Cant)
Other names: Nut grass, Coco grass, Chufa, Motha, "Fragrant support"; Kobu (Jap) Musta (San)
Habit: Perennial Eurasian herb from temperate central and coastal China; grows in marshes, on hillsides and roadsides, in fields and by villages; blooms in summer with compound spikes of terminal russet flowers.
Part used: the rhizome

Therapeutic category: mild remedy with minimal chronic toxicity
Constituents: essential oil 0.5% (incl. pinene, camphene, cineole, limonene, cymene, cyperene, selinatriene, patchoulenone, cyperone, rotundol, cyperol, copadiene, epoxyguaine, cyperolone, rotundone, kobusone), alkaloids, cardiac glycosides, flavonoids, glucose, fructose, starch
Effective qualities: pungent, a bit bitter and sweet, a bit warm, dry
    relaxing, stimulating, calming, astringing
Tropism: reproductive, digestive, cardiovascular, nervous systems
    Liver, Stomach, Triple Heater, Chong, Yin Wei channels
    Air, Warmth bodies

ACTIONS AND INDICATIONS

uterine relaxant: spasmolytic: spasmodic menstrual conditions with cramps before and during menses; spasmodic dysmenorrhea
estrogen stimulant: irregular menstruation, breast tenderness, prolonged or light menses, menopausal syndrome, abnormal PAP smears, infertility
nervous relaxant/sedative, spasmolytic, analgesic: PMS, neurocardiac syndrome, spasmodic angina; unrest, irritability; abdominal, epigastric and costal pain; abdominal pain from parasites, hernia, gastroenteritis
cardiovascular relaxant, hypotensive: palpitations, dysrhythmias, anginal pains, hypertension
antipyretic: fever
astringent, anti-inflammatory, antibacterial: diarrhea; dysentery, enteritis; peptic ulcer
antitumoral, interferon inducent: cervical cancer
anthelmintic: intestinal parasites

SYMPTOM PICTURES

uterus Qi constraint: PMS improved with menstrual onset, scanty or prolonged flow, cramps before or during flow

Qi constraint with **nerve excess (Liver Yang rising):** dizziness, ringing in ears, moodiness, unrest, stress, hypochondriac and abdominal pain, distension and lumps

heart Qi constraint: unrest, irregular heartbeat, palpitations, chest pains

Preparation

Use: The root Cyperus Xiang Fu is decocted or used in tincture form.
Dosage: Short decoction: 6-14 g
Tincture: 2-4 ml
Caution: Caution during pregnancy and in constipation. Not to be used in the following conditions: Qi deficiency without signs of stagnation, Yin deficiency and Blood heat.

Notes

The rhizome of the marsh-loving Purple nutsedge is an important *relaxant spasmolytic* remedy with prime use in painful menstrual disorders. Pungent-warm natured, it is a good *Qi circulator* for many types of premenstrual distress and other estrogen-deficient gynecological conditions.

Nutsedge root also releases constrained Qi in the digestive and cardiovascular zones, indicated by the key symptom spasmodic pain. The plant contains essential oil fractions, such as camphene, and alkaloids, that explain its *neurocardiac relaxant* and *analgesic* effects. The cardioactive glycosides contribute to its *relaxant* action on cardiovascular functions.

Many varieties of sedge were also used in Greek medicine for similar purposes, and today the Amazonian Jivaro tribe uses various sedge species for contraceptive, menstrual and child care purposes. The purple nutsedge is found in southern Europe, Arizona and California in ditch banks, cultivated fields, wet turf and ornamental areas.

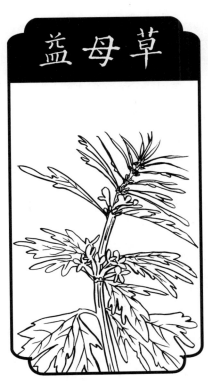

Leonorus Yi Mu Cao
Asian Motherwort Herb

Botanical source: *Leonorus heterophyllus* Sweet or *L. japonicus* Houttuyn or *L. sibiricus* L. or *L. artemisia* (Lour.) S.Y. Hu (Labiatae)
Pharmaceutical name: Herba Leonori
Chinese names: Yi Mu Cao, Chong Wei, I Ming Cao (Mand); Yet Mou Chou, Chong Wai (Cant)
Other names: Siberian motherwort, "Benefit mother weed"; Yakumoso (Jap)
Habit: Hairy annual or biennial Northeast Asian herb; grows in damp soil in sunny waste places, roadsides, hillsides and streamsides; blooms in summer with small pale pink or magenta axillary flowers.
Part used: the herb or herb and root

Therapeutic category: mild remedy with minimal chronic toxicity
Constituents: alkaloids (incl. leonurine, stachydrine, leonuridine), essential oil, potassium chloride, benzoic/lauric/linoleic/oleic acid, phytosterol, flavonoid, bitter glycosides, tannins, stachyose, calcium, trace minerals
Effective qualities: bitter, a bit pungent, cool, dry
relaxing, stimulating, decongesting, restoring, astringing
Tropism: cardiovascular, reproductive, urinary systems
Pericardium, Liver, Chong, Yin Wei, Ren channels; Air, Fluid bodies

Actions and Indications

uterine relaxant: spasmolytic, analgesic: spasmodic dysmenorrhea, PMS; difficult/painful labor, postpartum pain
uterine stimulant, emmenagogue, oxytocic parturient, estrogenic: irregular or late menstruation; prolonged pregnancy, stalled labor (uterine dystocia), uterine subinvolution, retained lochia, miscarriage; infertility
hemostatic: blood in urine or stool, menorrhagia, postpartum uterine bleeding
astringent: conjunctivitis, corneal opacity

Reproductive Relaxants

thyroid inhibitor: thyroid hyperfunctioning
hypotensive cardiac relaxant: neurocardiac syndrome, hypertension, menopausal syndrome
coronary restorative: cardiac/coronary weakness, angina pectoris, coronary disease
nervous sedative/relaxant: insomnia, stress, irritability
renal restorative, draining diuretic: kidney deficiency; generalized edema, oliguria, anuria, strangury, acute or chronic glomerulonephritis, acute renal failure, albuminuria, chronic prostatitis
resolvent detoxicant, dermatropic: eczema, pyogenic abscesses, skin ulcers
antibacterial, antifungal
Miscellaneous: night blindness

Symptom Pictures

uterus Qi constraint with **stagnation:** premenstrual cramping, tension, anxiety, abdominal lumps; delayed, irregular or heavy flow

heart Qi constraint: anxiety, tension, palpitations, stress

heart blood and Qi stagnation: stress, anxiety, chest tightness or pain, labored breathing

kidney fluid congestion: generalized water retention, leg or facial edema, scanty or obstructed urination

Preparation

Use: The herb Leonorus Yi Mu Cao is infused or used in tincture form. When part of a formula, it may be decocted along with other roots, etc., if added only 10 minutes before the end of cooking time.

Dosage: Infusion: 8-40 g
　　　　　Tincture: 2-4 ml
　　　For glomerulonephritis with edema, up to 120 g of the dried herb may be given.

Caution: Being a *uterine stimulant*, this remedy is contraindicated during pregnancy. Use with caution in Yin or Blood (metabolic) deficiency conditions.

Notes

Both the practical uses and chemical constituents of Asian motherwort herb correspond almost exactly to the Western *Leonorus cardiaca*. The two remedies may be interchanged with complete confidence in addressing tense or stressed conditions involving the reproductive and cardiovascular systems. Premenstrual distress is a prime example of such a condition. Another is chronic neurocardiac stress—expressed in the syndrome heart Qi constraint—accompanied by long-term stress, worry and emotional distress. In PMS displaying these symptoms, along with palpitations and sleep loss, (Asian) motherwort is also the right remedy.

Although nowadays also used highly successfully in clinics for conditions such as nephritis, hypertension and coronary disease, Asian motherwort remains as popular in China as in the West for women's menstrual and childbirth conditions due to Qi stagnation and Qi constraint with resultant pain, cramps and abdominal lumps. When this remedy is used postpartum, its *uterine contractant* effect has a slow onset, but is certain.

In traditional meridian energetics, Asian motherwort is one of several typical remedies for spanning the field of indications of both the Chong Mai and its coupled Yin Wei Mai, highlighted by Qi and Blood stasis in both the Lower Warmer (the pelvic area) and the Upper Warmer (the thorassic coronary circulation). However, with its use for urinary and dermal conditions, as well as for infertility, an influence on Ren Mai is also evident.

Asian motherwort seed, Chong Wei Zi (Mand.) or **Chong Wai Ji** (Cant.), has similar properties to the whole herb. It is especially *hypotensive,* and is traditionally used to enhance vision, strengthen the mind, gene-rate sperm and increase virility. Nebula and other superficial visual obstructions are also treated with it. Dose: 4-10 g of the crushed seeds in short decoction.

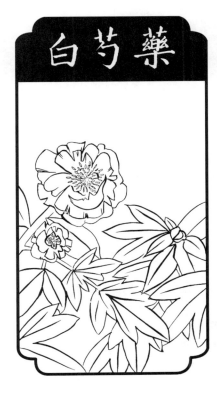

Paeonia Bai Shao Yao
White Peony Root

Botanical source: *Paeonia lactiflora* Pallas (Ranunculaceae)
Pharmaceutical name: Radix Paeoniae lactiflorae
Chinese names: Bai Shao Yao, Bai Shao (Mand); Baak Cheuk Yeuk, Baak Chat (Lai) (Cant)
Other names: Byakushaku (Jap)
Habit: Perennial herb from temperate Northeast China, Siberia, the Russian Far East and Japan; cultivated especially in Zhejiang and Sichuan; prefers warm, moist climates and loose, fairly sandy soil; blooms in summer with large white or magenta solitary flowers.
Part used: the root without its bark

Therapeutic category: mild remedy with minimal chronic toxicity
Constituents: essential oil (incl. monoterpene [paeoniflorin], paeonol), paeonin, triterpenoids, alliflorine, steroids daucosterol and sitosterol, benzoic acid 5%, tannin, glucosides, asparagin, tr. minerals (inc. iron, zinc, magnesium)
Effective qualities: bitter, sour, astringent, cool, dry
relaxing, restoring, astringing, decongesting, calming
Tropism: reproductive, nervous, digestive systems
Liver, Spleen, Lung, Chong, Dai, Yang Wei channels

ACTIONS AND INDICATIONS
uterine relaxant: spasmolytic: spasmodic menstrual conditions with menstrual cramps; spasmodic dysmenorrhea; hypertonic uterine dystocia
analgesic, spasmolytic: spasms or cramping of limbs, of calves; uterine, abdominal and intercostal pain, headache; intestinal colic
nervous sedative: PMS, unrest, dizziness
astringent, mucostatic: diarrhea, dysentery, leucorrhea, spermatorrhea
uterine astringent decongestant: congestive dysmenorrhea with heavy menses (menorrhagia)
antacid antisecretory: acid dyspepsia from hyperchlorhydria, peptic ulcer
anhydrotic: spontaneous sweating, night sweats
antipyretic, diuretic: low-grade fever
immunostimulant, antibacterial, antifungal
interferon inducent

SYMPTOM PICTURES
uterus Qi constraint: menstrual cramps, difficult onset of flow, headache, irritability, unrest

uterus blood congestion: heavy or early menstrual onset, irritability, downward pressure before onset

Qi constraint with **nerve excess (Liver Yang rising):** stress, unrest, headache, dizziness, abdominal or flank pain, cramping pain or spasms of hands or feet

Yin deficiency with **nerve excess:** hot spells, night sweats, unrest, sleeplessness, low-grade fever

PREPARATION
Use: The root Paeonia Bai Shao is either decocted or used as a tincture. The toasted root is more *astringent* and better for heavy menses due to uterus blood congestion and for sweating due to deficiency external wind cold.
Dosage: Decoction: 8-18 g
Tincture: 2-4 ml
Caution: Use cautiously in diarrhea from deficiency cold.

NOTES

Far and away the "popular favorite" garden ornamental of the Tang dynasty, the peony also was and remains a highly esteemed woman's remedy. Prolifically used in many types of Chinese herb formulations, the root of the white peony specifically has a versatile regulating effect in managing difficult and painful menstrution: It can relieve both spasmodic and congestive types of dysmenorrhea. Through its *nerve-relaxing* action White peony root treats uterus Qi constraint conditions, and with its *astringency,* uterus blood congestion.

The *nervous sedative* and *heat-clearing* effect of White peony root further indicates use for Qi constraint and Yin deficiency symptom pictures in general. These syndromes inherently entail nervous hyperactivity, found in types of PMS and menopausal disorders, for instance.

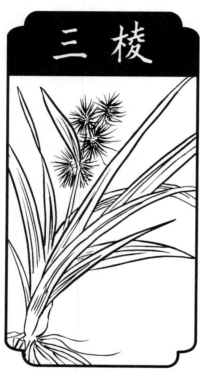

Sparganium San Leng
Bur-Reed Root

Botanical source: *Sparganium simplex* Hudson or *S. stoloniferum* Buchanan-Hamilton or *S. stenophyllum* Maximowicz (Sparganiaceae)
Pharmaceutical name: Rhizoma Sparganii
Chinese names: San Leng, Jin San Leng (Mand); San Ling (Cant); *S. stol*: Hei San Leng (Mand); Hai San Ling, San Leng (Cant)
Other names: "Three edges"; Sanryo (Jap)
Habit: Perennial herb from temperate East Asia, found in damp or marshy areas; in midsummer, terminal capitate flowers appear.
Part used: the rhizome

Therapeutic category: mild remedy with minimal chronic toxicity
Constituents: essential oil (incl. hexadecanoic acid, phenylethanol, benzenediol; benzopyranone in *S. stol.*)
Effective qualities: bitter, pungent, neutral
relaxing, stimulating, softening
Tropism: reproductive, digestive systems
Liver, Spleen, Chong channels; Air body

ACTIONS AND INDICATIONS

uterine relaxant: spasmolytic: spasmodic menstrual conditions with cramps; spasmodic dysmenorrhea
analgesic: postpartum pain, abdominal pain (all types), intestinal colic, IBS, abdominal lumps
uterine stimulant, parturient, abortive: amenorrhea, miscarriage, prolonged pregnancy, retained placenta
digestive stimulant: dyspepsia
anticoagulant: menstrual clots
galactagogue: insufficient breast milk
antitumoral: female reproductive tumors (incl. fibroids, endometriosis)

SYMPTOM PICTURES

uterus Blood congealed: painful, difficult menses with large clots, abdominal lumps, postpartum abdominal pain
uterus Qi constraint: severe menstrual cramps, painful clots
food stagnation with **intestines Qi constraint:** abdominal distension with dull or sharp pains, indigestion

PREPARATION

Use: The root Sparganium San Leng is decocted or used in tincture form.
Dosage: Decoction: 3-10 g; Tincture: 2-4 ml
Caution: Contraindicated during pregnancy; used with care in deficiency conditions and heavy menses.

NOTES

Containing a spicy-bitter essential oil, Bur-reed root has a strong affinity for the female reproductive organs in both *relaxant* and *stimulant* ways. The botanical's *pain-relieving* effect during menstruation results from both a *spasmolytic* and a *blood clot-dispersing* action—and the latter is said to be its specialty. Like White oxknee root (Achyranthes Huai Niu Xi) and others, Bur-reed root will also treat postpartum pain.

Modern research has confirmed *antitumoral* activity in this plant, which predictably has been applied with some success to gynecological tumors more than to any others.

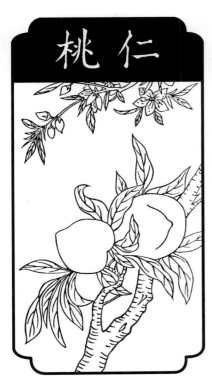

Prunus Tao Ren
Peach Kernel

Botanical source: *Prunus persica* (L.) Batsch or *P. davidiana* (Carr.) Franchet (Rosaceae)
Pharmaceutical name: Semen Pruni persicae
Chinese names: Tao Ren (Mand); Tou Yan (Cant)
Other names: Tonin (Jap)
Habit: Large deciduous shrub or small tree from temperate Eurasia; much cultivated throughout China; pink solitary flowers bloom in spring.
Part used: the seed

Therapeutic category: mild remedy with minimal chronic toxicity
Constituents: amygdalin, emulsin, oleic/glyceric/linoleic acid, protein, esential oil 0.4%
Effective qualities: bitter, sweet, neutral, moist
relaxing, stimulating
Tropism: reproductive, digestive, respiratory, nervous systems
Liver, Large Intestine, Lung, Chong channels
Air, Fluid bodies

ACTIONS AND INDICATIONS

uterine relaxant: spasmolytic: spasmodic menstrual conditions with menstrual cramps; spasmodic dysmenorrhea
analgesic, spasmolytic: pain of uterus, abdomen, intercostals; pain of injury or strains, myalgia, intestinal colic, abdominal lumps/spasms
uterine stimulant, emmenagogue: amenorrhea
bronchial relaxant, antitussive: asthma, cough
demulcent laxative: chronic constipation from dryness
resolvent: intestinal and lung abscess (early stage)

SYMPTOM PICTURES

uterus Qi constraint: difficult, painful menstruation, scanty flow, delayed menses
intestines dryness: small hard stool, constipation

PREPARATION

Use: The kernel Prunus Tao Ren is decocted or used as a tincture.
Dosage: Decoction: 4-10 g
Tincture: 2-4 ml
Caution: Being a *uterine stimulant,* this botanical is forbidden during pregnancy and in profuse menstruation.

REPRODUCTIVE RELAXANTS

NOTES
The peach tree is one of China's shamanistic-magical trees, its fruit a Daoist emblem of long life and immortality, and its crimson blooms the object of many a poet's paean.

The essential medicinal character of the kernel is *relaxant* and *analgesic*. Although also *emmenagogue*, Peach kernel primarily relieves pain and spasms in the chest, abdomen and, especially, the uterus. These conditions are caused by nerve irritation rather than blood clotting. Like most other remedies in the traditional class of "vitalizing Blood," Peach kernel has no literal *anticoagulant* action as such.

Lycopus Ze Lan
Bright Bugleweed Herb *

Botanical source: *Lycopus lucidus* Turczaninow and spp. (Labiatae)
Chinese names: Ze Lan, Di Sun (Mand); Yaak Aan (Cant)
Category: mild remedy with minimal chronic toxicity
Constituents: glycosides, flavonoids, saponins, amino acids, lycopose, raffinose, glucose, stachyose, fructose, essential oil (incl. phenol), organic acids, resin, tannins
Effective qualities: bitter, pungent, a bit warm, dry relaxing, stimulating, decongesting
Tropism: reproductive, urinary, cardiovascular systems; Liver, Bladder, Chong, Ren channels

ACTIONS: *Spasmolytic, analgesic, cardiotonic, draining diuretic, vulnerary, detumescent, antitumoral*
INDICATIONS: Spasmodic dysmenorrhea with uterus Qi constraint; PMS, hypertonic labor contractions, postpartum pain; palpitations, cardiac weakness; postpartum edema, facial edema, dysuria, pain and swelling due to traumatic injury and postpartum; boils, abscesses; gynecological tumors.
Dosage: Decoction: 4-10 g
Tincture: 2-4 ml
Washes, swabs, etc., are used for local traumata.
Caution: Use with care during pregnancy.
NOTES: Mainly a woman's remedy of a regulating nature, Bright bugleweed herb addresses uterine Qi constraint conditions with its *spasmolytic* and *analgesic* actions; it also reduces postpartum pain and water retention.

There is very little in common between the therapeutic applications of the Oriental and the American varieties of Bugleweed; the only places they overlap are in their *cardiac restorative* effect and in being both *relaxing* and *restoring*. Their tropism and symptom pictures differ completely.

Millettia Ji Xue Teng
Millettia Root and Stem

Botanical source: *Millettia dielsiana* Harms, *M. reticulata* Bentham or *M. nitida* Bentham, and *Mucuna birdwoodiana* Tutcher and *Spatholobus suberectus* Dunn (Leguminosae)
Chinese names: Ji Xue Teng, Shan Ji Xue Teng (Mand); Gei Hat Tang, Gei Hat Ting (Cant)
Category: mild herb with minimal chronic toxicity
Constituents: milletol
Effective qualities: bitter, sweet, warm, dry, relaxing, stimulating, restoring, astringing, calming
Tropism: reproductive, muskuloskeletal, nervous, vascular systems; Heart, Spleen, Chong channels

ACTIONS: *Spasmolgtic, emmenagogue, nervous sedative, analgesic, anti-inflammatory, reproductive sedative, leucocyte stimulant*

INDICATIONS: Uterus Qi constraint with spasmodic dysmenorrhea, delayed or absent menses; wind damp obstruction with weak or numb extremities, paralysis, muscular atrophy; menstrual cramps, lumbago, arthralgia, myalgia, neuralgia, unrest; acute rheumatoid arthritis; spermatorrhea, metrorrhagia; leukopenia from radiation treatment.

Dosage: Decoction: 10-20 g
Tincture: 2-4 ml

Caution: Use with care during pregnancy because of its *uterine stimulant* action.

Manis Chuan Shan Jia
Pangolin Scale

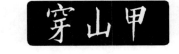

Zoological source: *Manis pentadactyla* (Manidae)
Chinese names: Chuan Shan Jia, Shan Jia Pian/Zhu (Mand); Chan San Gap (Cant)
Other names: Scaly anteater, "Penetrate mountain scale"; Senzanko (Jap)
Category: mild remedy with minimal chronic toxicity

Constituents: stearic acid, cholesterol, two aliphatic amides, butyltricosylamide, 2 diestereomers (cyclotyrosyls), 16 amino acids, 18 trace elements (incl. germanium)
Effective qualities: salty, cool; relaxing, stimulating
Tropism: urogenital, musculoskeletal, vascular systems; Liver, Stomach, Chong, Yin Qiao, Yang Qiao chan.

ACTIONS: *Spasmolytic, emmenagogue, antiarthritic, analgesic, galactagogue, leukocytogenic immunostimulant, diuretic, vulnerary, detoxicant, detumescent, hemostatic* (externally only)

INDICATIONS: Spasmodic and deficient menstrual conditions from stagnant uterus Qi with dysmenorrhea, amenorrhea; arthritic pain, stiffness and spasms of extremities, pain preventing movement, traumatic pain; insufficient lactation, leukopenia; traumatic injuries; urinary tract infections; boils, abscesses, scrofula, fistula, hemorrhage, blood in urine, bloody dysentery.

Dosage: Decoction: 3-10 g
Tincture: 2-4 ml
Powder: 1-1.5 g

This remedy is also applied topically for pyogenic and other skin conditions, breast abscess and earache (mixed with water.

Caution: Not to be used with draining abscesses, and only with caution when ulcerated sores and deficiency conditions are present. Forbidden during pregnancy.

NOTES: Pangolin scale is quite commonly seen in formulas treating various painful conditions such as dysmenorrhea and arthritis with restricted movement.

Recent experiments show that this remedy also acts to increase white blood cells.

Trogopterus Wu Ling Zhi
Flying Squirrel Dropping

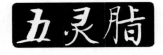

Zoological source: *Trogopterus xanthipes* Milne-Edwards and *Pteromys volans* and spp (Sciuridae)
Chinese names: Wu Ling Zhi (Mand); Ng Ling Ji (Cant)
Category: mild remedy with minimal chronic toxicity
Constituents: uric acid, urea, pyrocatechol, hydroxybenzoic acid, dicarboxylic acid, uracil, wulingzhic acid, protocatechuic acid, hypoxanthine, allantoin, tyrosine, resin, vitamin A
Effective qualities: bitter, sweet, warm, dry; calming, relaxing, astringing, decongesting
Tropism: nervous, reproductive, cardiovascular, digestive systems; Liver, Spleen, Chong, Yin Qiao channels

ACTIONS: *Spasmolytic, analgesic, emmenagogue, anticonvulsant, hemostatic, coronary restorative, antivenomous*

INDICATIONS: Spasmodic and deficient menstrual conditions with pain; uterus Qi stagnation; spasmodic dysmenorrhea, amenorrhea, lochial retention (lochioschesis); menstrual, postpartum, (epi)gastric, muscular, joint, chest pain; seizures; uterine bleeding (metrorrhagia), bloody sputum; coronary deficiency/disease; scorpion, centipede and snake bites; chronic childhood nutritional impairment with abdominal bloating; conjunctivitis; swollen/compound fractures

Dosage: Decoction: 3-10 g
Tincture: 2-4 ml

This remedy should be first wrapped in cheesecloth before adding to a decoction. When toasted, its *hemostatic* property is increased, treating menorrhagia and chronic infectious leucorrhea.

Caution: Use cautiously during pregnancy, and do not combine with Asian ginseng root.

NOTES: Flying squirrel dropping from North China is a secondary remedy frequently included in formulas for relief of pain from smooth muscle spasm, especially in menstrual and postpartum conditions.

Litsea Dou Chi Jiang
Cubeb Root and Stem

Botanical source: *Litsea cubeba* (Lour.) Persoon (Lauraceae)
Chinese names: Dou Chi Jiang (Mand); Dau Chek Geung (Cant)
Category: mild remedy with minimal chronic toxicity
Constituents: essential oil (incl. citral, laurotetanine, isocorydine, magnocurarine)
Effective qualities: pungent, bitter, warm, dry; relaxing, stimulating, calming
Tropism: reproductive, musculoskeletal, digestive, nervous, circulatory systems; Lung, Liver channels

ACTIONS: *Spasmolytic, analgesic, circulatory stimulant*
INDICATIONS: Spasmodic dysmenorrhea with lower abdominal cramps (uterus Qi constraint syndrome); lumbar pain, rheumatic and arthritic pain (wind/damp/cold obstruction syndrome), headache, epigastric and abdominal pain, tissue trauma pain; influenza or common cold with chills, muscle aches and headache.

Dosage: Decoction: 15-30 g
Tincture: 2-5 ml

Caution: None.

Rosa Mei Gui Hua
Japanese Rose Flower

Botanical source: *Rosa rugosa* Thunberg (Rosaceae)
Chinese names: Mei Gui Hua (Mand); Mak Gwai Fa, Mak Gwei Fa (Cant)
Category: mild remedy with minimal chronic toxicity
Constituents: essential oil (incl. linalool, geraniol, aldehydes, citral), paeonidin, paeonin
Effective qualities: sweet, a bit bitter, dry, warm; relaxing, stimulating
Tropism: reproductive, nervous, digestive systems; Liver, Spleen, Chong channels

ACTIONS: *Spasmolytic, progesteronic, carminative, hemostatic, hepatic, choleretic*
INDICATIONS: Spasmodic dysmenorrhea from stagnant uterus Qi with cramps, irregular menses; abnormal PAP smears; epigastric pain, acute dyspepsia with distension; coughing up blood; hepatitis.

Dosage: Decoction: 2-6 g
Tincture: 1-3 ml

Caution: None.

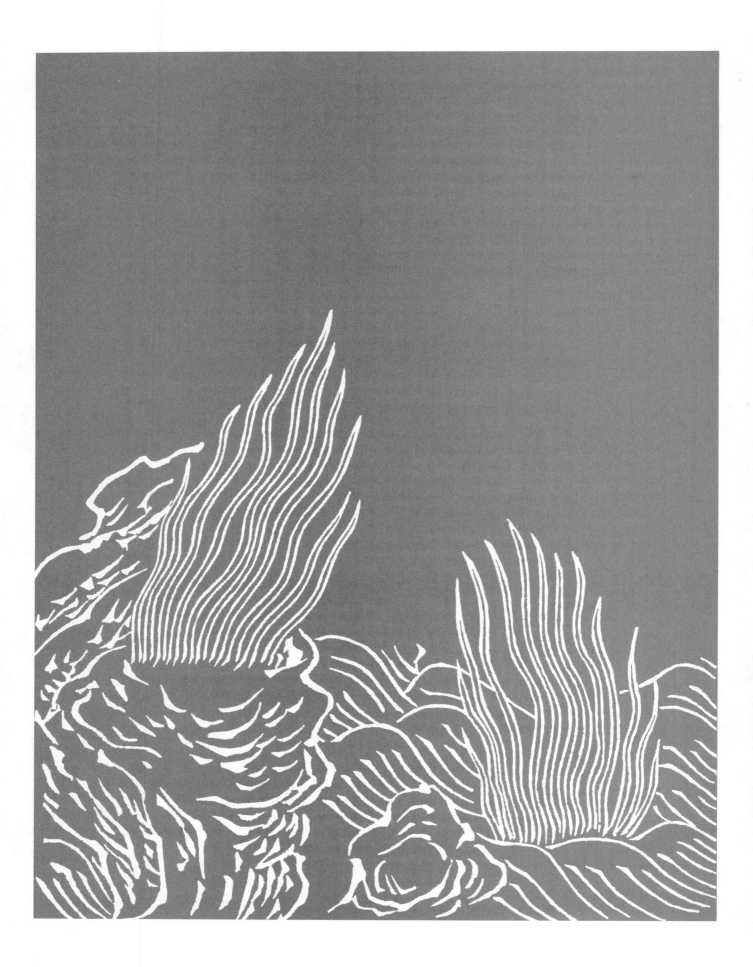

Index to Vol. 1

Abutilon Qing Ma, 368
Acanthus Lao Shu Le, 346
Achyranthes Huai Niu Xi, 420
Aconitum Fu Zi, 221
Actinolitum Yang Qi Shi, 408
Adenophora Nan Sha Shen, 148
Adenophora Ji Ni, 149
Agastache Huo Xiang, 292
Agrimonia Xian He Cao, 211
Ailanthus Chun Pi, 315
Akebia Bai Mu Tong, 390
Albizzia He Huan Pi, 247
Alisma Ze Xie, 371
Allium Cong Bai, 122
Allium Jiu Cai Zi, 363
Allium Xie Bai, 309
Alpinia Cao Dou Kou, 285
Alpinia Gao Liang Jiang 283
Alpinia Yi Zhi Ren, 362
Amomum Bai Dou Kou, 289
Amomum Cao Guo, 309
Amomum Sha Ren, 302
analgesics, 121, 152, 270, 272, 280, 282, 355, 366, 383, 384, 385, 390, 400, 402, 404, 409, 411, 413, 417, 419, 421-434
anastative nutritives, 258-265
Anemarrhena Zhi Mu, 143
Angelica Bai Zhi, 121
Angelica Dang Gui, 417
antacid antisecretories: 155, 167, 174, 187, 233, 258, 273, 310, 370, 413, 429
anthelmintics (see *antiparasitics*)
antiallergics, 118, 119, 152, 157, 159, 163, 165, 289, 343, 409, 418, 419
antiasthmatics (see *bronchodilators*)
anticatarrhals, 118-123, 165
anticonvulsants, 178, 184, 233-237, 241, 242, 244, 245, 335
antidiarrheals, 270-278, 356-358, 366, 370, 411, 412, 426, 429
antienuretics, 174, 355-365, 403, 404, 405

anti-infectives, 118, 119, 121, 128, 129, 130, 152, 164, 165, 167, 171, 175, 177, 186, 203, 220, 227, 228, 270, 280, 282, 294, 311-315, 335, 336, 341, 390, 400,
anti-inflammatories, 124-134, 144, 145, 149, 152, 167, 171, 177, 180, 181, 186, 205, 206, 211, 212, 223, 225, 226, 229, 238, 242, 269, 335, 340, 341, 343, 355, 383, 387, 390, 419, 432
antilithics, 174, 184, 198, 297, 345-347, 386-390, 411, 420, 422
antioxidants, 196, 201, 206, 358, 359, 361
antiparasitics (incl. *anthelmintics*), 164, 211, 217, 282, 285, 286, 288, 290, 306, 309, 313, 314, 336, 340, 375, 380, 382, 384, 386, 409
antipyretics, 144, 167, 178, 184, 238, 240, 266, 276, 283, 286, 336, 337, 340, 341, 344, 383, 390, 391, 416, 419, 425, 429
antitumorals, 145, 150, 157, 162, 163, 167, 169, 171, 173, 180, 181, 182, 183, 201, 215, 216, 261, 305, 339, 342, 366, 374, 376, 378, 384, 412, 417, 423, 424, 430, 432
aphrodisiacs, 363, 400-408
Apocynum Luo Bu Ma, 231
Aquilaria Chen Xiang, 307
Arca Wa Leng Zi, 310
Arctium Niu Bang Zi, 126
Ardisia Zi Jin Niu, 160
Areca Da Fu Pi, 290
Aristolochia Guan Mu Tong, 383
Aristolochia Ma Dou Ling, 171
Aristolochia Qing Mu Xiang, 308
Artemisia Ai Ye, 409
Artemisia Qing Hao, 337
Artemisia Yin Chen Hao, 336
arterial stimulants, 156, 218-224, 434
Asarum Xi Xin, 152
Asparagus Tian Men Dong, 142
Aster Zi Wan, 162
Astragalus Sha Yuan Zi, 363
astringents, 208-217, 270-278, 340, 342, 356-364, 385, 386, 411, 421, 429
Atractylodes Bai Zhu, 261

Atractylodes Cang Zhu, 294
Angelica Dang Gui, 417

Benefit the fluids and drain damp, remedies to, 370
Benefit the Spleen and tonify the Qi, remedies to, 258
Benincasa Dong Gua Ren, 184
Biota Bai Zi Ren, 246
Biota Ce Bai Ye, 415
Bladder damp heat, 144, 177, 186, 345, 346, 366, 368, 369, 372, 373, 383-391
Bladder Qi constraint, 366, 383, 385, 388
Bletilla Bai Ji, 213
Blood deficiency, 172, 259, 324-329, 418
bronchial demulcents, 141-151, 206, 240, 326, 328, 368
bronchodilators, 161-173, 196, 220, 223, 225, 226, 237, 272, 301, 311, 331, 332, 361, 366, 375, 381, 409, 416, 431
Borax Peng Sha, 132
Buddleia Mi Meng Hua, 132
Bufo Chan Su, 222

Caesalpinia Su Mu, 424
Calcitum Han Shui Shi, 236
Callicarpa Zi Zhu, 215
Callorhinus Hai Gou Shen, 408
Campanumoea Tu Dang Shen, 264
Campsis Ling Xiao Hua, 425
Campsis Ling Xiao Gen, 425
Canna Mei Ren Jiao, 344
Cannabis Huo Ma Ren, 267
Caragana Jin Ji Er, 171
cardiovascular relaxants, 225
cardiovascular restoratives, 196
cardiovascular sedatives, 232
cardiovascular stimulants, 218
Carthamus Hong Hua, 202
Cassia Jue Ming Zi, 229
Catharanthus Chang Chun Hua, 231
Celosia Qing Xiang Zi, 132
Celosia Ji Guan Hua, 217
Centipeda E Bu Shi Cao, 123
Cephalanoplos Xiao Ji, 215
Cervus Lu Jiao, 406
Cervus Lu Jiao Jiao, 406
Cervus Lu Jiao Shuang, 407
Changium Ming Dang Shen, 265
Chimonanthus La Mei Hua, 129
cholagogue laxatives, 167, 330-340, 411
Chrysanthemum Ju Hua, 128
Chrysanthemum Ye Ju Hua, 227
Cimicifuga Sheng Ma, 242
Cinnabarum Zhu Sha, 237
Cinnamomum Rou Gui, 218
Cinnamomum Zhang Nao, 219

Circulate the Qi and vitalize the Blood in the Lower Warmer, remedies to, 417
Circulate the Qi in the Lower Warmer and release constraint, remedies to, 426
Circulate the Qi in the middle and release constraint, remedies to, 301
Circulate heart Qi and release constraint, remedies to, 225
Circulate and lower lung Qi, remedies to, 161
Cirsium Da Ji, 212
Cistanche Rou Cong Rong, 403
Citrus Chen Pi, 330
Citrus Ju Hong, 331
Citrus Qing Pi, 331
Citrus Fo Shou, 308
Citrus Zhi Ke, 338
Citrus Zhi Shi, 333
Clear damp heat from the bladder, remedies to, 383
Clear damp heat from the large intestine, remedies to, 311
Clear damp heat from the liver and gallbladder, remedies to, 340
Clear deficiency heat, remedies to, 141
Clemastra Shan Ci Gu, 173
Clematis Chuan Mu Tong, 384
Clerodendrum Chou Wu Tong, 225
Codonopsis Dang Shen, 258
Codonopsis Yang Ju, 264
Coix Yi Yi Ren, 366
cold and flu remedies, 118-134, 152, 152, 154, 156, 165
Cool and transform phlegm heat, remedies to, 177
Cordyceps Dong Chong Xia Cao, 175
Cornus Shan Zhu Yu, 359
coronary restoratives, 196-207, 335, 361, 400, 417, 428
Crataegus Shan Zha, 198
Croton Ba Dou, 377
Curculigo Xian Mao, 402
Cucumis Tian Gua Di, 339
Curcuma E Zhu, 305
Curcuma Jiang Huang, 338
Curcuma Yu Jin, 334
Cuscuta Tu Si Zi, 358
Cyathula Chuan Niu Xi, 425
Cyclina Hai Ge Ke, 187
Cynanchum Bai Qian, 159, 214
Cynomorium Suo Yang, 405
Cyperus Xiang Fu, 426

Daphne Yuan Hua, 379
Daphne Zu Shi Ma, 205
demulcents (see *bronchial/gastric/intestinal/urinary demulcents*)
Dendrobium Shi Hu, 266

Desmodium Guang Dong Jin Qian Cao, 346
detoxicants, 169, 355, 375, 378, 380, 384, 386
Dianthus Qu Mai, 384
diaphoretics, 124-134, 152, 154, 156, 165, 219, 242, 293, 294, 337
digestive stimulants, 120, 156, 279-301, 330-339
Dichondra Ma Di Jin, 347
Dioscorea Bi Xie, 355
Dioscorea Huang Yao Zi, 216
Dioscorea Shan Yao, 262
Dioscorea Shu Liang, 214
Diospyros Shi Di, 288
diuretics, 165, 168, 170, 177, 181, 182, 184, 186, 261, 268, 290, 291, 294, 311, 345, 346, 347, 355, 366-391, 420, 428
Dolichos Bai Bian Dou, 276
Drain downward, remedies to, 299

eczema remedies, 169, 174, 258, 261, 280, 314, 334, 341, 343, 355, 362, 375, 379, 380, 384, 385, 386, 428
Elsholtzia Xiang Ru, 276
emmenagogues, 145, 150, 152, 154, 158, 181, 280, 282, 304, 376, 377, 384, 390, 411-413, 417-417, 432
Enrich Liver Yin, remedies to, 324
Ephedra Ma Huang, 165
Ephedra Ma Huang Gen, 364
Epimedium Yin Yang Huo, 400
Equisetum Mu Zei, 133
Equus E Jiao, 327
Eriobotrya Pi Pa Ye, 179
Eriocaulon Gu Jing Cao, 133
Eugenia Ding Xiang, 282
Eupatorium Pei Lan, 337
Euphorbia Gan Sui, 380
Euphorbia Jing Da Ji, 375
Euphorbia Qian Jin Zi, 376
Euryale Qian Shi, 356
Evodia San Ya Ku, 134
Evodia Wu Zhu Yu, 280
expectorants, 141-173, 179-187, 244, 245, 289, 291, 301, 330, 331, 378, 379, 381, 389, 400, 416
Expel fluids downward, remedies to, 377
eye and vision remedies, 132, 133, 227-9, 234-236, 311, 361, 384, 387

Ferula A Wei, 286
Ficus Bi Li, 422
Fluoritum Zi Shi Ying, 237
Foeniculum Xiao Hui Xiang, 287
Fluid congestion (general), 169, 194, 261, 268, 290, 336, 366, 370-376, 378, 380, 381, 428
Food stagnation, 286, 290, 296-298, 309, 430
Fraxinus Chin Pi, 311
Fritillaria Chuan Bei Mu, 149
Fritillaria Zhe Bei Mu, 180

Galla Wu Bei Zi, 313
Gallus Ji Nei Jin, 297
Gallbladder and stomach Qi stagnation, 279, 330-338, 375, 411
Gardenia Zhi Zi, 340
gastric demulcents, 142, 143, 204, 239, 258, 266, 329
gastrointestinal relaxants, 301
gastrointestinal restoratives, 258
gastrointestinal sedatives, 311
gastrointestinal stimulants, 279
Gecko Ge Jie, 176
Genitourinary cold, 400-408
Genitourinary damp cold, 263, 271-274, 283, 355-365
Genitourinary damp heat, 343
Genitourinary Qi deficiency, 360, 361, 363, 364
Gentiana Long Dan Cao, 343
Ginkgo Yin Xing Ye, 196
Gleditsia Zao Jiao, 158
Glehnia Bei Sha Shen, 147
Glycine Dan Dou Chi, 249
Gossampinus Mu Mian Hua, 315
Gossypium Mian Hua Gen, 412
Gossypium Mian Zi, 413

Haematitum Dai Zhi Shi, 172
Halloysitum Chi Shi Zhi, 277
Harmonize the Liver and Spleen, remedies to, 330
Head damp cold, 118-123
Heart and Kidney Yang deficiency, 218-224
Heart blood and Qi stagnation, 128, 197-209, 208, 226, 335, 401, 418, 428
Heart Qi constraint, 146, 225-231, 401, 418, 426, 428
Heart Yin deficiency, 225, 238-248, 274
Hemerocallis Xuan Cao Gen, 347
hemostatics, 151, 162, 208-217, 312, 324, 335, 340, 342, 361, 372, 385, 386, 389, 409-416, 419, 421, 423, 425
Hemsleya Xue Dan, 313
hepatic nutritives, 324-329
hepatobiliary relaxants/sedatives, 340
hepatobiliary restoratives, 324
hepatobiliary stimulants, 330
Heleocharis Bi Qi, 150
Hippocampus Hai Ma, 407
Homo Xue Yu Tan, 217
Hordeum Yi Tang, 265
Hordeum Mai Ya, 296
Houttuynia Yu Xing Cao, 177
hypotensives, 128, 198, 199, 203, 204, 206, 225-233, 241, 244, 340, 358, 426

Ilex Gang Mei, 129
Ilex Jiu Bi Ying, 130
Ilex Mao Dong Qing, 226

Ilex Si Ji Ching, 207
Impatiens Ji Xing Hua, 423
Impatiens Ji Xing Zi, 422
Imperata Bai Mao Gen, 372
infertility remedies, 400-404, 426, 426
intestinal demulcents, 266-269
Intestines damp cold, 270-278, 342, 356, 357, 366, 370, 372, 409
Intestines damp heat, 144, 168, 311-315, 342, 388, 415, 416
Intestines mucous damp, 157, 261, 281-295, 301, 303
Intestines Qi constraint, 301-310, 332, 333, 334, 409, 430
Inula Xuan Fu Hua, 170
Iphigenia Shan Ci Gu, 173

Juncus Deng Xin Cao, 369
Juncus Deng Xin Hua, 369
Juglans Hu Tao Ren, 174

Kidney dryness, 366-369, 388
Kidney Qi deficiency, 360, 361, 363, 364
Kidney Yang deficiency, 174-176, 358, 400-408
Kidney Yin deficiency, 143, 144, 151, 274, 325, 358
Knoxia Hong Da Ji, 376

Laminaria Hai Zao, 170
Lasiosphaera Ma Bo, 131
laxatives, 299, 300, 342
Lemna Fu Ping, 134
Leonorus Chong Wei Zi, 428
Leonorus Yi Mu Cao, 427
Lepidium Ting Li Zi, 381
Ligusticum Chuan Xiong, 199
Lilium Bai He, 146
Limonitum Yu Liang Shi, 278
Lindera Wu Yao, 303
Litchi Li Zhe He, 310
Litsea Dou Chi Jiang, 286
Liver and gallbladder damp heat, 279, 335, 336, 340-347
Liver and Kidney depletion, 360, 404, 405, 406, 421
liver decongestants, 330-347
liver restoratives, 258-261, 324-329, 339
Liver Qi stagnation, 330-347, 411
Liver Yang rising, 204, 225-236, 240-247, 421, 426, 429
Liver Yin and blood deficiency, 259-261, 324-329
Lobelia Ban Bian Lian, 374
Lopatherum Dan Zhu Ye, 391
Lung and Kidney Yang deficiency, 174-176, 235
Lung fluid congestion, 375, 376, 377, 378-382
Lung heat (dryness), 144, 145, 146, 151, 168, 169, 182
Lung phlegm cold, 152-160, 220, 244, 281, 378, 380, 381, 401, 412
Lung phlegm damp, 157, 158, 161, 166, 170, 291, 301, 330, 333, 334, 378, 380, 381
Lung phlegm heat, 177-187, 388, 389, 416
Lung Qi constraint, 159, 161-173, 197, 301, 308, 309, 311, 333, 416
Lung Yin deficiency/dryness, 141-151, 176, 260, 328
Lycium Di Gu Pi, 151
Lycium Gou Qi Zi, 326
Lycopus Ze Lan, 432
Lygodium Hai Jin Sha, 390
Lygodium Hai Jin Sha Teng, 389
Lysimachia Jin Qian Cao, 345

Magnetitum Ci Shi, 234
Magnolia Xin Yi Hua, 118
Magnolia Hou Po, 301
Malva verticilata, 367
Manis Chuan Shan Jia, 433
Massa Shen Qu, 298
Melia Chuan Lian Zi, 306
Mentha Bo He, 125
Meretrix Wen Ge, 187
Millettia Ji Xue Teng, 432
Mirabilitum Mang Xiao, 269
Moisten the intestines and unblock the bowels, remedies to, 266
Momordica Luo Han Guo, 185
Morinda Ba Ji Tian, 404
Morus Sang Ye, 127
Morus Sang Bai Pi, 168
mucogenics, 141-150, 204, 206, 238, 239, 258, 256, 343, 403
Musculoskeletal deficiency, 360, 404, 405, 406, 421
Myristica Rou Dou Kou, 270

Nardostachys Gan Song, 245
nasal decongestants, 118-123, 152, 167, 219
Nelumbo He Ye, 277
Nelumbo Lian Fang, 216
Nelumbo Lian Geng, 277
Nelumbo Lian Xu, 364
Nelumbo Lian Zi Xin, 248
Nelumbo Lian Zi, 274
Nelumbo Ou Jie, 21
Nerve and brain deficiency, 197, 220, 244, 260, 289, 326, 363, 401, 404
nervous restoratives, 197, 220, 244, 260, 289, 326, 363, 401, 404
neurocardiac restoratives, 196, 219, 259
neurocardiac sedatives, 146, 232-249, 369, 428
neuromuscular stimulants/restoratives, 400, 404, 405, 406
nose, throat and eye relaxants/sedatives, 124
nose, throat and eye restoratives/stimulants,

118
Nourish the Blood, remedies to, 324
Nourish the Heart and calm the Spirit, remedies to, 238
Nourish the Yin and moisten dryness, remedies to, 141,
Nourish the Yin and Blood, remedies to, 324

Ophiopogon Mai Men Dong, 141
Oryza Jing Mi, 264
Oryza Gu Ya, 298
Oryza Nuo Dao Gen, 365
Oroxylum Mu Hu Die, 131
Ostrea Mu Li, 233

Paeonia Bai Shao Yao, 429
Paeonia Chi Shao Yao, 413
Paeonia Mu Dan Pi, 419
Panax Xi Yang Shen, 259
Papaver Ying Su Ke, 272
Paratenodera Sang Piao Xiao, 364
Perilla Zi Su Ye, 119
Perilla Zi Su Zi, 161
Peucedanum Qian Hu, 153
Pharbitis Qian Niu Zi, 382
Phaseolum Chi Xiao Dou, 376
Phragmites Lu Gen, 184
Phyllostachys Zhu Ru, 178
Phyllostachys Zhu Li, 185
Phyllostachys Zhu Ye, 179
Phyllostachys Zi Zhu Gen, 185
Phytolacca Shang Lu, 378
Pinellia Ban Xia, 156
Pinus Hu Po, 237
Piper Bi Ba, 286
Plantago Che Qian Cao, 186
Plantago Che Qian Zi, 387
Platycodon Jie Geng, 154
Pleione Shan Ci Gu, 173
Pogostemon Guang Huo Xiang, 293
Polygala Yuan Zhi, 243
Polygonatum Yu Zhu, 239
Polygonatum Huang Jing, 206
Polygonum Bian Xu, 386
Polygonum Ye Jiao Teng, 248
Polyporus Zhu Ling, 373
Poria Chi Fu Ling, 371
Poria Fu Ling, 370
Poria Fu Ling Pi, 371
Poria Fu Shen, 371
Portulacca Ma Chi Xiang, 314
Prunella Xia Ku Cao, 228
Prunus Tao Ren, 431
Prunus Wu Mei, 275
Prunus Xing Ren, 163

Prunus Yu Li Ren, 268
Pseudostellaria Tai Zi Shen, 263
Psoralea Bu Gu Zhi, 361
Pteria Zhen Zhu Mu, 235
Pteria Zhen Zhu, 236
Pteris Feng Wei Cao, 314
Pueraria Ge Gen, 204
Pulsatilla Bai Tou Weng, 312
Pumus Fu Hai Shi, 186
Punica Shi Liu Pi, 277
Pyrrosia Shi Wei, 388

Qi constraint, 200, 201, 301, 419, 426, 429
Qi deficiency, 258-265

Raphanus Lai Fu Zi, 291
Rauvolfia Luo Fu Mu, 230
Reduce food stagnation, remedies to, 296
Rehmannia Sheng Di Huang, 209
Rehmannia Shu Di Huang, 324
Release the exterior and dispel wind cold, remedies to, 118
Release the exterior and dispel wind heat, remedies to, 124
reproductive relaxants, 426
reproductive restoratives, 400
reproductive stimulants, 417
Rescue devastated Yang, remedies to, 218
respiratory relaxants, 161
respiratory restoratives, 141
respiratory sedatives, 177
respiratory stimulants, 152
Restrain leakage from the intestines, remedies to, 270
Rheum Da Huang, 341
Ricinus Bi Ma Zi, 300
Rosa Jin Ying Zi, 357
Rosa Mei Gui Hua, 434
Rosa Yue Ji Hua, 424
Rubia Qian Cao Gen, 410
Rubus Dao Sheng Gen, 363
Rubus Fu Pen Zi, 360

Salsola Zhu Mao Cai, 231
Salvia Dan Shen, 201
Salvia Shi Jian Chuan, 202
Sanguisorba Di Yu, 210
Sargassum Hai Zao, 169
Santalum Tan Xiang, 307
Saussurea Xue Lian, 423
Saussurea Yun Mu Xiang, 332
Schizonepeta Jing Jie, 124
Sedum Chui Pen Cao, 347
Senna Fan Xie Ye, 299
Sepia Hai Piao Xiao, 273

Scrophularia Xuan Shen, 238
Serratula Guang Dong Sheng Ma, 243
Settle and calm the Spirit, remedies to, 232
Skin damp heat, 355, 375, 380, 385
Sonchus Ku Cai, 215
Sophora Huai Hua, 414
Sophora Huai Hua Mi, 415
Sophora Shan Dou Gen, 167
sore throat remedies, 124-134, 167
Sparganium San Leng, 430
spasmolytics, 121, 152, 200, 201, 203, 218, 270, 280, 281, 301-312, 331, 332, 362, 387, 409, 426-434
Spirit Instability, 232-237
Spirodela Fu Ping, 134
Spleen damp, 157, 170, 261, 289-295, 301, 303
Spleen Qi deficiency, 258-265, 270-278, 370, 372
Spread Liver Qi, remedies to, 330
Stabilize the Kidney and retain urine and essence, remedies to, 355
Stalactitum E Guan Shi, 172
Stegodon Long Gu, 232
Stellaria Yin Chai Hu, 214
Stemona Bai Bu, 164
Sterculia Pang Da Hai, 130
Stichopus Hai Shen, 407
Stomach and intestines cold, 270, 280-289, 303, 307, 309, 377
Stomach and intestines dryness, 142, 143, 163, 266-269, 329, 368, 431
Stomach and intestines Qi stagnation, 289-291, 296, 297
Stomach and small intestine Qi deficiency, 258-265
Stop bleeding, remedies to, 208
Subdue Liver Yang, remedies to, 225
Summer heat, 276, 386
Swertia Dang Yao, 279

Talcum Hua Shi, 385
Tamarix Xi He Liu, 134
Tagetes Wan Shou Ju, 130
Terminalia He Zi, 271
Thevetia Huang Hua Jia Zhu Tao, 224
Thuja Bai Zi Ren, 246
Tremella Bai Mu Er, 151
Tetrapanax Tong Cao, 368
Tonify Lung and Kidney Yang, remedies to, 174
Tonify the Kidney and fortify the Yang, remedies to, 400
Tonify the Qi, remedies to, 258
Tonify the Yang and dispel cold, remedies to, 218
Transform accumulation, remedies to, 296, 330
Transform Spleen damp, remedies to, 289
Tricosanthes Gua Lou, 183
Tricosanthes Gua Lou Pi, 183
Tricosanthes Gua Lou Ren, 182

Tricosanthes Tian Hua Fen, 145
Trigonella Hu Lu Ba, 287
Triticum Fu Xiao Mai, 249
Trogopterus Wu Ling Zhi, 433
Tulipa Shan Ci Gu, 173
Tussilago Kuan Dong Hua, 166
Typha Pu Huang, 208
Typhonium Du Jiao Lan, 157

urinary demulcents, 366-369
urinary restoratives, 355
urinary sedatives, 383
urinary stimulants, 370
uterine stimulants (see *emmenagogues*)
Uterus blood congealed, 305, 335, 414, 419, 430
Uterus blood congestion, 315, 409-416, 429
Uterus cold, 280, 281, 304, 401, 403, 404, 409
Uterus Qi constraint, 305, 335, 414, 418, 423, 424, 426-434
Uterus Qi stagnation, 411, 417-425

Venous blood stagnation, 415, 416
Vaccaria Wang Bu Liu Xing, 421
Vitalize the Blood and disperse Blood stasis in the heart, remedies to, 196
Vitalize the Blood and disperse Blood stasis in the Lower Warmer, remedies to, 409
Vitex Huang Jing, 156
Vitex Mu Jing Zi, 155
vulneraries, 167, 201, 203, 205, 212, 213, 212, 228, 232, 237, 247, 305, 313, 335, 338, 344, 361, 406, 411, 419, 421, 422, 432, 433

Warm and transform phlegm cold, remedies to, 152
Warm the interior and dispel cold, remedies to, 218
Warm the middle and dispel cold, remedies to, 280
Wind cold (external), 118-124, 152, 154, 155, 156, 165, 220, 293, 294
Wind/damp/cold obstruction, 119, 152, 294, 311, 315, 354, 366, 401, 402, 404, 433, 434
Wind heat (external), 124-134, 154, 155, 227, 336, 344

Xanthium Cang Er Zi, 119

Yin deficiency, 141-147, 266, 267, 429
Yang deficiency (see Heart Yang deficiency, Kidney Yang deficiency, Lung and Kidney Yang deficiency)

Zanthoxylum Chuan Jiao, 284
Zingiber Sheng Jiang, 160
Zingiber Gan Jiang, 281
Zizyphus Da Zao, 328
Zizyphus Hong Zao, 329
Zizyphus Suan Zao Ren, 241

STILL AWESOME

The Trials and Tribulations of an Egotistical Maniac

JASON ELLIS
WITH **MIKE TULLY**

PUBLISHED BY GREY BOOKS

Some names and characteristics of individuals have been changed to protect their privacy. Any resulting resemblance to persons living or dead is entirely coincidental and unintentional.

Book Design: Tim Harrington

Race Photo: Major Impact Photography

Fight Photo: Dave Mandel

Cover Photo / Back Cover Photo: © Mike Blabac

All rights reserved. No parts of this book may be reproduced in any manner without the express written consent of the publisher.

Copyright ©2019 Jason Ellis and Mike Tully

Print ISBN: 978-0-9982180-1-4

PRINTED IN THE UNITED STATES OF AMERICA

November 2019

First Edition

LEGAL SHIT:

This is the part where I cover my ass.

First off, I am not a doctor. I am a retired professional skateboarder who talks on the radio for a living. Any advice in this book is my opinion and might well be completely wrong.

In other words: "This book is written as a source of information only. The information contained in this book is based solely on my personal experience and observations of others and should by no means be considered a substitute for the advice, decision or judgment of the reader's physician or other professional adviser. My publisher and I expressly disclaim responsibility for any adverse effects arising from the use or application of the information contained herein."

Furthermore, legally I have to tell you that "I have changed the names of some individuals and the identifying features, including physical descriptions and occupations, of other individuals in order to preserve their anonymity. The dialogue has been re-created to the best of my recollection, which can vary given the circumstances of the moment."

All of the stories and quotes in this book are the way I remember them...not necessarily the way they actually happened. I am punchy as fuck. Also, I have changed details about some people in the book so no one gets embarrassed and no one gets angry and sues me.

But for the record, the story about me getting a standing ovation at an adult movie theater was not altered at all. That shit was real, and it was fucking awesome.

STILL AWESOME

The Trials and Tribulations of an Egotistical Maniac

Chapter 1

"Ladies and gentlemen. After submission by guillotine choke..."

I smiled. I shook my head a little, too, in disbelief. I'd heard those words so many times when I was watching fights on TV. But it was crazy to be hearing them in person, about myself.

Sal Masekela dug deep for his best ring announcer voice and continued. "...at two minutes 21 seconds, in the second round! In his professional fighting debut, the winner...Jason 'Young Wing' Ellis!"

The referee raised my hand. This ref was a legit dude. I'd seen him work real fights on TV. I was standing beside him and the guy I had just choked out in a legitimate cage on the floor of a legitimate venue, in front of a huge crowd. This was the real deal—or as close to the real deal as a guy like me had any business being. It was official. After months of training and suffering and an insane weight cut, I had won my first pro MMA fight. This was the moment the MMA fan inside of me, the little kid, had been waiting for.

When you're training at the gym, everyone tells you to visualize your fight. All the combinations you're going to throw. "I'm gonna fake with this to set the guy up for that." That kind of stuff.

But they also tell you to visualize getting your hand raised. I did all of my training exactly the way the guys in my camp had told me to, so I had done that, too.

Right, I told myself as soon as the ref grabbed onto my wrist. *This is the part where I should think about the thing I told myself I would think about.*

I looked up at the ceiling of The Grove in Anaheim. I thought, *Oh fuck, that's a pretty high roof.* There was one of those huge metal fans up there, spinning around. I guess I hadn't looked up there until then. That place was massive.

But I was also thinking about my dad. I knew I would be. That was the plan.

He hadn't been gone for that long.

I did it. I wanted him to see this.

I amped out hard on that for a second.

A couple years later, when I was back in Australia, Gregsy, my skate buddy from back in the lean years, brought that up. "You were thinking about your dad in there, weren't you?" It's crazy that he knew exactly where my mind was going during that moment. Gregsy can be spot on sometimes, when he's not shit-faced.

With all the spotlights shining in your face, you can't really see the crowd when you're inside the cage. But now that the house lights had come up, I could see my old friend Colin McKay and some other people from skateboarding. There were a lot of them there. It was Ryan Sheckler's event, for his charity. They were all freaking out.

Greg Lutzka, one of the top five street skaters in the world at that point, was pumped for me. He was like, "Dude, you won on behalf of skateboarding!"

If you think about it, I guess that means that if I had gotten knocked out, that would have meant skateboarding got its ass kicked because of me, too. Good thing I didn't realize I had that weight on my shoulders until afterward. I was shitting myself enough as it was.

STILL AWESOME

Chad Reed grabbed my back on the way out of the cage. If you're reading this book, I probably don't have to explain who Chad Reed is. But just in case: Chad Reed is the greatest Australasian motocross rider of all time. He's a really lovable guy and over the years me being a fanboy of his has taken on a life of its own on my radio show. We've made an annual holiday for him and we write theme songs in his honor.

I didn't know he was there. It wasn't like I was out there mingling and hobnobbing before the fight. Not even close. Everyone else might have believed I had transformed myself into a stone-cold killing machine, but by the time it was my turn to make my entrance, I was regretting ever taking the fight in the first place.

"You fucking mad cunt!" Chad said.

That's hilarious, I thought. *Chad Reed thinks I'm tough now.*

I don't think my own corner was quite as impressed with my accomplishments as the non-MMA people in the crowd. King Mo was happy for me. Mayhem Miller was too. He loved me. But I think he also needed to remind me that compared to a real fighter I was fucking pathetic. You can see it in his face in the pictures we took after I won. It was a bit of a joke to him. And when you compare what I did to what guys like him and Mo have put themselves through? That's fair enough. I was a little bit of a tourist in that world compared to the killers they've gone up against.

I know my trainer, Ryan Parsons, was proud of what I had done. Right after the fight, he was like, "You know, you could have more fights now." (And that was true. A couple weeks later, I even got a legit offer to keep fighting. A three-fight deal in Canada.)

Andrea, my wife at the time, nipped that in the bud. "Oh, that's not gonna happen," she said.

And that was that. I was informed by my wife that I would be retiring from MMA with a perfect 1-0 record.

I know Andrea was happy for me. She was definitely happy I was leaving the arena on my feet and not in the back of the ambulance. Going in, everyone knew that was a real possibility. But mostly by that point in the night she was just ready to get back to the hotel. I don't blame her. It was a long card of fights, and to this day I would not describe Andrea as a hardcore MMA enthusiast. Plus, she was very pregnant at the time with our son, Tiger.

Andrea had made all kinds of sacrifices for me to be able to train as much as I did leading up to the fight, and she had to live with me as I went through a brutal weight cut. And now, just like my long journey to fight night was over, in a way, so was hers. She was done.

I got my gym bag from the dressing room, received a delightful bag of cookies from a radio show listener known as the Cookie Lady, and Andrea and I made our way toward the door.

Somewhere along the way I caught wind of an afterparty Ryan Sheckler was throwing. "You should go," people told me. "You should sit at Ryan's table." I realized I was kind of the man of the hour.

As humongous as Sheckler still is now, at that point, he was truly a force to be reckoned with. I think he still had his MTV show. And Anaheim was his backyard. At that time and in that neck of the woods, he was the P. Diddy of skateboarding. He was P. Sheckler. Chances were this party would be going off.

And in a roundabout way, Ryan was the reason I was fighting in the first place. I was with my trainer Kit Cope at the Supercross and we ran into Sheckler. Ryan mentioned this MMA event he had coming up for his charity, Sheckler Foundation. Kit was already the main event.

Ryan was like, "You should fight, Ellis!"

And Kit was like, "You could totally fight, Ellis!"

And I was like, "Yeah! I could totally fight!"

And just like that I was having a pro fight. That wasn't my

plan. I didn't *have* a plan. I was just filling the void of not being a skater anymore, and of not being on cocaine.

There was no way in hell my pregnant wife was going to be hitting the club for the afterparty. And I wasn't entirely shocked when she informed me that I wasn't going either.

Most married people who are reading this would understand. Anyone who's ever had a pregnant wife would *definitely* understand. Jason had had his fun and now Jason's night was over.

But that doesn't mean I didn't try.

I argued with her in the car on the way back to the hotel. I worked on her in the elevator. I worked on her in the hallway on the way to the room, and then in the room, too.

At first, I tried to be pleasant. "Come on, baby. I won the fight! All my friends are going! Everyone's gonna be there!" She told me she didn't want to be alone in the hotel room. I moved on to more bullshit angles. "It's kind of weird for me to win the fight and not show up," I argued. "It's almost disrespectful."

"Just go then," she said. But needless to say, she was not sending me with her blessing.

Andrea knew who she was dealing with. I had been sober for a little while at that point, but at the end of the day I'm a loose cannon.

"You're gonna drink," she said. "You're gonna get loose. Who knows what you'll do with all those people boosting your ego." She had an argument. I had been sheltered from all of that for a few years.

Truthfully, at that point, I wasn't even thinking about drinking. The only thing I really wanted to put in my body was cheeseburgers. I was starving. I had been starving for weeks leading up to the fight.

But you know what can happen when you go the club and get too excited. I might have downed seven shots in 20 minutes and then been completely obliterated before I even saw food.

There were these three girls at the fight who I knew from my skateboarding days. They were going to be at Sheckler's party for sure. Those three were around a lot when I was a pro skater and I was the funny guy that everybody knew. Now that I was a radio guy and I got all jacked and had won a cage fight in front of a big crowd, maybe they would want to get reacquainted with me again. Andrea had seen them at the fight, and she knew full well how they rolled.

And then there was a guy from that world who really didn't like me. He had been at the event and he was going to be at the party, too. If I got drunk and started spracking off because I just won a fight, maybe that guy would beat me up.

Maybe Andrea was saving me, from him *or* from myself.

Relationships are about compromise. There isn't a right or wrong answer for every question. I had my angles for why I should go and she had her reasons for why I shouldn't. In all fairness, maybe she was right. I might have woken up the next morning hungover, mangled, and divorced.

But I doubt it. I was far from the greatest husband, but I'd like to think I could have kept my shit together out of respect for my pregnant wife. I think I could have stuck to Shirley Temples and stayed out of trouble.

I don't really like nightclubs. It's always the same thing at those places. If you've seen one you've seen them all. It's kind of boring, really, once you're a grown up. All I really wanted was the entrance. Walking in that door and seeing everyone get psyched for me, because I had won. Like a kingpin.

So, I decided to go.

I put all my shit on and closed the hotel door behind me. I made it all the way to the elevator. The door opened just as my guilty conscience kicked in. I realized I couldn't do it and turned back.

STILL AWESOME

At least food was still my friend.

I was hungry in a way I have never known before or since. Truthfully, in a way I don't think most people reading this book can understand.

I had lost 30 pounds getting down to weight for my fight. Nowadays there are ways to cut weight that aren't really all that bad. But my camp was old school. The old school way was how the guys in my camp did it, so that was how I did it, too.

That was the worst part of training. Not all the hours and all the effort. Not getting hurt all the time. Not balancing the training with a full-time radio show and a family. It was the weight cut.

I would never go on that diet ever again. It changes you. In a way, I would compare the experience of cutting weight to going to jail. If you go to jail for a night, that's pretty gnarly. That's a story most people will never forget. If you go to jail for a week, then even more so. But if you go to jail for three months? Six months? That changes who you are. Forever.

Thirty pounds is a lot to lose for anyone. But not all pounds are created equal. When you start cutting down near fight shape, your body starts talking to you. All day long, it's telling you that what you're doing is a really bad idea.

Put it this way: If you starve for a day, it's bad. Your stomach hurts. Your body keeps reminding you that you need to eat. It's a weird sensation. But try doing that for two days…and then three days…and then keep it up for six weeks. It adds up to something different. You hit these plateaus and you think you're used to it, but then you find new levels of hunger, over and over again. Food starts to literally look different. It looks kind of weird, actually.

You know how I said I had visualized my fight, and getting my hand raised after? Well, I also spent a lot of time visualizing all the food I was going to eat the minute I was out of that fucking cage. Pizza. Burgers. Milkshakes. Apple pie. I was going to give that room service menu a good going-over.

I went back to the room, took off whatever I was planning to wear to the club, picked up the phone, and called room service. If I wasn't going to the afterparty, then I was going to have a massive food party, all by myself.

The phone rang.

And rang.

And rang.

It was too late. Room service had ended. I was shit out of luck.

Even though we had just been arguing, Andrea still felt bad for me about that. She knew as well as anyone how hungry I was. She did for a minute, anyway. And then she fell asleep. Carrying a small human in your uterus all day will take a lot out of you, I am told.

All I had was that bag of cookies from the Cookie Lady. They were very good cookies. I will say that. But cookies don't help much when you're hungry. You need food.

I turned off the light, got into bed next to Andrea, and looked at the ceiling. The fight was still running through my head. Even though I had won, it didn't go down the way I had wanted it to. At all. I was thinking about how many mistakes I'd made. I had started off pretty shit. I had done a bunch of dumb things which could have cost me.

I thought about how valuable my corner was, and how much they had helped me. I hadn't really taken any damage. The other guy kicked me in the leg a couple times. And I got punched in the ear pretty good one time. All in all, though, I had walked out of the cage feeling fine.

But I had kind of panicked in there. I had needed to show up in killer mode from the start, and instead I let my opponent bring the fight to me.

STILL AWESOME

I felt like I had gotten a better understanding of what kind of a man I was. And the verdict wasn't good.

That's how the night of my first fight ended. By myself. Laying in the dark. Thinking dark thoughts. Scarfing down cookies.

Chapter 2

Around the time I had my first fight, if you were on the outside looking in, my life with Andrea would have seemed like it was moving in the right direction.

Right before that fight we had been living in a house in Temecula, about 60 miles north of San Diego. Being the real estate mastermind that I am, I bought the place when houses were super expensive. Then prices immediately went down. Way down.

It was a brand-new neighborhood. They had built a whole bunch of houses at the same time. A lot of them never sold. There was never anyone in the house next door to us the whole time we were there. I used to ride my dirt bike around that place because it was empty.

For a while there we had a little neighborhood going. At Christmastime there were lights on a bunch of places. But then even some of those houses started emptying out. And then one day my manager informed me that I was going to keep losing all kinds of money if I held on to my house.

He told me, "You're going to foreclose."

I was like, "What's that?"

And the next thing I knew we didn't have a house anymore and Andrea and I moved into a one-bedroom apartment in Santa Monica.

Living space was tight there. My daughter, Devin, slept in

the living room. And then when Tiger came along he was in a crib in the bedroom.

The last time we had lived in L.A. was when Devin was little. We were in Hollywood. People who have never spent time in Los Angeles might think Hollywood is a fancy, uppity place, but actually most of it is a giant shithole. One night when we lived there, a guy stuck a gun in my face and stole the bike I had been riding home from the radio show. That bike had been given to me by Mat Hoffman, the greatest BMX rider of all time. The guy who stole the bike probably had no idea who Mat Hoffman even is. I bet he turned around and sold it for 20 bucks.

So for the kids' sake, instead of Hollywood, this time around we moved right by the beach. That alone made my life way better. Although our old house in Temecula was less than 100 miles from Los Angeles, the traffic to and from the city was hellacious. On a Friday night, I could be looking at a six-hour drive home after the show. Just soul-crushing. So now, when work was over I no longer had to choose between rotting on the freeway for hours or staying in a sketchy hotel room in Koreatown.

From that point of view, things seemed to be looking up.

In some ways those years were hard times. Hard because Andrea and I didn't have tons of money. Hard because we were all crammed together in that one little spot. Hard because anyone who has ever raised kids knows what a challenge that can be.

But it was also a great time. As tough and as annoying as children are at times, they're beyond worth it. I love my kids. They're the best.

Seeing my son for the first time was glorious. I was really hands-on when Tiger was born, straightaway. I was like that with both kids. While Andrea recovered from giving birth, I got right in there, bro-ing down one-on-one. Changing diapers. All that shit. Trying to do as much as I could without getting in the way.

STILL AWESOME

I felt like my life at that point was a mission. Things were looking up professionally, and even if day-to-day life could be frustrating and if Andrea and I didn't click as well as some other couples seemed to, well, we were on our way to bigger and better things as a family. Remembering that struggle would just make it that much sweeter when we got there. That was the vision I had sold myself on. I was amped up.

But something always felt a bit off. Having a new baby on the scene kept Andrea and me busy. We spent so much of our time chasing around two little maniacs, there was no time left to think about how we weren't spending much time together as a couple. It was pretty easy to not analyze the relationship.

The truth was, her and I weren't in a very good spot at that point. But honestly, I had gotten used to not being in a good spot with her. At that point in my life, I had never been in a solid, healthy relationship for any stretch of time.

So did Andrea and I fight? Sure. But I didn't necessarily think that was really bad, or really unusual. I had fought with all my exes. My first wife used to physically beat me up. And Andrea would never, ever do that.

After Andrea and I fought, oftentimes I would think, *Man, it would be way better for both of us if you never had to deal with me again.* But that was also nothing new. When you suffer from low self-esteem on the level that I do, you think that kind of shit pretty much every day. I thought that was normal. I thought that was something people thought about from time to time in every relationship.

When you believe that you suck as a person, that doesn't make you want to leave your wife. It's the opposite. It makes you afraid of what will happen the day she finally figures out how lame you are and dumps your ass.

I really, truly did not want to get divorced. I was committed to making it work, if only for the kids.

Plus, I was terrified of being alone.

Let me be clear about something right off the bat: Everything that went wrong between Andrea and me was my fault.

Andrea wasn't perfect. No one is. But I don't blame her at all.

It was me. I was the bad guy in our marriage.

Andrea and I had split up for the first time before my MMA fight. Before she got pregnant with Tiger.

Having Devin and becoming a father changed me as a person. It changes you forever. But it seemed like it changed Andrea even more. It changed the kind of wife she was. And it didn't change the kind of husband I was. At least, it didn't change me enough.

I was a cheater when I met Andrea. When we first met, I was doing everybody. She knew that.

The world will let you play around as much as you want when you're single. But once babies and marriage come and it's time to settle down, you're expected to flip a switch and change. It seems like a lot of people have that switch inside them, waiting to be activated. I don't.

There was a guest on the radio show. She was a BBW—a Big Beautiful Woman. She did BBW porn or modeling or something. I forget. I find lots of big girls extremely attractive. But this particular lady was not the most attractive BBW I have come across. She was 300 pounds, easy. Maybe 400. She had a bit of a crooked eye, too.

That was kind of the point. I figured no one would suspect I would hook up with her. Most people wouldn't believe I would be down for that.

But at the same time, it was also a bit of a stealth kamikaze mission. I figured if I *did* get caught, Andrea would leave me and then she wouldn't be stuck with this hideous mess of a man anymore. Yes, in those days I really did think like that.

This lady came on the show as a guest and then she hit me up after. She invited me to her house. She made it really easy. Whatever I wanted to do, whenever I wanted to do it. No strings attached. No one would ever know.

I didn't want to cheat. We all know there are some guys who are married or in relationships who get off on pulling girls on the side, the kind who brag to their scumbag buddies about it. "Hey bro, look at this awesome Tiger Woods phone I got! It hides all the nude selfies from my side bitches! I am the James Bond of adultery!"

That life does not appeal to me, at all. Living that way must make your day-to-day existence such a struggle. You have to be wired a certain way to want to do that, and for all my faults, that's not me. It just sounds stressful.

That has to take a toll on your mental health—to say nothing of your wife's mental health. You kind of have to not give a shit about her to go around doing that. Because if she finds out—or more like *when* she finds out—that's like mentally punching her in the face.

If you know that having sex with other people is something you need in order to be happy, then you have no business getting married. Unless your wife knows from the start that you are that person, and she is okay with it.

To hide it is the sneakiest thing ever. If that's the kind of guy you are, you owe it to everyone to get the hell away from her and to let her start a new life.

I think there were plenty of other girls I could have slept with in those days. But I would have had to go after those girls. I would have had to work for it. And I sincerely didn't want to do that. I at least had the self-control to avoid those situations.

I'm not proud of some of the things I've done. I wanted to be a good husband. I was just weak.

The truth is, I can't be monogamous. It's not in me. In my whole life, I never met anyone where I thought, *This is all I need. Forever.*

If I was being honest with myself, I always knew deep down that it was insane to think there could ever be one person who could be the only person I'd ever want to sleep with for the rest of my life.

But I never faced that fact. I wasn't lying to Andrea about that. I was lying to myself. I wanted to believe I could change. But I couldn't.

The thing with that BBW wasn't the only time I had cheated on Andrea after Devin was born. I also hooked up with a porn star who came on the show. It was one of those nights I stayed in a shitty hotel in Koreatown so I didn't have to drive all the way back to Temecula after work.

I was really, really into her. She also made it really easy. She kept hitting me up.

"We should hang out sometime," she'd say.

She was always direct, but in a pleasant way. She didn't make it seem sleazy or evil.

"Yeah, sure," I finally replied. "We can hang out. Just not... like that."

"Just come on over," she said.

She was 100% the instigator. But I didn't put up much of a fight. I couldn't help it. I'm just an asshole.

Shit happens, as they say.

To me, it seems to happen a lot.

Andrea never found out about that one. That might have been the one time I got away with it. But it wasn't long before Andrea found out about my big beautiful friend.

She checked my phone for some reason or another and found

text messages. I didn't try to cover my tracks or defend myself. I'm not much of a liar.

"You talking to this chick?" she said.

And I was like, "Yeah."

"How could you?" she asked.

I had no answers. "I don't know. Because I'm a piece of shit."

Andrea didn't have to think twice. "That's it," she said. "We're fucking done."

The next thing I remember, I was standing in a parking lot next to Swing House, the rehearsal studio where the Sirius studios in L.A. used to be. It felt like my world was crashing down on top of itself. I felt my heart skip a beat. Literally. *Ooh, we're in deep today, buddy*, I remember thinking. My thoughts raced around. Where was I gonna live? What was I gonna do?

Then my phone rang. It was her dad. Andrea had told him everything.

"How could you do this?" he asked. He was furious. And rightly so.

I had no comebacks. I just took it.

At that moment in time, divorce seemed like a pretty appealing option. It seemed like the silver bullet that would get a lot of people who I had wronged and who were now extremely angry at me off my back.

So Andrea and I separated.

At the time, I thought we were done for good. I was pretty positive that sleeping with a 300-pound, one-eyed lady had sealed that deal permanently.

Andrea moved back to San Diego, where her family was, and got some kind of office job. I had Devin every weekend. I tried to be around as much as I could, whenever I wasn't working. Andrea went out a lot—I think sometimes just to get back at me a bit—and left me to be super dad.

I tried to embrace single life. I didn't have much of a choice. I went on a couple of dates. But I was really just going through the motions. My heart wasn't in it.

Right from the get-go, breaking up my family felt wrong. As a child of divorce, I was well aware of how much divorce can mess with your kids. That was hard for me to swallow. I kept telling myself, *You're fucked up because your parents split up. And now you're passing that down to your daughter.*

Over the years, I'd heard people say that it's better for kids to have parents who are happy apart than miserable together. But my gut was telling me that was bullshit. That it was something people told themselves so they could sleep at night when they knew they had mentally scarred their poor defenseless children. It just sounded too good to be true.

It seemed selfish to even think about myself. All I wanted was to get the team back together and fix everything.

So I dedicated myself to winning Andrea back. I really dug deep. I would pick her up at her place and take her out on dates and then drive her home and drop her off afterward. Like a proper gentleman. I wrote straight up love letters. Now mind you I am dyslexic and pretty much illiterate. These letters were totally pathetic. But I know Andrea appreciated them. If you had already been in love with me at one point, then you were already pretty okay with me not being able to spell. I think it's like if you're a parent and your kid writes you a big, long letter. It doesn't matter what it says or whether it makes any sense. You just love that they made the effort.

I pulled out all the stops. I really put on a show to win her over. And not just for a week or a month. For a long time. I was super committed. I could tell I almost had her. I had worn her down. We were talking about having another kid. She was gonna take me back.

STILL AWESOME

But then she heard about Chyna. By the time Chyna came on the show, her pro wrestling days were behind her. She had moved on to what some people might call the celebrity train wreck era of her career. While I was interviewing her, I noticed she was looking at me a lot. Right in the eyes. Really locking in. I was surprised by how forward she was, but I'm always up for a challenge. So I stared right back at her.

Afterward I asked her for her number. I think part of that was just seeing how she would react and how far I could take it. But I wasn't just asking her as a joke or so I could talk about it on the radio. I was genuinely interested in taking her out, if I could.

We texted back and forth a couple times. Just from those texts she was already coming across a bit flaky, to put it gently.

She invited me to dinner.

Saying yes to that had everything to do with where I was in my life. If I was single nowadays, I wouldn't even answer that text. A night out with her was guaranteed insanity.

But I was still in the clueless phase of being single again. I didn't know what I wanted or what I was doing. I just knew that for the first time in a long time I was free to do whatever I felt like doing. So I went for it.

I pulled up to the restaurant in my Ford F-150. This was the truck that later became the A6K, immortalized in song by my band, Taintstick.

But this was before it got customized. At this point it was a piece of shit.

I had gotten in an accident. Someone had hit me. Something was broken with the wheel. Every time I hit the break, it would squeak.

So that's how I rolled up to valet for my big date with a C-list celebrity—with my car grinding to a squeaky halt. It was quite an entrance.

I went inside. Chyna was already at the table with all of her friends. There were a bunch of gay dudes and a couple of weird-looking chicks. It was a motley assortment of people. Every one of them was a character. Just a really odd bunch of people.

Chyna had come in hot that night. She had on leather pants and high heels and she was wearing a big fluffy scarf thing. She looked like a gigantic party monster, ruling over the table.

By the time I got there, everyone was already pretty loose. They were laughing and carrying on and everybody was drinking a lot. It was like they were in a hurry to get wasted.

I wasn't drinking at that time so I didn't really join in on the action. Everyone was so busy raging that they weren't all that concerned with me. I was more of a fly on the wall.

After a while, she was like, "Let's get out of here."

That was fine with me. We got in my truck. I was following her lead.

"Let's go to the bowling alley on Sunset," she said.

We were in the Valley at the time, north of Hollywood. I took the freeway to drive us down there, but on the way she pointed to a spot on the side of the road and said, "Pull over in that parking lot."

Before I could do that, she straddled me.

Now Chyna was a substantial woman. She had big arms and big shoulders and she was still wearing that humongous feathery boa. And I was still on the freeway.

It was chaos. I was like, "I can't see the road!"

But somehow I pulled off the freeway and into the parking lot.

I don't remember how far things went there. She's a big human and I'm a big human and there's only so much room in the front seat of an F-150. Logistically it was challenging to get much accomplished.

So we just wrestled each other there for a little bit and then we continued to the bowling alley.

Truthfully, I don't think Chyna was all that much of a bowling enthusiast. I don't remember either of us rolling a ball. I think she was there more for the bar.

She rented a lane and then came back with a full tray of shots. "Let's do lemon drops," she said.

I told her I didn't drink.

"Oh, okay, then I'll do them."

I ordered a beer, to be social. I was just holding it. It didn't matter. She was so busy with her tray of shots that she wasn't keeping tabs on my Corona.

After a while she wanted to go home, so we went back together.

I remember waking up in the middle of the night and hearing another voice in the darkness, outside her bedroom.

When I came to, it took me a second to remember that I was in her apartment.

The voice I heard wasn't Chyna's. It was another girl. I didn't know who she was or what she was doing there, but she sounded sort of motherly.

From what was being said, I pieced together that Chyna was in the bathroom throwing up. I gathered that the other girl was Chyna's assistant. I think the assistant lived there, too.

You could guess from the tone in her voice that this wasn't the first time she had had to "assist" in some middle of the night drunken barfing. She was being helpful and supportive, but in a way that also said, *I'm only putting up with this shit because someone is paying me to do it.*

I had already started to regret the evening. Maybe if I had been drunk too it could have been a bit of a weird, messy adventure. Instead it was like being the only sober guy at the party, watching everybody else get dumber and dumber.

I didn't have anything against Chyna. If anything, being around her that night made me feel really sympathetic toward her. I felt bad for her. I could tell she was super innocent and super gullible. I felt like I could have taken her for a ride if I wanted to. I felt like lots of people in her life already had. And that's how she ended up where she was when I met her.

The next morning, I woke up to the sound of her voice. She was on the phone and she was completely naked. Her bedroom window faced the outside and the curtain was wide open. I could tell from how she was talking that she was doing an interview with some radio show. She was babbling into the phone about whatever she was promoting at the moment. It was probably the same thing she had been on my show for.

I saw my opportunity to make a break for it. I pulled myself together in a hurry. She got up and started grabbing on to me, trying to hold me there. She was gesturing to me to wait a minute while she finished the interview.

I made a move for the door. While the radio guy was asking her a question, she was mouthing *Don't leave* to me.

She followed me into the living room, still on the phone. I gave her a little wave, like, *Okay, bye, I'll see you later*.

While I walked down the corridor, she got off the phone. As I got on the elevator, she ran up to it, still completely nude.

"Wait, don't go!" she said.

Just as the elevator door shut.

Again, there was a time when having a naked bodybuilder chick chasing me down the hall would have been awesome. And it's weird, because I would probably be okay with it now, too. A fair amount of weird stuff with naked people happens in my life these days. If Chyna was still around and she still hit me up once a month to go paint the town red, I would probably take her up on it. She meant well. She had a good heart. Compared to a lot of other people in her life in those days, I would have been a relatively good influence. I could have sipped a beer or two and watched her go off.

But the timing wasn't right. I was a newly separated sober dad. That just wasn't my scene at that point in time.

It wasn't like I cut her off cold turkey after that. We still texted back and forth a couple times. I think she might have even called in to the radio show again, later that day.

That night definitely became a topic of conversation on the show. Everything from my life does, sooner or later. How was that going to be the exception?

But this was before social media was really popping off. Whatever was said on the air definitely didn't make it back to her like it would have nowadays. I'm glad about that. Lord knows she got bashed enough without me and everyone else on the show piling on, too.

Unfortunately, the story of my wild night with Chyna *did* make it back to Andrea.

Andrea didn't listen to the show. But she had friends whose husbands did.

Even when Andrea and I were together, that kind of thing bit me in the ass on more than one occasion. Maybe because of something I did in the past that came up on air. Maybe just because of a dumb conversation we had on the show. It would get filtered from the husbands to their wives and then over to Andrea. A lot of times, what she heard was way worse than what was actually said. And then I'd get in trouble.

I guess the news that Andrea's ex had gone out with Chyna was too exciting for those guys to keep to themselves.

I get it, kind of. Because Chyna was supposed to be a joke. She was this famous train wreck that people made fun of. It wasn't just Andrea who saw her that way. One time, years later, I was pitching a TV show and the producer of the show kept asking the network people, "Did you know Jason slept with Chyna?"

Eventually I remember asking him, "Dude, why do you keep saying that? Is this a thing that is somehow gonna guarantee me a show?"

And he was like, "I just can't help it! It's so funny!"

When I told the story of our date on the radio, everyone had their joke about it. I knew it was funny, too. But I also liked it. I liked her. As I have already mentioned, I like women in all shapes and sizes. I'm pretty equal opportunity. I wasn't doing it as some kind of sadistic radio bit so we could all laugh at her afterward.

I can't really speak for Andrea, but I don't think she truly cared that much. She knew who she had married. And while Andrea and I were split up, I slept with a lot of people. I don't think Andrea assumed I'd been celibate the whole time. But Chyna was the story that came up on the radio.

I think what she really hated was that people could turn on the radio and hear all those details of her husband's life—and therefore of her life, too. If you've seen the movie *Private Parts* you know exactly what I'm talking about. Just one more way in which my career is Howard Stern Light.

The Chyna thing stopped me in my tracks for a couple of months. I had to dig deep all over again, to convince Andrea to get over that and take me back.

Finally, I wore her down enough that she was willing to give us another shot. As long as I had been exposed as a cheater and as a guy who would sleep with Chyna and BBWs and whoever else, I figured I might as well put all my cards on the table. If we were going to repair the relationship, start over, and make things work this time, there was some stuff I wanted her to know about me.

Before Andrea and I met, I had sexual experiences with both men and with trans women.

STILL AWESOME

"I've kind of done gay stuff," I told her, after we were finally back together. "And I don't feel like that part of me is totally switched off."

I wasn't sure exactly what I was trying to say or how to say it. When something has been buried that deep for that long, it doesn't come out easily. This wasn't the most comfortable topic of conversation—for either of us.

"I'm not trying to tell you I'm gay," I continued. "I'm just trying to tell you that it's in there."

She didn't want to address it.

"I don't need to hear about that," she said.

That was the one and only time I brought that subject up to Andrea. If she didn't need to hear about it, then I didn't need to drag it out.

I tried. But we both agreed to sweep it under the carpet. So for all the issues in our marriage, that wasn't necessarily one of them—at least not one that we ever discussed.

Chapter 3

Tiger was three by the time Andrea and I got divorced. So I can honestly say that we gave it a good shot.

I tried as hard as I could to be a team player. But as we all know, a lot of times when you call yourself a team player, what you really mean is that you're doing a bunch of stuff you don't want to be doing because it's for the greater good and because you want to avoid confrontation. Nowadays I'm very, very free. It's pretty hard to get me to do anything I don't want to do. But for as long as Andrea and I were married, I tried to be a good soldier.

The truth is that, for me, the fun times with Andrea happened before the kids came along. When we first met, we would hang out and get high and have sex and play video games. Those are all things that I like. And when those things got taken away, being in a relationship was nowhere near as cool for me.

It's lame. It's pathetic. I know it. But it's true.

Andrea wasn't the same person she was when we met. Neither of us were.

The Andrea that I met was 20 years old. She was a little girl who got a fake ID and went to a bar one night. She stared at me across that bar for hours, and she fell in love. We planned to meet back at my house afterward, but I got so shitfaced I was passed out by the time she got there. So she left a cheeseburger on my back for me to find when I woke up.

Right before she met me, she was a kid working behind a counter at Hot Dog on a Stick. For those of you who are not familiar with the Hot Dog on a Stick corporation, it's this chain of restaurants they have in food courts at a bunch of malls in Southern California. They sell corn dogs. The corn dogs are pretty sick actually. We didn't have those in Australia when I was growing up. I was all about those the first time I got my hands on one.

No one works at Hot Dog on a Stick because it makes you look cool. Girls who work there wear these ridiculous old school blue, red, and yellow uniforms. There's also this big stupid hat they have to put on their heads. The uniform makes everyone look like a gigantic piece of candy.

Andrea was working at Costco when she met me. That's a step up from corn dog girl, but it's still not the most glamorous position you can hold. But working jobs like that tells me something about you. It tells me your parents raised you with a work ethic. They taught you to hustle.

Andrea probably got some of that work ethic from her dad, because he used to be in the military and was kind of strict. But by the time I met her, she was also rebelling against what her dad stood for and the way he had raised her, too. She was partying and sowing her wild oats a bit, like people do at that age.

Meanwhile, when we met, I owned a house and had two cars in the driveway. If you could see my bank account you would know I wasn't balling, but what I had probably looked pretty impressive to someone who until recently had a Hot Dog on a Stick uniform hanging in their closet.

To be clear: I did have an actual, real job. When you see videos of me and other skaters from that era, there's a lot of laughing and fucking around and smoking joints in the parking lot. But we were still putting in six hours a day at the ramp, every day.

Still, from the outside looking in, I know I seemed like a guy who sat back and got free money. A guy who everybody in that area knew about and who had a bunch of checks coming in.

When Andrea and I got together, our relationship was about fun, plain and simple. But then she got pregnant. She believed we could make it work and I wanted to believe that she was right and do the right thing, so we gave it our best shot. But everything changed, in a hurry.

Pretty soon I wasn't a pro skater; I was a guy who was desperately trying to get some shit started on the radio. We weren't living where she grew up; we were in Hollywood, where grown men pull guns on other grown men to steal their bicycles.

And she wasn't a Hot Dog on a Stick girl. She was a mom.

When Andrea had Devin, our sex life ended almost completely. And that was the beginning of the end of our relationship.

I'm sure there are some people reading this who can relate. Based on the people who have called in to my radio show over the years, that chain of events is not all that uncommon for married people.

Apparently, for some people that doesn't have to be a deal breaker. From what I've seen, there are some people who can motor along in a basically happy relationship that has little to no sex.

I'm just not one of them. Not at all.

I have an abnormally high sex drive. Sex was probably always more important to me than it was to Andrea. Sometimes it seems like it's more important to me than it is to almost *anyone*.

But something definitely changed in her. It seems like the same thing changes in a lot of women.

Having a human being grow inside your stomach—making a life and seeing it come out of your body and then interacting with a brand-new person that used to live inside you—can affect the way you think about everything. Not for all moms, obviously. But for some, having a penis in your mouth, for example, suddenly seems a bit rude. I don't pretend to understand the exact dynamic of it because I don't have a vagina, but for a lot of women, being a mom means you no longer want to do anything that might be considered a bit slutty.

Becoming a mom is a gigantic experience. I get that. It's bound to change you. But maybe things between me and Andrea didn't have to stay that way. Maybe if I had been more nurturing and more understanding and more present, maybe that would have just been a phase our sex life went through. Maybe it could have come back around a little.

But when things aren't working the way I want them to in a relationship, I can just switch off. I had done it before, and at that point with Andrea I did it again. We just didn't discuss it.

Even when sex did happen, it felt like more of a favor. It was almost like tactical sex. Especially once the radio show started to get bigger. People started to think that I was funny or special again, like they used to when I was a skateboarder. Andrea knew there were going to be opportunities. She knew who I was. She knew that if she didn't sleep with me from time to time, there was only so much Jason could take before he scaled the walls and went AWOL.

I wanted to be good. I wanted to be noble. But I'm not disciplined. And so eventually, as I have already told you, that's exactly what had happened. I never hid that I was married and a father from anyone. I wasn't going around slipping my wedding ring in my pocket after I left the house. Unfortunately, that doesn't scare every woman off.

Other men can say no and walk away. I would love to be one of those guys, but I'm not.

I tried to pretend that I could change and that our relationship could change, but all of the issues that made Andrea and I separate before Tiger was born were the same reasons we eventually broke up for good.

Maybe it was inevitable. I'm not sure Andrea and I were all

that compatible in the first place. Maybe the people we were when we first met had some stuff in common, but so much had changed since then. I think we both felt like if we tried hard enough we could *make* ourselves compatible.

Again, it's all my fault. She wasn't doing anything crazy or asking for anything unreasonable. I was the one who was hard to deal with.

I was definitely not ready to have kids. I could have told you that before Andrea got pregnant. It happened and I did the best I could. I told her I wasn't cut out to be a father. I said I would give her as much money and support as I could, but at the same time I was clear with her that I didn't know how much I had to offer beyond that.

But Andrea was delusionally in love with me. She had a vision of how things could be. And to someone like me who had such a chaotic childhood, that vision sounded awesome. I wanted to believe in it too.

You need to think long and hard before you commit to big stuff like marriage and parenthood. You need to have a plan. But I never thought about anything in those days. I just did stuff.

Over the years, tons of people have called the radio show to tell me they're thinking about getting married or having kids. Sometimes it sounds like they have a good head on their shoulders and they know what they're getting into. But other times, by the way they talk, I can tell they haven't really thought things through. Get out now, I tell them. Before it's too late. If I had called in to my radio show way back when, I would have told me the exact same thing. For everyone's sake.

Those years after we got back together were really just a slow downward spiral.

Andrea was changing into someone I was finding it harder and harder to relate to. A part of me is glad she changed. The kids needed someone to be the sane adult in the room, and at that point you couldn't always count on that person being me.

But as she was evolving into a sensible, respectable member of society, she was well aware that I was not. I think that, to her, everything I was and everything I stood for gradually became kind of gross and offensive.

I was definitely gross to a lot of her friends. If you've heard my show—especially in those days—it makes sense. To a normal person, a lot of the stuff we talked about *was* gross. I might spend four hours making a top ten list of the World's Greatest Human Slam Pigs. Or I might talk about how my balls are constantly moving. The list goes on and on. I didn't just say my penis was six pounds soft—I recorded a fucking metal album about it that went on the *Billboard* chart.

It was all kinds of things. Maybe I shared a few too many details of our personal life. Maybe I would get too flirty with a female guest.

We couldn't get a lot of famous celebrities to come on the show, so a lot of times I just talked to porn stars. They would come on and talk about how sucking cock was their number one passion in life. Some of them were probably being more truthful about that than others, but they would all still butter me up and hit on me. It was part of their schtick. And even when they didn't give me their number, that was one more thing making my marriage more difficult.

Many times, I would feel like I had done a really good show, but then I would come home to find Andrea angry at me because of something a friend of hers told her I had said on the radio.

I get it. It's a rare woman who would be totally unaffected by that stuff. But my job was definitely an issue.

And that for sure didn't help the way I felt about her friends. I obviously didn't appreciate them calling Andrea and stirring up shit. That made me turn against them, and me not liking her friends became another log on the fire, all by itself.

There were many, *many* logs on the fire.

There was for sure some jealousy. Andrea knew I liked certain kinds of girls. I liked party girls—the kind of girl she was when we met. And she knew I liked even more extreme types than that, like strippers.

She would get mad if that type of girl was on the radio show, or even just around us in public. If we were at a restaurant and some rowdy tattooed hot chick walked past, I knew I had to make it my business to pretend not to notice, or else Andrea might be salty for the next hour.

I see the angle for her jealousy. I mean, I cheated on her. But once Andrea knew I had slept with a 400-pound lady with a crooked eye that made her look like Shaquille O'Neal, she treated me like I could not be trusted to be on my own anywhere for more than 30 minutes.

When I would go to New York to do radio shows at the Sirius headquarters, Andrea would send me with a warning about specific people she thought I was planning to hook up with. "You're gonna meet up with so-and-so," she'd say. "I know you are. So I'm just gonna watch what you're both doing on social media to make sure that you don't see each other."

I wasn't having sex with my wife. And that was driving me crazy. But my wife was also keeping tabs on me to make sure I wasn't getting it anywhere else. I felt like I was surrounded by booby traps. I was like a mouse living in a world full of cheese. But I knew that if I touched the cheese I would get cracked on the head. So I just sat and looked at cheese all day and thought, *I'm such a bad person! All I want is cheese!* It was no way to live.

The first time I went on *The Howard Stern Show* was a huge moment in my career. Anyone who has ever hosted the style of show I do is following a path that he invented.

To be honest, half the reason I got booked on *Stern* the first time might have been because of the stuff I was doing on the radio, but the other half was probably just because I was willing to shove a bunch of M&M's in my foreskin. (Shout out to the Reverend Bob Levy for suggesting that bit. Couldn't have done it without you, Bob.)

But when I went to New York for that appearance, I think maybe 20% of Andrea was thinking, *Good luck on the* Stern Show. The other 80% was just thinking, *Don't fuck anybody.*

Having Howard Stern acknowledge that I exist was a huge deal. It made me feel pumped about what I had accomplished. It made my bosses see that my show was on the right track. It for sure brought me all kinds of new listeners. It was a sign Andrea and I were getting out of a one-bedroom apartment and moving on to bigger and better things. It was a big milestone in my career, and it should have been a big milestone in my relationship with my wife.

But I don't know that she ever considered talking on the radio a real skill. Sometimes when we were at dinners and stuff and people would ask what I did, she'd say, "He just talks for a living." Like that's an easy thing to do.

Did I feel like Andrea was really lame a lot of the time when we were married?

Yes.

Looking back, do I still feel that way?

I do.

But here's the thing: That was also my fault. I brought that on myself. I cheated on her and I hurt her. I made her be that way.

She wasn't being crazy and suspicious for no reason—I was suspect. I made her be the lamest wife ever. She had no choice.

I didn't make her mistrustful. I couldn't be trusted, and she knew it. There's a difference.

Did she go through my phone behind my back? Yes. But you

know why? Because she thought I was up to no good...and she was right.

She'd go in there and find messages from porn stars that would say, "I think you're hot."

Now, I didn't write back and say, "You too! Now send me pictures of your holes!" I would just say, "Awesome! Thanks!" But it doesn't matter what I said. I shouldn't have been texting back.

There was really no reason why I needed to have a bunch of porn stars' phone numbers in the first place. Or why they needed to have mine. I had producers and they had publicists. If someone needed to tell someone what day and what time so-and-so was booked on the show, then there were other people who could have—and should have—been texting each other to handle that. And there was no other legitimate reason I needed to be in contact with the porn world.

When these girls would say, "Hey, you should come over," I didn't sneak out and do it. But I also didn't say no.

I would say, "I can't do that now. Maybe some other time."

I might have told myself I was just being polite or that I was just maintaining professional relationships. But I certainly wasn't telling Andrea that I was talking to those girls, or what they were asking me to do. And here's a good rule of thumb: If you're doing stuff that you wouldn't tell your wife about, then it probably counts as cheating.

I'm sure having to keep tabs on me wasn't any more fun for Andrea than it was for me. She's in a great relationship now, and I bet you anything she doesn't do that shit anymore. Why? Because she knows she doesn't have to.

At the bottom of it all, our biggest issue was my issues.

I've been in therapy for a long time, and because of that I can now tell you that I have what are known as mommy issues. My parents got divorced when I was very young. I kind of had a choice between which parent I was going to live with, and I chose my dad. My stepmum was obviously not my real mum, and pretty soon she had sons of her own. As far as I could tell she was not a huge fan of me in those days. I think she would have preferred if I wasn't around at all, to be honest. Meanwhile my mum was very young when she had me and she was an addict on top of everything else.

Because of therapy, I can see now that because I missed out on having someone to really mother me when I was little, I went into adulthood looking for girlfriends and then wives to do that job.

Two marriages in a row followed the exact same pattern: I would show up as this badass. I would be drunk and on tons of coke and be super irresponsible. But then somehow I would flip the script so that not too far into the relationship, the girl I was with would be getting mad at me if she so much as caught me smoking weed.

I didn't force that change directly. I never said, "You need to help me, lady! I'm out of control!" But somehow, some way, before too long they would be saying, "Jason you shouldn't be doing that," and I'd be like, "Stop telling me what to do, Mom!"

Andrea and my previous wife weren't like that when I met them. They weren't similar people at all, really. But by the end of my relationships with them, they both treated me exactly the same way. The way they talked to me was identical. Like the exact same mom, talking to the exact same child.

That was my pattern. I handed my wife the keys and put her in control of me. And then I got angry that she was trying to control me.

Andrea and I always made a point not to argue in front of the kids. We thought we were pretty good at keeping it under wraps, too. But kids are smart. They can tell when there's tension, whether you think you're hiding it or not.

One time, Devin told us she didn't like it when we fought.

STILL AWESOME

Tiger might have still been too little to notice. But obviously we weren't fooling her.

We argued about all kinds of stuff. Andrea had issues with me hanging out with my friends. Some of my old friends had grown up, but a lot of them were still hanging out all day, smoking weed and skating. Mind you, these weren't a bunch of dirtbags who had nothing going on in their lives. These dirtbags were some of the greatest skateboarders who ever lived.

But sometimes to avoid the argument I would agree to not hang out with them. And then I would sneak off and do it anyway. And then I would get caught. And then that would become an even bigger argument.

Starting in my mid-30s, when I looked into the mirror, I saw another person in there. Someone I aspired to be. And that person had a lot of tattoos.

I'd had tattoos since I was a teenager, but somewhere along the way something inside me changed. I got way more into them. They became a bigger part of how I saw myself.

One day, I told Andrea that I wanted to get my knuckles tattooed.

"Absolutely not," she told me.

She wanted me to keep everything above the elbow. At this point I was pretty sure there was very little future for me in corporate America. And I couldn't see how my getting tattoos was hurting anyone else. But for some reason that was the line in the sand she chose to draw.

"You're definitely not getting that," she said.

That was tough to hear. I felt like I had only scratched the surface of the person I was going to become. And my wife was shutting me down before I even got started.

A lot of times in those days I would sit around being bitter about stuff, thinking, *I'm not sure why exactly, but something about how today is going really bugs me.* I had a general sense that something was off. I couldn't always put my finger on what it was, though. But this one felt especially blatant. It was like our marriage was no longer an equal partnership. Her word had somehow become the law. I felt like I was being controlled.

I was like, "Wait, do you even know what you just said? You can't just say I definitely can't have something."

Needless to say, she won that argument.

I remember laying in bed by myself later that day, thinking that this was definitely not a good sign for our relationship.

Eventually I did get my way. After my brother passed away, Andrea was letting things slide for a while. I got *Fire* and *Rain* tattooed on my knuckles, after the James Taylor song.

But then I got more tattoos on the sides of my hands. I always went too far, because I always wanted more. And then she was mad at me for that.

Again, I was inviting a mommy to control me, and then getting angry when she actually did it.

Around that time, I started getting some outside help.

There was one day I was having a really rough time. I was just really dark. That wasn't all that uncommon back then.

Rude Jude from Shade 45 did his show in the studio right next to ours. He had a guest on that day named Devlyn Steele, a life coach. Mike Tully—who was the producer of my show at that point—caught Devlyn on his way out of Jude's studio and said, "Hey, do you want to come in and do something on this other show over here? Maybe talk to my friend?"

And then I did an interview with him that was really just him giving me therapy on the radio.

I kept in touch with Devlyn after that. At the start, he was just giving me basic positive affirmation kind of stuff. Waking up with a routine. Already having a plan for the first couple of moments in your day, to get yourself started on the right foot. Talking to the mirror and pumping yourself up a little. Just being positive, more than anything.

Until I started doing that, I didn't even realize how badly I needed it. At that point, I knew I had made mistakes in my marriage. I beat myself up a bunch over those. And if you talk to radio bosses for a couple years, plenty of them can convince you that you're a piece of shit, too. But I didn't realize just how low I had gotten until I started trying to pick myself back up.

Devlyn was a really good friend to me. I started seeing him all the time. I forget if it was free or if he was charging me fifty bucks a session or something, but he definitely wasn't getting rich off me. I think he genuinely wanted to help.

Eventually I convinced Andrea to come along to see him, too. Devlyn tried to help us communicate better and sort some things out.

Some of it was dumb little stuff. For example, Andrea and I would argue about how often I got to go to the gym.

That was not a lie either. I wasn't just saying I wanted to go to the gym so I could sneak off behind Andrea's back and do other stuff. When I was allowed to go to the gym, that's actually where I went. I just wanted to get punched in the face. That was pretty much my only idea of a good time back then.

If it was up to me, after my first MMA fight I would have picked up right where I left off and kept on training. Being sober was still a relatively new thing for me, at least compared to all the years I had spent getting wasted. Outside of work time and family time, I didn't have much else going on. If I didn't have the gym, I didn't have anything that was just for me.

Andrea needed gym time, too, when she could leave me with the kids and have some solo time of her own.

So as crazy as it sounds, Devlyn would listen to us argue

about gym time, and then help us work out an exercise schedule.

He also tried to help us with our sex lives. I was always angling to have more sex and to try new things. She would say, "Well, if you were nicer to me, then sure."

And then we'd go home and I'd try to be a little nicer and maybe things would change a bit for a little while. And then before long we'd wind up right back where we started.

Around this time the radio show really started taking off. You could tell there were people listening. My comedy boxing event Ellismania had made the leap. It had gone from being something we talked about on the radio to being something we did a couple times in a little boxing gym in Hollywood to being this gargantuan event that thousands of people flew to the Hard Rock in Las Vegas to attend.

I signed a new contract and finally really got paid. At the same time, I got out from under the house in Temecula and no longer had to pay anything for that. For the first time since my skating career was still popping off, I was no longer broke. Shit got good.

I had a business manager running my finances. Plus, I had my wife. So I had two people keeping tabs on my cash flow. For the longest time, both of them were telling me that I couldn't spend any money.

Then all of a sudden Andrea found a house for us to rent in Beverly Hills. No more one-bedroom apartment for us.

That was when I felt like I had really made it. Until we moved in, I was convinced I was penniless. I would be wandering around in the backyard of this really nice house in Beverly Hills, staring into a pool that was all mine, and thinking, "So, does this mean I'm rich now?"

Andrea and I were still trying at that point. I even got a face tattoo to save my marriage.

STILL AWESOME

OK, obviously I mostly just wanted a face tattoo. But Andrea was *part* of the reason I got a face tattoo, anyway.

It started as a joke. I was sitting there with Grant, my tattoo artist. I wanted to get something on my face, and I was asking myself, "What can we put on there without getting in trouble with Andrea?"

Grant was one of my "bad" friends in her eyes, which made things even trickier.

I thought maybe I could get away with it if it was just the letter "A." I thought she might be willing to make an exception if it was her first initial.

Obviously, I couldn't be sure that would fly, and as a guy who wasn't even supposed to get forearm tattoos, I couldn't afford to be wrong about something like that. If I played it wrong, that could be like a 'Don't come home tonight' kind of thing.

So Grant was like, "I'll do it with a marker. I'll put a little red paint around it and make it look legit. And if she goes for it, then we'll do it for real."

He drew it up and we sent a picture. And then we waited. I'd say my odds were 50/50.

Well, maybe a little less than that.

She texted me back. It said, "How adorable."

I was amazed she went for it. Grant and I both were. So we put it on for real.

Sure, I was getting a face tattoo out of it, but I honestly also thought that it would stop me from cheating again. I wasn't worried about chasing after girls. Like I said, I wasn't that bad. I was just worried about girls chasing after me. I figured if you saw an "A" on my face, you'd probably want to know why. And once you found out it was because of my wife, you would back off. There's no way you would fuck somebody who had that.

It's a big part of the reason I got elephants tattooed on my back, too. There's four of them. Two parents and two kids. I figured anyone who saw that would get the message.

It was advertising. I was trying to send a message to other people.

I was also trying to send a message to myself: *This is you, man. This is what you're going to do. This is your life.*

I tried. I really did.

I don't think I had that face tattoo for long before Andrea and I split up for good.

I went and talked to Devlyn Steele at his office. He and I agreed that I needed to get divorced. I just didn't know how to tell Andrea.

Devlyn had an idea. He knew that I was attracted to trans people. He was one of the first people I ever really opened up to about that. As I got to know him, I could see that his advice in other areas was really helping. Even Andrea noticed it. So he had earned my trust.

I don't know what I was hoping to gain by telling him about that. Having those kinds of urges had always made me feel like there was something wrong with me. Maybe I thought he could help me make them go away. Or maybe I just wanted someone to tell me that feeling that way didn't make me a monster.

Devlyn thought that I should tell Andrea that her and I needed to split up because I was contemplating sleeping with transgender girls. Not that I had already done that behind her back—just that I was thinking about it.

I think the idea was that everything would be easier if the reason I wanted to leave her was something she couldn't compete with. He thought that would make the separation cleaner.

I wanted to sleep with other females as well, and he knew that, but we decided to leave that bit out.

He said, "Bring her in and we'll tell her together. We'll do it in a way where she doesn't get angry, because trust me, if you get divorced, you want to keep things as friendly as you can."

That last bit was good advice. I'm not so sure about the part with transgender girls.

We sat her down and said what we had planned to say.

"Right," she said. "We're splitting up."

So I guess…it worked, kind of?

Andrea would have left me eventually, I'm sure. Even if I wasn't a cheating bisexual. The two of us were never really meant to be.

The things that neither of us liked about our relationship were never going to go away. She was always going to have to call and check up on me. I was always going to resent seeing that call come up on my screen. And she was always going to resent having to tell me it was time to come home—again—like I was an angry teenager and not her husband and the father of her children.

By the time Devlyn and I talked to her, I think she was already okay with it. She had been deeply in love with me for a long time, but I think by then she was already over it. I was so busy thinking about myself that I just didn't see it.

She put up with more shit than she ever would have if we didn't have kids. Coming from two parents who stayed together, she saw the value in giving the kids a stable home and she was willing to fight for any chance our kids could have that.

But that was the old school way. As I have already said, there are plenty of people who will tell you that it's better for two parents to be divorced and happy than to live under one roof and drive each other crazy. I think by that point in our relationship, Andrea felt like she had no choice but to test that theory.

And once she opened her mind to that possibility, there wasn't anything left to fight for.

I was living a dream I'd had since I was a little kid. I was successful. People cared about what I had to say. Dudes looked up to me and women wanted to have sex with me. People started naming babies after me. Like, more than one. I had signed the big contract and moved to a beautiful house in Beverly Hills.

And then, while Andrea and I figured out what happened next, I moved into the backyard of my dream home and started sleeping in the pool house.

I don't know what you're picturing right now, but where I was sleeping was probably way worse than that. Kato Kaelin definitely had a better set up at OJ's house. It was sketchy. There was asbestos and a bunch of mold stains on the walls. There were also a bunch of beehives I couldn't get rid of. If a pool house could have been haunted, then this would have been the one.

My set up back there was as basic as it gets. I definitely didn't hang any pictures or decorate. The place was really small to begin with, and then we had a bunch of pool stuff stored out there. I had a bed and a phone charger and that was about it.

Again, I don't blame Andrea for us breaking up. Sure, we had our differences. Every couple does. But once Devin came along, Andrea wanted to be normal and grown-up and respectable. And that's understandable. That's the way most people feel. Once kids are in the mix, you want to settle down.

But that didn't work for me. It's just not how I'm built.

People who listened to the radio show knew me as a guy who had a crazy past who was making the adjustment to life with a wife and kids. I think a lot of listeners could relate to that struggle. A lot of them were going through the same thing.

People would call me because they were having problems making it work. When I gave them advice, a lot of times I was telling them things I was also telling myself.

I was going through all the same stuff they were, replacing drugs and sex and being irresponsible with shitty diapers and mortgages and in-laws. That evolution works out for a lot of people. That life can be awesome. It just wasn't for me.

Sometimes you can do the right thing for the wrong reasons. I don't think Andrea and I should have ever been married in the first place. And it was ridiculous to think anything was going to change between us when we got back together. But because we tried to make it work, we have our daughter and our son, and that means in the end all of our efforts were worth it.

When my marriage to Andrea ended, I don't think I could have told you exactly where I was headed. I just knew that where I was wasn't working. I had been an indoor plant. Until I got put outdoors, I didn't know how many things I would be into.

But ready or not, I was about to start finding out.

Chapter 4

Splitting up with your wife and the mother of your children is always a bad time. For me it was even harder because I had let myself become so dependent on Andrea. I had always needed someone to take care of me, and I was losing that, too. I don't have a great track record when I'm on my own.

Of course, there was some potential upside to being single again. I was once again free to do whatever I wanted—for better or for worse.

As I got back on the dating scene, I quickly realized I was dealing with a new generation of women. Before I met Andrea, I slept with a lot of people. But things used to be pretty stock when you got laid.

The first girl I slept with after Andrea used to punch me and scratch me. Not in a mean way, mind you. These were horny sex violence maneuvers. "Punch me in the ribs," she'd say, while we were doing it. Or she would throw some fists at me herself.

It was pretty stupid. But I was so fresh back in the game that those moves seemed exciting. Even when I was a pro skater and I was traveling the world, no one ever asked me to do anything that tweaked. Sex punching is not something I have any desire to do, but still, I would have appreciated that kind of attitude. Back in the nineties, you would have definitely gotten an E for effort in my book for that.

It had been ten years since I'd been with (almost) anyone but Andrea. And now I could go completely HAM and this chick was telling me how into it she was? It was liberating.

I very quickly ended up dating someone else. There were warning signs right away. She wanted to go out a lot. Nightclubs and dinners and that whole thing. I remember trying to pull that off as cheaply as possible, because Andrea was still running the bank account and I was broke. And this girl liked to drink. A lot. That was kind of a red flag. Especially because at that point I was still sober.

Nonetheless, she still became my girlfriend. Right away. That's how I roll. Everybody I've ever met, if I go out with them twice, then it's a serious relationship. I don't fuck around. So I was madly in love with this person for about a week.

The final straw was the night her and I drove out to watch some MMA fights. When we got there, I went to get us some beverages. It was early. The event had just started. They were maybe three fights into a ten-fight card.

I didn't know anybody there, but while I was at the bar some guy came up to me in a hurry.

"Hey, Ellis," he said. "Your chick's in a fight, man!"

I assumed it was a dude who listened to the radio show, because I didn't know him but he definitely knew me.

"My chick?" I said. "I don't have a chick."

The relationship was that new. It took me a second.

Then I realized who he was talking about.

I turned around and saw her in the middle of a crowd. Somebody was grabbing her by the hair and another person had her legs. All in all, there were three or four girls working together to subdue my date.

By the time I started to put together what was going on, she was being hoisted up in the air by the other girls, flat on her back. She balled herself up—pulling her legs in toward her body—and then, boom! She straightened back out and kicked one of the other girls in the face.

That chick went down and then my date threw another one to the ground. She worked herself free, hit the floor, and then picked herself up and started fighting again. She landed multiple shots on people's faces. It was an impressive display, to be honest.

And the whole time I could see she had a smile on her face, like an absolute insane person.

At that point, a bunch of dudes moved in to address the situation. They all looked Brazilian and they all looked way tougher than me.

At the same time, I saw Bas Rutten in the vicinity. For those of you who don't know, Bas Rutten is a very, very nice man. He was also once the UFC Heavyweight Champion. And before that, he was a legendary bouncer and street fighter in Europe. He's like if Patrick Swayze in *Road House* was a real person... who after the movie went on to get a belt in the UFC. There is literally no one else on the planet you would want to tangle with less in this situation than Bas Rutten.

Bas started circling the perimeter. He was keeping tabs. Seeing if he needed to move in and regulate.

I stood back. I was not going in there. I knew that if I did, whatever the hell my chick was mixed up in would become my responsibility.

When they finally pulled her out, she licked some blood off her lips. She did it in a sexual manner. It appeared that fighting was some kind of aphrodisiac for her.

And she didn't do the licking thing to impress me. She didn't know I was watching. That came from her soul.

Someone tapped me on the shoulder. "Those chicks your chick was fighting are all Gracies."

The Gracie family basically introduced Brazilian jiu-jitsu to the world. They're like the royal family of MMA. These were serious people. And my girlfriend of one week had just tried to fight all of them.

It turns out my instinct to stay out of there was even more spot on than I had realized. Between Bas Rutten and several generations of Gracies, if I had gone in there, I could have died.

"That's not my chick," I replied.

I grabbed her and got her out of there.

I never did find out what started the fight. It doesn't really matter. I took her home and that was the end of that relationship.

My new single life soon involved spending a lot of time with a new friend, Benji Madden, of Good Charlotte fame.

Benji listened to Faction, the SiriusXM music channel my show was on at that point. My friend Carey Hart had told me I should get Benji in as a guest, and then him and I hit it off and started hanging out a lot.

We each had something to offer each other. Benji thought I was super motivated, and also that I was tough. He saw that I was a pretty good boxer (for a Hollywood guy anyway) and he wanted that, too. He came to the gym with me a whole bunch. He got really into boxing for a minute there and then eventually he knocked out Riki Rachtman from MTV at an Ellismania.

Meanwhile, I was kind of in awe of him. Benji and his brother, Joel, are super successful, super famous guys. They seemed to have it all figured out. I wanted to know how Benji had pulled off everything he had accomplished so I could copy his approach and do it for myself.

It made me feel cool that someone at that level of success was so ridiculously nice to me. We bro'd down really hard with one another. We were calling each other 'bestie' and he was tweeting about how much he loved me.

I know at least a couple people thought there might have been some gay stuff going on because of how lovey-dovey and over the top we were. I can assure you that was very much not the case.

Benji was single back then and the ladies loved him. He didn't even have to try. Girls would just throw themselves at him.

That was another reason it was awesome being friends with him. As a newly single guy, it was pretty exciting being around a dude who was a magnet for insanely hot women.

That New Year's Eve Benji and Joel took me to Vegas. There was a big party at some club. Benji and Joel were making an appearance there. Not performing, mind you. Just 'appearing.' That's what it's like being that famous. You can get paid a lot of money just to go to a club and be seen there.

The club put the two of them and all their friends like me up on some pedestal thing, up above everybody. There was loud club music blaring, of course—DOOF! DOOF! DOOF!—so it was really hard to talk. We kind of just sat there on display for everyone in the crowd. Like zoo animals.

I was like, "This is the worst thing ever. Everyone's just staring at us. Do you know that?"

To Benji and Joel, that was everyday life. "You just block it out," they said.

It got weird. I didn't like it. At that point, I really wanted to be famous. I assumed becoming famous was the most awesome thing that could ever happen to me. And sure, it was exciting rolling with them and getting in the club through some private side door and then being escorted to the VIP section to go hang out with a bunch of hot chicks. I won't lie. But that event was the worst. That was an eye-opening experience.

I was learning that being a single, eligible guy around that world was pretty overrated, too. I bet it would have been different if I had been ten or fifteen years younger. But I was too old to not be fully aware that every hot chick who wanted to fuck me only wanted to do it because I was Benji's friend, and because she was thinking that maybe, if she put up with me having sex with her for a while, she could stay in the game long enough to fuck him. (This was long before Benji was married, of course.) I could not get that out of my head. And that really took the fun out of it.

I finally started to understand that I actually didn't want to be a part of the fame game. I just wasn't that guy.

There was a girl I knew who lived in Vegas. She was skinny, had big boobs, and was covered in tattoos. For me, that's all it takes.

She hit me up that night when she saw I was in town. Before it was even midnight, I ducked out of the event with the Maddens to meet up with her at the Hard Rock. I had my first drink in a long while with her. And then another. And then after that we went up to her hotel room.

After we closed the door, she was like, "Do you mind if I do something in front of you?"

I'm not the kind of guy who's going to tell people not to do drugs. She took out some pills, crushed them up, and snorted them.

I asked her what she was doing. She told me they were called Roxies. (FYI I later learned Roxy is short for Roxicodone. It's a type of oxycodone. So, legal heroin.)

I could tell she was really enjoying them. And I guess I asked enough questions about them that finally she offered me some.

I can't really blame the alcohol for making me say yes. I'd only had a couple drinks by then because I was really trying not to overdo it. I'd had some weird heart problems back when I was with Andrea. That was one of the major reasons I stopped drinking in the first place. I didn't just think drinking was bad for me—I thought it might well *kill* me. Ever since my father passed away from a heart attack at 53, pedaling a bicycle up a mountain in Australia, I was convinced the same fate was waiting for me. It made me panicky about drinking at all.

But then this girl invited me to snort some off her ass. That was all the extra enticement I needed.

I have taken painkillers before. With all the skateboard injuries and broken bones I've had over the years, I've done more than my fair share. But snorting them wasn't the same. At all.

I got really high, really quick. It freaked me out. Which made me panic even more than the thought of drinking did. Which made me drink more, to make the drug panic go away.

It was a vicious circle. Long story short I ended up hellaciously hammered.

Later on that night I called Andrea from the Circle Bar, downstairs at the Hard Rock.

I knew she had already moved on from me. I think she was trying to keep me from knowing it, but Josh Richmond—my co-host on the radio show back them—saw a picture of her with some younger dude on social media and told me about it.

Still, I told her now that I loved her.

"I love you, too," she said. "But you need to move on."

I felt so bad the next day. I looked like shit. Benji and Joel had stayed at a different hotel, and by the time I got back there, they were like, "What the fuck happened to you?"

I woke up with the worst hangover, and the deepest regret. I believed that I had already dodged a bullet in my life. There had been a period of time back in Australia when I used to get really drunk at the bars, and then go get hookers and heroin. Not once. Many times. I built up a little habit of smoking heroin, and then one time I shot it up with a couple of sketchy hookers. They robbed me and left me for dead in a park.

I was a total mess back them. I easily could have died.

And then when I moved to America and my skating career

finally started making me money, I became a train wreck all over again. I truly believe that, by the end of my skating career, I could have killed myself with drinking and cocaine. I don't think anyone who knew me back then and saw me at my lowest would have been shocked if I had accidentally ended myself.

But I got out of it. I left that life behind.

I had been pretty much completely sober for four years. No drinking. No weed. And definitely no coke and no heroin—legal or otherwise. I had surrounded myself with people who did not live like that either.

Radio had given me a second chance. Being a husband and a father had given me a second chance, too. I knew how insanely lucky I was to have my skateboard career go to shit and then to land on my feet with a second career that was just as good. Arguably better. I didn't want to piss that away. I didn't see any third chances waiting for me if radio fell through.

Being sober was a big part of who I was on the radio. It was a big part of my life, period. It was important to me.

That doesn't mean it was easy, and that doesn't mean I was perfect. The whole time I was with Andrea, the desire to use was there, just like it is for all addicts.

And yes, there were windows of weakness. I'm sure plenty of addicts can relate. Here and there, I snuck a beer or a glass of wine and got a little buzz. Maybe on an airplane or something like that. That happened two or three times while I was married. I kept that to myself. I didn't tell Andrea. I didn't tell anyone.

But for the most part I was fully committed. I didn't trust myself with drugs or alcohol. Plus, I knew I was so bad at hiding it that Andrea would figure it out right away. It was always that way, even back when we first met. If I smoked weed, she would know. If I had two beers, she would know. It was too risky.

The closest I got to falling off the wagon had happened during a trip to Mexico. After my brother Stevie died, and not too long after my father passed away, my brother Lee and some friends of ours from Australia all went on a boys' trip down there. Those dudes went off, to put it mildly.

I know a lot of Americans think Australians wrestle giant snakes on their way to school every morning and drink humongous cans of Fosters for breakfast. For the most part Australia is not really like that. At least not now. It's really just like a shitty America.

But on this trip, Lee and our friends might have lived up to some of those stereotypes. It was an old school Ellis throwdown.

There was over-the-top drinking. There were drugs. There were arrests. I had every intention of being the sober guy on the trip, and then within four hours I was smoking weed. I was going to leave it at that, but then we were on a boat and everyone was encouraging me.

"We're not on American soil, Jase. And we're not on Australian soil, either."

That was the argument someone made for why drinking was somehow justifiable for me under the circumstances. Maritime law, I guess. As usual I didn't take all that much convincing. I had a margarita, ready or not.

But that was as far as it went. I still didn't get drunk.

Andrea was calling me the whole time, anyway.

"What the fuck? Where are you? Why didn't you pick up?"

With my track record I guess you couldn't blame her. But on that trip, she didn't have much to worry about. I didn't need anyone else to stop me or to slow me down. I was not interested in the slightest.

After my brother died, I became even more scared of dying than I already was after my father passed away. Now I was doubly sure that whatever got my brother and my father was coming for me, too. And whatever that thing was, it didn't need any help from my dumb ass.

I kept that up straight through my marriage. I was still on the straight and narrow even when Andrea and I were splitting up, straight through a bunch of sad sober nights, all by myself, out in the pool house.

And now here I was, a father, falling face first into that same shit all over again.

Laying there in bed in Vegas on New Year's morning, all I could think was, *I'm going to die.*

That might not have been the first time I've ever had that thought. But it was the first time since I had met Andrea that I might have been okay with it. I felt really sad about being here on planet Earth. I wasn't about to get a gun and shoot my brains out. But I thought that if something bad were to accidentally happen to me, that maybe that wouldn't be the worst thing. For everybody.

The radio show was doing really well at that point. Everything was looking up. And I felt like I was about to piss it all away.

In that moment, I felt weak. I felt like I could slip back to being the guy I used to be. I could feel the bad guy inside of me who might choose doing drugs over going to work. I felt like I could easily wind up jobless.

A part of the panic might have been a little exaggerated. You can get a hangover so bad that anxiety sets in the next morning and everything seems even worse than it is. But most of that depression had been there before that night, and it was still there long after the hangover wore off. I felt beaten down, and I didn't feel strong enough to pick myself back up.

That's why I decided I needed to go to rehab.

At least, that's what I told everybody. Maybe that's what I even told myself. I mean, I am an addict and that was a dangerous road I was going down. Nothing good was going to happen if I kept that shit up.

But secretly there was more to the story: I had a plan. I was going to get my wife back.

I didn't think I could survive on my own. The solo path I had set out on clearly wasn't working, so to me it made sense to try—again—to get back on the road I had been on before everything went to shit.

Get your shit together, I told myself. *You're not built to live that life. Not anymore, anyway. Get on the straight and narrow. Get sober. Get your wife back.*

I think most of us have similar thoughts from time to time. We bottom out, or maybe just get a little too loose. And then we decide to turn off all the bad stuff and put it behind us for good. Until we wind up back in the shit again. And then decide to turn over a new leaf yet again. That's how it was for me anyway. New leaf after new leaf. Just the same plan, over and over again. Believing, or maybe just hoping, that this time would be different.

I didn't tell Andrea I was planning to win her back. Not that I needed to. She knew how I thought. When we split up, she knew there was an excellent chance I wouldn't be able to survive by myself and that I would come crawling back. And she wasn't wrong.

"Don't try to get back with me," she said, when I told her I was going to rehab.

She was concerned that I would make the kids think their parents were going to work things out, and she didn't want me misleading them. So I didn't tell the kids about my plan. But that doesn't mean I gave up on it. I thought I had an ace up my sleeve.

I could picture it: After I was there for a while, Andrea would come in and sit down with me and a therapist. The therapist would tell Andrea that I was an addict, and that all the mistakes I had made were a result of my addictions. They would tell her that I had been doing the work and making progress.

They would say that they could cure me, and that I would no longer be the man Andrea was afraid I would be if we started over again together.

I thought they would give me a hall pass. I thought they would cosign my bullshit.

Right before I went in, some chick I had hooked up with posted a dick pic I had sent her on the internet. Andrea called me as soon as she saw it on Twitter. Not that she needed to. By that time, several hundred of my own social media followers had been kind enough to let me know it was up there.

I had already been on *The Howard Stern Show* with a bunch of M&M's shoved up my foreskin. Way more people had seen those pictures and they're still out there any time anyone gets bored and wants to Google my penis. At least this one was from a flattering angle.

I didn't really care. But that was still one last little kick in the balls on my way in to fix myself.

This was going to be my first experience with rehab in America, but I had been to a couple places back in Australia. The first one was a camp for people who had mental breakdowns and stuff like that. That one was run by a naturopath my mum knew. They sent me there when I was a teenager.

The naturopath said I had anger issues. But really I think I was sent there because I had been caught sleeping with my mum's best friend…and her best friend's sister. I think my mum just wanted a quick and easy way to put that behind us. She just thought, *I know how to handle this. I'll send him to a camp!*

I had not been on board with the plan. I was like, "I'm a teenager. Your friend and her sister are adults. *They're* the ones fucking *me. I'm* fine."

But it wasn't my decision. I think it was easier for her to treat me as the problem than to deal with what her friends had done, so off I went. That rehab experience memorably concluded with me and an old man naked in a pool taking turns cradling each other, for God knows what reason.

And then after that, the lady who was married to the naturopath seduced me, too, and then the naturopath physically threatened me because I had fucked his wife.

The next time I tried an Aussie rehab place it was for drugs and alcohol. I was in my mid-to-late twenties. I don't know if there was any one incident that sparked it. I was always getting wasted and doing insane shit, so it could have been any one of a million things.

My mother is a recovered alcoholic and so was her husband at the time. Both of them were always saying I was out of control and that I needed to get help.

I think I had temporarily broken up with my girlfriend or something. I drank a ridiculous amount of alcohol and took a ton of ecstasy, and then went to my mum's house to cry about my life. While I was shit-faced I agreed I had a problem and then she held me to it the next day, after I sobered up.

I checked in one night and had an appointment with a therapist the next day. I told her about my bisexual tendencies—I think because that secret had always weighed on me, and because I knew this was one place I could spill the beans and know it wasn't going to get back to my friends. When you're hiding a heavy secret like that, you look for opportunities to come up for air wherever you find them.

The therapist made it very clear she was not prepared to handle a conversation like that. It was a very different time. She was expecting to talk about drugs and alcohol and I had thrown her an unexpected twist.

She basically said, "I don't see why you're in here. It sounds like you just need to be more open with yourself."

My reaction was, "Oh, so…I'm fine then?"

And then I texted my brother and said, "Can you come pick me up?"

I don't remember if I hopped the fence to get away or if I just walked out the door. I know I didn't talk to anyone on my way out. No one tried to stop me. It was a government-run place. That was the problem. Nobody cared. If you actually needed help you probably weren't going to get it. You could just say, "I don't know why I'm here. I don't think I need any help," and they would say, "Then you probably don't. Off you go!" Because, as we all know, addicts would never lie to your face so they don't have to quit.

The place I went to this time around was way better. Devlyn Steele helped me find it, and so did Kevin Zinger, my manager at the time. Zinger ran the record label that my band Taintstick was on. He knew a place that gave a discount for musicians, so he hooked that up for me.

It was this really beautiful place up in Malibu. The house used to be owned by Pierce Brosnan. I got the biggest room, so I think I can officially say I have slept in the same room as the shittiest James Bond ever.

There were five or six other people at the rehab with me. There was a really young kid who took a bunch of Vicodin or whatever and fell asleep on his arm for so long it died on him. He was wearing a wrist guard the whole time I was there. They weren't sure if the arm was going to come back for him or not.

There was an old rich guy from the Midwest. His wife had left him and he was drinking himself to death. He would hang out in the backyard and smoke cloves continuously, all day, every day.

And there was some sex addict chick who kept doing the splits in front of me, trying to get me to fuck her. But that was never close to happening. I was on a mission. I was there to fix my life and win my wife back.

Despite the fact that I put my life on hold and checked myself into rehab, I wasn't really struggling with alcohol and drugs all that much. That night in Vegas had been a whopper, but unlike most people who get help at a facility, I went in sober. I had already been clean for three days. I even did a radio show right before I drove there. I wasn't stinging for anything. Looking back at it now, it was more like a safety precaution.

I'm sure lots of junkies would tell you they don't have a problem and don't need rehab. But I'm pretty sure if you took a poll of everyone I was in there with, they would have said I was the one who was most intent on getting out with a clean head.

When I showed up, they were like, "Do you need detox?"

I told them I already had. I don't think they hear that much.

I said, "I'm here to get the job done. Nobody forced me to come here. I begged to get in. I'm ready to move on with my life."

They told me I needed sleeping pills. I think they give those to everybody. Most people show up at rehab jonesing for something, so while you're coming off stuff, the sleeping pills help you go to sleep and wake up at a certain time. They start to put you on a routine.

They gave me Trazodone. I liked it. I'm still on it. It's great. If I want to stay up all night, I can. But if I don't want to stay up and my brain decides to fuck with me and keep me up anyway, I take that and I go to sleep. For once, Big Pharma nailed it.

There were certain things about rehab I didn't like. One big thing was all the smoking. I hate cigarette smoke and it was just constant in there. Everyone was smoking cigarettes all the time and chewing their Nicorette.

And everyone was bitching all the time. Everything was bad for everybody, constantly. And they loved to go on and on about it and wallow in their misery.

The worst part, for me, was when they put us on a bus and took us to AA meetings. I was rolling my eyes the whole time. AA can be great for many people. I know that. It has saved all kinds of lives. But not all meetings are great, and the program is not for everybody.

I would be looking around thinking, *Half you motherfuckers are lying.*

Maybe most of the people at that meeting who said they were sober were telling the truth. But I suspected a lot of the people who talked about how they'd stopped drinking had started doing something else instead. No one who's sober smokes that many cigarettes. If you've ever been anywhere near the vicinity of an AA meeting, I'm sure you know what I'm talking about. It's insane.

The religious part of AA was also hard to swallow. I got weird about that. I mean, I did it. I held people's hands and prayed to God to help keep me sober. I didn't think it was going to help. But I did try.

A couple of gay dudes at those AA meetings wanted to sponsor me. I got weird on them, too. I thought they probably just wanted to have sex with me. There's a decent chance I was wrong about that. They might have just been really nice guys who wanted to help. That's just where my mind naturally goes. If people are being nice to me, I assume it's because they want something.

But for the most part I liked rehab. I liked the routine. I liked going to bed early. I liked getting up early. I liked having my breakfast every day. I wanted to go for runs and go down to the beach and they wouldn't let me leave the premises. That pissed me off. But aside from that, if you really do want to do the work, it feels good to put aside the day-to-day bullshit and focus on fixing yourself.

All of the professionals there agreed I was addicted to drugs and alcohol. They diagnosed me with sex addiction, too. I was told that I couldn't have sex, and that I couldn't jerk off, either. I felt like they were trying to diagnose me with every addiction they could think of.

STILL AWESOME

A big part of being sober is helping other addicts, and in places like that they kind of overdo it. Everybody wants to help, partially because they're nice and because they care, but also partially because helping you helps them with their own recovery.

That's the way recovery works. The worse an addict you are and the more you're stinging to fall off the wagon, the more you want to sponsor other people. Helping other addicts can become your new addiction. Everybody wanted to sponsor me and give me phone numbers for all these other people who also wanted to help me. It was insane how many phone numbers I got in there.

I'm very gullible. I just said thank you and went along with every suggestion and every diagnosis anyone gave me.

In addition to the meetings, I was talking to three or four therapists a day. I had nothing to do all day but talk.

Slowly but surely, we started getting everything out in the open.

Everything.

Chapter 5

Therapists at rehab places want to hear everything about your life. In particular, they want to know about any traumatic circumstances that might have started you on the path to self-medicating with drugs and alcohol.

I barely knew where to begin. I've got so many demons. As far back as I can remember I was always trying to numb myself with whatever I could get my hands on, because I was always hurting.

When I first sat down with a therapist to talk about the source of my problems, I couldn't put my finger on any one thing. I started with my brother Stevie and my dad both dying. I've got issues about those. Those both fucked me up. Stevie's death was particularly at the forefront of my mind, because it was fresh.

I felt a lot of guilt. I had come to America to be a famous skate dickhead. It was always all about me. After my father passed away, I could have gone home and helped Stevie. Maybe I could have been there the night and the morning after when him and his wasted friends were making a bunch of dumb decisions that ultimately led to his death. Maybe I could have stopped it.

At times I was disgusted with myself. I felt like it was all my fault.

We talked about that. We talked about my dad, too.

The way I thought about my dad had changed a lot since he died. He was a crazy person. And he did a lot of bad things in his life. But when he passed away, he was still my hero.

As I had become a father and cleaned up my life, though, I started to look at who he was and some of the decisions he had made in a different light. And what's more, since he had passed away, I had heard more stuff about him that was crazy—even by my dad's already crazy standards.

I found out that at one point, near the end of his life, he owned a house that was used to grow a bunch of weed with hydroponics. It sounded like a pretty big operation. He was just a part of it. He was the guy who technically owned the house, because he had good credit (which is insane, since my father went bankrupt multiple times).

I think my dad was also shacking up part time with a stripper at that house. She worked at the same strip club where I met my first really serious girlfriend.

They had to shut that operation down. Apparently, the feds were getting wind of it so everyone wisely decided to walk away.

And that was just the tip of the iceberg. After Tiger was born, me and Andrea brought him over to Australia to introduce our new baby to his family. And while we were there, one my dad's old friends, a guy named Roger, started dropping some stuff on me. You could tell he was kind of enjoying it.

"You know the craziest thing, Jay?" Roger asked me one day, when me and him were alone.

I didn't really want to know the answer to the question, but he kept talking anyway.

"Your dad was available."

"What are you talking about, dude?" I said.

"He was fucking *available*. You could get him. On the internet.

You could look him up, and he'd fuck your wife."

The dude knew exactly where my mind went when he said that.

"I know what you're thinking, Jay," he went on. "That he did the gay shit. But no. I called him. I pretended to be a guy calling him to fuck my wife. I was like, 'Do you do gay shit, too?' He was like, 'No. Fuck off. I don't do that shit, mate.' Then I was like, 'Ah, it's Roger anyway.'"

Roger had a good laugh. It was a big joke to him.

I've been around enough to know that this story did not add up at all. My dad was 53 years old when he died. Even if my dad had been able to deliver the goods like nobody's business, absolutely no one is hiring a 50-year-old man to bang their wife. Even if you were the kind of husband who really wanted to watch that happen, there is no shortage of men half his age who would gladly do it for free. It's crazy.

On top of that, I was told my father was performing live sex shows. Like, up on a stage. For people to watch. This made even less sense to me than the idea that he had been a gigolo.

Here's a story to help explain why that is: Shortly before he passed away, my father took my brother Lee all around Australia so Lee could race moto and get a career started. My brother Lee was a privateer. In moto terms, that means a guy who isn't sponsored, and who has to pay his own way to every race and be responsible for maintaining his own bike.

Along the way, my dad won the Australia Motocross Championship in the Over-50 class. He wasn't the quickest dude. He was good. Probably top five-level ability. But while Lee was going around the country doing his races, my dad was doing all the senior races, too, and because he was at the most events out of all the Over-50's competitors, he was able to rack up the most points. That's really why he won.

Anyway, he won that championship and my brother also won Amateur of the Year. I flew back from America to go to the awards ceremony. There's a picture from that ceremony of me and Lee and my dad. The two of them look petrified because they both knew they were going to have to get up for five seconds when their name was announced and say thank you into a microphone.

I was like, "How are we all related?"

I couldn't understand how being the center of attention could not be fun for them.

I said, "I will go up there for both of you, and grab the microphone, and while I am up there, I will make up a fucking song about you, too!"

I love that kind of thing. Getting on a microphone in front of a group of people was even more exciting to me back then, before I had a radio show and got paid to ramble on about stupid shit for three hours every day.

But that's the way they were. My dad wasn't faking. He wasn't just trying to pretend he was the strong silent type. He hated the microphone. Hated the guy introducing him. Hated the people looking at him. Hated getting up when his name was called. And when he sat back down after he muttered his thanks, he was still in hell for 15 more minutes, just because he thought people might still be looking at him.

That's not just him. That's old school Australian stuff. A lot of older people in Australia, if you point a camera at them, they run away. Or they cover their eyes. Like the camera is going to swallow their soul or something. They really don't like it.

The point is this: You're telling me a guy like that got up on stage and put on a sexual performance?

I don't even know where such a spectacle would have taken place. I got up to some pretty shady shit in Melbourne in my day, but I never saw anything like that. If that happened, it had to be in such a grungy, dirty, creepy part of town.

A little while after that visit to Australia with Tiger, I also heard from the stripper chick my dad had been involved with. It was the one he was shacking up with in the hydroponic weed house. She tried reaching out to me on MySpace. She sounded like she had even *more* stuff she wanted to tell me.

I was like, "Thank you. I've heard plenty. Out of respect to my stepmum, please don't ever talk to me again."

I didn't need to know any of this stuff. Roger—the guy who was telling me all this shit—didn't get that. After everything, I was still my dad's son. He was probably thinking, *Jay's a tough guy. He lives in America. He's a big man now. He can take it.*

But you can't just hit somebody with that. For years that fucked with me. I didn't believe all of it. But I also didn't *not* believe it. Plus, I was sure there was more to the story than even Roger knew.

I really didn't know *what* to believe. I still don't. With my dad, anything was possible.

On top of all the therapists at rehab, there was also a hypnotist. One day she did that thing where they knock you out and control your mind, and then the therapist lady started running me back through my childhood.

Eventually she figured out that I had been abused when I was little. Obviously, she perked up when she heard that.

"Oh, you were molested?" she said. "Tell me a little bit more about that."

That had always been extremely difficult to talk about. When I was younger, I went years at a time without bringing it up.

Once at a skateboard contest I started drinking with another skater, a guy I considered a friend, and I guess I drank enough that it just came out.

The guy looked at me and said, "Why the fuck are you telling me that?"

People didn't know how to talk about that kind of stuff back then. A lot of people *still* don't. And me and this guy were kids.

Him and I were never really friends in the same way after that. I remember learning a big lesson from that. *Right*, I thought. *Don't tell anybody about that anymore.*

So for the most part I locked it away.

But the therapist dove in more and more. She made me retrace a bunch of moments in my life until I started seeing them in a different way. The therapist and the hypnotist both worked on me for a week, until I started seeing things in my memory that I hadn't been able to see before.

One time, way back in Australia, when I was skateboarding on the Big Day Out tour, I did a ton of acid and then started talking to an invisible friend about how I had been molested. I was basically blacked out, but when I came to, my girlfriend was freaking out about what I had been saying. She called my mum immediately.

I expected my mum to say I was imagining things.

Instead, she said, "I thought you forgot about that."

After I got home from the tour, I went back to my dad's house and he brought it up.

"So you think you got molested?" he asked.

I said yes.

"You think it was me?"

"Nah."

"Oh. Okay," he said.

And that was the end of that conversation.

That memory wasn't new to me. I even talked about it my first book. But as I told the therapist about that incident, something terrible clicked inside me.

I am a dad. If Tiger was abused and he mentioned it to me 20 years later, would I just ask if he suspected it was me and then leave it at that? That's insane.

After I talked to my dad that day, I remember I got right on the train and went to the skate ramp. My brain immediately shifted to a different subject. *What skateboard tricks am I going to be doing today?* I asked myself. Meanwhile, I shoved that conversation with my dad as far down inside my brain as it would go.

And that's pretty much where it stayed, for years.

Looking back to that from rehab, I started to see that I had pushed that conversation out of my conscious mind for a reason. I was doing it to keep myself from facing reality.

I realized there were only two possible scenarios: The first was that my dad knew someone had molested me and didn't do anything about it. And that option didn't really check out. This was the same guy who drove my brother Lee all over Australia for a year to help him with his moto career. He wasn't a hands-off father. For all his faults, he definitely gave a shit about his kids.

The second scenario was worse. And all of a sudden, that one seemed way more likely.

I was hysterical for a second. I immediately called my mum. I told her what I had remembered.

I thought she would tell me I was wrong. I thought she would say, "Look, that's not what happened. I know you think that, but you've got it all wrong. I know who did it."

But she didn't. She didn't even hesitate.

"I'm really sorry," she said.

She almost agreed too quickly, if that makes sense. Like she wasn't surprised I was telling her this. Like she always knew—or always feared—this day would come

Thinking back, she had reacted the same way when my ex-girlfriend called her from the Big Day Out tour, that day I had first remembered being molested.

"I thought he forgot about that," she had said then. Like she had *never* forgotten, and maybe just hoped *I* would.

Talking to her now, she was mostly just sympathetic.

"I'm so sorry," she said. "Now that I think about it, it makes sense. I had my suspicions," she continued. "But how can anybody think that anybody would do that?"

It hurts to hear your mother say that she should have known. That she could have—and maybe even *should* have—stepped in and stopped my dad from abusing me. I was thinking, *Yeah, I wish you had figured it out, too.*

But I appreciated that she was at least trying to understand my point of view and trying to believe me.

I called my stepmum next. Marn, the woman my dad married after he left my mum, who up until that point had been my mum's best friend. Marn is my half-brothers Lee and Stevie's mum.

She seemed more inclined to defend my dad. But she also started apologizing for how she had acted toward me when I was growing up.

"I was so mean to you back then," she said.

Which is true. Once her and my dad had my brothers, I had always got the very clear sense that she would have preferred if I wasn't in the picture.

But that wasn't what was important at that moment. She wasn't the reason I was in rehab talking to hypnotists and therapists all day. I guess you just never know what high-pressure conversations are going to bring out of people.

During those two phone calls both Marn and my mum both brought up another story from when I was four or five. One day I started saying that someone had done something to me. I said someone had put their penis in my mouth.

I said that it was my dad.

At that time, my mum had asked me, "Are you sure?"

STILL AWESOME

And I said, "He had red hair."

I was told that I was mistaken. We had a neighbor who babysat me sometimes, and he had red hair. I was told that the neighbor did it.

Supposedly after I said what I said, my dad went over to the neighbor's house and told the guy, "Stay the fuck away from my son."

And then he left it at that.

That didn't check out.

My father was a lunatic with the most insane temper I have ever witnessed. I've seen my father get into disagreements with total strangers over absolutely nothing, and then punch their teeth out.

Australia was a rough and tumble place when I was a kid. Fist fights weren't all that out of the ordinary. But even by local standards my dad was still really, really bad. At one point he had to get plastic surgery on his face because some bouncers put him in an alleyway and stomped on his head while he was unconscious.

Actually, that was probably the only romantic story I've ever heard my mum tell about him. Supposedly they were at a bar, and some dude said something to my mum, and then my dad jumped on his back and started punching him in the face until the guy fell on the ground. The bouncers came to break it up and so he fought them, too. Then they beat the fuck out of my dad and dragged him outside. I think they fucked with my mum a little bit too. They might have pushed her around a bit. That's why he took on everybody. They dragged him downstairs and pulled him out back and then stomped on his head. He needed surgery afterward to put his face back together.

I was 10 when she told me that story. It came from my mum, so it might not actually be true. But that's the kind of person we're talking about here.

The story her and Marn were telling me now about the neighbor just didn't add up. I'm not my father. I'm old and wise and I have never punched people for no reason. But if my son told me that a neighbor sucked his dick, that neighbor would be fucking gone. I would end him. Guaranteed.

When all this happened my father was 25 years old and not wise at all. He *warned* the guy? Come on. It sounded to me like he knew what he was doing when he went and scared the shit out of that poor guy. He was well aware that his warning was total bullshit.

It now seemed pretty apparent that everyone had switched the story around and made little four-year-old me believe that I had been wrong.

Maybe they tried so hard to change the truth that they almost believed it themselves.

I also talked to the therapists about feeling attracted to men and to transgender women. Like I have said, every time I talked to a mental health professional the subject usually came up pretty quickly because I knew it was a rare occasion to get it off my chest and to know it was going to stay in the room.

I started right at the beginning.

My first experience with a transgender woman happened at a dinner party in Australia when I was 19. The hosts were these people who controlled all the skateboard distribution throughout the country. I think they were on the list of the top ten richest Aussies. It was a big dinner for all the people that worked for them—in marketing and sales and all that—plus a whole bunch of skaters, including me.

There was this girl there. She was tall and skinny, and she was going for a Cindy Crawford-type look. I was super into that. This was the heyday of the Cindy Crawford era. Although she pulled that look off pretty well, I would still imagine it was clear

STILL AWESOME

to everyone in the room that she had not been born as a woman.

I don't really remember interacting with any transgender ladies before her. One time, when I was really young, there was a belly dancer at a restaurant who might have been transgender who seemed like she might be into me. I was with my mum and her friends at the time, and they were all drawing attention to it and making jokes. But I was just a kid at the time. Plus, I was there with my mum. That situation definitely wasn't going to escalate.

But now, a bunch of years later, this Cindy Crawford lady kept giving me the eye, and during the course of that dinner party someone gave me two E bombers. I had already been drinking, and this girl kept eyeballing me from across the table. So when the ecstasy kicked in, I was like, *It's on*.

I had a serious long-term girlfriend at the time. She was there with me at the party.

We were both sleeping with other people. I wasn't doing anything behind her back.

There was this other skateboard dude there. Me and my girlfriend had already had a threesome with him, so I knew my girlfriend was into him. I suggested that the two of them head off together while I made a new friend. That was fine by him and my girlfriend, so the four of us went our separate ways.

By then me and this girl were rubbing on each other. If I was trying to be smooth about what I was about to get up to, I definitely didn't pull it off. Drunk people on ecstasy never do. When the two of us left I think it was pretty obvious to everyone what was going on.

This girl and I got a taxi and she took me to some brothel and snuck us in a back window. She knew someone who worked there because at some point she had worked there, too.

Later that same night, I went back to my girlfriend's house. When I got there, I gathered that the skater guy she had left with had come in a little too hot. He was still trying to sleep with her, but by now she had changed her mind and wasn't into it.

She was like, "This guy's fucking still here. You fucking took forever. What the fuck?"

She always did have a way with words.

There was another skater there too. He was really drunk. He started saying, "Ellis is a fag," right in front of me.

I didn't know what to say. I definitely didn't play it cool or give him some inspiring speech about freeing his mind and becoming accepting of alternative lifestyles. I just froze.

I don't know if my response would have mattered anyways. This was the '90s. That's a long time ago. At that time, if you did gay stuff—even just one time—to most people, that meant you were gay. And gay was bad. End of story.

That was the beginning of some people in the skate world telling anyone who would listen that I was gay. My girlfriend did the same thing. At the party that night she might have pretended she was okay with it. But she wasn't, and as soon as she got the chance, she started telling everyone what I had done, in detail.

The Cindy Crawford chick and I became a thing after that. I started seeing her on the side, and my girlfriend started seeing some other dude on the side, too. Eventually my girlfriend fell in love with that other guy and left me for him.

That wouldn't be my only experience with gay men or transgender women in Australia. I used to do tons of ecstasy with friends of mine at clubs. And then afterward, sometimes, instead of heading down to where the whorehouses were, I would go to Melbourne's gay area, to the clubs there. Cross dressers would blow me in the bathrooms.

That wasn't necessarily my favorite thing to do or something I felt like I needed to do. It wasn't like, *Oh, I'm feeling kind of gay today!* It was just a way to get off quickly, without any effort.

There was no internet in those days. There was no Tinder or Craigslist. There was no other way to get anonymous sex in a hurry. I had stumbled into these places accidentally and then found out that there were guys there who were really into me.

In my mind, I was just trying to get off. I was an addict, and I was trying to get every hit I could. This was an easy source for me to tap into.

I wasn't doing anything *to* anybody. I wasn't making out with people. No penis ever touched my face. I'd just get jerked off or get some weird no-conversation blowjob. I wasn't taking anybody there seriously or looking for a boyfriend. I wasn't having heart-to-hearts with anyone. Not that there's anything wrong with doing any of the above, of course. That just wasn't why I was there.

And it only really happened when I was shitfaced. To this day, I don't know how I physically managed to pull it off. By the time I got there, I would be hammered. Just completely gone. Lost. I don't know how I stood up or walked around.

"Damn you, legs," I used to say. "How dare you keep me up?"

If only they had buckled. If I was laying on the ground, covered in my own vomit, then no one would have been willing to fuck me. But somehow I kept going, like some wasted useless sex zombie.

I don't know how I even made it look like I was aware of what was happening. I can't imagine how I talked, or what I talked about. Wasted me should have failed with 100% of the people I went up to 100% of the time. But that wasn't the case.

For whatever reason, that stuff didn't follow me all that much to America. When my radio show was still just getting started, we used to be on at nighttime. There was barely anybody listening. And one time we brought in two of the transgender prostitutes who hung out at a taco stand on Santa Monica Blvd., up the street from the studio.

We didn't have many guests in those days. And that taco stand was a full-on scene. You'd see a bunch of transgender girls hanging out in the parking lot, night after night. You couldn't help but be curious about what the hell was going on over there.

Knowing all this stuff about me, you might assume I was playing dumb when I asked those two girls who came on the show about what their lives were like. But I wasn't. At that point I had never picked up a transgender prostitute in Hollywood. I was really experienced when it came to some things with gay and transgender people, but in other areas I was just as ignorant as everyone else.

There was one time, years and years ago—way before I married Andrea—when I came to L.A. and got totally blacked out. When I came back to my senses, the sun was coming up, I was missing both of my shoes and one of my socks, and I was walking down Sunset Boulevard with a half a six-pack of Mike's Hard Lemonade. I don't know what I did that night, before I came to. But I know for sure I did something. And I'm fairly certain it was with a transgender girl.

But that was really it for me, as far as L.A. went. I felt like even if I was just talking to transgender girls hanging on the street in L.A., I was going to be seen. I was bound to get busted.

Hell, even if I just went through Boystown in West Hollywood, I was paranoid someone would see me and want to know what I was doing there—even though tons of straight people go to Boystown all the time. It's not a crazy thing to do. There's, like, good places to get burgers there, too. You don't have to go there because you're trying to get laid.

But I never wanted to take any chances and blow my cover.

Having said that, obviously I did keep certain parts of my past a secret on the radio for a long time.

If you listened to my show really early on, or if you read my first book, you might remember the story I've told of the time

STILL AWESOME

I went to Amsterdam, hired a hooker, and then found out that the prostitute I had hired had a penis. I joked about how I only put two and two together when an erection came in contact with my butthole and achieved 'suction.'

For the record, that wasn't a lie. I was really young when that happened. That was before I started hooking up with the Cindy Crawford chick.

I really did think that was a girl, and I really was shocked when she bent me over and started poking me in the butt. I honestly thought it was a thumb. Once I saw my mistake, I pulled up my pants and politely got out of there.

But in other instances, obviously I felt the need to leave things out or stretch the truth.

I definitely never mentioned any non-hetero behavior from back in Melbourne in my early days on the radio. And in my first book, I talked about how I used to get wasted and tell my first ex-wife, "I don't know if I'm gay." In the book, I blamed my confusion about my sexual orientation on me having been molested as a kid. But looking back at that now, obviously the way I told that story was just me bobbing and weaving around the truth.

I had already had encounters when I told her that. I only said that because, if I got drunk enough and honest enough, I already knew damn well that I wasn't completely straight.

I was seeing a bunch of different therapists at rehab, and they all had their own opinions as to what was wrong with me and how I could be fixed. The sex therapist definitely saw a big connection between my abuse by my father and my sexual orientation. Her basic message was: You're in here because of your sex addiction and your abuse. Your father molested you when you were a kid, and now adult you wants to have sex with strange women and men and transgender people because in a weird, unhealthy way it allows you to relate to your father again.

And she wasn't totally off base. There's definitely a connection. According to my current therapist—who's far wiser than I'll ever be—there are three factors that can affect sexual orientation. You can be born that way, you can have a certain kind of parenting that bends you in that direction, or there can be a sexual thing that happens when you're young.

That sounds pretty believable to me. I don't know the science behind that, but if I had to diagnose myself, I think it's most likely that I turned bisexual from being molested when I was a kid.

That still doesn't make it a choice. Believe me, for several decades my choice was to *not* be this way. I tried, for half of my life. It doesn't work that way.

But at the time I wasn't ready to face that. So I went along with what the therapist was telling me: It's not your fault. And if you can get a hold of it and go to sex therapy, then you'll be cured and you'll be straight and you'll be worth going out with again.

After two weeks of hard work and some brutal revelations, the day I had been waiting for finally arrived.

In a way, the therapists had given me exactly what I had hoped they would. It was all going to be okay now. They encouraged me to bring in Andrea so we could tell her the good news.

The door opened and Andrea walked in. She was all dolled up. She had pulled out all the stops. She was as beautiful as I had ever seen her.

The second I saw her I knew I was fucked.

We were over.

That was her way of telling me there was no fucking chance we were getting back together.

As my therapist broke down what she and I had been talking about and what the plan was going to be, I was cringing with every word that came out of her mouth. I knew there was no point.

STILL AWESOME

When we told Andrea it was my dad who had molested me, she did not give a shit. Her and I had tried so many times to fix so many things, and now she was just done.

I saw her disappearing that day. Really, she was already gone. I could see in her eyes that she was in love with someone else.

This was her payback. I'm sure she was thinking, *I've been trying to get you to love me for years, and now you're saying you want to get back with me?*

Her new guy was in, and I was out. She ended up with that guy for four years.

I do not blame her.

All in all, I was in rehab for three weeks.

On the last day, everyone gives you a hug. They tell you to come see them soon and to not forget to go to AA.

"Remember," they say, "Don't drink. Don't do drugs."

And because everything with me always has to be super over the top, they also added, "Don't jerk off!" Those were my marching orders. Go home and then don't do…anything, really.

There was no one there to pick me up. Someone gave me a ride home.

I moved back into the same apartment complex in Santa Monica where I used to live with my family. I am a creature of habit, to put it mildly. I wanted the exact same apartment I used to live in, but it was taken so I moved in to the one next door.

My business manager at that time was this nice middle-aged lady who helped me move in all my things.

Andrea had set up the space a little. She gave me some furniture and stuff. She'd been doing things like that since we broke up. She'd tell me I needed some towels or a bathmat or something and I'd be like, "Do I?"

She might have been over me, but she still knew I needed a functional home, if only for when our children would be coming over.

And she still had a little pity for me. She knew I needed all the assistance I could get. After all those years, she knew exactly who she was dealing with.

A helpless little child.

Chapter 6

Facing the reality that Andrea and my old life were never coming back was one of the hardest things I ever had to deal with. In its own way it was almost as hard as dealing with my brother dying.

I was so depressed. I was so freaked out. There was this relentless sadness. I didn't know who I was on my own and I didn't know what to do with myself.

As pathetic as it sounds to say it, I needed my mommy back.

My plan to go to rehab and win my wife back had failed miserably. It probably never had a chance in the first place.

And that wasn't all. People look at you differently when you've been to rehab, at least for a while. It's not a great look.

Ultimately, I'm still glad I went. Rehab can be helpful for anyone, even if you don't have a problem with addiction. Life is hard sometimes. It's easy for things to get out of control. If you're in a downward spiral for any reason, everyday life can be tough to deal with. And when handling your day-to-day shit gets overwhelming, it then becomes even harder to clear your mind and figure out the reason why you started spiraling in the first place and what you're going to do about it.

Rehab gives you time to think. You get to make everything stop. And you get to spend hours and hours sitting around talking about your problems with other people who are also dealing with their own shit.

If you're really trying to do the work, then I don't care how clueless you are—you are going to make some connections. You are going to see some bad patterns in your life. You are going to start putting two and two together and asking yourself how you might be able to make some changes.

You also have professionals there who have lots of training and experience. They can help you see the puzzle for what it is and suggest some strategies for putting all the pieces together in a smarter way.

Some of the advice I got in rehab was bullshit. But some of it wasn't. I was such a broken person and I had almost no experience with therapy. Some of my problems weren't that hard to figure out, so I was able to get some small results very quickly. It's like when you're really out of shape and you start going to the gym. Those first ten pounds are the easiest ones to lose.

Rehab made me see the value in therapy, and in working on myself. That carried over. I started seeing other therapists on the outside. It took a lot of trial and error for me to find someone who worked for me, but the journey to fix myself started in rehab.

I'm grateful for that. However, at this point that long journey was just getting started.

Andrea and I finalized our divorce right after I moved into my apartment.

Divorce is brutal. Both you and the person you're splitting up with see everything differently. Of course you do. That's the reason you're getting divorced.

And now, these two people who have decided that they need to get away from each other—and very often, who did things they regret on the road to deciding they couldn't live together—need to work together to split up everything they own.

It's a recipe for disaster. There are bound to be disagreements over who deserves what and why. You're bound to piss each other off.

On the scale of divorces, I had a great one. But that doesn't mean it was a cakewalk.

We didn't go through any lawyers. We figured it out ourselves. Anytime there was a disagreement about who should get what, we asked her parents what they thought and then I agreed to whatever they suggested. I wasn't angry at Andrea, and besides, she was still the mother of our children. I wanted to do right by her and her family.

Losing my in-laws was shitty in its own way. Other than my kids, at that time I didn't have a lot of strong family connections.

My dad was gone and one of my brothers was gone. My mum was weird toward me because she knew what my dad did to me. My stepmum was weird toward me because she didn't totally believe my dad had abused me and therefore didn't appreciate the shitty things I was saying about her late husband.

My in-laws were the closest thing I had to a mother and father, especially over here. And now they didn't like me either.

I also had a falling out with my brother Lee, on the phone from Australia.

"I heard you went to rehab," he said. "That's tough." And then he got to the point. "So, you think dad did that shit?"

I guess he had talked about one of my phone calls from rehab with Marn—his mum—or with my mum.

I told him I did.

"You know I don't believe you," he said. "It didn't happen to me, so it's pretty hard to swallow."

I could understand that argument. But it still didn't change what I believed to be true.

I said, "I don't blame you, dude. I almost don't believe it

myself. I wish that it didn't happen. I wish I could just pretend that it didn't and make everybody happier. I don't know what to tell you, man. I feel bad to have to tell everybody about this. But then again I'm the one that has to live with it."

And that was pretty much the end of that.

It wasn't as brutal as it could have been. It was a phone call. It wasn't face to face. Maybe that made it easier for both of us.

Of course, I would have preferred for everyone to believe me and be okay with me. I don't know why anyone thought I might lie. I certainly wasn't benefiting from it.

But it wasn't like Lee wanted to fly to the States to beat me up or anything. I just got the sense he felt let down by me. That my whole family over there did. My brother and I definitely became distant after that.

All I really had left was the kids. I got them every Wednesday and every other weekend. But at that point they were still little. I love Devin and Tiger dearly, but in those days, they didn't have much to offer in the way of conversation, unless you wanted to talk about SpongeBob.

Outside of work, there wasn't much of anything going on in my life. I was washing clothes like three times a day just to stay busy. I would put five or six things in the laundry at a time. As soon as something was dirty, in the washer it went.

I've always loved being a neat person, so even if my life was a mess, at least my apartment wasn't. Tidying up after myself wasn't hard. I only had like three cups in the cupboard to begin with.

But other things weren't so simple. Pretty much immediately I saw the financial reality of divorce. Basically, I was fucked. My business manager informed me that after alimony and child support I could barely afford my rent.

Sobriety didn't last long, either. When I went back to work, my co-host from the radio show, Josh, showed me a text. "Hey man, I'm not sure if you need to see this or not, but Andrea tried to score some weed from me the other day, when you were in rehab."

Andrea wasn't a big weed smoker, so I'm not surprised she didn't have a bunch of dealers in her phone that she could hit up. But I don't think it was a coincidence that, out of all the people she could have asked, she picked a friend of mine and someone that I worked with. I think she wanted that to get back to me. I think she wanted me to know that she was having fun with her new life and her new dude.

That was a little more payback.

That was when I started using again. I went home and got weed off somebody that day.

Just like the first time me and Andrea split up, I assumed that the silver lining of losing my marriage was gaining the freedom to date whoever I wanted.

I have a weird life. Hosting a radio show like mine can stroke your ego. There are listeners telling you you're awesome. There are female guests and female listeners telling you you're hot. I would have preferred to have still been married, but now that I was single I imagined there was a great dating life waiting for me to jump into.

Back when I was married, I thought I could have been banging every night if I wanted to. Especially once the radio show blew up a bit. But the grass is always greener. Sometimes the unattainable married guy might be a more attractive target than a broke divorced dude who owns three cups.

Plus, I was still seeing that same sex therapist from rehab once a week, and she was telling me I couldn't have sex or jerk off.

Sex therapy didn't last long after rehab either. As I have said, there are good therapists and bad therapists. Truthfully, in my experience they're mostly bad. Good therapists are really hard to find.

Things went south with the one I was seeing pretty quickly. She was constantly forgetting things I had told her. That made it seem like she wasn't really paying attention.

Therapists have a lot of education and training. They know stuff you don't know. That's why you're paying them. But that means that a lot of times, when they give you information or opinions, you kind of just have to take their word for it. You have to have faith in their training and their ability.

And with this therapist, there were one or two times she said something that I knew for a fact wasn't true. And that made me question all of her other so-called facts.

I also noticed that a big part of her plan seemed to revolve around me continuing to see her for a long, long time—and, of course, to keep *paying* her.

The vision she had sold me in rehab was that we could work through my issues with my dad and my abuse and cure me of being bisexual. I don't know if I still believed that was possible. But if it was, I came to the conclusion that she wasn't the person who was going to help me make that happen.

She also told me she thought Andrea was going to come back, and I was nowhere near delusional enough to fall for that.

I definitely think sex addiction is real, but despite what that therapist might have thought, I don't think I have it. I think it's possible to have a really high sex drive and to not be a sex addict. Those two aren't the same thing.

Sex addiction is when you have sex and afterward you feel really bad about it, and then you go and have sex again because you think it will make you feel better, and then you keep repeating that insane pattern over and over. It's when you start showing up late for work late because you just couldn't bring yourself stop banging. That isn't me. It never has been.

I added it all up and decided, *Fuck this, I'm gonna go home and jerk off.*

STILL AWESOME

Things did pick up somewhat in my single life after I dropped her. I used to eat all the time at this restaurant across the road from my place in Santa Monica. It was this raw vegan spot that sold a $30 smoothie. And yes, that is totally obnoxious.

There was a hippie chick that worked there. She was into yoga and all that stuff. Very high on life. She was really pretty and she had a great big dragon tattoo. Once again, I'm that easy.

She would ask me to hang out. I remember one time she told me she was a runner and asked me if I wanted to go for a run with her on the beach. I said sure.

Then later on she said, "Actually, do you just want to go eat instead?"

That's when the light bulb finally went off.

"Are you hitting on me?" I asked.

She was like, "Of course I am, you idiot. How did you not get that?"

It really hadn't occurred to me. I thought she just wanted someone to run with.

I was so bad at dating. You need to have the mojo. That's half the game. Of course, it helps to be handsome or funny or rich or successful. But you also need to have confidence. And I'd lost mine.

When you have confidence, you see a pretty girl and you think, *I'm gonna go over and sling some game.* But at that point, I would see someone I thought was cute and think, *I don't want to talk to her. I'm a loser.*

Looking back, it's crazy to think about how insecure I was. To not even realize someone is blatantly hitting on you? And then, when you find out she is, to ask yourself, *Why?* Holy shit, dude. Only a couple years earlier, there had been a *New York Times* bestselling book called *I'm Awesome* with my face on the cover. And now I had fallen to a point where I couldn't believe a girl would be interested in me.

Me and her dated for a little bit. She was really into me. That helped build my confidence up a little bit.

As I have said, if I go out on a couple dates with someone, I usually roll straight into a serious relationship. That's always been my pattern. But this time was an exception. I was so insecure that I considered myself undateable. I was sure that if we got more serious, I was bound to blow it. And I was also convinced that not blowing it might be even worse. I was positive that I was not relationship material. As far as I was concerned, if I liked you, then the nicest thing I could do for you was to get myself the hell away from you.

My friend Dingo felt bad for me. He knew how down in the dumps I was. One afternoon, still not long after I got out of rehab, we were at his house. We smoked some weed and then we sat there on his couch and laughed like idiots. It was the most fun I'd had in months.

He decided to give me a pep talk. He's Australian, and he knows me as an Australian, if that makes any sense. I feel like he understands me on a deeper level because we come from the same place.

His message for me was, *You don't have a drug problem. You don't have a drinking problem. You're not a sex addict. You're just this sad lonely dude who got divorced. You just need to let loose and have fun.*

He was like, "You're all right!"

I felt myself perk up immediately. I felt a weight come off me that I had been carrying around for I don't know how long.

I was like, "I *am* all right, aren't I?"

"Fuck it, you're fine!" he said. "Have a beer, smoke some weed, and fucking cheer up, you cunt!"

That argument made sense to me.

STILL AWESOME

What the fuck was I thinking? I thought, as I sat there enjoying a doobie. *This is living!*

Dingo invited me to join him and his friends out that night. He wanted to show me a good time.

He took me to Beacher's Madhouse. It was this ongoing nightclub event that used to happen at the Roosevelt Hotel in Hollywood. For a while there it was a hot thing to do for all the Hollywood bottle service wankers. A bunch of celebrities used to go.

It was this weird show with a bunch of unusual-looking people doing crazy stuff. There were characters dressed up in costumes and there was a gigantic lady and a bunch of little people. There was one guy dressed up like Chucky from *Child's Play* who was in a harness on a zipline. He would zip over to your table from the ceiling to give you drinks.

Dingo convinced me to take some molly at the beginning of the night. What I did not know—for like a year afterward—was that he continued leaning over and sprinkling more and more of it in my vodka tonics throughout the evening.

I woke up the next morning in Dingo's bed with a black chick on one side and a blonde on the other. Dingo had slept on his couch. I had officially gone off several wagons, all at the same time.

It was probably not what my therapists at rehab would have recommended. But Dingo seemed pretty proud of himself. *Mission accomplished. You're welcome.*

As someone in my position—just restarting recovery after blowing years of sobriety and a couple weeks in treatment—was it a good idea? No. Was it the most intelligent token of friendship that Dingo could have offered me? Probably not.

But I don't blame him in the slightest. I appreciated it then and I still appreciate it now. Dingo was my friend when I had no friends. I love him for it.

My heart was no longer in sobriety. I don't think I went to a single AA meeting after rehab. It just didn't appeal to me.

Besides, for years, I had been totally paranoid that if I got wasted my heart would explode in my chest, mostly because of my father dying. But now I had drunk all night at a club while Dingo had secretly fed me multiple rounds of ecstasy. Beforehand I would have predicted that would kill me. But it didn't. So my final reason to stay sober went out the window.

One crazy night out with ecstasy and a threesome was a welcome break from my problems, but it obviously didn't cure them. I was still so depressed. I got tired of staring at the walls in my apartment, so I started drinking alone.

One time I remember spending an entire Sunday lying on a floor, drinking wine, thinking about getting ready for work on Monday. Just a pathetic piece of shit.

Before I got divorced, I accidentally discovered rub-and-tugs. I can't say I had never heard of them or that I hadn't thought it might be fun to try one. I had been to some places like that way back when I lived in Australia. But I didn't know where to find them in Los Angeles.

To this day, I still can't tell when a massage place is a rub-and-tug and when it's not. They all look the same. They all have the same shitty New Age music playing inside. And it's not like there's a waiting room full of creepy dudes all sitting together waiting to get jerked off. Usually it's just you in the front until they walk you down the corridor, past all those same little fake rooms set up with temporary walls they have at every other strip mall massage place.

The crazy thing is, the cheaper the place, the better the chances you might get jerked off. If it's $150 for a massage, then no way. But if it's 60 bucks for a deep tissue massage, there's a decent chance a little Thai lady is rolling you over at the end and grabbing your dick.

But that's just a rough guide. Sometimes at the end you ask for a hand job and it's all good, and then sometimes they get offended that you would even ask them the question. If there's a way to tell the difference, I can't tell you what it is. For me, it's a crapshoot.

I am told there's an app that can tell you which massage places are rub-and-tugs. But back when I was married, I don't think I had any apps on my phone at all. I might have had a moto video game or something like that, but that was the extent of what I knew how to get from the app store.

But one day, when I was still with Andrea, I found one not far from the Sirius studio. I honestly thought I was just going for a massage. I think it was forty bucks. The place looked like a normal spot, and I did get a proper massage. But then at the end the lady jerked me off.

I truly did not see it coming. I didn't even tip extra the first time, which is obviously the polite thing to do when someone gives you a happy ending. I'm not sure if me stiffing a stranger who just gave me a hand job makes it any better, but it should show you how unexpected it was.

When I left I asked myself, *Wait, was that even cheating?* Because I didn't do anything to her. And I didn't ask her to do anything to me, either.

Of course, anything can be cheating if you wouldn't tell your wife about it. And I can assure you that, when I gave Andrea a rundown of my day, I definitely left out the part where the nice Asian lady surprised me with a handy. But I let myself live in denial and even went back there a few more times.

Now that I was single there was nothing stopping me, so I started going to that same place again.

Every time I went, the guy at the front desk asked me, "Man or woman?"

And every time I asked for a woman. Until one day, for whatever reason, I said, "Man."

I saw him flinch hard on that one. He clearly did not see that coming.

And then he said, "All right."

He walked me into one of the little rooms. Then a dude came in and that was that.

I didn't know how to meet gay guys back then. If Grindr was around, I wasn't aware of it. Rub-and-tugs were one of the only options I knew how to pull off. It was easy.

There were the Korean spas, too. Just like with the rub-and-tugs, I was genuinely surprised to find out what dudes got up to in there. Because just like with massage parlors, a lot of Korean spas are straight up legit establishments. I've been to super expensive day spas in a bunch of different cities around the world, and there's one place not too far from K-Town that has the best steam room I've ever seen. They've got a legitimate cold plunge. It's awesome.

But every now and then in the steam room, someone jerks off. And then sometimes, somebody next to them will say, "Oh, let me help you there."

And then sometimes you walk in the steam room and there's like eight dudes in the corner, all getting along with each other. You never know what you're going to get.

There's an etiquette. When you come in with your towel on, everybody stops. You give yourself a nudge on your dick through the towel, to let everyone know you're a part of the club and that it's okay to keep going. A guy like me especially has to give the okay since I come across as super straight. If you don't give the okay sign, then everything stops. It's understood that it's not appropriate to make a straight dude who just wants to steam hang out and watch that.

I can't imagine what happens in these places is a great big secret in the Korean-American community. There are so many Korean spas around K-Town, and even though tons of Korean guys go there, I bet 80% of the money they make is from gay dudes jerking each other off. If they banned that stuff, these places would go broke.

There are always old Korean dudes there and they totally know what's going on. The gay guys just don't do stuff in front of them. When an old Korean guy comes in there and sits down with no towel and no shame, with a huge bird's nest of pubes and his little knob poking out, you can see all the gay guys putting their dicks away, back in their towels.

They'll wait. They're in for the long haul. Guys will ride it out for twenty minutes while he's in there, then get back into it when he leaves.

But nothing happens while Old Guy sits there and sweats and loudly hucks up loogies from his throat. Everybody respects his ass.

No matter what was going on in my personal life, I still had to go to work every day and keep the radio show moving forward. And eventually that meant another Ellismania came around.

Up to that point, Ellismania had been a pretty triumphant time for me. For a weekend I would pack out the Hard Rock with hardcore fans. People flew in from all over America and Canada. I would get to stay in some ridiculous VIP suite at the Hard Rock the whole time. There would be thousands of people at the fights and then our band Taintstick or Death! Death! Die! or whatever we were called at that point would play a concert and everybody from the radio show would get to pretend we were shitty rock stars, too.

But this one was different. It was the first time I ever drank at an Ellismania. I was in a really dark place, and instead of using Ellismania to try and lift myself up I drank myself into a worse depression.

I was so sad about being divorced. I felt like such a failure, even though the event was a huge success, just like it always had been.

One night that weekend, one of the fans came up to me as I was leaving the Circle Bar, downstairs at the Hard Rock. He was crying. He gave me a hug, just because he knew how sad I was. And the fact that he did that for me made me cry, too. Misery loves company.

That Ellismania happened around the time the show had made a few friends from the transgender porn community. I don't remember if Foxxy or Morgan Bailey came on the show first, but pretty soon both of them were friends of the show on air and friends of mine off air.

And friends was all we were, by the way. I think people suspected things were happening with me and transgender girls way before anything actually did.

Having them on the show really just started as a way to make up new radio bits. Howard Stern and everyone else had done porn stars to death. And then I came along and started beating that dead horse, too. Having transgender girls just seemed like a new wrinkle on that. A way to escalate things.

We did games involving putting your face really close to their dicks or holding on to their tits while a snake bit you. Stuff like that. The joke, obviously, was that their private parts were things that none of us super macho hetero guys in the room would ever want anything to do with.

Looking back, I'm not proud of that. We were making a joke out of transgender people. I didn't see it that way at the time, because Foxxy and Morgan were in on the joke and they were my friends. And I can now admit that—even if nothing was happening between me and those girls off air and even if I thought nothing was *ever* going to happen between us—I did not think that it was gross to hold on to those titties while the snake bit me. Not at all.

STILL AWESOME

But that doesn't automatically make it all right. I'm not proud of those bits. I have evolved. We wouldn't do that now.

That night at Ellismania, when I got back to my room after hugging it out and having a good cry at the Circle Bar with a fan, a transgender girl I knew was waiting for me. We had dinner together.

I wasn't planning for anything to happen. Up until that point she had just been my friend.

But I was crying my eyes out to her. Literally crying in her arms. And then one thing led to another.

That was my first time in a long time, hooking up with a transgender girl. And that was the last time, for a while anyway.

Looking back, that was a real dark time in my life.

I was still a dad. I did my best to shield my kids from my problems and depression and drinking and all that. I definitely kept my dating life away from them. They met one girl I was seeing in a park one time, when I thought me and her might have a future together. But I was very careful where they were concerned.

I'd love to tell you that, as far as they knew, I was the same old dad I'd ever been and that they had no idea anything was wrong. I tried to keep it together as best I could. But kids are smart. They can sense things. Devin had been able to tell when things went south between me and her mother, and I bet she had some inkling that her dad was a bit off now, too.

On the radio, I went from always talking about how awesome I was to shooting myself down all the time. I was dark. I was angry. I thought I was a bad person. I started to jeopardize my career.

Everything I thought about myself shifted. My taste in music shifted. All I wanted to listen to were songs that were dark and sentimental and sad. I didn't just want to listen to Slipknot—I wanted to listen to the saddest, angriest songs Slipknot had. Over and over again. Just wallowing in it.

Just like that New Year's morning at the Hard Rock, after taking those roxies, I began to question how necessary I was to my kids' lives. Was there a chance they might be better off if I just didn't exist? I wasn't sure I knew the answer to that question.

I was stuck.

I came up with a new intro to play at the beginning of the show. The song that played underneath all the talking bits and radio sound effects was "You Gotta Move" by the Rolling Stones. I put it there as a daily reminder to myself. Keep moving. Just keep going. Don't stop. Don't look back.

Cross your fingers and hope that if you keep doing that, eventually you'll see some daylight at the other end of the tunnel.

Chapter 7

One night, I invited some friends over my house to watch some UFC fights. This was years ago, at the Beverly Hills house. Back when I was married to Andrea.

Benji Madden came over. He brought his brother Joel and some of their friends. One of those friends was Joel's assistant, Katie.

Katie and I had actually been at a party together once before that. But this was our first proper introduction.

Benji told Katie, "This is Jason. He ate a shark's heart while it was still beating."

I think he wanted to shock her a little bit and make me sound hard. No one in their right mind thinks that is cool. (Not even me, by the way. It happened a long time ago. I was drunk and I regret it.) But he knew Katie would be into that. She is what you might call a blood enthusiast.

And then that was pretty much the last I saw of her that night. My daughter Devin cornered Katie and dragged her upstairs to her bedroom. As I later found out, while the rest of us watched fights in the living room, Katie spent the next couple hours meeting all of Devin's princess dolls.

The next time Katie and I saw each other, Andrea and I were in the process of splitting up. I was still at the Beverly Hills house, but by now I was spending my nights in the pool house. This time it was a birthday party for Nicole Ritchie—Joel's wife—on the roof of the Roosevelt Hotel in Hollywood.

By that time, my tattoo artist Grant had told me I should get to know Katie if I ever got the chance. Grant was also Katie's tattoo artist. We both talked to Grant about personal shit from time to time while he was working on us, and because of that he knew Katie and I were both pretty tweaked in the sexual department.

Her and I made out at that birthday party. I could already tell there might be a spark between us. Some kind of a connection.

She gave me a ride home afterward. We drove up the driveway, all the way to the pool house in the back.

She was like, "I'm not coming in."

And I was like, "Yeah, no shit."

And that was that.

I started texting her here and there. She shot me down every time.

Her message to me, in a nutshell, was: *I really enjoyed your company that one night. But you have an "A" tattooed on your face to symbolize your wife's name. And also, you are a goddamn mess.*

See—getting a tattoo of Andrea's first initial *did* keep women away from me…as soon as I no longer wanted it to.

After I had bottomed out for a while on weed and alcohol, Devlyn Steele told me I needed to get on antidepressants. I had always resisted them. But I was at such a low point that I didn't see how I could keep saying no. Devlyn took me to a doctor and they gave me a prescription.

The pills did mellow me out. When I was on them, I didn't get quite as down. They didn't work miracles. They're not happy pills. Believe me—if they were, I'd still be on them. But I did feel like they helped me manage the day.

STILL AWESOME

There were side effects, though. They made me feel tired. My dick didn't work for a couple of weeks after I started taking them. I didn't really like them, to be honest. I just thought, *Okay, this is a more steady me. People seem to be more pleased with the more steady me. End of story.* And so I stayed on them. For years.

Devlyn was really there for me at that time in my life. He encouraged me to look on the bright side of being alone.

His take was, "You have been in a bunch of relationships before. And you are a good-looking dude. You are going to be in a relationship again. Don't worry about that. Instead, think about how much time in your adult life you are going to spend with another person. And then think about how little time you truly spend by yourself. You should appreciate this time and make the most of it."

I didn't love hearing that at the time. I certainly didn't walk out of that session happy. That message didn't fix any of my problems right then and there. But for some reason, it stuck with me.

That talk made me start to go to the gym again. I needed that. I *always* need that.

When you go to the gym, you knock down that first domino. That one move gets the ball rolling. It helps you start to get the other parts of your life on track. When you go to the gym consistently, it always seems like the bullshit in your life doesn't pile up as much. And I seem to have more bullshit than most people. And also, when my shit starts piling up, it seems to get out of control faster than it does for other people. I overdo everything, both good and bad.

So I started overdoing it at the gym again. That was a positive first step.

Katie and I had lost touch by then. We'd gone quiet for a while. But then one day I tried her again.

Hey, seriously, what happened? I texted. *It's been a long time.*

And lucky for me she texted back.

All in all, I wasn't on my own for all that long. Maybe eight months. Less than a year for sure. By that point I had put myself together enough to be worthy of a date in Katie's eyes. I was officially divorced. And I no longer had my ex-wife's first initial tattooed on my face. So that was a start.

I showed up for our date in a station wagon. After Tiger had been born, I got rid of my truck and replaced it with a sensible family vehicle. Needless to say, that car was the end result of an argument that Andrea had won.

It was an Audi, so it went fast and it handled. That was the bit that I got to pick. It wasn't a bad car. A lot of people would be stoked to have it.

But it wasn't what I wanted. It was just as rebellious of an automobile as I had been allowed to get. I had to choose a dad car, and that was the one I settled on. Looking back, I was such a bitch.

Anyway, I showed up in the dad-mobile. Katie asked where we were going. I didn't have a plan or anything, so she suggested a spot called Jumbo's Clown Room.

Jumbo's is basically a strip club in Hollywood, except the girls there don't get nude. It's like a classic old-school dive bar, only with benefits. Instead of the cookie cutter chicks you get at a lot of strip clubs, the girls at Jumbo's have more of their own vibe. It's a tattooed goth kind of thing. Courtney Love danced there way back when, before she started Hole and ruined Kurt Cobain's life.

Jumbo's has been there forever and it has all of my favorite kinds of girls under one roof. But I had no idea it existed. I don't know where anything is. I'm a lone wolf most of the time.

But Katie was a cool person. Before we met, she hung out at cool places and got wasted with people like Dave Grohl. She knew about all kinds of stuff like that. Still does.

I remember staring at her that night while we were sitting at Jumbo's, in awe. I remember thinking, *Who is this person who is totally covered in tattoos, and yet can form full sentences when she speaks, and be witty and a smart ass in text messages?*

Who gets Ol' Shitty *tattooed on their knee? And then* Fun *on the other? Like, you know those things are forever, right?*

I couldn't figure her out at all. And I liked it.

When we left Jumbo's we decided to head out to the beach in Venice. I had a blanket in the back of my car. We found a spot near the pier.

At that point in my life, I had been all around the world. I had seen and done many, many crazy things. When you are in your late 30s and you have two kids and a station wagon, you figure you've already seen all of the crazy sex stuff you're ever going to see. But that night, on that beach, was one of the most exciting times I've ever had.

A lot of stuff was happening, very quickly. It was dark. I was really just along for the ride. Doing my best to keep up. I felt like a kid again.

After that, it was on. Katie and I stayed together that night and then went for coffee the next morning. We became a thing right off the bat.

Everything came together pretty easily. I'd never dated anyone who had so many of the same interests as me. The same opinions, too. Obviously, we're two different people and we're not identical. Who wants that? But all of our shit just meshed together really well.

I could tell we had the same sarcastic, smartass sense of humor. We both have a very 'fuck the world' way of looking at things. I'd like to think that when it comes down to it, we're not super jaded as people. But having little jokes about strangers we pass on the street and just the normal world in general—that's our shit. That's fun for us.

We'd talk shit to each other, too. That was one of the ways we bonded.

For example, we both love metal. That's something we have in common. But we like different kinds of metal, and we'd make fun of each other's music. In general, I don't appreciate people fucking with my metal, but we hammered each other's bands in such an awesome way that it became fun.

There's the tattoo thing, obviously. We both love tattoos and generally speaking we do try to get good ones. But we're also both fond of ones that are incredibly stupid. You can tell a lot about a person from their shitty tattoos.

I'm a guy who has a tattoo of a shrimp on top of a Barbie doll. (Shrimp on the Barbie—get it?)

Meanwhile, *Ol' Shitty* and *Fun* are just the tip of the iceberg for her. Katie got a tattoo of bacon coming out of a piggy bank while she was working on the Warped Tour. Why? Because she loves bacon. That's the whole story. On another tour she got a tattoo of the fucking Kool-Aid Guy. Who does that?

There was more to our relationship than just insulting lame strangers behind their backs and enjoying stupid tattoos, of course. We bonded over animals. My mum used to rescue all kinds of animals, so I've always found it very normal to live in a house that's covered with fur. Katie's really into creepy crawly things plus weird deformed cats.

Her cat, Prince, liked me the first time we met. And Katie is one of those people where, if her cat likes you, you know you have a chance with her too. I think the fact that I love animals went a long way toward showing Katie that I'm not some cold, hard son of a bitch. It shows that I do have a heart.

We had similar takes on society. We see things our own way. In our eyes, a lot of people who get treated like they're super respectable are really full of shit. And a lot of people who might be considered outcasts are actually the people who are worth knowing.

A lot of people don't respect strippers, for example. They're cool with them existing and everything. But they wouldn't want

STILL AWESOME

to be friends with one. I think deep down inside most people believe that strippers are bad people.

I dated a stripper for years in Australia. I bought her an engagement ring and I would have married her if she hadn't already fallen in love with someone else by the time I did it.

In Melbourne, at least at that time, stripping was not a glamorous profession. You didn't get to just rub against a pole with a bikini on and then watch the money come flying at you. If someone there gave you 20 bucks, that meant they expected to see inside the hole. It was a rough and tumble world.

But I remember later on this girl stopped dancing and started doing yoga, and then all the sudden she thought that strippers were below her. I remember thinking, *Of all people, how could you think that?*

What makes a stripper bad? Or a porn star? Everyone seems to be jerking off pretty often, and it seems like porn stars are pretty handy for the mainstream world when it comes to that? So why do you have to turn around after you're done jerking off and shit on them?

Katie and I saw a lot of things the same way because in some ways our backgrounds were pretty similar.

Her family moved to Alaska when she was an itty-bitty baby, and then stayed there right through her teenage years. She got in a car accident when she was 16 and broke her back.

If you know anything about teenage girls, then you know that is the worst possible time to have to wear some big, uncomfortable brace every day. I think wearing that thing made her feel like an ugly, broken duckling who had been forced to live up in this dark, cold, desolate place.

And so she rebelled. She went dark. She developed a 'fuck you' attitude toward the world. At some point, she decided she was getting out of there, so when she was old enough she moved to L.A. and made a new life for herself.

In a lot of ways, I could relate to that. I understood her in a way most people probably couldn't.

And she understood me. We both had a dark side. And so we both knew how to deal with it when the other one went dark. If you've lived a normal, well-adjusted life, you're not always prepared to roll with it if your boyfriend or your girlfriend wakes up on the wrong side of bed some days and can't just snap themselves out of it. But we knew how to put up with that, because we'd been there so many times ourselves.

Katie appreciated the stuff that I'm good at. And that made me feel good about myself. A lot of people seem to think that any jackass could talk on the radio for a living. But if you've flipped through a radio dial recently—or listened to 98% of podcasts—I think you'll agree that it's harder than it looks. I think Katie thinks that I have a gift.

But at the same time she doesn't blow smoke up my ass. It's not like everything I do is automatically awesome to her. Even though I have technically appeared on the *Billboard* chart, I know she doesn't think I'm much of a musician. And in that case, I respect her for not respecting me.

Have you heard me sing? She's got a point.

I never dated anyone who was as open-minded as Katie. I have always been the crazy one in any relationship I've ever been in. But if anything, in the beginning she was almost too open-minded for *me*.

When we first met, she had this painting in her house. It was a legitimate painting, except it looked like it had been made with this really shitty red paint.

I asked her about it. It turns out she had painted it herself. With her menstrual blood.

She didn't have any deep and meaningful reason for doing it. Just a rainy day arts and crafts project, I guess. Something to do.

Nowadays I've been around Katie enough to know that she's

not the only person like that. There's this whole little scene of goth-type people who own hairless cats and enjoy doing taxidermy on dead things and making art with their blood when they get bored. They're out there. But Katie was my crash course in that weird little world.

Blood became a thing in our relationship, early on. It was a sex thing. It's called blood-play.

We started cutting each other. That was definitely her idea. Just one more thing Katie was aware of that I knew nothing about.

I would not say that I am into pain or that the sight of blood turns me on. But early on, for me and Katie it was just about trying stuff out. Doing crazy shit for the fuck of it. Seeing what kind of weird shit we could get up to.

But one morning, we were at a diner drinking coffee, and she decided to cut her arm with a knife. And not just a little bit.

Deep. *Too* deep.

I went off on her. I told her I was not a fan of that, and that I never wanted to see her do that again.

Like I said, at that point we were pushing the limits with each other. I don't think she was trying to prove a point or anything. I think she was just thinking, *Hey, you think you're a crazy guy? Well watch this!*

I can respect a little light insanity over breakfast. But I'm actually not that crazy. She pulled back immediately and apologized.

Katie's younger than me. Maybe that's part of it. I think most of us were crazier in our 20s than we are in our 40s.

But she was also a real deal punk rock crazy bitch. When I met her, she wasn't planning for the future. She was living day-to-day. She was wild.

But I had kids, man. I owned an Audi. I know everyone looks at me and expects me to be this untamed crazy person, but most of the time, I actually just want to go to the movies and eat food and act normal.

Katie wasn't there yet. And if her and I were going to work—especially since there were kids in the mix—it meant that she would have to change her act a bit.

When you have kids, you look at relationships a lot differently. Every step of the way—right from the start—you have to proceed carefully, because you know that what you're doing could potentially affect your children as much as it affects you. Maybe more.

From the very start, I made it clear that I had no intention of getting married again. Katie was able to see firsthand how painful and complicated divorce can get while I was splitting up with Andrea. In the scheme of things, Andrea and I had an easy and peaceful split. And it was still absolute hell.

Katie knew I was not keen to ever put myself through that again. And that was fine with her. Marriage wasn't high on her agenda either.

Having kids was also off the table. Personally, I'm kind of old school when it comes to that. When I fall in love with someone, it feels natural to me to want to make a baby with them.

But for me, the worst part of getting divorced was feeling like I had let down my kids. My parents got divorced. Some pretty fucked up stuff happened to me when I was a kid, but if you ask me to list all the things that affected me for the worse, my mum and dad splitting up would be right up there. That's how bad it is.

With my track record, how could I have another kid and risk splitting up with Katie some day and repeating that failure all over again? Or on the other hand, what if I *did* stay together with Katie after her and I had kids? What an insult that would be to Tiger and Devin, for me to make it work with their stepbrother or stepsister's mom when I couldn't make it work with theirs.

I wanted to do everything I could for my kids moving forward, to try and make up for the divorce. And it seemed to me that having a new kid would make that way more difficult. I don't have my kids all the time. And since we don't get to hang out every day, it's a struggle for me to stay really connected to their lives. I knew that having a new little human being crawling all over the place and shitting in its pants all the time might well make it impossible.

But right off the bat, Katie let me know that she was not interested in motherhood. I know some girls might be tempted to say that to a divorced guy with kids even though they don't really mean it, because they're afraid of scaring him off. She certainly wouldn't have been the first girl to say that at the start of a relationship and then change her tune later on. But I believed her. She's not even that great of a kid person, to be honest—which makes it that much funnier, thinking back to the first time we met, when she got trapped having a tea party with Devin's princess dolls.

Still, Katie accepted from the start that being in my life meant being in my kids' lives. She quickly rose to the challenge. When we first started dating, I wasn't all that great at taking care of myself, much less my children. So Katie got thrown into helping me handle kid shit whether she liked it or not. She became an accidental stepmom. Immediately.

One of the first days we had together with the kids, we all went out to breakfast at this diner in Santa Monica called Swingers. We were all walking back to the apartment afterward. Tiggy was on a balance bike. He was so good on it that he was like a freak. Everywhere we went, people would stop and point at this three-year-old that could ride a balance bike.

The walk back to my apartment was downhill. It was pretty steep. And all the sudden Tiger took off, straight down the sidewalk.

I sprinted after him. Devin ran. And I remember looking up and seeing a reflection in a store window. There was Katie, a couple steps back, hauling ass, too.

Just a couple weeks earlier she had been hanging out smoking cigarettes with rock stars at four in the morning. And now it was 7:30 AM and she was running down the sidewalk in Santa Monica, chasing after a fucking toddler on two wheels.

I remember thinking how funny that looked.

There she was, right behind us, making an effort to be part of the family.

Chapter 8

Needless to say, on top of all the other things we had in common, Katie and I had an extremely strong sexual connection. That was a huge reason why our relationship clicked. I have a really high sex drive. Until I met Katie, I had never had a relationship with someone who could keep up with me. Or who really cared to try, for that matter.

I think some of the girls I dated after I got divorced *tried* to seem crazy in bed for me. But I'm not sure that was who they really were. I think they might have just acted that way because they assumed that was what I wanted. They would see a shaved head and a bunch of tattoos and they'd think they had to whip out some extra badass Hollywood movie sex to impress me. They figured I must be into that because I look like I'm the bass player from Mötley Crüe or something.

But I never doubted that Katie was on the level. She might be crazier than I am. If anything—like when it came to the blood stuff—*I* was the one who wanted to pull it back.

Despite what many people seem to think, I'm not some weird vampire metal sex guy. That's not my sweet spot. But I am pretty adventurous. And I had found my partner in crime. The best way I can describe Katie is this: Imagine someone with the same attitudes toward sex as a gay man, only in the body of a really pretty girl.

As soon as we got together, all bets were off. We wanted to try everything. A fun day for us was to say, *Let's go to the sex store, and if there's anything there we haven't seen before, let's buy it and shove it up inside one of us.*

Everyone has a bucket list. Owning a Lamborghini is on my list, for example. I know that it will probably never happen. But it's fun to imagine.

Before Katie and I met, both of us had always imagined trying all kinds of extravagant sex stuff. But we both assumed a lot of those things were just fantasies. We never really expected them to happen. But after the two of us got rolling, it dawned on me that a lot of the stuff on my sexual bucket list was suddenly very achievable.

I realized, *Wait, this doesn't just have to be a fantasy. I have a job. I have money. We can go buy supplies and then go get a hotel room. We can do whatever the hell we want, whenever we want.*

And that worked both ways. I don't think Katie ever had such a willing partner before me, either.

We got into bondage for a while. We learned how to tie people up and all that. As it turns out, that's not my favorite thing to do. It's cool. If someone wanted to invite us to a bondage sex party, we'd probably go. But it's not like I have a gimp suit in my closet just waiting to come out.

I also wouldn't say it was a lifelong dream to have sex in a hot air balloon, and yet one day there Katie and I were, half a mile above the ground, with a hot air balloon operator who had promised to look the other way while we executed our mission. That was dumb. It was really just a stupid thing to do so I could joke about it on the radio afterward.

But for both of us, it felt so liberating to have the freedom to explore any ridiculous idea that popped into our heads.

And it wasn't just that we could try anything—it was that we could do it without guilt. If things got heated in the moment and we pushed the envelope, it didn't become this taboo thing that couldn't be discussed afterward.

STILL AWESOME

The first time she tried to put her finger in my ass, I got a little weird about it.

She was just like, "So what? People stick fingers in butts. Get over it."

And that was the end of that.

Neither of us had to be ashamed of anything we did, or anything we wanted to do, or anything we might have done in the past. I'm pretty sure Katie would not have personally chosen to sleep with Chyna. That is not her scene. But I never had to explain why I had wanted to do it. She got it. She got me. She knew exactly who she was dealing with.

From the very beginning, Katie and I had an open relationship. By the time she came along, I had finally faced the fact that I needed that in order to be happy. I love Katie. If I got to design my perfect partner, she is exactly the person I would create. But if she needed me to be monogamous for our relationship to work, I don't think we'd still be together.

I'd tried in the past. Man, had I tried. But I'm just not built for it.

Luckily, Katie didn't want that either. And again, I knew she wasn't just agreeing to an open relationship because she felt like she had to. She was the one who brought it up, actually.

Right from the start, she was saying, "I don't think it's right for a person to only sleep with one person for the rest of their life. I personally wouldn't want to do that."

It didn't feel like she was just giving me a pass. It felt more like she was asking for permission to do it herself.

I told her that if she really believed that, then that was great, because I agreed with her. I had always looked at monogamy the same way that she did. As long as you're committed to the person you're in a relationship with, then what's the harm in having some fun with other people, as long as everyone knows what's going on and is okay with it? No harm, no foul, I say.

I had been with women who told me they were okay with threesomes and that kind of stuff, but I could tell from the start that Katie was different. She knew herself, and she knew what she wanted. Truthfully, I think she knew herself more than I knew myself.

Even with the green light, it was a challenge arranging a threesome that worked out for everybody. You can't just snap your fingers and have willing partners who are down for the cause.

You have to start somewhere, so I started by going through my phone and hitting up girls I either already knew or who had hit me up online. That strategy didn't always work out so well.

One day I was leaving work, driving my Porsche. I had only recently gotten it. That was the best. I loved that car. I bought it from Thomas Haden Church, the actor.

Thomas listens to the show and is a friend of mine. One time, a long time ago, before we met, he was at the SiriusXM studios in New York doing some interviews, and he was talking to people there about my show. He was looking for me, not knowing at the time that I broadcast from L.A. So him and I got in touch after that and the relationship grew from there.

The Porsche was his car, but he wasn't using it. It was sitting in a garage in L.A. So he hit me up and offered to sell it to me.

It was a bad idea on my part. I couldn't afford it.

But Thomas listened to the show and realized I was depressed. He thought, *Fuck it. I feel like this dude is going to rally. He's going to make money later on.*

That dude loves me like a brother. He wanted to help.

I called my manager and my business manager, and basically said, "Please, can I have it?"

I think my manager went and found some company to sponsor me so I could get the car. Or at least to get me close enough to where I could be in the ballpark of being able to afford it. Because truthfully, I did not have the money, at all.

I went from the Audi dad-mobile to that Porsche. And to this day, it's still the highlight of my driving life.

So anyway, I was in that car one day leaving work and I passed this chick. She had big hair extensions, a big ass, big tits, and this really over the top orange fake tan. She blatantly checked me out as I was driving by.

I remember thinking, *This car rules.*

And then later on I saw a tweet from her saying, "Jason Ellis just drove by me in a Porsche." So I DM'd her.

I don't want to get too graphic in describing what came next. I'm well aware that no one wants to hear about the actual in-out, in-out. (Well, a couple of you might. Sorry creeps, this chapter is going to be a letdown.)

But at one point during the proceedings, she put her hand over Katie's vagina and said, "Look, I'm a DJ!" And then she moved her hand back and forth and made that 'Wicka, wicka' record-scratching noise.

That was a mood killer, to say the least. It was funny to joke about later on but in the moment that was hard to bounce back from.

The bigger problem was that the girl wasn't really interested in having sex with women. As a result, it wasn't really fun for Katie.

That was a problem with a lot of the girls we hooked up with in the beginning. I had already slept with some of them before I met Katie. And I got the impression that, if Katie wasn't in the picture, most of them would probably have been happy to start a relationship with me themselves.

Those were a little awkward. That kind of girl isn't coming over for the right reasons. She's not there because she wants to have a good time and then go home. She has other intentions.

In those cases, it was basically just two girls having sex with me. If the girl wasn't truly bi, there wasn't a lot there for Katie to get excited about.

That type of experience is very overrated. At the end of the night, you get to say you had a threesome. But that's really the only good part. No one goes to bed happy or as satisfied as they hoped they would. Someone probably ends up a little bummed out or has a little bit of regret.

Or even worse, when the party is over, someone doesn't want to leave, or just can't take the hint that it's time to go. Another one of our early misfires was with a bigger girl. Again, she was a nice lady, but I don't think she was all that into women, and so once again I don't think it was all that great for Katie. But everyone was pleasant and polite.

The girl stayed over. The next morning, Katie was feeding the dogs. And she was saying all the stuff that you say to dogs in that situation.

"Are you hungry? Do you want some food?" You know, *who's a good boy* kind of stuff.

And our new friend popped up from the couch and said, "Yup! I'm starving!"

So just like that, instead of feeding the dogs and starting our day, we were feeding the girl we'd had a threesome with the night before.

Once again, funny to look back on afterward. But not really what Katie and I were looking for.

There were a couple early victories. One night we met up with two girls at the Rainbow. I knew one of them and she brought her girlfriend.

At that point Katie and I were expecting to be disappointed. We were learning just how many ways these hookups could go wrong.

But both of the girls were extremely attractive, and both of them turned out to be super cool. One of them was into me and one of them was into Katie, which worked out well. So we had some drinks and then went back to our place.

We had so much fun that night we saw those two again. We actually had a little relationship going on between the four of us for a minute there. It wasn't even just about sex. We really enjoyed each other's company. Sometimes we'd just go meet up for food and hang out and totally keep our clothes on the whole time.

Unfortunately, those two broke up and then one of them started dating the bass player in a nu metal band and that was that. Foiled again by butt rock.

Very early in our relationship, Katie found a calendar laying around my apartment. One of the trans girls who had been on the show was in the calendar and had given me a copy, so I took it home and dropped it on the counter.

Katie flipped it open.

"You're into trans girls?" she asked.

Based on my past experiences with other girlfriends (not to mention the impression I have gotten from most of the human race), I thought this might be a trap. So I proceeded carefully.

"Uh, I don't know," I said. "Why, would that be a good thing?"

She said, "It would be super hot."

I thought she was fucking with me. But she wasn't. She wasn't just *not* turned off by it, she liked it. She told me she was into trans girls, too.

It's hard for me to explain how huge it was for her to say that. It meant I didn't need to hide that part of myself. That was big, all by itself. But even more than that, it meant that I truly didn't have to apologize for *anything* else that I'd done in the past or that I would like to do in the future. Anything I'd ever done that made me cringe when I remembered it—and trust me, I had a pretty good list going—no longer needed to be cringe-y. What a humongous weight off my shoulders.

I had told all my serious girlfriends that I had gay tendencies. And none of them welcomed that information. None of them even knew what to do with it.

I don't blame them. I didn't know how to handle it myself. Where I come from, if you've ever done gay stuff or wanted to do gay stuff, that means you're gay. End of story.

I remember hearing Artie Lange on *Howard Stern*, saying, "If you touched a dick, you've got the homo."

I said similar stuff on my own show, too. Years ago, we did a recurring bit called "Dude, Is It Gay?" We would tell guys if we thought they were straight or not, based on the stories they told us. We told many dudes who had been in heterosexual relationships for their entire lives that if they hooked up with one man one time, that made them gay.

That was the way we looked at things. It wasn't just us—that was most of the world. And not that long ago.

Back in the '90s, when I was still a pro skater and living in Hollywood with my girlfriend at the time, I would sometimes take ecstasy and hang out at gay clubs.

One night I asked two guys I'd been talking to, "Am I gay? What do you think?" because I didn't act gay, but I had come to accept that I did enjoy gay acts.

One guy was saying, "Oh, you're totally gay."

And the other guy was like, "Relax. You are not gay at all."

That was a white-knuckle conversation. I remember talking to those guys like they were these two gay angels on my shoulder, giving me two different options to choose from. I was totally willing to believe whatever verdict they came up with. Like they could see through me and somehow figure me out better than I could understand myself.

The answer, of course, is that I'm bisexual. Duh. It was pretty fucking obvious the whole time.

Once I figured that out, I told the whole world on *The Howard Stern Show*.

I could have done it on my show. I'm pretty sure everyone who works on the show was at least kind of aware of it by then.

I just didn't feel comfortable going on air one day and saying, "Everybody, please, if you don't mind, I'd like to take a quick break from the dick and fart jokes for a minute so I can make a very serious announcement." For some weird reason, my show didn't feel like the right place for that. It felt awkward.

But I did want to get it out there. Once it was an open thing between me and Katie, I didn't want it to be a secret from anyone anymore. The few people who knew about it behind the scenes had all been really supportive, and I took a lot of empowerment from that. It made me feel like what I am maybe isn't so bad.

And after I went public, almost everyone else was supportive, too, right from the start.

There are a couple of old skateboarder friends who may or may not be cool with me anymore. These were guys I wasn't really in contact with. I might not have had a face-to-face conversation with a couple of them in 20 years. But right around when the news about my sexuality came out, they unfollowed me on social media. To me that didn't feel like a coincidence.

But for the most part, no one really seemed to care all that much. And that made it easier for me not to care so much about it either.

Katie was just as enthusiastic about bringing guys into the mix as she was with girls. But the same problem kept popping up: Finding someone who was equally into both of us.

Again, I just started with names that were already in my phone. I invited a guy I knew from that massage place over, but he was super gay, so he wouldn't touch her.

That happened with more than one guy. They didn't even want Katie to watch. I was so new in that scene I didn't know how anything worked.

In my experience, most gay dudes react to naked women the way a vampire would react to a footlong garlic sandwich.

There were a few times when a gay guy would come over and him and I would be chatting a bit and getting to know each other, and then when Katie came in the room they'd be like, "Who's this?"

And as soon as I would tell them she was my girlfriend, you could see their faces drop. Not only were they out on her, I could see from their reaction that my stock had also dropped dramatically, simply because they now knew that I also enjoyed having sex with this lady. It's pretty amazing how angry some people can be at vaginas, considering we all came out of one.

I couldn't blame them. These guys moved to L.A. so they could live in West Hollywood, AKA Boystown. For their entire lives, wherever they grew up, they had to live in the straight world and play by the straight world's rules. But then they got themselves to L.A. It's like the gay capital of America. And now if you wanted to come into their world, you had to play by their rules. It's their own little bubble. I get it.

And then there I was blindsiding them with the last thing in the world they wanted to see. I can see how it was a big shock. And I get why they weren't into it. I never thought any of them were out of line. It was a learning experience. And truthfully, it was pretty funny, too.

Things weren't any different at first when we tried bringing trans girls into the mix. There was one girl I knew who Katie and I were both interested in. I thought she was into both of us, too.

But then we started to notice that she only wanted to hang out when Katie wasn't around. That was a red flag, so that was the end of that.

We went to a trans girl night at a club one time, and it became apparent really quickly that Katie wasn't welcome there. She tried to get a dance and the girl gave her the whole 'Hold on a minute—I'll be right back' routine and then disappeared.

Katie was cool about it. She was like, "I don't belong here. It's fine. You stay, but I'm out of here."

Just like it had been with a lot of gay dudes, when Katie entered that room you could see it was a game-changer. I think sometimes trans girls see it as a bit of a pissing contest when she's around. I think they compare themselves to women who were born looking like women and they get competitive.

I think a lot of them are thinking, *I grew up trying to be a pretty girl. And it was way harder for me than it was for you because I started as a boy. I put 40 grand into looking like this, and now you're just going to come in swinging around your natural titties?*

Again, I get it.

There were a lot more fails than wins when we tried hooking up with other people. But as I have said, even the fails were fun, in a way. Anyone who's ever gone out and gotten drunk and had one-night stands—or even just tried to have one-night stands and got shut down—would know what I'm talking about. The good times make the bad ones worth it. And even when the bad ones happen and you go home empty-handed, you might be bummed but you still had the thrill of the chase. And you have a dumb story to laugh about the morning after. It sucks, but in a funny way.

We definitely got some stories out of Grindr, the gay hookup app. I heard about it from Katie. She has a friend that's super plugged into the gay scene. We were all hanging out one day and Katie and her friend were like, "Start an account. See what happens."

It was hilarious. As soon as I signed up, the three of us gathered around my phone and watched all the dick pics come flying. I was fresh meat on the scene.

Can you imagine what it's like being a really pretty lady on Tinder? The kind of reaction she gets? How many guys hit her up, constantly? Well, that's what it's like being a dude on Grindr. The only difference is I'm guessing a decent amount of guys are too intimidated to go after the hottest of hot chicks on Tinder. They figure they don't have a shot so they don't risk the rejection. But Grindr is a goddamn free-for-all.

At first, I could hardly believe it was real. Guys would come over and do whatever I wanted. As someone who loves all kinds of sex, Grindr was a huge win.

I'm not a full-on gay dude. I don't want to do too much to dudes. But it turns out there are tons of guys who would love nothing more than to come by, blow a 'straight' guy, and then leave.

They'd thank me for the privilege. Literally. Guys would come over, have at it, thank me for the opportunity, and then walk out backwards—facing me the whole time—close the door behind them, and disappear. They weren't just being polite—they were being *overly* polite. Like an old-school Japanese geisha in a movie or something.

It's hard to describe, but it happened more than once. Katie wouldn't believe me so one day I told her she could see it for herself. She hid in the dog cage. I put the blanket on top at the perfect angle so she could see out but no one would ever be able to see her crouched down in there watching. We didn't just do this once. We did it like ten times. That might not be everyone's idea of a good time, but we were having a blast.

STILL AWESOME

Around that time I got another raise from SiriusXM. After all the money I had to give Andrea every month for the divorce and for the kids, I finally had enough left over for Katie and me to move out of the apartment.

We rented a house in a town called Tarzana. As usual, I did a shit ton of research on my new home before I moved.

I was like, "What's Tarzana?"

Katie said, "It's in the Valley."

I said, "What's the Valley?"

And then I signed the lease.

In case you are wondering, the Valley is the bit of L.A. that's north of Hollywood. You know the Hollywood sign? The Valley is what's behind that hill. It's basically the suburbs.

I got a big house and a backyard and a jacuzzi and a great big pool. That's really all I've ever wanted in life. It didn't even cost that much. I was like, *Why doesn't everybody live out here?* And then the first time I drove the kids to school, there was so much traffic the drive took two hours. The house was only maybe 20 miles north of where they went to school, but hey, that's L.A. for you.

Katie didn't really like it out there. Again, she's younger than me, and at that point she was more motivated than I was to go out and do nighttime stuff. If you wanted to go out and drink it was a really long Uber ride back. On top of that, our neighbors were all old people, plus we were so far out that no one wanted to come out and visit us.

But we made the best of it. That's the house where I discovered waterproof lube. That stuff is crazy. You can't use it all the time. Even though it makes pool sex amazing, you're still smashing a bunch of pool water into someone's vagina, and that's kind of dangerous. You need to save that move for special occasions.

Katie and I started to really hit our stride as a sexual team out in Tarzana. We'd had enough threesomes with enough people that we'd figured out how to work together. Whether it was a guy or a girl or a transgender lady, Katie was the Robin to my Batman. We were teaming up on people. We were almost *too* into it. It became like a sport.

As long as the kids weren't around, we could spread our wings and party a little bit. I don't mean that we were doing cocaine or anything like that. There wasn't even that much alcohol involved.

Truthfully, alcohol probably hurt our cause more often than it helped. Although sex and alcohol can frequently go hand in hand, in my experience, the kind of person who would want to come over to someone's house to get shit hammered and then fuck tends to be an idiot.

There was one girl we were going to hook up with, but then she started drinking and, in the course of a couple of hours, turned from a nice lady into a complete psychopath. That night wasn't especially pleasant.

But again, for the most part, most of the fails were funny. At least, funny to people like me and Katie.

One time a friend of mine came out to Tarzana with his new girlfriend. The four of us were all going to hook up. *What could go wrong*, I figured.

My friend's chick got in the jacuzzi.

"Jump in with her," he told me.

I did, and to my surprise I discovered that my friend's lady friend had a rather large lump, right smack in the middle of her groin region.

Katie was out getting tattooed. She was planning to join us at the house after she was done.

I texted her at the tattoo shop and said, "Just so you know, this guy's girlfriend has a ball."

She was like, "What? What does that mean?"

I repeated that the woman in our jacuzzi seemingly had a testicle.

Katie and I are both into trans girls, but this was an entirely different story.

Katie said, "Well, then I'm not getting in there."

I said, "I completely understand that. I don't think you would want to be involved if you saw what I just saw."

I had to have an awkward conversation with my friend.

"Katie's not feeling it," I said.

He was like, "What? What are you talking about?"

I said, "I don't really want to get into it, dude."

What was I going to say? "She's got a ball, dude"?

He put me in a tough situation. I couldn't tell him why to his face.

So…I just went into work the next day and said it on the radio.

That was not the only suspect genitalia I have encountered in the course of my free-wheeling bisexual open relationship life, by the way.

I was in Palm Springs one time by myself. I had done some GHB and I was floating around in a pool, looking at clouds and tripping out on them. Then I hopped in the jacuzzi and some dude started chatting me up.

We had a beer and made some jokes with each other. He seemed like a fun guy. And then he started groping me, kind of out of nowhere.

I didn't see it coming but I didn't want to ruin my mellow vibe and get aggro with him. Most of the time with men I'm not going to reciprocate, and the dudes go in knowing that. So if someone wants to do something to me, a lot of times it's easier to let them do it, even if I'm on the fence about them.

In this case I did go back at him a bit. But when I reached

down for his crotch, something seemed off. It seemed like there was something…extra down there.

I wasn't positive, so I grabbed again.

And sure enough, this man had three balls. Not even like two regular ones and one little one. Three equal-sized testicles.

That ended it. I consider myself open-minded, but I *was* a little deterred by a three-balled man.

I get to be kind of picky when it comes to dudes. I get to call the shots a bit more in that realm. With every day I grow older, I may be growing more and more hideous to women. But in the gay world, I'm still like an 8.

When hookups did work out, they made all the bad ones seem worth it. There were girls I wanted to sleep with who wanted nothing to do with me, but who were into Katie. Some of those times I got to watch from the sidelines while my hot girlfriend had hot lesbian sex with a hot chick. I would maybe get to grab some stuff, too. I'd call that a pretty decent Saturday night.

And if anyone wants a juicy behind-the-scenes tidbit from Ellismania, Katie and I had a three-way with a trans girl at the Hard Rock, right before I went out and beat Gabe Ruediger.

I didn't finish that time, because I was under the impression that you're not supposed to finish right before you have a fight. A lot of fighters will tell you that's true. I'm pretty sure it's bullshit, but at the time I was buying it. I didn't want to risk losing my mojo.

And then there was one I never saw coming: One time, Katie and I went to the Abbey, which is probably the most famous gay bar in West Hollywood. I was sitting there talking to a gay couple, but when Katie came over and sat next to us, instead of making the vampire garlic sandwich face, one of the guys went straight in for the kill and made out with her.

She made this face when he was done.

"Damn, that guy tastes like cocaine," she told me.

We didn't really make anything of it. We invited the guys back to our house, but on the way, Katie was looking at her phone and started seeing tracers.

She was like, "I think I'm high."

It turns out the guy had given her a mouthful of ecstasy when he kissed her. Not a little, like residue or something. Not accidentally. He full on molly-mouthed her.

I gather that guy was extremely high himself, because he had definitely been gay back at the Abbey but by the time we got in the hot tub he was going at my girlfriend like he was a full-blooded heterosexual. It was confusing.

Everybody had a great time that night. We all had fun, and then when we were done, they were like, "Okay, we'll see you later." We didn't have to give anyone the hint to leave. It was a clean exit. Just 'see you around' and off they went, into the night.

Another time Katie and I thought it might be fun to cruise around in the Porsche and pick up a lady of the night. That seemed like a fun thing to try.

We drove around until we found this black chick we were both really into hanging out by a taco stand. (Not the one the trans girls used to hang out at, by my old radio studio. That place was gone by this point. L.A. just has a *lot* of shady taco stands.)

We rolled down the window and were like, "Hey, wanna come with us?"

And she didn't hesitate. She was like, "Hell yeah!"

She told us her name was Chocolate or something crazy like that. She had these crazy long acrylic fingernails. And she was a bigger girl. Katie had to move to the back seat of the car because Chocolate was too substantial to fit back there. She hopped in up front and suggested a cheap motel we could go to.

Katie just watched. Chocolate was saying all this weird shit to me while it went down. She was talking to me like I was a little kid, calling me 'honey muffin' and stuff like that the whole time. That was a bonus. I have had my fair share of experience with prostitutes—at least back when I was younger—and she was putting in way more effort than I ever remember seeing back then.

That was the last one you would have expected to work out. She easily could have tried to rob us or something. But it was awesome. We liked her. She was really nice. I think she liked us, too.

Afterward we took her back to the taco stand. She was like, "Take care, sugar." And that was the end of our adventure together.

The best one of all happened after a transgender award show. Katie and I rented a Hummer limo, just to be funny. And then when it was over, tons of people piled into it to come back to the house. We turned on the pool heater and people started drinking and getting naked. Pretty soon everyone was boning everyone.

Katie wasn't even trying to get involved. She was like, "I'm gonna go to bed now."

But our guests weren't having it. She went inside to go take a shower and they all followed her. By the time I walked in the room, everyone was naked and on the bed.

As I said earlier, over the years a lot of trans girls have told me they are turned off by straight women. Well, that night I found out a couple of them were lying.

For the first year or two after Katie and I got together, we took the good experiences with the bad ones. They were all part of the adventure. But gradually, over time, the bad ones stopped being quite as funny to us.

Looking back, the bad threesomes and foursomes we had were really me and Katie's fault. When we first got together, we were both so excited to have a partner in crime. We couldn't wait to try a bunch of stuff and hook up with other people. And

STILL AWESOME

because of that we were forcing it. We were trying to make it work with the wrong people.

For example, we met these two strippers on the internet. They were friends who were also kind of dating each other. We flew out to Vegas to meet them and rented a room.

It sounded like a dream come true. And at the start everything was great.

One of the girls was a squirter. I wouldn't say squirting is something I am especially into. But hey, it wasn't my house. I didn't have to clean up after her. So who cares? It was something different.

But then Katie and I started to notice that one of them was energetic. *Very* energetic. *All* the time.

On our last night in town, we went to a club and she got in an argument with some people. I think she tried to sit on their lap or something and caused a bit of a ruckus. She was all worked up.

All the sudden it hit us. We were like, *Wait, are we hanging out with a junkie right now?*

Sure enough, later on I met up with those same girls in New York when I flew there for work. I went to smoke weed out of a pipe that was laying around in my hotel room and when I did I could taste something different. Cocaine, to be specific. Turns out the chick had been smoking coke the whole time.

So that's how I ended up accidentally freebasing a tiny bit on my way into the office. I thought my heart was going to explode during the opening hour of my show that day.

It was terrible. That was the end of me and those two.

But it wasn't always something big or dramatic that made hookups go bad. Katie and I just became pickier about the people we wanted to hang out with. Things that might not have been problems for other people were total deal-breakers for us.

During the height of our craziness, we also became friendly with this really hot porn star. She was in a relationship at the time and introduced us to her boyfriend. Her dude told us that the two of them wanted to hook up with me and Katie. We were totally into that, but then somehow when the time came he showed up without her.

The three of us hooked up, but then later on we learned that he had come over behind his girlfriend's back. She didn't know anything about it. They had some big fight and broke up, and in the end, we never got to hook up with her.

After that, the ex-boyfriend would still come over from time to time. And when he did, he would say the dumbest shit. One time he was bragging to me about how great he was at jiu-jitsu. I am not the biggest jiu-jitsu enthusiast, but I know enough to know when someone is bullshitting me about how much *they* know.

This guy told me, "I'm either a blue belt or purple belt. I can't remember." Which is beyond moronic. If you really do jiu-jitsu, you know what belt you have. Obviously.

And more importantly, why are you lying to me about that? No one ever said you needed to be an elite mixed martial artist to be eligible to fuck me and Katie. It's insane that you would feel the need to make up a lie that dumb. It makes me wonder what else about you might be weird and sketchy.

Katie thought he was really good-looking, so I looked the other way on that one on her behalf. But then another time he was listening to the Red Hot Chili Peppers, and he said something like, "If you don't think they're the best band in the world, you're a moron."

That was the straw that broke the camel's back. Even Katie was out on him then. How could you sleep with someone after they told you that? The whole time I would just be picturing Anthony Kiedis swinging his junk around and singing about keeping it like a Kaiser.

STILL AWESOME

Slowly but surely, Katie and I started to realize that it only really worked out when we hooked up with someone we knew and that we liked. If someone seemed like they might be a kook—or even if something dumb like their taste in shoes rubbed us the wrong way—that was probably a sign. If we didn't go into a sexual situation already being friends, then in the end, it usually wasn't going to be worth it.

That's why we don't do it anymore. It just took us a while to learn that lesson. But for about two years we really went for it. We tried everything that either of us had ever been curious to try. Nothing was off limits.

Like the times we went to Studs, for example. Not too many couples I know have that on their to-do list.

I will explain: Studs is a movie theater in West Hollywood that caters to older gentlemen. It's been there forever. It's like a regular old movie theater, except instead of *Captain America*, the posters out front are all of shirtless dudes with pecs.

Inside, the layout is the same as a regular movie theater. (I'm sure it *was* a regular theater at one time.) There are three screens, for gay, straight, and trans porn. Every color of the porn rainbow, pretty much.

It's open day and night, but it's never packed. There's usually ten or 20 people there. Thirty at the most. Every now and then you'll see trans women who are working girls taking a break from the street and coming in there to take a rest.

The place is pretty eye-catching. A lot of places of that nature would keep a low profile, but Studs is loud and proud, right there on Santa Monica Blvd. Anyone who's ever driven past it—straight, gay, whatever—has definitely wondered what it is and how it exists and pays rent every month.

So one day Katie decided she was going to go in and find out. That's just Katie.

We went in together. It was the middle of the afternoon. It

was really dark inside. It took your eyes a while to adjust.

For the first couple of minutes I couldn't see shit. There were dudes reaching for us out of the shadows, like a bunch of gay zombies. That might have deterred most couples, but we went back a second time.

If you sit down in one of the seats in the theater and unzip your pants, someone will come out of the darkness and start blowing you. So, for fun, we dressed Katie up in my clothes and gave her a baseball cap and a fake dick.

We went in and sat together and then we both pulled our pants down. Somebody grabbed her dick and knew it was fake, and then after that no one would touch her.

We were just sitting there like that for a minute, and then, from the row behind us, suddenly a penis appeared, right between my head and Katie's head. There was a dude standing there presenting himself to us, so to speak.

We tried our best not to laugh. It's their place and we had basically laid a booby trap and fucked with them. But it's hard to keep a straight face when you take your date to a movie theater and a stranger sticks his dick between your face and hers.

Needless to say, there are mostly gay dudes in there. But there are straight dudes, too, jerking off to the straight porn. And to be honest, I think a lot of the 'gay' dudes in there would be pretty excited if a girl ever walked in. They just do gay stuff out of necessity.

It's kind of sad. A lot of times, what I see in there are people who are just horny and lonely and bummed out. It seems like the world has judged them unfuckable, so they're making the best of it the best way they can. Some of the guys don't even jerk off. It's like they just want to be there, to be part of any scene that will have them.

One time I started having sex with a trans lady (who was also a weight lifter) in there. I was in the trans room at the time.

And very quickly the whole fucking place was looking right at me. I pulled her top off to the side and I leaned around. I wasn't sure they all knew exactly what was happening, so I gave everyone an angle with a clear view. But that did not deter anyone from watching. At the end, when I finished, everyone cheered.

Yes, I got a standing ovation at Stud's.

I put my arms up in the air to celebrate. I felt like I had no choice under the circumstances.

I think the owner's been trying to clean up his act a little and attract a slightly more sophisticated clientele. I notice he's brought the lights up a bit recently.

I saw a hetero couple in there the other day. The chick looked scared. Come to think of it, the dude looked a bit unsettled, too. I don't blame them.

Shit is happening in there. There's this old guy who always hangs out. He dresses like an old Italian wife, I guess you'd say. She has fake tits and wears black lingerie and a black skirt and she's got a little bob haircut, but she's obviously a dude.

If people sit next to her, she does poppers and starts jerking them off. But I've also seen her before with her skirt over her head, running a train on people. That's how wild it can get.

I also saw four drunk white chicks in there recently. One of them was like, "I can't do it. I've got to get out of here!"

And another one was like, "Oh, relax!" Like her friend was lame because she was making a big deal out of a bunch of old dudes jerking off.

I definitely saw the lame friend's angle. It's not for everybody. Katie and I are just tweaked.

For a while there when we first met, the two of us really tried anything and everything. All bets were off.

Let's see who we can get to come over the house, we'd say. They can jerk you off and then I'll lick your butt at the same time. Whatever. Who cares? What can we think of next? It was something new every day. We would do stuff just for the fuck of it.

I'd find myself hanging upside-down for some reason or another, completely naked, laughing at my own penis, and thinking, *I've been around. Nobody on Planet Earth is doing this right now besides the two of us. No one but us would be okay with all of this. This is a special bond we have here.*

There's no way any of that stuff would happen nowadays. I have no desire to invite more strangers over to the house while Katie hides in a cage and watches us.

But I don't regret doing that. I don't regret any of it. Both of us had always wanted to push the limits, and once we found each other we owed it to ourselves to go off.

For the most part that's over now. But while it lasted, we had a good run.

Chapter 9

I started getting tattoos as soon as I was legally old enough. I got my first one in Amsterdam when I was still a teenager. But I don't know that I really considered myself a full-fledged tattoo person until right before Andrea and I split up. That's when I started looking in the mirror and seeing a new me wanting to come out.

At that time in my life, I wanted to feel like a warrior. I wanted to look at myself and see someone that no one was going to fuck with. And that someone was a person who had lots and lots of tattoos.

I got the knuckle and hand tattoos before Andrea and I were divorced. After I started dating Katie, I added a bunch more stuff. And then I decided I wanted to get a head tattoo.

As a bald guy who hates being bald, I wanted to cover my whole head so it would look like I had hair. I also just love wolves and tigers and I wanted to put some pictures of them on top of my skull. It's really that simple.

Andrea may have had strict ideas about what kinds of tattoos I could and could not get, but Katie has never told me what to do. And as someone who once paid a stranger to draw the Kool-Aid Man on her body in permanent ink, she certainly wasn't going to try to give me any tattoo advice. There was nothing stopping me, so I decided to go for it.

I was halfway through getting my head covered when Katie and I split up.

If you know me at all, you know that you should never underestimate my ability to fuck myself over.

Everything was going great between us for the first several months. But then slowly but surely I started doing the dumb things I had always done when I got into serious relationships. I started shutting down. I started closing myself off.

I have this thing I can do to people who are close to me. If I don't get my way on something—maybe even something small—instead of addressing the issue and making myself heard and finding a compromise, I grow resentful. I switch off and stew on it and become miserable. And after I've done that for a while, then I *really* won't talk about the issue, because by then I've gotten so salty that I know if I open my mouth, I'll only make it worse. So instead I just sit there in silence.

When I'm pissed off, it ruins everybody's day. It's a disease that I have.

There was a therapist Katie knew about. One of her friends used to see him and found him to be really helpful.

She was like, "You need to go talk to that guy."

"I'm not seeing a fucking therapist," I told her.

Instead, I did absolutely nothing to address the situation, and so things kept getting worse.

Finally, one day, about a year after we started dating, I went so dark on her that she started coming at me. "I feel like you're not there anymore," she said. "I don't know if you even care about me anymore. I can't get in. And because of that, I can't trust you."

I didn't have a good answer for what she was saying, so I didn't say anything at all. And I mean that literally. I went silent.

STILL AWESOME

"What is it?!" she asked.

And I just sat there, stone-faced.

"After all this?" she asked. "After I move in with you? And after everything we've done together? This is how you're going to treat me?"

She had a point, of course. She more than had a point—she was dead fucking right. But I'm stubborn, and I was in too deep. So I didn't say a word.

Katie moved out. She owned her own house, but she had rented it to some friends, so she moved into her own garage.

She left angry, and then she stayed angry. For the longest time she wouldn't even talk to me.

I started seeing this model chick. She had a rose tattoo. When I added a rose to my head, Katie popped up to DM me and say, "You got a fucking rose on there because that dumb bitch you're with has a rose tattoo?"

I hit her back and said, "No, I did not get a fucking tattoo to copy somebody else."

And that was pretty much the extent of our communication for a couple of months.

During that time, I kept thinking about how things had gone down between us at the end. I ran that last argument through my head over and over again until finally something clicked.

I realized that my girlfriend in Australia had given me the very same speech about me shutting down and shutting her out. And I remembered another time when Andrea had told me the same thing. All three times had been exactly the same. Almost word for word.

If I had heard that speech two times? Maybe that could have been a coincidence. But three? No way.

I realized that the point where I had shut down on Katie was the exact same point where all my other relationships had also started to die. I had to face the facts. I had a pattern. And I had to ask myself, *do I want to repeat this shit again and again for the rest of my life or do I want something different?*

It was my fault. I needed to get help. My experience with the sex therapist had left a bad taste in my mouth. It convinced me that therapists were all a bunch of bullshit artists who just wanted to steal your money.

But I decided to give the guy Katie recommended a shot. I didn't have much to lose. And sure enough, talking to him was different. He put things in ways that made sense to me. Instead of telling me I should never jerk off again or suggesting anything ridiculous or impossible like that, he suggested little adjustments I could actually pull off. And I could see that those first few small changes made a noticeable improvement in my life.

I never gave up on wanting to get back together with Katie. In fact, the longer I was apart from her and the more other people I went out with, the more positive I became that I had well and truly fucked up. But I kept my distance. I wanted to keep working on myself. I wanted to take my time and really plan out my comeback.

Eventually I thought I had let sleeping dogs lie long enough that I could attempt to contact her. I knew she was still angry at me. But I thought she'd cooled off enough that if I tried to hit her up, she probably wouldn't key my car. That still wouldn't have shocked me, but I figured that was a risk worth taking.

I decided to write her a love note. The letter was different from the ones I used to write to Andrea when I was trying to get back together with her. With Andrea I basically just said, "I'm sorry I was shitty to you. Take me back and I'll try to be better this time." With Katie's, I said, "I'm going to therapy to fix myself. And if it doesn't work, then you can just leave me."

I really felt that way. I knew I was the problem. If this therapist couldn't fix me, then I was unfixable and had no business being in a relationship. I still stand by that, to this day.

STILL AWESOME

My letter to Katie was also different from the ones I had written to Andrea because this one had little knives and daggers drawn all over it. Plus, I had cut myself and leaked a bunch of blood on it.

I went out in the middle of the night and stuck the note on Katie's car windshield. Looking back, that probably would have appeared pretty suspect to an outside observer. If a cop saw me sticking a bloody note covered with crude drawings of weapons on some lady's Prius, he would have assumed I was a deranged stalker. My first phone call to Katie in months would have been from a holding cell.

Lucky for me, Katie got the note and it did the trick. For a guy who didn't go to school, I seem to write a mean love letter.

I give a lot of the credit to therapy. It didn't just save my relationship with Katie—it changed my life. Really, it changed both our lives.

The more I go to therapy, the more I see my mistakes. I see how, when someone is emotionally damaged, it affects so many things about the way they act. Your childhood comes with you in ways most people would never notice without professional help.

And the more I understand why I am the way I am, the more I am able to see why Katie and I fell in love with each other. We both have a lot of scars.

After all these years, this guy is really fixing me. And as a result, he's kind of fixing Katie, too. She comes in with me every now and then, but more importantly I think just being around me makes the lessons I'm learning about myself trickle over to her.

Ironically, by helping me, my therapist has made me lose interest in a lot of things that used to seem really fun and important to me. Not because he forbids me to have them, like the sex therapist who outlawed me jerking myself off, but because I don't need them anymore.

Just as soon as I finally got the head tattoo I had wanted so badly, I no longer felt it was necessary to cover myself in tattoos so I can try to convince strangers that I'm a badass. I guess I would still do it all over again. I don't regret any of my tattoos. I'm very happy for my body to be covered in cool pictures. But it's more of a hobby now.

I don't feel a deep psychological need to get tattoos anymore. I no longer feel like I need to cover myself in armor like I used to. Sometimes nowadays I look in the mirror and just think, *Aw, look at you. You tried so hard to be scary.*

Therapy also shut down a lot of the craziness in my sex life. Looking back, I think it's fair to say I was out of control, at least for a while there.

At the beginning of our relationship, I had the full green light. Katie was like, "Why don't you sleep with everybody you want to?"

Those were words I never dreamed I might hear from a girlfriend. And so for a while, that's exactly what I did.

I probably needed to do that to get it out of my system. But I took it too far. I always do, with everything.

Eventually Katie asked, "Do you realize how many people you've been sleeping with? What's going on with you? Do you think that's a good idea?" I don't think she was mad. She was just concerned. It's like if you have a drinking buddy, but then all of a sudden you notice that guy has started ordering tequila shots at lunch on a Wednesday.

I was like, "Fuck. Should I talk to my therapist about it?"

So I did. And my therapist broke it down for me. He walked me through all the different kinds of people I was sleeping with. He said, "You like some of these people. They're your friends. Those ones are fine."

"But this other group," he asked me, "Do you think you're doing those things for the right reasons?"

He was referring to strangers, and to what many people would call risky or unsafe situations. The times when the contact was completely anonymous, and where my attitude toward the other person was just, 'get me off and then get out of here.'

I would meet people on Grindr and invite them over my house. Obviously, I was not running background checks on any of these dudes.

"You realize they now have your address?" my therapist asked.

And I said, "So? I'm me. What the fuck are they going to do to me?"

And he said, "But Jason, your kids live there, too."

I didn't have an answer to that. I hadn't considered the fact that some sketchy Grindr guy could come back another time when I wasn't there. In my mind, the whole thing was harmless. Everyone was winning. But that's because I was only thinking of myself.

That conversation took a lot of the fun out of Grindr.

And on an even deeper level, my therapist showed me that, while some of the things I was doing were healthy and fun, some of the other stuff was just me acting out because I was abused as a child.

Basically, my therapist explained: During the times I was molested, I had felt powerless. But now, to be an adult and to be able to hook up with strange people and call all the shots made me feel like I was taking that power back.

It makes a lot of sense when you think about it. I was like, *Well, there goes that scenario forever. No more dudes showing up at the house and then bowing and thanking me when they leave a half hour later.* With a couple of sentences, my therapist had ruined that completely.

He took a lot of fun out of glory holes, too. I used to be a fan of those. And yes, they are out there.

There's a place in Hollywood called The Zone. It's this maze of glory holes. And not just a couple—there are multiple floors of them.

It's not some underground illegal club, either. It's a legitimate business, as far as I can tell. There's a big sign outside. I'm assuming they pay taxes and everything. You can find it on Yelp.

You pay 15 bucks to enter. But they won't let girls in. Not even trans girls. Believe me—I've tried. Inside they sell poppers and lube and rubbers and shit. There are sex cages and sex swings, in addition to all the glory holes. It's like a great big playground for people who are tweaked.

In case you've ever wondered, here's how glory holes work: People lay their finger in a hole cut inside a wall. That's the cue for a person on the other side to stick his dick inside it.

And also, in case you were wondering: No, the mouth never belongs to a girl. If you've got a buddy who says he went to one and it was a girl, your buddy is either dumb, lying, or kind of gay.

Actually, I have come across one exception. People make their own personal glory holes in their houses sometimes. They'll drill a hole in their cupboard door or something like that and then go on Grindr, give out their address, and say, "Just walk in, shut the door, and put your dick in the hole." I used to go to those every now and then. And one time it was different.

I was like, "Fuck, that feels like a girl." Girls don't have stubble. I think that's what it was.

I was trying to look through the little crack. I pulled myself back a little bit so she would lean in, and sure enough, there she was. But trust me—that is the exception by far.

Needless to say, just like inviting Grindr dudes over your house, doing things with strangers at glory holes can also be a little risky.

I was in New York once to go on *The Howard Stern Show*. There was a place I knew about in Times Square that I had stumbled on during one of my first *Stern* appearances, back when I was still married.

The first time I had gone there, I went into a little room, paid some cash, and then a blind opened up with a naked lady on the other side. She opened a slot on the wall and told me to put my hand inside. She put my hand on her titty while I watched her through the glass and jerked off.

It was awesome. I was like, "This isn't even cheating!" because I didn't ask her to do that. Even though technically, duh, of course it was.

Anyway, I went back to the same place a couple years later, but instead of a naked lady, now there was a video screen. I figured it had become a little jack off booth. But there were also these holes in the wall on the side. Someone put their finger into the hole and gave it the tap, so I went for it.

I'm not sure exactly which *Stern* visit this was. It was definitely one of the times I got naked in front of George Takei. But then again, I've had my dick out in front of George Takei so many times—really who can keep them all straight?

Anyway, by the time I went on air, I had a funny feeling in my crotch region. I didn't know for sure if something was wrong, but I definitely had an inkling. I also don't recall if it was gonorrhea or chlamydia I got that time, but whichever it was, it was inside my dick when George was jerking me off.

I doubt George Takei will ever read this. If he does, I sincerely apologize. It was an honest mistake. I'm sure he was fine. No one ever caught anything from a couple little love tugs. But still—my bad, homey.

I flew home and it was another day or two before I really started to feel it.

This wasn't my first rodeo getting an STD from a blowjob. Once, when I was a young'un, I caught something after getting a BJ from a hooker in Perth on some skateboard tour. It started to hurt when I peed. I was married to my first wife at the time, so I went to the doctor on the down low and took care of it myself. Then the bill came to the house three months later and I got busted.

I was with Katie by the time I caught whatever I got in New York. I told her when I got back to L.A. I was like, "I got the clap in a fucking glory hole." And quite sensibly, she said, "You've got to stop doing that."

This wasn't even the first time that had happened since Katie and I had been a couple. I had also gotten it from some guy at a spa. You would think blowjobs would be safe, but it turns out you can't just put your penis in random mouths. It took me a while to learn my lesson, but the third time was finally the charm.

Because of therapy, having sex with other people in general started slowing down, a lot.

I used to make these big plans. I used to try to dream up some new scenario and then try to make it happen. But they almost never worked out the way I imagined. There were so many letdowns.

It's still nice if there's a couple Katie and I can hook up with. Katie gets to enjoy one of them and I enjoy the other. But even then, we'll only do it if we know for a fact that the other couple are also in love with each other. Then, at the end of the night, everyone goes back to their own house and is happy to wind up in bed with the person they showed up with. There's no drama.

We rarely do threesomes anymore. There's too big a risk of one person becoming the odd man out. If someone comes along who's really into both of us and we're both really into them, then sure. Why not? But that's not a common situation to come across. We don't go looking for it and it doesn't fall into our laps very often. If it doesn't work for everyone all the way, then our answer is thanks but no thanks. We've had our fun. We'll skip it.

STILL AWESOME

Even if I hook up with someone on my own, it's gotta make sense. I'm still up for anything, but only if I know there is basically zero chance it might end badly. The same goes for Katie and the people she wants to sleep with.

Neither Katie nor I would do half the shit we used to do. We've learned a lot of lessons, and more importantly we're not as motivated to push the limits. We're pretty normal now. Normal for us, anyway.

The more I worked on myself, the more I wanted to get to the core of my issues. It's a natural progression. I didn't just want to learn how to *deal* with my problems—I wanted to *solve* them. Luckily, on top of therapy and prescription drugs and stuff like that, there's a whole new universe of treatment options popping up. Some of them are new. Some were just new to me.

Aubrey Marcus—the founder of Onnit—is a friend of mine. He's also one of the smartest, most passionate people I know. Onnit sells supplements and workout equipment and stuff like that. Everything they do is part of one larger goal, which they refer to as "Total Human Optimization."

Onnit's thing—and also Aubrey's thing—is combining tried and true strategies for mental and physical health with more cutting edge, outside of the box kinds of stuff. Every time you talk to Aubrey, there's always some new training regimen or new supplement or whatever that him and his people are getting excited about. Those guys never stop.

Around this time I first heard about ayahuasca, a traditional psychedelic medicine they've been using in the Amazon for literally thousands of years. My first exposure to ayahuasca was a video of Aubrey. He was in Peru trying it alongside another guy I didn't know. That guy was wide-eyed the whole time, and seemed really happy and free-spirited. The experience looked intense. Truthfully, it looked straight up scary and, to me, the other guy seemed creepy as fuck.

I had dinner with Aubrey a while after I saw the video, and sure enough that creepy guy came to the dinner with us. That's when I met Dr. Dan. (His full name is Dr. Dan Engle, but everyone just calls him Dr. Dan.)

In general, I get suspicious of people like Dr. Dan. I don't trust them. Maybe it's because I think that if you act happy all the time you're probably just hiding something. Or maybe I'm just jealous that some people get to be carefree, laidback hacky-sack motherfuckers while people like me are so dark and fucked up.

But as usual, Aubrey's instincts were correct. Dr. Dan is a great guy and he has the heart of a champion.

That night at dinner, I talked to Dan and Aubrey about ayahuasca. Aubrey said it had done amazing things for him. He said it made him confront death and that he was better off because of it. That was very appealing to me. I have always been terrified of death. I guess most people are, but I think my fear goes above and beyond.

They say ayahuasca "calls" to people who really need to take it. I usually call bullshit on that kind of stuff. I don't think ghosts are real and I think Bigfoot is a fucking bear. But I have to say, I think ayahuasca started calling to me from the moment Aubrey and I had that dinner.

Still, I was nowhere near ready to commit. I may have been afraid of death, but I was also afraid of ayahuasca.

That conversation also turned me on to some other kinds of therapy. DMT was one they talked about. MDMA was another. I took lots of ecstasy when I was younger, so I wasn't afraid of that. Unless you take tons of it for days on end, I knew it's a fairly mellow experience. And that long-ago night at Beacher's Madhouse with Dingo had shot a hole in my theory that taking drugs was going to kill me. So under Dr. Dan's supervision, I decided to give that a go.

STILL AWESOME

I didn't have any specific goal when I decided to do MDMA therapy. I just wanted to get to the bottom of everything. For as long as I could remember, I had felt broken. And as I got older, that feeling never went away.

I had periods when I was younger where I got really dark. It seems like most people grow out of those phases once they reach adulthood, but after I split up with Andrea for good, I had gotten really dark on myself again. I became filled with anger. I started listening to the darkest metal songs I could get my hands on, over and over.

It was just like when I was a teenager and first became obsessed with Metallica. You know that age? When you could listen to a song and it would motivate you in this over-the-top irrational way? Like, *This song makes a great point! I'm gonna change my whole life, because of this one lyric!* I had been like that again. And not in a positive way. During that time, I felt self-destructive. Not toward my body necessarily, but toward my career. I believe that deep down I was afraid of success and so I subconsciously started to wreck my own shit.

Since then, I had moved on with my life and met Katie and moved myself out of that headspace. But I knew I hadn't addressed that darkness. I knew it was still inside me, ready to come back if I let it.

As I made more progress in therapy, I arrived at the conclusion that I needed to break myself open. I felt like I had to end the old me entirely. I needed to get rid of all my shit once and for all and then put myself back together. Only this time, finally, I would do it the right way.

When I initially agreed to do MDMA therapy with Dr. Dan, I told him I wanted to deal with anxiety and depression. But just like with the therapists at rehab, it pretty quickly became apparent that we were going to be zeroing in on me being molested.

Honestly, I was still holding out hope that the MDMA therapy could show me that I was mistaken about what I believed had happened when I was a kid. There was still a shred of doubt in the back of my head. What if I was wrong?

I was hoping that afterward I would be able to call my brother Lee back and apologize. "Guess what? I took some ecstasy with some weird, happy guy, and it turns out it *was* the babysitter the whole time!" I would have been really happy to have been wrong.

I had made a pretty massive accusation and I didn't have a family anymore because of it. The only proof I had were some foggy memories. This seemed like one last chance to get a good look at the shit that happened when I was a kid and to maybe change my mind.

Dr. Dan came over to the house and gave me the pill. The first one didn't kick in strong enough, so he gave me a second one and then we waited for something to happen. I felt a familiar sensation kicking in. There's a reason I used to take so much ecstasy. I could easily see how I could have kicked back, let my brain fry, and had a good time. And for sure, after he left—when we were done—I did get to enjoy it a bit.

But Dr. Dan knew exactly what he was doing. And for the next three or four hours, I wasn't thinking about having fun or getting laid. He was steering my brain—and not in fun directions. At all.

I could see inside my childhood bedroom. It looked so real. I could see little things laying around my room—things I had totally forgotten about until that moment. It was crazy how many details were coming back to me.

And that was just the tip of the iceberg. That MDMA experience ended up being about rediscovering all kinds of things from when I was a kid that were still hiding out in the corners of my mind.

Over the years, I had tried to keep the abuse I went through out of my mind as much as possible. For obvious reasons, it was something I didn't want to think about. But every now and then

STILL AWESOME

I would get a little flash of it in my mind.

I could remember a heat lamp. It would happen during nighttime, so it was always dark. My dad would carry that thing around so he could check on the three of us in our bedrooms. The lamp wasn't that bright. It didn't light up the room. I would just see the circle of those neon orange-red heat things glowing in the dark, right in my doorway. And then he would come in.

Before I did the MDMA therapy, I could remember the voice and I could remember the dick. I know that's a gross, weird, uncomfortable thing for me to say. But what can I tell you? That's the truth.

But I never saw a face. It was like my brain couldn't even handle thinking about that part.

Another thing I already remembered about my childhood was times when I would get scared and go under my bed. I would hold onto the bed springs with my fingers and my toes and lift my body off the ground so it would be harder to see me.

Because I had been keeping all these memories at arm's length, I didn't put all the pieces together. Before I took the MDMA with Dr. Dan, I would have told you I used to do that because I had night terrors or something. The way I remembered it, it was something a kid might do when they're scared of the boogeyman. You know—your kid brain figures maybe it's hard for the monster to find you if you're under the bed and off the ground.

But when I took the MDMA, I remembered that it wasn't a monster I was hiding from. Actually, I would see that fucking heat lamp coming, get super scared, and then cling to the bottom of my bed for dear life.

I also remembered some other times that had happened earlier, before I started going under the bed. I recalled a couple times when I was on top of the bed and things were happening to me. I don't mean that anything was going inside me. Just that

I knew something was happening on my back. I remembered clenching my hands on the sides of the mattress.

And finally, that night I took the MDMA I remembered the last time I was underneath my bed. I remembered saying, "No. Please stop," and then seeing the heat lamp going away.

In my mind's eye, still on the MDMA, my thoughts started to wander. I wasn't exactly remembering things that had happened anymore. I was imagining things that I thought might have happened next. I saw my dad go back down the hall, past Lee's room, past the kitchen, past the living room, and into his bedroom where Marn was. I saw him realize that what he had been doing was fucked up.

I don't think it ever happened again after the night I said no. I don't think my dad had the information or the intelligence to know the damage he was inflicting on a child. But I think right there, at that moment, it had to have finally hit him that what he'd done was unforgivable. And I saw that once he came to that realization, he had to carry that knowledge with him for the rest of his life.

I believe knowing what he had done affected the way my dad saw himself. It affected the way he saw me for sure. My whole life, my dad always treated me kind of weird. The relationship I had with him was very different from the relationships my dad had with my brothers. It was like I was never a kid to him after that.

My dad cleaned up his act a lot after my brothers were born. (Or at least that was the way he made it look.) But heavy conversations would still come up from time to time, about the old days. Like how this friend of his might have killed a guy. Or how this girl he knew went to jail and then got burned alive in her cell. No one was talking about those things in front of Lee or Stevie. No fucking way. But when conversations got dark like that, Jason was okay to hear them. Our father never told Lee, "I didn't even want a kid." Lee never heard the word *accident* when the story got told about how he came along. But I did.

STILL AWESOME

There were things my dad and I did together that he would never have dreamed of doing with my brothers. When I was 18, or maybe even younger, him and I went out on a river on a speed boat with these two chicks. Later that day, we docked the boat and jogged to his business, Ellistronics. He went inside, opened the till, pulled all the money out, and then walked away. We all went and got a hotel room together and drank champagne and then he fucked one chick and I fucked the other.

These were not traditional father-son bonding activities. Because we didn't have a traditional father-son relationship. That wasn't possible because of what had happened when I was little. And he knew it.

I didn't get what I was hoping for from MDMA. Instead of finding out that all of these horrible things I had come to believe actually weren't true, I was finally convinced that they were.

Dr. Dan hit me up later and asked if I wanted to do another session. I never even hit him back. I was done. I felt like if there were any more memories still locked away in my brain, I didn't need to let them out. I knew as much as I needed to know. Finding out more shit wasn't going to help me fix myself any faster.

I now knew for sure that the person I should have been able to rely on more than anyone in the world had taken something from me in a way that was so earth-shattering, it almost made me want to die just to think about it. But I also knew there was no need to dwell on it any more than I already had. Now it was time to get to work and to start figuring out how I was going to live with everything I knew. And how I was going to rise above it.

By that time, I was overdue to bring the kids back to Australia. Things may have been weird between me and my relatives, but that's Devin and Tiger's family, too. The kids deserved to see their Australian family and their Aussie family deserved to see them as well. I want my kids to have that relationship.

In the past we probably would have stayed with relatives, but under the circumstances I got me and the kids and Katie a hotel room in Melbourne.

We were there over Christmastime. One night was set aside as a boys' night. We went to my friend Tom Payton's house. There was drinking and arm wrestling and other assorted forms of dude stupidity.

I started to notice that this one guy I had known forever was going out of his way not to talk to me. Over the course of the next couple hours, I realized he was also giving me looks. He actually started mad dogging me.

I asked my brother Lee, "What the fuck is going on with him?"

And Lee said, "I got something I need to talk to you about."

I could tell by the way he said that that he had been saving up something for a good long while, so I said, "Oh, yeah? What's that?"

We moved into one of the bedrooms and he let me have it. "You just made up that you got molested to be on *The Howard Stern Show*," he said.

If it was anyone else, I would have thought he was joking. But my brother isn't that guy. This wasn't sarcasm.

And meanwhile that other guy was standing right there in the bedroom with us, eyeballing me the whole time, just to let me know that he backed up whatever Lee said. As if I gave a fuck about his opinion.

Maybe this conversation would have gone differently if I hadn't just done the MDMA therapy. Up until that point, I still had a tiny bit of doubt. Until I relived all those memories I had blocked out for decades, a small part of me still suspected that my mind was so evil that it wanted to destroy me, and that it may have convinced me of something that wasn't true.

But now I had confirmation. Those couple extra pieces had completed the whole puzzle. And in my mind, that knowledge had opened the door to other frightening possibilities. What if it had happened to Lee, too? If something so seemingly insane had happened to me, how could I rule out anything?

Lee kept coming at me. He was mad at me for writing that my dad had molested me in my first book. The only problem was I never *said* that in my first book. When I made that book, I still thought the neighbor did it.

I was like, "Wait, have you even *read* my book?" He admitted he hadn't.

I was like, "Dude, you're my brother, and you're going to chastise me about what's in my book when you didn't even bother to check it out for yourself?"

I gathered that Lee had gotten most of his information from conversations that happened on *Howard Stern*. But I knew that Lee had for damned sure never listened to *The Howard Stern Show*. You can get books sent over from America as long as you're willing to pay a crazy amount for the shipping, but you can't get SiriusXM in your car in Australia. You'd have to go out of your way to find *Howard Stern*. You'd have to go listen through the internet. And I knew there was only one person Lee knew who would ever bother to do that.

There was this girl in Australia I used to sleep with. Katie and I had seen her earlier on that same trip, as a matter of fact. Katie didn't like her straight away because she was super clingy toward me. She came in too hot. She was always like that, every time I went back there.

Andrea had had the same problem with her. As I have said, Andrea had a problem with anyone she thought might be interested in me. Anyone who she considered a potential threat. All in all, Andrea was a composed, rational adult person, but I'd have to say this was the most immature side of her.

Andrea knew me and this girl had hooked up a few times. But by the time Andrea met her, that was already like ten years ago.

And obviously it was no secret that I had a past. There was no reason to make it weird.

We were out at a bar one night with Stevie and Lee's friends and Andrea was vibing the fuck out of this chick. She was gnarly like that. If Andrea thought a girl might have any interest in me sexually, she had no problem saying, "Fuck you, I don't like you."

That was how she rolled. Another time, in America, I was talking to a girl somewhere and all the sudden a glass came whizzing by our heads. Andrea had had a couple drinks and when she saw me with another woman, she didn't give any warning—she just chucked her cocktail at the poor girl.

That kind of attitude doesn't go over well anywhere. But Australians especially don't like it when a pretty lady from America comes over and tries to run that game. It didn't make Andrea any friends.

I suspected this Australian chick might have remembered that shit with Andrea. Maybe she wanted a little revenge. Or maybe she was just bored and wanted to stir the pot a bit. Who knows?

But out of everyone I still know in Australia, this chick was the one person who would listen to my show on the internet or Google me and then pass whatever information she found along to Lee. Unfortunately for me, she hadn't bothered to get her facts straight.

And there was no one else over there who was going to stick up for me. Maybe my mum believed me at that point, but that's not Lee's mother. They don't have a super tight relationship. They wouldn't ever have that kind of conversation.

And Marn—his mother and my stepmother—didn't believe me. She thought my father was faithful to her at the end. She didn't know that, after all of his cheating and getting caught and promising to do right by her if she took him back, he then turned around and cheated on her even more...*and* allegedly sold weed...*and* did live sex shows...*and* that you could hire him to come to your house and fuck your wife (and maybe the husband, too, is how it seems to me, if I'm being honest).

All Lee had was a bunch of secondhand information, but he decided it was enough to get his boy and confront me over it. I was like, "I'm out of here, man. I'm never coming back."

I went back to the hotel, and I haven't been back to Australia since.

I first heard of DMT several years back, from some skateboarder guys. Apparently, it was the hot new psychedelic drug in their world at that time. The trip was way shorter than acid or mushrooms. It lasted less than 30 minutes. But it was also way more intense. These guys were telling me it had given them the worst trip they had ever had. And these were dudes with plenty of experience with drugs. So I made a mental note to never ever try it.

But then years later, my accidental psychedelic medicine guru Aubrey Marcus started talking it up. DMT is known as "the spirit molecule." Unlike acid and mushrooms, our body naturally makes DMT. Supposedly your brain releases it when you die. You know those people who almost die and then afterward they about going toward the light? It turns out those people might not be getting a sneak preview of the afterlife after all. They might just be tripping balls on DMT.

Aubrey invited me to a DMT ceremony. Aubrey is the kind of guy who does his homework, and at this point he obviously had put a lot of research into mind-altering drugs.

It took a little convincing, but eventually I agreed to join him and his friends. Just like with the MDMA therapy, DMT was presented to me as a learning experience. Otherwise, I wouldn't have been a part of it. Despite how it might sound, it definitely wasn't Aubrey saying, "Hey, you guys wanna come get fucked up with me?"

Unlike MDMA, I had no prior experience with DMT. But by this point I was totally past that nagging fear that taking drugs would kill me. I had been getting back into boxing and MMA training at that point. I was going at it hard. I would do four straight minutes of punches at the gym. My heart rate would get up to like 195 for half an hour. If that kind of training didn't get me, then I figured that 30 minutes of tripping balls probably wasn't going to take me out either.

You can take DMT a couple different ways. In our case, we were smoking it. The guy who went first took a massive rip and then just like that he was off on another planet. I took a way smaller toke, but still, the second it went in my body, I was immediately launched into a totally different reality. I was gone.

A few moments later a friend of mine tapped my chest. I was holding my breath in. That was the only thing that reminded me to breathe. It was scary. I panicked a bit. I worried that my brain might forget to make me breathe again, and that next time no one would catch me. And at that point I knew it was too late to back out. The roller coaster was already out of the gate and on its way up that first big hill. I was past the point of no return.

I saw a room, inside my imagination. There were all these weird people inside. They had these big smiley faces, but in a scary, evil, Satanic kind of way. It was clear they weren't friendly.

They wanted me to join them. They were doing that creepy 'come hither' thing with their finger, trying to get me to come inside where they were.

And then just like that, my little starter puff of DMT wore off and I got pulled back into reality.

The stuff I had seen in there was really freaky, but then again, I'm pretty used to having dark thoughts and living with weird shit inside my head. That doesn't shake me like it might shake other people. I knew there was nothing fun waiting for me back inside that room, but I still wanted to find out what it was. I was on a mission to get to the root of my problems and it looked like some of the answers might finally be right in front of me. This wasn't the time to run away.

I took another puff—much bigger than the first one—and then instantly I was in this crazy white room inside some big building. There was a maze of people and all this stuff to look around at.

I took that all in for a few minutes. I didn't like it in there. It's hard to explain. Being on DMT is kind of like being in a waking dream. In the end nothing happened, but I got the vibe that the place did not intend good things for me.

And then the second dose wore off. By that point I did not care to go back inside wherever I had been anymore. I was done.

I didn't really get any big insights or learn anything about my past from DMT. But I'm still glad I did it. It was part of a journey. It brought me one step closer to ayahuasca. It let me dip my toe into what ayahuasca might be like. DMT was the starter kit. It made me a little less scared of the big trip that I was one day destined to take.

Whether or not you consider yourself an addict, many of us who enjoy drinking and smoking weed occasionally have nights—or maybe even weeks—where you push it into the red a little bit and go overboard. You do a couple of stupid things while you're wasted or you get a couple of bad hangovers and then you decide to dial it back a little bit. Around this time, I felt like I had been going too hard on weed, so I decided to take a break from it.

Shortly after I started that break, I got invited to something called the Bass Player Live! Awards. Jason Newsted—formerly of my all-time favorite band, Metallica—asked me to come. Obviously, I was very excited to take him up on his offer.

I hadn't eaten anything when I arrived. And since I wasn't smoking weed, I might have started off drinking a bit faster than I usually would. I got buzzed pretty quick.

Newsted and his wife had this big private area to themselves on the balcony, because...he's Jason Newsted. Me and Katie were hanging out there, and then some insanely rich billionaire guy with a button-down shirt and a crazy watch recognized me and Jason, invited us to the bar, and ordered a full tray of shots. I was planning to stick to my rum and pineapples, but then someone said, "Do these shots, Ellis!" And then that's kind of the last thing I remember.

I am told that after drinking God knows how many of those, I was talking to Jason Newsted's wife. I have no idea what I was talking to her about, but apparently I was very passionate about the subject. I am told I was speaking very vigorously.

Later on in the night, there was an all-star jam thing where a bunch of celebrity rock stars went on stage and performed with each other. Geezer Butler from Black Sabbath was there. So were Zakk Wylde and Corey Taylor from Slipknot and a bunch of other legends. It was a whole big thing.

Sebastian Bach was up there at one point. Sebastian had been on the radio show a couple times by then so him and I knew each other a bit. Naturally I don't remember this happening, but he tells me that I was screaming at him from up on the balcony. He seems to recall that I knew the words to a lot of the songs and that I was loudly singing them back down at him. I'm pretty sure I was just screaming nonsense.

Whatever I was doing, he seemed to think it was great. He might well have been the only person there that night who felt that way, but anyway afterward he joined me on the balcony to hang out. Based on what I heard the next day, our conversation seemed to mainly involve me yelling "Fuck you!" at him at the top of my lungs.

After I did that for a bit, for my final act of the evening I fell down a flight of stairs. Then Katie and I went home.

I woke up with a rug burn from taking that tumble. I could feel that I had hit my head pretty good, too. Katie filled me in on most of what I had forgotten. I told her I didn't need to know all the details. Obviously the gist of it was that I had acted like a complete and utter moron.

I haven't spoken to Newsted since. I'm sure he's a busy guy, but I don't think that's a coincidence. I think he thinks I'm an animal.

Oddly enough, I managed to become even better friends with Sebastian Bach that night. He thinks I'm an animal, too. The difference is that's cool in his book, because Sebastian Bach is even more of an animal than I am.

Katie was never going to tell me to stop drinking. She was never going to stop me from doing anything. She knows how people work. She knows how *I* work. She's always known that you can give people help and support and advice if they ask for it, but if someone isn't going to take the steps to help themselves you can't do it for them. If anyone was gonna check me, it was going to have to be me.

That night wasn't rock bottom. It wasn't the final straw. It was just a dumb, regrettable accident. I still went to work on Monday. I still went to the gym that week. My kids were still being properly supervised and all that. I wasn't off the rails by any means.

But by coincidence this was when I met the actor Dax Shepard. He was a guest on my radio show. Dax is a big Howard Stern fan. He had heard me on *Stern* and was very complimentary about my most recent appearance. He thought I was really brave for talking about being molested and all that stuff.

While I was interviewing him, he said, "I'm surprised you're not an addict."

"I am," I said. I believe that at that point in my life, I had drinking and weed under control, at least for the most part. But I still knew who I was.

He said, "So do you go to any meetings?"

I told him I didn't. AA had never appealed to me. And I felt I had given it a decent shot when I was in rehab.

Dax talked to me a bunch after that radio show ended. He is a very wise man. He didn't have the most stable upbringing either, but he's gone to therapy and gotten sober and he does the work. As a result, instead of being a massive fuck up he has a great career and a great wife and two amazing kids. He's living proof that AA really can help.

I immediately felt like I could trust him. If he thought going to meetings was a good idea, then maybe I was wrong? I was at least open to the possibility. There are lots of different meetings, after all. Just like there are lots of therapists. I had seen how much good the right therapist could do. Maybe I just hadn't been to the right meeting?

So I decided to stop drinking.

By then I had started smoking weed again. I figured the first 'A' in AA just stood for alcohol, so I assumed that was okay. I wasn't trying to hide it or anything. I openly admitted it to Dax.

He was like, "You're still smoking weed?"

And I was like, "Fuck yeah—I'm high right now!"

He told me I had to stop that, too. Truthfully, I didn't feel like quitting weed was necessary. Alcohol might have been getting in the way here and there, but I really didn't feel like weed was a problem. Still, I took his advice and went along with it.

I knew from past experience that getting off weed will make me pretty edgy. I was fine with quitting, but I didn't want it to affect the show or my children.

Dax asked me if I had a window of time where I could get away from my responsibilities. And as it just so happened, I had a week of vacation coming up where I wouldn't have the kids. It almost seemed like it was meant to be.

I rode it out through those first few days and made it to the other side. And after that I started feeling pretty good. I felt like I was hitting my stride.

STILL AWESOME

It wasn't the first time in my life that I had been sober for an extended period of time. But for once, I wasn't on the straight and narrow out of fear that I might die or because I had bottomed out and had nowhere else to turn.

I felt happy. I felt motivated. It seemed like this time it just might stick.

Maybe this is the new me? I wondered—*the me I was destined to be all along?*

Chapter 10

Sometime, a while back, when Katie and I were still in the midst of sowing our wild oats, we went to a swinger party out in Palm Springs.

We went to more than one of those. We found them to be kind of fun and also kind of funny, all at the same time.

Those things always advertise themselves like there are going to be all these sexy adventurous young naked people fucking each other left and right while getting down to today's most cutting-edge hit music. I may be in my late forties, but I take care of myself. And Katie is super hot. So we figured we could probably hang in that scene. Instead, we arrived to find that everyone was out of shape and over 50. I'm not even bragging when I say we were the most attractive couple...by a lot. And the whole time, DJ Dickhead was playing nonstop mashups of hip-hop beats and really shitty mainstream butt rock.

I am sorry to report that the swinging scene is kind of a bust, at least compared to what we expected. Nonetheless we still had fun dabbling in it, and by the end of the night we always found someone decent to hook up with.

Anyway, at this one particular party, Katie and I were kicking back in the jacuzzi, sipping champagne, looking at saggy old naked people, and enjoying an insane mix of rock and beats. I don't remember how the conversation led up to it, but at one point, Katie casually mentioned she would be open to getting married. It just kind of slipped out. I didn't make a big deal out of it and we didn't discuss it in detail. Just as quickly as that had come up, the conversation moved on to some other topic.

But I filed that one away. If I wanted to ask her, now I knew she would definitely say yes.

I think about a year went by before I was finally ready to pop the question. It wasn't because I wasn't sure about Katie. I had already been divorced twice, but there wasn't a doubt in my mind that her and I were meant to be together forever.

I just wanted to do it right. I wanted to really plan it out. I needed to save some money to get a ring. And most of all I wanted to make sure that Katie really knew what she was signing up for. As open as I had been with her throughout our relationship, I wanted to share everything about myself—good and bad—before we got engaged. I may have even exaggerated some of the bad stuff to make myself seem worse than I really am. I wanted her to know everything about me that might potentially be hard to deal with, just to make sure there were never going to be any surprises that would make her regret or rethink being married to me.

Once I got that out of the way, the last piece of the puzzle was finding a way to pop the question. Mike Tully—my co-host on the radio show (and the guy who wrote this book with me)—came up with the answer.

We played a game on the show. It was me against Katie. The idea was that we would both look at pictures of bad tattoos and then try to guess which celebrity they belonged to.

Katie and I made a bet on the game. We each had to secretly think of a horrible tattoo idea for each other, and then the winner would get to surprise the loser by personally giving them the shitty tattoo they had chosen.

I'm pretty surprised Katie didn't see through the plan. It was the dumbest idea for a radio bit ever. I think she might have figured out that my producers were feeding me the answers to all the questions to make sure that I won, but I knew she wouldn't care about that. As I have probably made clear by now, she wasn't afraid of going home with a shitty tattoo.

Nonetheless, I think she was genuinely surprised when she looked at her leg and saw that it said, *Will you marry me?*

Those things are permanent. Once I got that bad boy on her, she pretty much had no choice.

I got a phone call shortly after that, out of the blue. It was from King of the Cage, a fight organization. They asked if I was retired from MMA.

As it just so happened, I had been thinking about taking another fight.

In many ways, my first fight had been great. I loved the training. I loved testing myself. I wouldn't say I loved the weight cut, but I was proud of myself for having the discipline to endure it. I loved that I had faced my nerves and had stepped into a situation very few people ever choose to put themselves in. And obviously, I was happy that I won. It was cool to know that if you looked up Jason Ellis on Sherdog—the big official MMA website—you saw a 1-0 pro record next to my name.

But the fight itself was kind of lacking. It was all too much. It's so hard to keep your composure in your first fight, especially when you're the main event at a great big venue. I didn't feel like I had followed my game plan or used my training nearly as much as I had hoped to. And because of that, I felt like I still had some unfinished business.

When King of the Cage called, I was still training all the time. And even though I was getting older, I felt like I was getting better. I was more well-rounded than I had been the first time I fought. And that wasn't just my opinion. I trained with pro fighters—like my friend Mike Jasper—and they all told me the same thing.

I was a little bit inspired by CM Punk, too. He's the WWE

guy who quit fake wrestling to try to become a real fighter and then got his ass kicked in the UFC. (Twice.) I knew I didn't belong in the UFC, either. But I also knew for damn sure that I was better than him and I wanted a chance to prove it.

I was ready for another test. I am always at my best when I have a challenge in front of me. And while King of the Cage isn't the UFC or Bellator, it's a completely legit MMA organization in its own right. So pretty much immediately, I was in.

I threw myself into training. One day I was out in the garage with Katie, starting to work myself into fight shape. We were both doing a kettlebell workout to a video that Aubrey Marcus made for Onnit.

I finished the workout and noticed that my heart rate was way up. I don't remember the exact number, but it was definitely higher than usual for a workout like that. I sat down and took some deep breaths, but instead of slowing down, my heart just kept going.

"Something's wrong," I said.

I headed inside to the kitchen. My heart started thumping even faster and then I got dizzy. I think I blacked out a bit. My head bobbed down for a second. After all the years of fear and doctors and false alarms with my heart, I assumed that this was death, finally coming for me.

The kids were at the house that day. Devin was in the kitchen with me. I told her to go get Katie. I knew I needed help, but I also wanted to get my daughter out of the room because I was afraid I was about to make her witness her father dying.

Katie drove me to the hospital. When we got there, they told me I was experiencing an episode of AFib (which is short for atrial fibrillation). I was informed that they were going to have to knock me out and operate.

By that time, I was very familiar with the term AFib. Way back when Devin was a baby and Andrea and I were still living in that apartment by the SiriusXM studio in Hollywood, I had started having panic attacks. One day I woke up feeling like something was wrong. I felt dizzy and weak and panicky. And then a pro skater named Stevie Williams came on the radio show, and while I was talking to him things went from bad to worse.

After I finished the interview, I told my boss, Will Pendarvis, what was going on. He said, "You should go to the hospital."

Andrea was away at a wedding in Italy with a friend, so I drove myself to Cedars-Sinai. I started feeling really sad on the way over. I had a feeling that something really, really bad was happening. I walked into the hospital and said, "Something's wrong with my heart."

I could tell they thought I was imagining things. I'm sure every hospital in the world sees hypochondriacs every day. And Los Angeles has an especially large number of crazy people and drug addicts and people who just generally have their heads up their asses.

They humored me and put me on a heart monitor. I don't know what they saw on there, but within a couple minutes they all started shitting themselves. It was very obvious they had started taking me seriously.

They put me in a hospital bed. I was scared. Obviously, I wouldn't have gone to the hospital if I didn't think something was wrong, but at the same time, I was still a little surprised to find out I had actually been right.

As I was laying there listening to the heart monitor beeping, one of the doctors said, "Keep breathing."

Keep breathing? I thought. *Are you genuinely concerned that I might stop?* In my mind, that was a pretty clear indication that I was about to die.

I thought of my friend Sluggo. We'd been tight—like brothers—going all the way back to the early skateboarding days. Him and I weren't cool with each other at that point. It doesn't matter why. It just bummed me out that I might die without having a chance to patch things up and tell him I loved him.

I remember praying. I have never believed that there's an old dude with a long white beard sitting up on a cloud listening to me. But as someone who's had my fair share of close calls, I have noticed that seems to be a thing that you do in these types of situations. It comes pretty naturally when all hope seems lost.

For a while after that, things got pretty confusing. The doctors gave me a stress test. That was the first time I ever heard about AFib—when they told me I had it. Then later on they told me the test had been inaccurate, but that I still definitely had some kind of heart disease.

They put me in the hospital for three days and stuck me on this crazy diet. They told me I had to become a vegetarian for life and that I could no longer lift weights.

I went through three months of living like that—and thinking it was forever—plus I went through a bunch more tests before they finally decided that my heart was fine. They prescribed me anti-anxiety medication and then that was the end of it.

Or at least, that was the end of it until the day of that kettlebell workout.

All of a sudden, I was back at Cedars-Sinai. Back in the exact same emergency room. I fucking hate that hospital, man. Nothing good happens there, at least for me.

My heart rate wouldn't go down. The doctors gave me a great big *Pulp Fiction* needle, right in my chest, but that didn't do anything. Katie was crying. It was terrible.

My heart kept doing something. I have no idea what it was, but apparently it was a really bad sign. Every time it happened, I could feel all the medical professionals in the room get really concerned all over again.

Once again, I started praying, to no one in particular. I was talking to a God that, in my heart of hearts, I was positive wasn't there.

STILL AWESOME

You're not there, I said. *I know there is no God. But if anyone can hear me right now—the ghost of my brother Stevie, whoever—I don't want to die. I'm not done. There's so much more for me to do.*

Eventually they had to knock me out and put me on a machine to make my heart go back to normal. When I came to, I was once again diagnosed with AFib. Only this time the doctors stuck with that conclusion.

They told me I needed something called an ablation. They go in through your groin and then all the way up to your chest, and then they fuse a valve in your heart.

I'm not a professional, but I believe an ablation works something like this: AFib makes your heart think there's something wrong, even though there isn't. And then your heart starts beating faster as a result. When they do an ablation, they literally burn the part of your heart that the AFib uses to transmit that message. It's like they cut the phone cord so the part of your heart that's sending dodgy information can no longer communicate with the other parts.

In theory, the ablation cured everything. But after all I had been through, it was kind of hard for me to believe that. When the doctor told me about an optional heart monitor they could put in my chest for a few weeks, I was so paranoid I insisted on getting it.

The problem with the monitor, I soon found out, was that it meant I would have to back out of my fight. The athletic commission has to approve every fighter before they license them to compete. They make you work out in front of them and prove that you're up to it. And it's not some bullshit test. It's not just a couple jumping jacks. It's a real thing. As a guy in my forties, I knew they were going to scrutinize me extra hard. And understandably, a heart monitor that had been surgically implanted in my chest was probably going to be a deal-breaker for them.

I had no choice but to take it out and hope for the best. Besides, I figured if my heart was going to fuck me over, there was probably nothing I could do about it anyway.

At first, I wanted to just pull the monitor out myself. Like, with my bare hands. On the radio. The procedure to remove it ended up being a bit of a nightmare, so ultimately I was thankful I left that to the professionals.

I went to the gym right after I got that thing taken out of my chest. I just had a band-aid over the hole where the monitor had been. My coach was like, "Dude, get the fuck out of here. You'll get staph in that." That was definitely good advice. I love MMA gyms, but they are fucking disgusting.

That was pretty much the end of the heart thing hanging over my head all the time. I think it will probably always be in the back of my mind. My heart still jumps from time to time. I really do have an irregular heartbeat. Sometimes it's *really* irregular and in those moments, I feel like I might be getting a sneak preview of what the end will look like. That's never fun.

And obviously there is a psychological element to this. I will always suspect a heart attack is coming for me because a heart attack is what got my dad.

But I honestly don't believe it's coming for me today, and I don't believe it's coming tomorrow, either. I have a really good doctor. "You're solid," he would tell me. "Stronger than an ox. Go out there and do your thing."

Finally, for the first time really since the tail end of my career as a pro skater, I didn't wake up every day convinced that I was a heart attack waiting to happen. I trained harder and harder, just to hammer that point home to myself. I trained harder than people at the gym who were literally half my age.

There are no guarantees in life. No matter how well you take care of yourself, we could all get sideswiped by some idiot driver at a moment's notice. So fuck it. You might as well make the most of today.

STILL AWESOME

Training for my second fight was very different from the first time around. It was easier. I was surrounded by so many knowledgeable people, and I was way more knowledgeable myself.

The first go-round I had split my time between my MMA trainer Ryan Parsons and Team Quest and my boxing trainer Justin Fortune. But my weight cut was done 100% the old school boxing way. It basically amounted to starving yourself while you pushed yourself harder than you had ever pushed yourself, for weeks on end.

Justin's regimen basically amounted to, "Eat a fucking sweet potato and shut up, you weak cunt." That was the way Justin had done it throughout his career, and he fought Lennox Lewis. And his approach hadn't been some hard-ass throwback exception to what everyone else was doing. At that time, Lennox Lewis was the champ, and his dietician might not have been telling him anything a whole lot smarter. It wasn't that long ago but compared to what we know now about training and diet, it was the dark ages.

By the time of my second fight, I was friends with Mike Dolce. Mike designs diets for UFC champions, and now he was telling me exactly what to eat and when. People used to believe they had to starve to cut weight. (Actually, you occasionally still see a guy or a girl pass out at their weigh-in. So clearly some people still do.) But under Mike's guidance, I was eating five times a day. Sometimes it was actually a challenge to eat all the food I was supposed to eat. And I still lost all the weight I had to lose. When you see how easy it can be, it's amazing anyone still misses weight. It's not like Dolce is keeping this stuff a secret. He wrote a book about it.

King of the Cage gave me a choice of a couple different opponents. I picked the toughest guy they offered me.

I wanted to fix everything that I thought had gone wrong in the first fight. And one of those things was the opponent. The guy I had been supposed to fight didn't end up getting cleared by the commission. He gassed out during the final workout so they wouldn't allow him to fight. That was only a couple of days before fight night, so instead I fought a last-minute replacement. With all due respect to the replacement guy, I thought he was a bum. I respect anyone who steps in that cage—especially on short notice—but that fight was too easy.

In my experience, everybody wants to fight someone they know they're going to beat. And that goes double for people in the public eye. I don't know how many celebrities over the years have told me they wanted a fight in Ellismania, only to back out once they confronted the reality that there was a chance they'd get their ass kicked and be embarrassed in front of a bunch of strangers. Their egos couldn't handle it.

I didn't want that. I wanted a fight I could lose. Maybe even a fight I *should* lose.

Ever since the radio show got popular, I have always gotten to be a spoiled, shiny pants motherfucker. I get to cut to the front of the line. If I want to race cars there are sponsors ready to hook me up with more money and support than most people who devote their life to that sport will ever get. I know some of the core people in that sport have looked at me and thought, *Fuck you, Ellis. You're not worthy.* I can't argue with that. I'm really not, at least compared to them.

My first MMA fight, I trained with Dan Henderson's team and I had multiple pros in my corner. And then I made my pro debut as the main event in a big, nice venue in Anaheim. So once again, fuck me. I didn't pay my dues.

For my second fight, I wanted as much as I could handle. If I won, I wanted it to take everything I had. And if I lost, good. I'd been around other guys in the gym who had taken losses and I saw how it builds character. I've lost a lot in my life and I know firsthand that losing has made me a better person.

The guy I fought in my second fight—Gabe Rivas—was older and kind of fat and washed up. But you know what? I'm in my 40s and my body is trashed, too. At one point, that guy fought for the WEC championship.

I showed my buddy Mike Jasper videos of my prospective opponents. I told him I was leaning toward Gabe. Mike is such a sweetheart. He knew my athletic ability and my skill level more than anyone and so he knew more than anyone what I was signing myself up for. "You don't have to take this fight," he said. Obviously, what he meant was, 'You *shouldn't* take this fight.'

My coach said that maybe I should work my way up to Gabe. He suggested I think about doing three fights and making Gabe the last one.

I was like, "So you think if I beat this guy, it's a solid fight?"

He said, "You beat this guy, that's a solid win."

For me, that settled it. "Then I want that guy," I said.

Looking back, it was a bad call. I should have thought it through more. But in the end, that's exactly what made it the right decision, you know?

That wasn't the only iffy decision I made going into that fight. Around that same time, I was competing in a series of short course off-road races. For those of you who aren't familiar, it's like motocross, only in cars. It's pretty much buggy racing.

By total coincidence, I had a race scheduled the same exact day as the fight.

As much as I enjoyed being a part of racing, obviously I should have backed out of that commitment and focused on the fight. As a matter of fact, several people whose opinions carry a lot of weight with me recommended I do just that. They strongly encouraged me to focus on the guy who would be trying to break my bones and knock me unconscious later on that same day.

But it occurred to me that in all probability, no one in the history of humankind had ever podiumed at a race *and* won a pro MMA fight in the same day. Nowadays, I don't think I would give a shit about that. But at that point, that sounded like a very awesome thing to shoot for—even if no one was going to give a shit if I pulled it off but me.

I knew there was next to no chance I could actually full-on win that race. There was a lady in that class who was basically untouchable. She had all the best sponsors and her husband made these amazing race cars, so every race was hers to lose.

I just wanted to make the podium. I had never done it, but I knew I was getting closer. I had been steadily improving, but when push came to shove, either my car broke down or I just flat out wasn't good enough. So I went to sprint car school. I paid extra money to do extra practice. I put my fucking work in.

And that day, when the race got started, I hunted her ass down. She was in second and I was in third, meaning I was already in a podium spot. That alone had never happened. With two turns left, I managed to pass her and then I held that spot until the checkered flag. I had spun out earlier and I still finished second, which meant that all in all I was actually the fastest person on the track that day.

I was pumped. I had envisioned being up there on that podium and there I finally was. My son, Tiger, was even there to see it. It was a really cool moment.

And that's how long that feeling lasted—about a moment. I got to savor it for all of about five seconds. A bunch of Ellisfam—what the super hardcore listeners of my radio show have named themselves—had come out to see me. They were cheering me on and taking pictures while I got my trophy. Then one of them said, "Hey, Ellis! Your fight is starting soon! You gotta go!"

I drove my race car off the podium and to the tent, ripped my helmet off, put it in the backseat of my regular car, and said, "Katie, can you drive?" Then she took off as I tried to meditate in the passenger seat. It was an hour or two from race location to the fight location. That was all the time I was going to get to transition my mind and put my game face on.

STILL AWESOME

I realized I needed to eat so I called my friend Keith Jardine, who was already at the venue. When he was in the UFC, Keith was known as the "Dean of Mean." But outside of the cage, he is one of the biggest sweethearts you could ever meet. I asked Keith to get me some food. He said there was nothing to eat there. That was my first clue that the scene around my second pro fight was going to be a little more rugged than my first.

When I got there, I found out that no one had brought wraps for my hands. My coach, Julio Trana from Saekson Muay Thai, got his hands on some material and made some, and then we hit some pads. I still hadn't eaten. That would have to wait until after I fought. Because just then, one of the guys who was running the event came backstage and told us it was thirty minutes until fight time.

Mike Jasper and my other friend Eddie Jackson—a pro fighter in his own right and also one of my trainers—both gave me funny looks. Who the fuck races a car on fight day? Who the fuck shows up for their fight 45 minutes before it starts? Some fighters have specific routines they follow from the moment they wake up on fight day. Meanwhile, everyone backstage could tell by looking at me that mentally, I wasn't even there yet.

They were right. Even as I walked toward the cage, I was thinking, *I can't believe I just got second in that car race!*

The next thing I thought was, *Man, this is a shit place to fight.*

And it was. The King of the Cage people were great to me and I appreciate them giving me that fight. But when they said the fight was at some Indian casino, I assumed they meant *inside* the casino. Instead we were out in the open air. And it was freezing. I know people think it's always 70 degrees in southern California, but it can get pretty chilly at night, especially out in the desert. That didn't affect me. Between the pre-fight jitters and my warm-up, I was perfectly comfortable. But I know it was a different story for anyone in the audience who hadn't realized ahead of time that they needed to bring a coat.

Lastly—and most importantly—while I was making my entrance I was thinking, *I can't believe how many people are here to see me fight.* So many people had made the trip out there to the middle of nowhere. I saw so many familiar faces on my way to the cage. I may live in Hollywood now, but my roots are straight up bogan, so that whole scene felt weirdly perfect to me.

The one thing I *should* have been thinking about—the fight that was about to happen—was far from my mind. It didn't even register that my opponent, Gabe, was already in the cage until I climbed in and saw him there.

While the ring announcer did his bit, I was just moving my shoulders around a little bit. I was very casual. *Too* casual. "Hey, man!" I remember my coach Julio saying. "This is a fucking fight! Get ready!"

I tried to turn on the anger. I think I even started snarling a bit. I could feel the adrenaline start to kick in.

We touched gloves, the bell rang, and I came out with this weird soft jab, to measure him. It was way too calm and relaxed.

He threw a counter right-hand over the top of it, straight away. He hit me with a one-two. Both of those punches landed clean. One on the temple, one on the chin. I stepped to the side to move out of the way and I felt my left leg turn to jelly for a second.

This guy had had dozens of fights. He was a veteran. He was calm, cool, and collected, and he understood everything that was happening in there, right as it happened. He saw my leg buckle. I smiled at him a bit. It was a smile that said, *Whoops*. I had fucked up massively and now we both knew it.

Before I even threw a kick or really did anything, he was moving in to finish me. I was covering up to keep from getting hit, but I was still taking damage on top of what he had already done with those first two shots. I was disoriented. At one point I couldn't even see where he was.

The next thing I knew I was on the ground. My butt was

up against the cage. All I could think was, *Oh man, everybody is here to watch me and I'm about to get knocked unconscious.*

To my friends from the fight world that wouldn't have been that big of a deal. That shit can happen. But a couple of my Hollywood actor friends like Dax Shepard and Rob Corddry were there, too. I'm assuming neither of them had ever watched one of their friends get beaten to a pulp right in front of them. *Why did I invite them?* I thought. *It's going to be really uncomfortable the next time I see them.*

I wiggled around and then Gabe mounted me. At that point I was definitely concussed, and now I was under the mount. *This is where it ends*, I thought.

I ripped my left arm out to roll over. You're not supposed to do that. You're supposed to give up your back. But I figured either I would get my arm out somehow, or else I was going to keep getting smashed in the head. And I was already half unconscious.

I gave him my arm, but luckily he wasn't that good at jiujitsu, so as soon as he went for it I spun around and got on top of him. I thought I could rest a bit at that point, but then he started popping off from the bottom and hitting me.

I don't know how long I had him down there. It might not have been that long. But I was so tired from getting beat up that I could barely keep holding him. I could feel him getting up, so I got up with him.

I think I threw a spinning elbow at him. Or at least somewhere in his general direction. He may not have even been in my vicinity. That was not a move that I have in my core arsenal. That was just desperation, really.

I was going on instinct at that point. When you get hit really hard there's this ringing or buzzing inside your head. You're still conscious and in the moment. But you're not really making decisions anymore. Your body—and hopefully your training—sort of take over.

Lucky for me, the cobwebs cleared out pretty quickly. All of a sudden I snapped back into reality. We traded a couple punches and I was like, *Oh! Okay! We're fighting now!*

I felt like I had already taken his worst. And I was still standing. *You're not going to finish me*, I thought.

The first round finally ended. I was so goddamn tired. I sat down on the stool and my corner gave me a look that told me they all thought I was done.

Just from the look in his eyes, I could tell my friend Eddie was thinking, *I am trying to give you props right now because you survived. But mostly, I am just sad for you, because I'm pretty sure you're going to go back out there and then he's going to really fucking finish you.*

But thankfully, no one gave up on me. No one was thinking of throwing in the towel. I remember Julio saying, "He's fucking tired, man! He gassed himself out on you. I know you're tired, too, but dig deep, dude. Go back to your wrestling. Mix it up. Confuse this guy. Don't give up!"

My brain felt very motivated by that. "Okay!" I yelled. "I will not give up!"

I stood up from the stool, threw a couple of jabs at the air, and experienced what is known in the MMA business as spaghetti arms.

I got angry at myself. Once the next round started, I willed myself to land a couple of shots, but they had no effect on him. I had nothing in the tank.

Looking back at the tape later on, I think I might have lost the second round, too. He caught me a couple more times. But I also started to find my confidence. I started to throw leg kicks. If he hit me, I hit him back. I started to take some shots at takedowns. At one point in the second, I even started to apply a Kimura thing. I didn't get it, but I did feel like the tide was starting to turn in my favor.

In the corner before the last round, Julio said, "We're even, man. That's one each. This is the whole fight, right here. Who wants it the most?"

I had to take a good hard look at myself. Did I have what it was going to take? I truly didn't know the answer. But starting in less than 60 seconds, I was about to find out.

Before the third round started, my opponent Gabe was yelling over to me. "Do you want to hug it out?" he asked. I knew he was saying that because he had fucked me up in the first but somehow I was still standing. I thought it was really cool that this guy was giving me props.

We bumped knuckles and then we hugged when we came out for the third round. After that, it was war.

I'm going to get that fucking key lock, I thought. I felt really positive about that.

We traded a bit at the start. I double-legged him against the cage and then I put him down. I had him in a mount for a second but then he rolled out. I was so tired. I knew I needed to put my knee on top of him, get him back in the mount, and then start raining punches. But that takes cardio. I needed a minute to catch my breath and gather my strength, but I didn't have a minute.

He bucked again and I put him on his back yet again. That took everything I had. I again had him in a perfect position to ground and pound and finish him. The problem was, it had taken everything I had to put him in that position. And there were still three minutes left.

I knew I couldn't take him trying to throw me off again. I didn't have the strength to stop him. If he had tried, he would have rolled me over and I would have been done.

I kept working that Kimura, and then a key lock. I don't know how many times I tried to get that key lock in. He wrenched his arm back so many times. But he was just as exhausted as I was.

I finally got it. I cranked it to the point where everybody taps. That should have been it. Only he didn't tap.

I was yelling at him. "Tap, dude! Tap!" I must have said it five times.

I wrenched it even further. I could hear things pinging and ponging inside his arm. Little bits of tendon or cartilage tearing. It was gruesome. But the guy still wouldn't give up. He was as tough as it gets.

Finally, the ref tapped me on the back and pulled us apart.

Gabe never physically tapped. It was a verbal submission. I didn't know those existed until after that fight. Basically, if your opponent unleashes a bloodcurdling scream because of how much pain he's in, that's considered a verbal tap.

My first instinct was to help Gabe. I was like, "Dude, I broke your fucking arm." He indicated that he did not care for any help from the likes of me. Under the circumstances, that was understandable.

Then my friend Eddie got right in my face. He was so excited. "Dude!" he said. "You got him with one second left!"

The ref came over to me afterward. His name is Mike Beltran. MMA fans know who I'm talking about. He's the ref with the huge Fu Manchu moustache that hangs off his face in braids. If you've seen him once, you probably know who I mean. He's pretty memorable.

It turned out he listens to the show. He's a solid dude.

"That was a fight, guy," he said. "I let you go in the first round. I thought you were in trouble, but I knew you had something left so I let you go."

I told him I appreciated that. It wouldn't have been the craziest stoppage ever if a ref had decided he needed to bail out the dumb radio guy who was in over his head and taking a bunch of brain damage.

When they raised my hand after my first fight, all I could think about was my dad. But a lot had happened between that fight and this one. I had figured out a lot of stuff about him, and about myself, too. I had changed, and the way I thought about him had changed, too.

Whether I realized it or not, I had devoted my whole life to trying to measure up to my father. But now, finally, it wasn't about him anymore.

I had forgiven him for who he was and for the things he'd done to me. I'd be willing to bet you there was some stuff about his childhood that was pretty fucked up, too. I understood that now.

But more importantly, I just couldn't be mad at him anymore. That takes a lot of energy, and for the rest of my life, I choose to devote my energy to myself and my kids and Katie. My life isn't about my past anymore. It's about me finally being happy and making the most of whatever time I've got left on this planet.

This time around, when Beltran raised my hand, I was thinking about my brother, Stevie. For a second I thought I was going to start crying. When you see people cry after winning a fight, you would always assume those are tears of joy. But in that moment, I was wondering how many of them cry because there's one person they wished could have seen them, but who isn't around anymore.

I feel like I won that fight for me *and* my brother. I felt like I showed everybody something—about both of us.

When I got out of the cage, the King of the Cage doctor looked at me and said, "You need stitches." I was so pumped when he said that. That was another thing I had wanted from an MMA fight. I wanted to bleed. Some people might go in the cage visualizing themselves landing a knockout without breaking a sweat. But to me, seeing my own blood was a critical part of my dream fight.

"How bad is it?" I asked. "How many stitches do I need?"

"Two," the doctor replied. "Maybe three."

"I'll be all right," I said. "I'll glue it when I get home."

He okayed that and sent me on my way. I didn't actually see my face until I got back to the dressing room, so I had no idea how fucked up I looked.

"Yeah, dude!" Eddie said. "Why do you think I've been looking at you the way I've been looking at you since the first round? You got so fucked up. I can't believe you're still here!"

The way I looked also attracted some attention when I got back to the hotel. It was this cool old brick place with fancy architecture, somewhere in the Inland Empire. Katie and I had stayed there with the kids before.

When we walked in the lobby, security came over immediately. The guy looked extremely concerned. "Sir," he said. "Do you need me to call the police?"

He assumed I'd been assaulted. Which was true, come to think of it—just not in the way he was thinking.

I had a towel on my face, but I was dripping a lot. By that time the fight had ended over an hour ago, but for some reason I seemed to be getting even bloodier. Maybe my face just got tired of clotting. In my face's defense, it had been a long day.

I tried to explain, but everything I said just made it sound worse and worse.

"No, I was in a fight," I said. "But it was an organized fight. But not like a gang thing. It was in a cage."

"Look," I finally said. "I'm fine. Can I please just have my key so I can go to my room?"

Katie loved all the gore pouring out of my face, of course. Her and I had talked about that possibility way ahead of time. She considered it a very horny thing for me to have a bunch of blood dripping off of me. So that day was pretty much mission accomplished for everybody.

That night was very different from the night after my first fight. For one thing, room service was still open. Believe me—I had made sure it would be ahead of time. I ordered a cheeseburger, but then I had trouble opening my mouth to get it in. I had to take these little baby bird bites but I managed to get the job done.

Our friends Leigh Raven and Nikki Hearts came back to the room. Those two and Katie were drinking a bit and smoking weed. I was still sober at that point, but it was still a fun, festive atmosphere to be around.

I had some time to sit there and reflect on the fight. There was a good chance it would be my last one. And not because Katie had informed me I was going to stop, like Andrea had after my first fight. If I woke up tomorrow and told Katie I was quitting radio to devote my life full-time to going to the UFC, I believe she would be okay with that, regardless of how insane that plan might be. But in reality, the only reason I would do another MMA fight is if the opportunity was too amazing to turn down. CM Punk, if you are reading this, I am still available to kick your ass whenever you want me to.

Assuming this was it, I knew I could walk away in peace. I was aware that I had made mistakes in the cage, just like after my first fight. But this time around that didn't bother me. Who gets to fight a perfect fight? Everybody makes mistakes. That's part of the game.

And who the fuck ever raced a car in Temecula before they had a fight? That's some Roy Jones Jr. shit, if you ask me.

It was a terrible idea. I almost lost the fight because of it. If I hadn't done that race, the fight might have gone very differently, and way more smoothly.

But the way it went was still cool. I love the way I won. The night after my first fight, while I laid awake in bed with my pregnant wife lying next to me, I looked deep inside myself and I wasn't impressed with what I saw. This time, I felt like I had gotten hurt about as badly as I could without losing consciousness, and I knew that not one part of me thought of giving up for even a second.

I really wish I could become an amazing martial artist. I wish I could pull off spinning back flips and all that flashy shit. But I don't have that. For the most part I believe that people can accomplish anything they set their mind to, but there are limits. I'm not Anderson Silva. I just don't have those skills.

But you know what? I have the heart of an Anderson Silva. That night I proved to myself that when push comes to shove, I will not quit. And that is something I can be very proud of forever.

That's what my quest in fighting was really about. I still love going to the gym. I still love working on stuff and getting better. I still love to spar.

But ultimately it was always about that test. I finally got it. And I'm happy to say I passed.

When I came out of the ring that night, Dax Shepherd was one of the first people who came over to congratulate me. At that point in time, I really looked up to him. He was kind of like a father figure to me. It was really cool of him to drive out into the desert and sit on a metal folding chair in the cold, just to support me.

AA and sobriety were the things that Dax and I had bonded over. But by then, my faith in AA and sobriety and a lot of things Dax believes in was already pretty shaky.

Truthfully, as much as I wanted AA to be the answer to my problems, it never felt right to me. The guys you meet in there get in your head. They talk a good game. And I'm very gullible. When they tell you what a mess they used to be and you see how put together and happy and successful they seem now, it's very tempting to hope that the same thing might happen for you. So I went along with it. I tried to do the steps. It seems to work for lots of people, but it never really clicked for me.

Just like the meetings I went to in rehab, I found that a lot of people seemed to go there mainly to complain about their problems. I get the value of venting and sharing the challenges you are facing in your life with people who are going through similar stuff, but there was way too much of that for me. It was way too negative. I'm not sure the best way to try to maintain a positive attitude is to spend that much of your day bitching.

And I felt like some of the rules they had didn't really add up or make sense. In my experience, smoking a little weed here and there has always been harmless fun. If you take one bong rip and then an hour later find yourself with a crack pipe in your mouth and a needle hanging out of your arm, then I would agree that you shouldn't smoke weed. But that wasn't me.

To AA people, marijuana is a big no-no. But then they all turn around ask you if you want a piece of nicotine gum. I don't know if you've ever tried that stuff, but it is strong. I bought some of that gum because everyone else in the program seemed to think it was great and after five minutes of chewing a piece my face went gray. I felt like I was going to vomit. I can smoke pretty much as much weed as I want and be fine on the radio, but if you made me chew that gum, there would be no way I could do my job. It's the worst high ever. But it is for sure a buzz. Those guys yank on that gum all day, every day. And none of them see it as a problem.

Also, in my experience, a lot of those guys spend a lot of time talking about getting on antidepressants. And guess what? Those are drugs, too. It seems like everyone in AA is sad about how they aren't allowed to take drugs anymore, yet it's somehow acceptable to let a doctor prescribe them more drugs. It doesn't add up.

But most importantly, I just felt like my problems with drugs and alcohol weren't nearly as crazy as a lot of people I was seeing at the meetings. I will freely admit that I am an addict. But I felt like a lot of guys at that meeting were on a whole other level.

There would be guys in there one week saying, "I've been sober for ten years." And then the next week that guy's story might be that he fucked up and had a drink. And then the week after that, that same guy might have totaled a sports car or done a ton of blow or spent more money on hookers than most people make in a year. (I'm making up the details here, out of respect to Alcoholics Anonymous, but I am not exaggerating. There were some serious high rollers at the meeting I went to.) And then for the rest of that year, that guy was a train wreck who was quickly pissing his whole life away. There were people I saw who went from three decades of sobriety all the way down to the lowest of rock bottoms.

Compared to those guys, I just didn't feel like blacking out one time at the Bass Awards really compared. Once those guys relapsed, they were at it all day, every day. I can look at myself in the mirror and know that is never ever going to be me.

Everyone has to find the answers in life that work for them. There's no one-size-fits-all. The answers at AA just didn't feel like they could be my answers. I was already on antidepressants, and at that point, I was already pretty sure that I wanted to be done with them. When I have a weekend free with my kids and I'm barbecuing in the backyard, something is missing if I don't have a beer. When I was in AA, *that* was my biggest problem with alcohol—that I wasn't allowed to have a beer while I grilled some cheeseburgers.

At the end of the day, you've got to figure out what makes you happy. If your idea of being happy is being shitfaced 24/7, then I hate to break it to you, but unless you're the lead singer of Motörhead, that plan probably isn't going to work out. But can you be stoned all the time and do your job? For some people, I believe the answer is yes, as long as you pace yourself. Can you drink a six pack on a Friday night without robbing your kid's piggy bank to go get smack? If that's what you want to do, I say do it, even if it means you are sometimes going to be a full-grown adult with a hangover.

Some people get really into the sober lifestyle. After a while, self-discipline becomes a thing they get off on. It's almost like their new drug. I've seen several people go down a similar path. It's not enough they're sober, now they're not going to use their smartphone, either. And then after that, they have to eliminate sugar from their diet, too. And so on.

Discipline is cool. At certain times in my life, like when I've trained for fights, I have been very, very disciplined. I know I could be that guy all the time if it was really important to me. I could have a six-pack when I'm 60 years old and all of my Instagram followers could be incredibly motivated by me. But I don't want that. I'm not living my life to impress social media. Whatever I do from here on out, I do for me.

I mean no offence to hardcore sober guys. I have been around a lot of them and they are very admirable and inspirational. Dax is a great guy. I still love him. He was really trying to save me. But somewhere along the way, I stopped believing that I needed to be saved.

I think people who are in AA look at people who leave the program and think, *He had a chance but now it's over*. But it's not over for me. It's just that they have their way and I have mine.

I don't think I'm that broken anymore. I like me. I'm actually becoming fonder of myself by the day. Maybe for the first time in my whole life.

A few years ago, Katie and I went to one of Benji and Joel Madden's record release parties at a mansion in the Hollywood Hills. It's this cool old spot on a big piece of land that used to belong to Harry Houdini. There are handcuffs all over the place and there's a big chain link staircase, because…well…it was Harry Houdini's place. That stuff appealed to the metal part of us. We both thought it was the sickest place ever.

When it came time to pick a place to get married, we thought doing it at that house would cost an impossible amount of money. But it turned out it wasn't any more ridiculous than any of the hotels we had looked at, so we booked a date.

I wouldn't say wedding planning is a hobby of mine, but planning my wedding with Katie was way more fun than the first two experiences had been. The process was pretty stress-free. Katie put a lot of work into making it great, and as a result everything came off without a hitch. But even if things had gone to shit, I went into the big day knowing that also would have been fine by both of us. We both find cringe-worthy social catastrophes pretty hilarious. So basically, we couldn't lose.

Unlike my other two weddings, there wasn't any clash between what I expected the day to look like and what my wife expected. My first wedding was held in this sick old castle, but that night, after the reception, my wife made me stay in our room while all our friends raged and took mushrooms and scaled the walls like medieval warlords.

It definitely helped that I didn't go into my third marriage with the feeling that I might be making a humongous mistake. Before I met Katie, I was with too many other girls for the wrong reasons. I was always looking for women who would mother me, because of the way my childhood went down. But because of the therapy I had started while Katie and I were split up, I had finally broken that pattern.

And before Katie, I always started relationships with women primarily because they were hot and because I thought it would impress other people to see them on my arm. I figured that everyone who knew me when I was young believed that I was destined to become a loser. So I looked for girls I could show off, girls who would prove that everyone who ever doubted me had been wrong. That was the main objective for my dating life.

Many of those girls weren't really my type. What I really wanted the whole time was a badass metal chick with a bunch of tattoos. What I wanted the whole time was…Katie. I had finally allowed myself to be in a relationship with the kind of girl I was genuinely most attracted to. And so as a result, marriage finally felt right.

I didn't marry Katie for anyone else. And I didn't marry her because that's what society says you're supposed to do once you've been living with a woman for a certain amount of time. My business manager tells me there's some kind of tax break for married people, and it's cool that now Katie gets to be on my health insurance, but we didn't do it for The Man either. We didn't need the piece of paper. Katie and I are never breaking up, whether or not there are rings or a marriage license involved.

Katie had never been married before, and if that was something she wanted, then it made me really happy to do that with her. End of story.

Our friend Dingo got a license to marry people. He put on a big white robe and then we made it official in front of both of my kids and a bunch of people we love.

The first two times, I had no business getting married.

The third time, I had no doubt.

Chapter 11

Ever since Aubrey Marcus and I had dinner with Dr. Dan, our conversation about ayahuasca had been rattling around in my brain.

I remember Aubrey telling me how it worked: You fly to Peru and go into the jungle, and then you throw up and shit yourself for a week while you see dead people. Oh, and while that's happening you feel like you also died, too. The end.

At the time, I told Aubrey that ayahuasca sounded very interesting. I also told him I would probably start shooting up speedballs before I ever paid good money to go to South America so I could drink a bunch of black shit some shaman gave me. I had zero interest.

But for some reason, I kept thinking about it. In particular, I kept remembering how Aubrey said he took ayahuasca and then he saw his grandmother, who had passed away.

And yes, I know that's ridiculous. I have called bullshit on so many mystical things that other people believe in—aliens and psychics and floating magical old guys with white beards in the clouds. Aubrey's grandmother is not alive. She's gone. Did I believe he was actually speaking to her? No, I did not.

But more and more I realized that it didn't matter if he really saw her. It was real to him. And it helped him. So he could give a fuck what the rest of the world thinks.

And I have to admit, there was also a little part of me that kept saying, *Who knows?* I call bullshit on ghosts and Bigfoot and all that stuff because I've never seen them myself and because, in my opinion, most of the people who claim to have encountered them are kooks. (Sorry, Corey Taylor.) But I had never tried ayahuasca. And I don't consider Aubrey a kook. So who was I to say? Maybe he really *did* connect with her spirit.

His story just hit me so hard. I wondered if ayahuasca could make me see my brother, Stevie. I would do anything to see him again and to know that he's okay.

I knew there was only one way I was going to find out. Slowly but surely, that sliver of hope was enough to make me contemplate giving it a go.

My interest in ayahuasca had been one more thing that made me realize that AA wasn't for me. Back when I was still sober, the recovery community, or at least the part I was in contact with, made it very clear that ayahuasca was not an approved part of the program.

Just like with smoking weed, I didn't feel any need to hide my curiosity about ayahuasca from them. Because, same as weed, I didn't see it as a potential problem. Anyone who has ever tried ayahuasca will tell you that it's not a drug. It's medicine. No one in their right mind would take it for fun. That would be insane. But to people at AA, if you take ayahuasca then you're using again. No grey area. No ifs ands or buts.

It was one more reminder to me of how rigid the AA lifestyle is. To the best of my knowledge, no one at my meeting had ever tried ayahuasca. And yet they all knew for a fact that it was bad.

I was like, "What if it helps me solve some of my problems? Aren't my personal issues potentially part of the reason why I'm an addict? So if I fix myself, won't that help fix my addictions, too?"

Suffice it to say, no one went for that argument.

Meanwhile, as I have already said, those same people in AA

would turn around and encourage me to keep using antidepressants. I had been on those for a while at that point, and I didn't like them. I had never liked them.

It could be my imagination, but I always thought they made me a little fatter than I would have been without them. No matter how hard I worked out, I always felt a bit chunkier than I should be. For someone as self-conscious and insecure as I am, looking in the mirror and always thinking I looked fat was a pretty shitty side effect for pills that were supposed to make me happier.

And antidepressants made me feel lazy. I really thrive on using my body, but those pills made me just a little more likely to skip the gym and stay on the couch.

It's a proven scientific fact that physical activity improves your mental well-being. A good, solid workout literally releases happy juice in your brain. And exercise has all these positive ripple effects that fight depression. Going to the gym gets you on a routine. It also helps you sleep. If antidepressants kept me from going to the gym as often as I would have without them, in my book that alone was a major strike against them.

More importantly I thought they made my brain work slower. I never felt as sharp as I could be. On top of the radio show, I was doing a solo podcast every week. And for the first time since I had started getting paid to talk into a microphone, I felt like I had nothing to say. That had never happened before. No matter how tired or depressed or even hung over I might have been, I had always found that if I dug deep, I always had something at least mildly interesting to blather on about. But now it felt like the well was running dry. I felt stupider. I questioned why anyone would want to listen to me. A couple of those episodes didn't even get posted because I thought they were so shitty.

And in a way, I felt like I had been duped by the people who gave me antidepressants. In the beginning, I thought it was understood that I wasn't going to be on them forever. I thought they were just supposed to be a crutch to get me through a bad time, and that if I kept going to therapy and making positive adjustments in my life, eventually I'd get off them.

But then when my situation started to improve, the story seemed to shift. If I was feeling better, my psychiatrist asked, why would I want to change anything? To me, that hadn't been part of the deal.

Every six months I had to go see this guy. He asked me the same questions every time, and every time he would charge me 500 bucks and then give me the exact same prescription all over again, no matter what I said. It felt like a scam.

And here's another thing they don't necessarily tell you when you start taking antidepressants: It's not always easy to stop.

More than once, I decided to try to wean myself off them. But whenever I did, I always started to go dark. So I felt trapped. I didn't like the way the pills made me feel, but trying to get off them made me feel even worse. Doesn't that sound like the exact same story junkies tell you about trying to get clean? It was like I was technically a sober person…but at the same time, I also had something that sounded an awful lot like a drug problem. And to AA, that was okay.

Meanwhile, I was watching documentaries of people who were going to Peru and trying ayahuasca. Some of them had been on antidepressants for years. Some of them were straight up heroin addicts. And then they took ayahuasca, and months later they weren't on anything anymore and they were talking about how they were happier than they'd ever been.

I was jealous. I felt like the people in those videos had started off a lot like me, and by the end they had found what I wanted. They had been fixed.

I didn't want to put Band-Aids on my problems anymore. I didn't want to just lean on a bunch of strategies my therapist taught me so I could make my life more manageable. I wanted to get rid of the darkness that had followed me around for as long as

STILL AWESOME

I could remember. I wanted to get to the source of it, get control of my life, and end the pain once and for all. And as much as ayahuasca scared the shit out of me, I decided I was willing to confront death in order to have a shot at that.

To be clear, even after I decided to do it, I was still fucking terrified. Everyone who's ever done ayahuasca agrees the first time is the most brutal. The first time is when you really have to face your worst demons head on. And I felt pretty certain that my demons were especially bad.

I know one person who tried ayahuasca, and the biggest problem she faced was that she'd never been sure if she wanted to start a family. She took the medicine, and it made her realize that her friends were already her family, so it didn't matter if she had kids or not.

If that's your big revelation, that's great. I'm sincerely happy to know that's what your worst internal dilemma looks like. It sounds like you've got a great life, all in all.

But I felt like I carried a darkness around with me that very few people could comprehend. Maybe everyone confronts death when they take ayahuasca, but I was pretty sure that death meant something far different and far worse to me than it does to a typical person. If you're a dude who has a normal life and does CrossFit with your bros and shit like that, then I'm sorry, but I'm pretty sure your hell is my fucking picnic.

Katie was also interested in trying ayahuasca. She's fucked-up, too. I mean, why do you think she's in love with me? We're two fucked-up peas in a pod.

But she was even more scared of it than I was. So she had decided to use me as her guinea pig. If I did it and made it out to the other side in one piece, then she would consider trying it herself. That meant that I was going in solo.

I called Dr. Dan and asked him to help me make the arrangements to go to Peru. Katie wasn't even making the trip with me.

If she didn't want to come barf and shit herself while she tripped balls in the jungle, then she sure as hell didn't want to fly a thousand miles to watch me do it either.

Dr. Dan told me that the shaman he knew had retired, but that, as luck would have it, the shaman's protégé was planning a trip to L.A. Whatever ayahuasca had in store for me, it turned out I wouldn't have to go to South America to find it. It was coming to find me, right inside my very own living room.

You can't go into ayahuasca cold. At least not if you want it to work the way it's supposed to. I spoke to the shaman on the phone a couple weeks out. He told me I had to eat really clean for a couple of weeks. Nothing processed at all. I don't eat much of that stuff anyway so that was no big deal. I also wasn't allowed to smoke weed for a full week beforehand. That's always made me pretty edgy and grumpy, and this time was no exception.

But worst of all by far was getting off the antidepressants. After I stopped taking them, I got these little brain zaps out of nowhere. They're hard to explain. It's like every now and then, without warning, someone takes a little baby Taser to your brain. There were also these weird dizzy spells. And I started to feel depressed. This feeling of hopelessness set in, and then my brain started saying, *You know, if you took those pills again you wouldn't feel like this.*

The more I found myself having those thoughts, the more convinced I became that I no longer wanted anything to do with those things. The harder the withdrawal got, the more obvious it became that they were fucking with me. That they had *always* been fucking with me. And the anger I felt toward them made me more driven than ever to get off them for good.

Having a reason to not take antidepressants really helped me stay the course. Even when I had a really bad day, I had extra incentive to resist the temptation. I knew there was a light at the end of the tunnel. There was a larger goal. I just had to make it through.

STILL AWESOME

All of these little challenges were valuable in a way. They helped get me in the right frame of mind. The plan was for me to take ayahuasca for three days straight. I knew that if I was going to get what I wanted out of that experience, I was going to have to crawl through a whole lot of shit to get there. And the weeks leading up helped me prepare for battle.

The last three days before the shaman came over, I also had to give up sleeping pills. As a result, I didn't sleep very much. Maybe four or five hours a night. The night before the first day reminded me of the night before a skate contest back in the day, or the night before a fight. You tell yourself, *I'm not going to think about it*. And then you just lay in bed and think about it the whole time. I went to bed nervous as fuck, and I was still nervous as fuck when the guy came by the next morning.

We got to work setting up our space. I put a bunch of MMA mats down on the living room floor. He set up a bunch of blankets, and he had a cushion for himself, too. Him and I were going to be camped out there for five or six hours at a time, so we were making the room as comfy as possible.

He brought buckets with him, too. Those scared the fuck out of me. He set them up in the bathroom and said, "We're going to keep our area dark, but we can have a candle in the bathroom. You might need to go in there and use these."

I wasn't scared of shitting and vomiting at the same time. I mean, I didn't exactly *want* to do that, especially in front of a virtual stranger. But given the life I've led and the kind of person I am and the kind of radio show I do, that part didn't flinch me. The buckets just made it hit home that today was the day. This was really happening.

Once the sun went down, Katie gathered up all the supplies she needed for the evening and headed upstairs. That was the last I saw of her until the shaman and I were done for the night.

Once it was just me and him in the living room, he poured out that evening's dose. He kept the ayahuasca in this little plastic container. The container was white but kind of see through, and I could see the dark black liquid swishing around inside. He spilled it out into these little shot glasses. One for me and one for him. The shaman took the ayahuasca with me, all three nights. He goes in there with you.

He said, "You need to get all of it. After you've drank it, run your finger around inside the glass and then lick it. Get every single bit out."

People will tell you that ayahuasca tastes like shit. They're not totally wrong, but they are being a little dramatic. It looked like a liquid form of Vegemite, and that's pretty much what it tasted like. If you've ever taken Echinacea or Goldenseal or any bullshit like that, you would know what to expect.

After we drank it, the shaman started chanting and smoking a bunch of tobacco and blowing it all over me. He had warned me and Katie ahead of time that the house was going to be full of smoke, so we knew to expect that. It was a slightly different tobacco smell than a Marlboro Light or something. It was a little more pleasant. The guy is actually a professional tobacconist as well, so he for sure had the good stuff.

The shaman had told me a little bit about what I could expect. He told me it would take about forty minutes for the drug to kick in. During that time he would be chanting and I would just be hanging out.

That was a little awkward at first. I've never had a man chant at me before. He was sitting cross-legged in the corner, singing his little songs, and I knew Katie was upstairs. I was thinking, *I wonder if she can hear this?* It must have sounded insane.

The shaman made me smoke some tobacco. He told me to take a big rip, then he said, "Swallow it and hold it in there." I think that was supposed to make me puke a little bit. I got a bit dizzy, and I held the bucket and spat up a bit, but that was all that happened.

STILL AWESOME

Then he changed up his chant. That made the trip kick in. I thought that might have been a coincidence, but he did the same thing the next two nights, too. By the end of it all I had a lot of respect for this guy's skills. I realized he could totally control my trip.

All of a sudden, when I closed my eyes, there was this blackness. I felt like I had entered a big, dark room. I could tell something was about to happen.

I started seeing patterns. I have done enough acid and mushrooms in my time to know that the shit was starting to go down. *Here we go*, I thought. Usually, in the past, seeing visuals from drugs would be a cool, exciting thing. But under these circumstances it just made me scared of what might be coming next.

I hadn't done any psychedelics in a long time—not since my 30s—and all the reasons why I had stopped were coming back to me. I didn't like how it felt to be in that headspace and I didn't like knowing that I couldn't get out.

It was making me think too much, about stuff I didn't like. There was nothing specific happening that I could really put my finger on—I was just hearing eerie voices and feeling generally uncomfortable while a guy I didn't know kept chanting and smoking in my living room.

At one point I realized my body was moving in unison with his chant. I didn't feel like I was doing it. I felt like he was moving me—or really, that the *chant* was moving me. Like he was a snake charmer or something.

Not all that much happened that first night. The shaman had told me we were going to take it easy and start off slowly. "We'll do the work the next day," he said.

But it wasn't nothing, either. All in all, it was kind of like a bad mushroom trip. If you've had enough of those you know how to ride them out, but that doesn't mean they don't suck.

Katie and I didn't talk much when I went upstairs afterward.

I just told her that I was okay and that was about it.

I slept well that night. I actually got my first really solid night's sleep since I had stopped taking the sleeping pills.

I wasn't allowed to watch TV or look at my phone the whole next day. I didn't do much of anything until it got dark again and it was time to take my second dose, but I never felt bored. The anticipation made the day go by really fast. Before I knew it, Katie got all her stuff again and disappeared upstairs.

My dog Burger stayed downstairs with me. She was next to me all three days.

The shaman and I sat there and meditated together and then he started chanting again. It was maybe an hour before he pulled the ayahuasca out. I noticed he poured out almost twice as much as the night before.

He kept doing the chanting and then he made me smoke more tobacco. I could see the patterns and the blackness again. And then, just like the night before, he switched up his chant and everything changed.

I put my head down and started to look between my legs, into the black. I had instantly lost touch with reality. I was still sitting on my living room floor, but all of a sudden, I felt a million miles away. I was in a whole different realm.

Out of that darkness, I saw a big gray being floating up at me. It had a giant head with big horns that looked like a ram's. Then the body came up after it. The body just kept coming and coming, without ending. It was like those ships at the beginning of *Star Wars*.

I noticed it had tits. In general, it looked like something H.R. Giger—the guy who designed the creature for *Alien*—would have made. Only it was way darker, so you could barely make out all the details.

There were all these crevices, and inside of them there were demons and evil-looking clown-faced people hiding out. I felt like I had seen them before. I don't know if they were the same faces I saw when I was on DMT, but the evil grins and come hither gestures were exactly the same. They were all giving me looks like they knew something I didn't know. And whatever it was, it was something really bad. They were all trying to get me to come inside where they were.

And then I felt a big wave of nothingness wash over me.

Wait, is this death? I thought. *I didn't even catch the bit where I died.*

And I realized that if I was dead, I didn't care. I had spent my whole life in fear of death, and now that I was looking at it—or, for all I knew in that moment, now that I *had* died—it didn't bother me. It wasn't that bad. There was no pain. There was nothing to be afraid of.

I sat with that feeling for a long time, while that H.R. Giger Ram-Man Tit Monster hovered over me.

I don't know how long I stayed like that. But then I started seeing flashes of things. There were flashes of porn. And then flashes of a phone. Over and over, back and forth. I would see the porn and then I would see myself trying to use the phone to make it stop.

The porn started off basically normal, but then it started getting more and more evil. The people in it were killing each other while they were fucking. And they were both okay with it, like it was murder porn. Then the people started to have tails and stuff.

I didn't want to watch it anymore, but I couldn't get it to go away, and the ayahuasca just kept showing me worse and worse stuff. It was making me feel sick. At one point, I know I said, "Make it stop. I just need it to stop."

The shaman never once asked me what I was seeing. I know I said some random words or phrases here and there—enough that at certain points throughout the evening he probably had some clues. But he didn't ask any questions. He just said, "You've got to face it. You've got to go through it."

And that encouragement actually helped. I started to understand what was going on. There was a reason behind everything I was seeing. It wasn't just random shit. I started to ask myself, *Okay, what is it that ayahuasca is really trying to show me here? And why?* It was stuff that was in my life. Stuff that maybe isn't totally good for me. Stuff that might actually be a problem.

Then ayahuasca started taking me back to my childhood and showing me things like I was a fly on the wall. I saw the most horrible things happening to me. There was nothing all that surprising, but it still wasn't easy to watch. It made me sad to see what had really happened and who had done those things to me. The whole trip that night probably only lasted four hours, but at the time, that part alone seemed like an eternity.

Eventually the ayahuasca moved on and started showing me a bunch of things having to do with addiction. I saw still photos of drugs. Then I saw videos of drugs, and then videos of people using drugs. And then it was just me using drugs. I saw myself drinking. I saw myself injecting things. I saw myself intentionally overdosing. Killing myself, on purpose.

I was still a fly on the wall for all these things. It was like my brain would think of the worst shit it could come up with and show me that. And then it would say, *You think that was bad?* and then zoom in and show me something way worse.

Sometimes the visions didn't even make sense. I watched myself shooting up when I was maybe seven years old. I was like, *Come on, that didn't even really happen. Why are you showing me that?*

And then the ayahuasca would say, *Oh yeah? Well what about the same thing, only now you're a baby?*

And I would stall on these images and have to look at them for a really long time. I was like, *I got it, man. Can we fucking move on now?*

STILL AWESOME

It was like I had to live with this uncomfortable stuff until I could really feel the hurt, and until I could fully realize what I had been doing to myself.

Back in reality, in my living room, I was rolling around on the floor. Every now and then I'd be somewhat conscious of that. It was like my body was trying to pull me away from what was happening in my brain. I would pick myself up off of one side and say, "Stop!" And then I would roll over to my other side and the ayahuasca would show me more.

At certain points I think the shaman knew I had done enough time looking at whatever was happening at that moment. He would get up close to me and then spit some stuff on me.

The first time he did that it took a second for the reality to sink in. I was seeing and experiencing so many things that were only happening in my mind that it took a moment for me to piece together that yes, this dude really did just spit on me. But I would only be back in reality for a second before the ayahuasca would take me to another place, where a totally new and different scene was waiting for me.

At one point he gave me a big cigarette thing. I was really in the shit by then. I was literally moaning as I took a puff.

"Swallow it," he said.

And as soon as I swallowed the smoke I felt all hell break loose inside me. I grabbed a bucket and started vomiting so hard. My eyes were closed, but I could swear that a big, black, nasty tar thing came up out of me. It was like all the darkness and bad stuff inside of me was physically getting purged out. When I opened my eyes I could swear I even saw the black stuff in the bucket, even though later on I looked in there and it was just regular puke.

I started to be able to see a bit again. I started to come back down into reality, slowly but surely.

The visions didn't end immediately, but I became more and

more aware that what I was seeing wasn't real.

"You feel a little better?" the shaman asked. And then he did more chanting.

As I sobered up, I started to reflect on my life and on all the problems I have had. I felt a whole new sense of clarity and perspective. I was able to see how events from my childhood have affected the way I've reacted to things in my life.

The solutions to a lot of problems I had carried around with me for as long as I can remember suddenly started to seem kind of obvious. It was like my whole life, I had only been seeing half of a picture. But now all of a sudden my eyes were open and for the first time I could see the whole thing. And that instantly made a whole lot of my issues a whole lot easier to understand.

I wasn't really pumped for day three. I felt good about where the second night wound up, but it was so hard getting there. It was so uncomfortable and so painful, and it took so much out of me. I felt tapped out. I didn't know how much more I had left. But I had signed up for three days, so I was determined to follow through.

I was more familiar with the shaman by then, and with how the process worked in general. We drank the ayahuasca again and he started to chant, and when he changed what he was chanting, I knew we were off to the races again.

I was sitting on the floor, facing him. It was me and him and my dog Burger in the room. But I could feel someone else floating behind me.

One of the biggest reasons I took ayahuasca was because I wanted to see my brother Stevie. I thought for sure if I was going to see someone it was going to be him. In the back of my mind I was always afraid that I would see my father instead. I wasn't sure how I might handle that.

But I didn't even have to turn around to know that my dog

Fifty was there. Fifty had been gone for about a year at that point. He came over and was next to me.

The shaman knew somebody was there. He said something like, "Listen to what he has to say." I don't know if that meant he could see Fifty, too, or what. But that was one of the weirdest little details of the whole three days.

I couldn't talk to Fifty, obviously, because he's a dog and dogs don't talk. But I knew that Fifty knew that I knew he was there. The connection I felt with him was really intense, even deeper than on the day he died.

I felt so sad that he was gone, but also so happy for the friendship we had. He meant a lot to me. Him and I went through a lot together. I started to cry a bit. It was a happy cry and a sad cry, all at the same time. It was all the emotions I felt for him, all put together. To this day, I still can't talk about that moment without getting choked up.

Then something changed. I was still crying, but I started to feel angry. About the people who have been taken away from me. About a lot of things. I started screaming. I was just venting all of this primal rage. And I felt a lot better when I got it all out.

But then, something told me that was just the tip of the iceberg. I could tell that I was still holding more stuff in. And that I had to get it *all* out.

That led me to a terrifying realization. I was going to have to do more ayahuasca. Probably multiple times. I was going to have to go through way more horrible nights, facing the worst shit my brain and the medicine can come up with.

I probably have to see my father again. That sounds like pretty much the worst day ever. But something tells me it has to happen.

I had come to the end of a journey a couple years in the making, only to find out that it was just the beginning.

Chapter 12

I got a call from Australia one day not that long ago. It was my stepmother Marn. She told me she had something she wanted to talk to me about.

My father, she said, had done live sex shows.

From the sound of her voice, I could tell that was news to her.

Marn had known what kind of man my dad was when she met him. But after my brothers came along and the family moved to the suburbs, she truly thought that he had changed. When my father passed away, she believed that he had died as a faithful husband.

In reality, for a long while there he had gotten even worse. He had just figured out how to get away with it. When he passed, I was well aware of some of the shady stuff he was up to (although, as I found out later, not nearly all of it). I was never shielded from things like my brothers were. At times, my father and I were partners in crime, doing things his wife would not have approved of.

By the end, though, even I would have told you that he had at least partially cleaned up his act. I wasn't over there and I wasn't paying attention as well as I could have. I fell for his bullshit, too.

The first clues Lee and I had that we were wrong came right after my dad died. Lee still had his phone. My dad died so suddenly that a lot of people who knew him—or who were maybe just clients of his—were still trying to contact him.

Lee saw the texts coming. Lee is an upstanding member of the community. He is not a scumbag. So he didn't know how to interpret what he was seeing. The messages led him to believe that my dad owned a brothel or maybe a sex shop.

It all made sense a little while later, when I flew back to Australia and that guy Roger told me that my dad had been a gigolo.

I assumed that Roger had told Marn about all that stuff way back when he told me, but apparently that wasn't the case. Marn had been in the dark the whole time. Until now.

Clearly, this information had made a strong impression on her. "When I heard that," she said, "It made me wonder what else he might have been capable of. I wouldn't have believed he was doing half of that stuff Roger told me about. So now, I don't see how anything is impossible."

She told me she was sorry for doubting me. She didn't flat out say she believed my father had molested me. But her words made me think she had started leaning in that direction, or at least coming around to the idea that I might not be making things up.

I'm not quite that far along in the process with Lee yet. I don't think my stepmum has ever told Lee what she told me. Marn is old-school Australian. They don't want to talk about anything. For them, a lot of times it's easier to just let things go and move on.

Lee and I are not all the way to where I'd like us to be, but we're getting better. In his clearer moments, I think he believes at least *I* believe what I'm saying. In the beginning, he accused me of making things up to be famous. I know he doesn't think that anymore.

It's difficult for him. I understand. It was hard for me to believe something so terrible about my own father, too. It took me decades to get there. It's maybe even harder for Lee, since he didn't experience it firsthand like I did.

Lee's father and his brother are both gone. He loved them both so much and he doesn't want anything to change the way

STILL AWESOME

he remembers either of them. My dad did a lot for Lee. He put his own life on the back burner and spent his own money flying Lee around the country to get Lee's moto career started. Lee has a tattoo of our dad. Their connection runs deep.

But Lee and I talk, at least. Maybe once a month. We're both parents, so we talk about our kids. His daughter is racing BMX now. And she's good. The next generation Ellis lunatic is here, only this time it's a girl. It's awesome.

For as long as I can remember, my life has been one drama after another. I've dealt with so many problems. So much darkness. It's such a huge relief to feel like that is finally coming to an end. And I truly believe that it is.

I think a lot of people who knew me a long time ago would be surprised to see me now. Some of them would probably just be surprised I'm still alive. But they might also be surprised that I'm successful. And most of all, I think they'd be surprised that I'm happy, and that I'm enjoyable to be around, at least most of the time.

More and more every day, I'm starting to feel something that's pretty new to me: Peace. Things are really coming together on all fronts.

My ex-wife Andrea and I have never been better friends. We were never meant to be together as a couple. But we got two amazing kids out of our relationship. And now I'm with the person I'm supposed to be with and she's completely and utterly in love with the person she's supposed to be with. So that's a happy ending for everybody. The drama was well worth it.

Katie and Andrea are friends. Things might have been a little rocky at the start, but nowadays everyone's cool. They like each other. And I know they're not just making nice to keep the peace. I see group texts where Katie and Andrea are friendly and joking around with each other and it warms my heart. It's so good for them and for me and, most of all, for the kids.

It definitely helps that Andrea has seen Katie really step up and have a relationship with our children. For someone who genuinely wanted nothing to do with kids when we met, she's come a long way. When I have the kids during the week, Katie's there in the kitchen making them breakfast before they go to school. It's like a normal, all-American family situation. Just me, her, two kids, three dogs, three cats, and a pet dragon.

Thanks to therapy, the man Katie married is very different from the one Andrea and all my other exes had to deal with. I'm still needy. And I'm still pretty useless around the house. Katie makes the bed and stuff. I'm not much help there. But I think I can honestly tell you that my mommy issues are a thing of the past. It took a lot of work, but I am proud to say that I recognized the unhealthy pattern I had forced all my previous relationships to follow and then took the steps to break that pattern.

No one wants to be a nightmare to live with. No one wants to be undateable. And no one wants to be alone. I don't, anyway. And to have Katie in my life, it was well worth making the extra effort.

I didn't see her coming. I never would have believed I would ever want to get married again. But it's like we were made for each other. I truly believe that if Katie had godlike powers and she could have created a guy to spend her life with, that guy would pretty much look like me. That guy would like the things I like. That guy would even come with the same baggage I come with, as crazy as that might sound. And I feel the exact same way about her.

It feels good for my kids to see both of their parents in happy relationships. Now that I've lived it, I think it actually is true what they say: it's better for the kids to see you happy apart than miserable together. It's kind of obvious, when you think about it.

The kids could sense the tension between me and Andrea, no matter how hard to we tried to hide it. But Katie and I don't have any tension to conceal, so there's no reason for us to argue in front of them. I mean, of course we'll get a little chippy over which one of us lost the car keys. But that's the extent of it. Katie and I don't argue much at all.

The few minor fights we've had have mostly involved me doing something stupid with my penis. I am allowed to do pretty much whatever I want and yet sometimes I have still stepped over the line. I need to get permission to sleep with anyone else. That's one of the only rules. It's really just about being considerate and polite. But sometimes I'll still fuck up and say yes to someone without checking with Katie first. That bums her out. And she's right, of course. If she did that to me, I'd be heartbroken.

I definitely push it way further than Katie does. I'm an asshole sometimes. But I'm getting better. I'm learning.

I know it might be hard for some people who don't know us personally to understand how our relationship works, but most of the time I swear it's pretty mellow. We're just wired a little different, I guess. It's not a big deal.

When one of us comes home from being with someone else, it's not weird. It's not awkward. We're not secretive. We can talk about it. We can joke about it. If something stupid happened, we can laugh about it.

It's like if your boyfriend or girlfriend had a weekly bowling night. We have the same conversation that you would have when your significant other gets home from the local bowl-o-rama. Only instead of talking about how one of us bowled a mean strike or "Man, Jimmy was really putting back the Jim Beam tonight," one of us just got laid.

Am I going to tell you that having an open relationship is perfect all the time and that there is never any jealousy? No. Nothing's perfect. Monogamy sure as hell isn't. In my experience, you can be in a totally monogamous relationship and still have plenty of jealousy. I'm sure some people reading this are nodding their heads right now.

Katie has one other guy that she likes to sleep with from time to time. I'm not gonna lie. It took me a while to handle that. But fair is fair. You take the good with the bad and when it comes to our relationship there is a lot more good than bad.

And anyway, sexually speaking, things have slowed down a lot for us. Outside of just me and her, it's mostly just one-off things every now and then. I've mostly gotten that out of my system. Life's too short to organize orgies every weekend. They're kind of a headache, to be honest.

Not that Katie and I will ever stop doing stupid shit entirely. Not too long ago, I rented a Lamborghini Aventador S for a weekend. I've always wanted to own that car. It's 100% because of my dad and I know it. He always wanted that car, back when that model was called the Countach. I have always felt like to own one was to beat my father, because he never managed to get one.

To this day, my therapist recommends that I buy the Countach. I'm like, "It wouldn't even go up my driveway. And besides, I don't even own a house and you want me to buy a $300,000 sports car?" He gets it, but he also thinks it might help me get over the hump psychologically. He thinks I would enjoy my life more if I got to drive that around.

Truthfully, having that car was overrated. I don't really feel the need to defeat my father anymore.

But don't get me wrong—it was also really fucking fun. I went as fast as that thing could go.

I almost wrecked it. I was driving with Katie on Mulholland Drive—this big winding road that goes through the Hollywood Hills. It was dark. I was doing 60 around a turn, which is about as fast as that car could handle that curve, and there was a giant metal plate sticking up a little too high in the middle of the street, covering up some road work.

I tried to avoid it, but I still clipped the side of it. I thought for sure I blew a tire, but somehow I miraculously dodged that

STILL AWESOME

bullet. That would have been an expensive fuck-up for sure.

And then Katie and I headed up the 101 Freeway into Malibu and had sex on top of the car and took a bunch of stupid photos. We filmed a porn on it, too. Not for any reason. It's never going to see the light of day. It just seemed like the thing to do.

I may be calming down a bit and finding a little inner peace, but make no mistake, I am a lunatic. I am never going to stop doing random stuff like that. I am always going to want to do dumb shit. And not just driving irresponsibly at times and making amateur pornography on luxury rental cars.

Should I stop fighting? You could make that argument. Am I going to? No. At least not yet.

Over the last few years, I have taken some really dumb fights at Ellismania. Shane Carwin. Kyle Kingsbury. Retired UFC fighters who were way bigger and stronger than me. People I had absolutely no chance against. It was like being an unarmed bullfighter squaring off against a bull. The only appeal of those fights for the people watching was seeing how long I could go before I got hurt.

I don't see myself doing anything like that again. But if it's more of an even competition and it sounds like an exciting challenge? Then sure. I like having stuff like that in my life. I need excitement. I'm willing to risk a small amount of brain damage in the pursuit of glory. I don't want to live if I have to be perfect and safe all the time.

The same applies to drugs and alcohol. To a lot of things. The overall attitude I found in AA was that once you admit you're an addict, you have to lock yourself down completely. You have to stop doing everything forever or else eventually you'll wind up in a ditch somewhere.

I tried that life, and I can't be happy living the way those guys live. And honestly, when I look in the mirror, I just don't think that's how it ends for me.

Am I an alcoholic? Probably. Am I a weed addict? Yes. But I also love doing things that don't go well with being fucked-up all the time. That keeps me in check. If alcohol or weed ever made me not want to go to the gym or not go skateboarding on a Saturday, then alcohol and weed would have to go. But that isn't the case. I think I can balance them.

I am an addict, but I'm also really sensible and lame. I will drink and sometimes I will even drink too much. But I still go to the gym at nine in the morning. Especially since I got off antidepressants. I swear, those things sapped my energy way more than a couple beers ever did.

I know I might live five or ten years longer if I got sober and started juicing every day, but I don't want that life. I enjoy beer and weed. I enjoy the occasional cheeseburger. I like ice cream and candy. And I'll live with the consequences.

Everyone's got to live the way that makes sense for them. I've added it all up, and this is the version of me I choose to be.

When I met Katie, after me and Andrea split up, I had already started trying to find out who I really was. But then a lot of things changed. I got stopped dead in my tracks.

I came to the horrible realization that my own father had abused me, and I had to deal with that. And then I realized that being molested wasn't the only shitty thing about my childhood. When I called my stepmother from rehab to talk about my dad, she brushed over that subject. Instead, she immediately apologized for the way she treated me when I lived with her and my dad and my brothers. Until then, I had never really analyzed our relationship. But as I started thinking about it, I realized it for sure had an effect on me, too. If Katie ever told my kids that she hated them, she would be fucking gone. Out of my life. Just like that. No matter how happy she makes me. But my dad didn't have my back like that.

I'm past all of that now, but it took years. It took therapy and time and MDMA with Dr. Dan and then finally ayahuasca. I had to relive my whole childhood again. It was like my brain had shielded me from the reality until I was old enough and mature enough and wise enough to handle it. And then I went all the way back to the beginning with my adult brain and made sense of it all.

Now I am able to see everyone else's perspective. My dad was a troubled guy. He had a real problem. And he hated himself for it.

I forgive him. But that forgiveness didn't happen in a day. It takes time.

I still don't like talking about my experience on ayahuasca. It's difficult. The emotions still seem so fresh, even though I took it months and months ago. On a day-to-day basis, that experience is not something I sit around bullshitting about.

I only talked about it once in detail on the radio, the first day I got back after taking it, and then we left that segment up in the SiriusXM On Demand section. If anyone wants to hear it, it's still there. But I don't want to have to repeat the story on air. It's way too heavy.

I also wanted to include it in this book because it's a big part of where I am in my life right now and because I know people are curious about it. And I want other people to know about ayahuasca.

If you are interested in potentially trying it, let me be clear: You have to be very careful what you take and who you take it with. There are some tourists who have died in Peru because they got some sketchy shit off some sketchy guy. And for all I know, that could happen in America, too. Once the word gets out like the word's getting out on ayahuasca, there are going to be con artists and morons trying to get involved with selling it (especially as long as it's basically illegal in America). You've gotta do your homework. You've got to be sure you're doing it right.

But there are people in my life who I know for a fact could benefit from it. For friends of mine who have inner demons, I feel like sharing the ayahuasca experience can one day be my gift to them.

It's a legitimate tool to help people. It really is medicine, just like they say.

Psychotherapy is legit. It helps a lot of people. If it helps you, then use it for all it's worth. The same goes for AA. But personally, I think before you try any of those things, you need to give ayahuasca a shot.

You have nothing to lose. In my opinion, you're not going to come out worse. If you try it—again, under proper supervision, with a legit shaman—and you come out on the other side feeling just as shitty, then psychiatrists and AA aren't going anywhere. You'll still have those options to explore. But I would bet you're at least going to come out with a little more clarity.

I would especially think about giving ayahuasca a go before you try antidepressants. Before you start taking those pills every single day—maybe for the rest of your life—you owe it to yourself to see what ayahuasca can do for you. There are a bunch of different antidepressants, and every one of them works differently for different people. Maybe you'll get lucky and find one that fixes your problems with no side effects. I'm sure there are people out there who have that story. But then again, maybe you'll be like me and get stuck on one that never lets you feel like your full, true self.

I am finally living my life the way I have wanted. I am so grateful that I got to really be me before it all ends.

I'm so happy to finally be open about my sexuality. Katie made it so much easier for me. I'm very thankful for that. I think eventually I would have opened up about it, with or without her. Secrets that big don't stay hidden just because you want them to. They want to come out and see the light of day. One day I would have stopped running from it. I just think it would have taken a lot longer, and I'm not entirely sure that info would have ever made it on the radio. I believe that would have been a massive missed opportunity.

When I first started talking publicly about being bisexual, I second-guessed myself a lot. I definitely had days where I regretted it. I opened myself up to a lot of jokes and a lot of criticism. I was afraid my kids would get picked on later in their lives, when their friends realized that Devin and Tiger's dad is maybe a little different from their dads. I'm sure I lost a couple listeners over it—although not as many as I might have feared. I think all in all most people in my world are open-minded.

But not everyone is so lucky. After opening myself to the gay world and the trans world and following new people from those communities on social media, I started to understand how tough the world can be for people who are not heterosexual. Trans people make up a really small portion of the overall population, but the percentage of them who commit suicide—or at least try to—is off the charts. It's so sad, and so unnecessary.

I started putting two and two together. Over the years on the radio, I've talked about being an alcoholic. I've talked about being abused. I've talked about just being a general fuck-up. And I know that's helped other people. Listeners tell me all the time. They call me on the show, or they DM me, or they tell me face-to-face when I meet them at Ellismania.

I didn't set out to help people. I just wanted to make funny radio that would make somebody's shitty commute a little more bearable. But along the way, talking about my problems has helped a lot of other people face their own problems, and start fixing them. That wasn't my intention, but I believe it's the most important thing I've ever done or ever will do.

And now, once again by accident, by talking about my sexuality I have opened myself up as an example to a whole bunch of other people who I believe I can also help. The guys who follow me on social media look pretty much like what you would expect the guys who follow me on social media to look like. But you should see the messages I get.

There are more people in the closet than I ever would have guessed. Not all dudes who are closeted are full-on gay, of course.

Some of them are bi, and some are just interested in doing stuff here and there with guys, or maybe with trans girls. Whatever the individual cases may be, it seems very obvious to me that lots of the most manly-looking 'no homo' bros you run into are straight up lying to the world about who they are. And maybe even lying to themselves.

My message to all of them is the same: Don't die lying. Life is too short to never be yourself. Be honest about who you really are. It might be hard at first, but guess what? Living in the closet is pretty hard, too.

Coming out was easier for me than it is for a lot of other people. I had a lot of things going for me when I decided to tell people the truth. My wife loves me for who I am, and I have friends who stand by me no matter what. I live in Los Angeles and I have a job where no one is ever going to openly frown on homosexuality.

But I am well aware that my show reaches people who live in very different situations. I understand why some people might not want to come out loud and proud over a Facebook announcement. But at least try being honest with yourself. Or even better, be honest with one friend you know you can trust. Even if you can't talk to people in your life, see if there's any way you can talk to people anonymously on the internet. Trust me, it feels good just to hear somebody else say, "Hey, man, I'm totally like that, too."

By taking small steps, you can start to feel how liberating it is. You might start to realize just how much stress keeping that secret to yourself has been causing for your whole entire life. And once you hear yourself say it out loud, you might realize that it doesn't sound like as big of a deal as you always thought it would.

In my experience it's a big relief. You might not feel that relief straightaway, but eventually you'll feel better. You'll feel lighter. I don't think anybody who's hiding their true self is a happy person. Not entirely happy, anyway.

Everyone's situation is different. Coming out can cause different kinds of issues for different people. In a weird way, I have found that being bisexual sometimes presents more challenges than if I had gone on *Howard Stern* and announced that I was just a regular old gay guy.

Society has evolved. For the most part, people have opened up a new category in their minds to fit gay people in. But a lot of people still don't know where to put bisexuals. *So wait—you're married to a girl, but then sometimes you're also into dudes?* That's too messy for a lot of people to handle, at least at this point in time.

I get it. I'm new to this, too. Even I feel like it sounds kind of weird.

Most people can wrap their heads around gay parents. But when you say you're bisexual, you still hear, "But think about the children!" Trust me, I have thought about my children more than anybody else ever has or ever will. And I choose to look on the bright side.

I don't think kids care what their parents do behind closed doors. I think most people would prefer to pretend their parents aren't having sex at all, regardless of whether it's a rowdy Saturday night threesome or a stock night of eyes-closed lights-off missionary.

But I do want my kids to grow up knowing that people like me exist, so they can have a better understanding of all the different kinds of people out in the world. I want them to see firsthand that it's not that big of a deal. I know I came from a weird family, but if I was a normal person and I had a normal family and then years later I found out that my mother and father enjoyed having sex with other people from time to time, how exactly would that turn me into a bad person—or retroactively make my parents bad people in my eyes?

And then to take it a step further, if the person mom and dad are having fun with happens to have a dick instead of a vagina, then how does *that* change things, exactly? Again, it doesn't. Nobody's hurting anybody.

Obviously not everyone sees things the same way I do. I accept that. My skin has gotten a lot thicker over the last few years. To a lot of people, until recently I was a cool guy with a badass life. I have tattoos and I talk on the radio and I fight MMA and I have a hot chick who lets me fuck other hot chicks, too. All of that stuff was true. All of that stuff is *still* true.

But now everyone knows I also like doing stuff with guys. And I know that, to some of the people who thought I was cool, that last bit nullifies all the other stuff.

That's where we are right now. Maybe that will change someday. I think it will. But maybe I'm wrong.

The cool part is, I finally don't care what other people think. I'm just doing what comes natural to me. I'm living my life.

I see things so much brighter these days, for a lot of different reasons. I am eternally grateful to Aubrey Marcus for starting me on the path that led me to ayahuasca. But it's not just that. It's everything. It's getting older and wiser, and being open about who I am with the world, and going to therapy, and being in love, and watching my kids grow up, and getting to do what I do for a living, and a whole bunch of other stuff, too. It all adds up.

I can see so many improvements in myself. I'm way less insecure. I used to need a pat on the back to feel good about myself. But I don't need anyone else's approval anymore. And I'm more accepting of my flaws. I know I'm not perfect, but I also know that nobody is. It's just part of the deal of being a person.

I am so in love with my life sometimes. That never used to happen. When I was a skateboarder, there were some days in there where I was really on fire. I was accomplishing things that I never could have imagined the first time I went to a skate ramp. But I don't remember really rejoicing over those accomplishments at the time.

Nowadays, I feel true joy from something as simple as hanging out with my kids. Making jokes with my daughter and seeing

STILL AWESOME

her develop her own little wiseass sense of humor. Going to buy stupid limited-edition cool guy sneakers with my son. I'm just living in the moment and soaking it all up.

I'm not saying all my problems are totally cured. I'm still a sad, dark, bitter dude too much of the time. I'm better, but I've got a long way to go.

All of my life I have been an emotional person. I overreact to stuff. I've been jealous and envious. It has often bothered me to see other people have things that I don't have.

I'd see something I resented or envied about someone else, and I'd automatically think, *Fuck them*. I still do sometimes. It's a bad habit.

The difference is, before I didn't see any problem with it. I let myself believe that was a reasonable response. Now at least I'll catch myself. I'll question myself. *Fuck them? What did they do to me? So what if they've got something I don't have?* For one thing, I see that a lot of things other people have—like fame, for example—might look way more exciting from the outside than they really are. And more importantly, I am able to remember that I've got a lot of stuff going for me as well. I've come a long way, especially when I consider where I came from.

I don't need to beat myself up anymore. It took me a long time to realize that.

It's been almost ten years since my first book. A lot of shit has gone down between then and now. Will there be another one in another ten years? I fucking hope not. If ten years from now you hear me talking about how incredibly excited I am for everyone to read my next big tell-all book, you'll know things either got amazingly good for me or something went horribly wrong. But I sincerely doubt that's in the cards. I expect the next decade to be pretty boring, at least compared to the ride so far.

I'm starting to think that my body isn't going to take a total shit on me anytime soon. Maybe I can be one of those freaky

60-year-old men who can still do crazy stuff. They have amazing therapies and treatments nowadays and I know I'll keep going to the gym and training for as long as I physically can. So maybe that's part of my future.

I still feel like I have a lot of ayahuasca and therapy that still needs to be done in the years to come. Life is full of problems, but I see now that a lot of my biggest problems are all in my head. I have already lost a lot of baggage, but I look forward to carrying around even less of the fantasy weight that I still carry around every day. There's still a lot of room for me to grow and I am ready to do the work.

I look forward to finding new ways to be more helpful to other people. I look forward to becoming more stable and more relaxed with my day-to-day life. I look forward to just being way happier. This is an amazing life that I have been given and I want to enjoy it.

I'm in my late 40s, man. And I've put a lot of miles on my body. My father was only five years older than me when he died. I don't know how much longer I've got. Nobody does. If I'm not going to find a little peace in my life sometime soon, then when the fuck am I planning to do it?

I finally understand that every day is a gift.

And I intend to make the most of every single one of them.

Acknowledgments

Thanks to skateboarding. I love you forever.

Thanks to the listeners of *The Jason Ellis Show* and SiriusXM. Because of you I have this amazing platform that reaches so many in a positive way. It's been a very fulfilling career. Thanks to all of you.

Thanks to Will Pendarvis for always being a friend and for his awesome radio skills on the show.

Will has always been there as the voice I trust on how well both me and the show are performing on a day-to-day basis. This means the world to me. Thanks, Will.

Thanks to Tully not only for writing this book but also for being a giant part of the show. He is the rational intelligent part of the show, not to mention he is incredibly handsome with beautiful feet. We have created so many great things together and I'm very proud of almost all of it. Haha.

Thanks to Kevin Kraft. Your contributions to the show have been vital to our success over the years and I'm honored to call you a friend.

Thanks to my friend Aubrey Marcus. The things you have opened my mind, heart, and soul to can never be repaid. I am forever in your debt. Thanks for everything! I love you, man.

Thanks to my kids, Devin and Tiger. I love you guys so much. I hope this book doesn't make you too uncomfortable. Dad is into some crazy stuff, but he's happy and free being himself and I really feel like everybody needs to be themselves in life, even if that's not what most people do. You are the greatest—so beautiful inside and out. I'm so proud of you guys.

Thanks to my wife, Katie. You are the greatest, most beautiful, fun, fantastic, warrior-friend-human I have ever met in my whole life. And I see you every day! This is why I'll die smiling. This life with you has been everything I've always wanted. I love you and my life so much. Thanks, baby.